Advances and Technical Standards in Neurosurgery

Volume 44

For further volumes
http://www.springer.com/series/578

Yoko Kato • Ahmed Ansari
Editors

Cerebrovascular Surgery

Controversies, Standards and Advances

Springer

Editors
Yoko Kato
Department of Neurosurgery
Banbuntane Hotokukai Hospital
Fujita Health University
Nagoya-shi, Aichi, Japan

Ahmed Ansari
Department of Neurosurgery
Jawahar Lal Nehru Medical College
Aligarh Muslim University
Aligarh, Uttar Pradesh, India

Department of Neurosurgery
Banbuntane Hotokukai Hospital
Fujita Health University
Nagoya-shi, Aichi, Japan

ISSN 0095-4829 ISSN 1869-9189 (electronic)
Advances and Technical Standards in Neurosurgery
ISBN 978-3-030-87651-7 ISBN 978-3-030-87649-4 (eBook)
https://doi.org/10.1007/978-3-030-87649-4

This Springer imprint is published by the registered company Springer Nature Switzerland AG
The registered company address is: Gewerbestrasse 11, 6330 Cham, Switzerland

Dedicated to Prof. Majid Samii and Prof. Hirotoshi Sano,
and
the numerous patients who have kept their faith and are the best teachers.

Foreword

It is a privilege to write a foreword for *Cerebrovascular Surgery—Controversies, Standards and Advances*, authored by a truly international group of authors who have all been recognized for their excellence and for being at the forefront of our specialty. It has been an exceptional professional journey for me personally as I have observed the spreading of excellence in our specialty to all corners of the world during my lifetime. Through technical hands-on courses, digital media, and a plethora of presentations, our young trainees can learn first-hand from the leaders in our field and apply their knowledge for the benefit of their patients wherever they may reside. So many colleagues of our art have given their time and knowledge tirelessly to accomplish the goal of educating all neurosurgeons on our planet. The authors and editors of this volume are prime examples of this level of dedication.

Professor Kato is an exemplary model for sharing her knowledge and skill and for her tireless efforts towards educating our young neurosurgeons and trainees. She is a role model for what neurosurgeons can aspire to, and she must be applauded for having risen to the top of our specialty despite the many obstacles that she had to overcome in a specialty dominated by male neurosurgeons. This volume is just another example of her willingness to go far beyond the call of duty to the benefit of our specialty. Professor Kato's former fellow and co-editor, Ahmed Ansari, is another tribute to her dedication to training young neurosurgeons. Although still in the early years of his career, Dr. Ansari shows promise for contributing greatly to education and the advancement of our field.

I applaud the authors, the editors, and Professor Concezio di Rocco, the series editor, for creating a timely and well-written volume that addresses the critical issues in cerebrovascular surgery in a cogent manner.

Department of Neurosurgery
Barrow Neurological Institute,
Phoenix, AZ, USA

Robert F. Spetzler

Preface

Cerebrovascular surgery, as a specialty, has grown leaps and bounds in this era. Indications of endovascular neurosurgery have grown significantly, though clear indications for open cerebrovascular surgery are very much intact. Proponents of both specialties linger on the pros and cons of their respective subjects.

The present work has been carved out of the desire to get multiple stalwarts in the field, and get their experience regarding standard approaches, advances in the field, and then further discuss the complications that may ensue.

Whilst there are classic texts in the field that describe in detail indications, outcomes, and controversies in cerebrovascular surgery, we endeavoured to contribute a volume that focuses on standards, advances, and complications in the field that would be readily available to senior neurosurgeons and those in training. We believe this text will serve justice to its very purpose and be a ready reckoner in the field.

Nagoya-shi, Aichi, Japan — Yoko Kato
Aligarh, Uttar Pradesh, India — Ahmed Ansari

Acknowledgements

We are thankful to Prof. Concezio di Rocco for his trust in this wonderful project. We would like to acknowledge Donatella Rizza and Sasirekka Nijanthan at Springer Nature for their continuous support in the project.

Yoko Kato

Ahmed Ansari

Series Preface

Advances and Technical Standards in Neurosurgery (ATSN) represents the successful achievement of the wish of Jean Brihaye, Bernard Pertuised, Fritz Loew and Hugo Krayenbuhl to provide European neurosurgeons in training with a high-level publication to accompany the teaching provided by the European postgraduate course. The project was conceived during the joint meeting of the German and Italian Neurosurgical Societies in Taormina in 1972, and the first volume was published in 1974. The English language was chosen to facilitate the international exchange of information and the circulation of scientific progress. Since then, the ATSN has hosted chapters by eminent European neurosurgeons and has become one of the most renowned educational tools on the continent for both young and experienced neurosurgeons. The successive editorial boards have maintained the ATSN's high scientific quality and ensured a good balance between contributions dealing with advances in neuroscience over the years and detailed descriptions of surgical techniques, as well as analyses of clinical experiences. Additional appeal has been added by the freedom granted by the Editor and Publisher in the length, style and organisation of the published chapters.

The current series aims to preserve the original spirit of the publication and its high-level didactic function, but intends to present itself not only as a historic European publication, but as a truly international forum for the most advanced clinical research and modern operating standards.

Hannover, Germany

Concezio Di Rocco

Contents

Chapter 1
Tailored Skull Base Approach to Management of Intracranial Aneurysms

Imad N. Kanaan

Surgical management of intracranial aneurysms (IAs) remains one of the most challenging and dynamic tasks for neurosurgeons. The introduction of tailored skull base approaches facilitates IAs microsurgical treatment. The merits of these approaches rest in providing short, versatile avenues for excellent exposure of the aneurysm complex and its intimate neurovascular structures with minimal brain retraction and free surgical maneuverability.

The recent innovation in microscopic and endoscopic technology, intraoperative 3D and ICG video-angiography, high-quality aneurysm clips, and refinement of cerebral bypass techniques enhance IAs neurosurgical management and foster more successful surgical outcomes. The selection criteria of a proper skull base approach include anatomical location of the aneurysm, its orientation and configuration, size, and presence of rupture or multiplicity. This chapter describes the two main "power horse" skull base approaches referred to as pterional and retrosigmoid approaches and highlights their variants along with other innovative interventions.

1.1 Introduction

Management of intracranial aneurysms (IAs) is one of the most challenging tasks for neurosurgeons. During the early years of the past century IAs were referred to as "noli me tangere" (do not touch me) lesions; however, Avant-garde neurosurgeons (Dott, Dandy, Norlen and Olivecrona) were able to challenge this conviction and reported their successful surgical intervention [1–3]. The promotion of

I. N. Kanaan (✉)
Department of Neurosciences, King Faisal Specialist Hospital and Research Center "General Instituition", Alfaisal University - College of Medicine, Riyadh, Kingdom of Saudi Arabia

Y. Kato, A. Ansari (eds.), *Cerebrovascular Surgery*, Advances and Technical Standards in Neurosurgery 44, https://doi.org/10.1007/978-3-030-87649-4_1

microsurgical treatment of IAs in the 20th century was credited to the masterwork of Drake, Yaşargil, and Sugita [4–9], pioneers who ignited the path for future successful surgical management of intracranial aneurysms with excellent durable outcome.

Rapid advancements in endovascular therapy have provided a competitive but complementary treatment option for cerebral aneurysms, transforming neurovascular referral patterns with compromise of neurovascular surgical exposures and training opportunities. Consequently, neurosurgeons now strive to treat more complex aneurysms, giant aneurysms, blister aneurysms, and small aneurysms, in addition to handling post-endovascular intervention failure.

The selection of tailored skull base approaches is a crucial step toward proper surgical exposure of IAs complex including their neck and adjacent perforators. The merits of these approaches include providing proximal and distal control of parent vessels, access to basal cisterns and release of CSF, ability to evacuate hematoma with minimal brain retraction and free surgical maneuverability. Modern microscope and endoscope technology, intraoperative 3D and ICG video-angiographic control, design of high-quality aneurysm clips, and the refinement of cerebral bypass techniques pave the way for a versatile, time-honored, and durable treatment option of IAs with excellent neurosurgical outcome.

Aspects influencing the choice of skull base approach include anatomical location of the aneurysm, its orientation and configuration, size, and the presence of rupture or multiplicity. The author adopts a simple classification of skull base surgical approaches into anterolateral and posterolateral approaches. The former includes pterional approach, fronto-orbito-zygomatic (FOZ) approach and variants, and the latter embraces the retrosigmoid approach, presigmoid combined approach, and far-lateral suboccipital approach.

1.2 Anterolateral Skull Base Approaches

1.2.1 Pterional Approach

The original description of pterional approach was credited to Heuer [10] in 1918, modified by Dandy to clip an anterior communicating artery aneurysm in 1941 [11], and later refined and popularized by Yaşargil in 1969 [8]. This versatile approach provides excellent functional exposure and allows clipping of most anterior circulation aneurysms including contralateral proximal carotid and rostral basilar aneurysms.

1.2.1.1 Intervention

The surgical approach starts with the patient placed in supine position, uplifting the ipsilateral shoulder and elevation of the trunk 25° to assure gravity-supported venous drainage. The head is fixed in the Mayfield head clamp, extended and rotated 25° to the contralateral side. Elevation of a standard frontal skin flap using a vertical incision above—but within 1 cm anterior to—the tragus that slowly curved behind the hairline, and just passing the midline. It is important to preserve the frontal branch of the facial nerve using the inter-fascicular dissection at the anterior attachment of the temporal muscle to fronto-zygomatic line, as described by Yaşargil, and to maintain the integrity of the superficial temporal artery for its potential use in EC-IC bypass. Mobilization of the temporal muscle basally and posteriorly after sharp incision of its anterior attachment exposes the pterion and part of the temporal squama and leaves a muscle cuff at the temporal line for future re-suturing of the muscle.

The bony exposure proceeds with fronto-temporal sphenoidal craniotomy using two burr holes: one at MacCarty (thinking point) and the second at the bottom of the temporal squama. Flattening of the orbital roof, resection of the greater and lesser wing of sphenoid enhances the exposure and minimizes brain retraction. Anatomical location, complexity and configuration of the aneurysm, and the need for proximal control dictate the need for extradural or intradural drilling out of the anterior clinoid process. In such cases, the author advises to complete the extradural anterior clinoid resection after the opening of the dura first for a better bilateral inspection (Fig. 1.1).

The way to open the dura is parallel to the orbital rim in a slightly curved fashion with a relaxing slit over the Sylvian veins. Early introduction of microscopy for inspection and prior to any retraction to open the proximal Sylvian cistern and other regional skull base cistern including Lilliquist membrane or lamina terminalis releases the CSF for relaxation and/or lavage of blood collection. Next, identify the parent vessel for potential proximal and distal control, to check the feasibility of

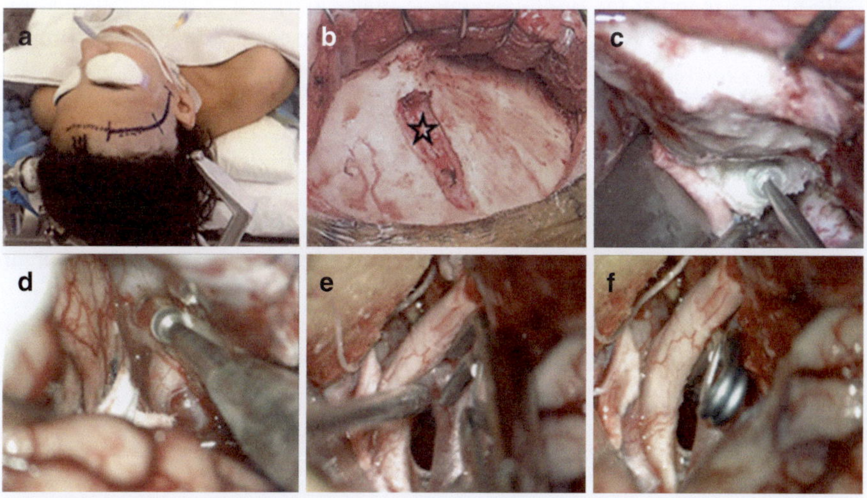

Fig. 1.1 Right pterional approach. (**a**) Frontal skin incision "solid line". (**b**) Fronto Pterional Craniotomy "dotted line" leaving a muscle cuff *. (**c**) Extradural drilling of sphenoid wings and anterior clinoid process. (**d**) De-roofing of optic nerve. (**e**) Exposure of an ophthalmic aneurysm neck. (**f**) Clipping of the aneurysm "Kanaan-Baldocini"

applying a clip to the aneurysm neck without compromise of the surrounding perforators or other important vessels in the vicinity "en-passage" and to maintain the integrity of adjacent cranial nerves such as the optic nerve or oculomotor nerve. The author recommends drilling of the anterior clinoid process and the roof of the optic canal and releasing the falciform ligament in order to provide proximal control, clip an ophthalmic artery aneurysm or a low proximal internal carotid artery aneurysm, and prevent traction injury to the optic nerve during manipulation.

In recent years, we have reverted to using the simple pterional approach for clipping of most anterior IAs. The list includes P-com A, A-chor A, MCA, A1, A-com A, bilateral proximal A2, bilateral ophthalmic A, and rostral basilar aneurysms. The less invasive variant is the trans-eyebrow or trans-ciliary mini-pterional or FOZ approach; it may be adequate to treat some selected anterior circulation aneurysms [12–14].

1.2.2 Fronto-Orbito-Zygomatic Approach and Variant (FOZ)

The fronto-orbito-zygomatic (FOZ) approach welds several surgical avenues and satisfies the philosophy of skull base surgery by removing bone obstacles in favor of better exposure with minimal brain retraction. Historically, this approach evolved from the pioneering work of avant-garde neurosurgeons. McArthur 1912 and later Frazier 1913 were the first to remove the supraorbital ridge as part of frontal craniotomy [15, 16]. Jane et al. revived this approach to include the anterior orbital roof osteotomy in a single flap to approach orbital tumors and vascular lesions [17]. Pellerin [18] reported the orbito-zygomatic-malar approach in 1969 followed by Hakuba [19] who first described a newer version in the early '80s labeled as orbito-zygomatic subtemporal approach to central skull base lesions. This approach was eventually adopted and modified by Al Mefty and others as fronto-orbito-zygomatic (FOZ) approach [20–23].

The FOZ approach provides an excellent neurosurgical avenue for safe removal of skull base tumors and management of complex vascular lesions around the central skull base, cavernous sinus, and upper clivus. Several publications quantified this approach and highlighted its advantages in the contemporary practice of skull base surgery.

The FOZ approach represents an extended version of the pterional approach that includes removal of the superior and lateral orbital rim (zygoma) medial to the supraorbital notch and down to the malar eminence.

1.2.2.1 Intervention

The frontotemporal bone flap of pterional approach will include the anterior part of the orbital roof and the lateral wall of the orbit; hence, it negates the need for later orbital reconstruction. This step may be performed as a single or two-piece

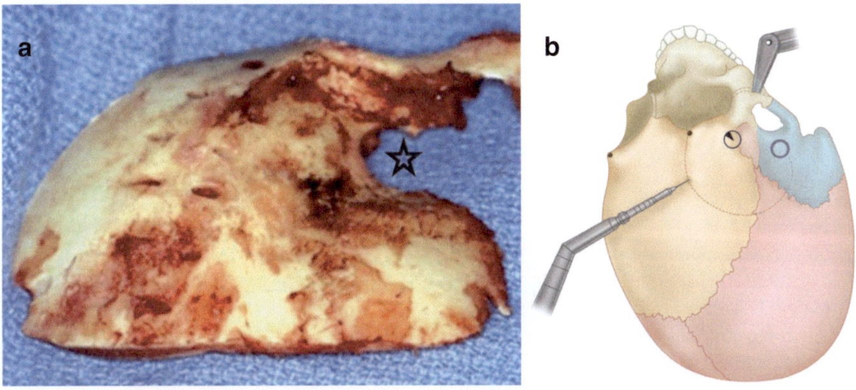

Fig. 1.2 Right FOZ approach. (**a**) Frontotemporal bone flap including superior and lateral orbital rim and its anterior roof. "Resected pterion*". (**b**) Highlights of FOZ: Fronto orbito zygomatic approach including orbital rim, anterior roof and its lateral wall (zygoma)

flap using a pediatric oscillating saw or fine bone cutter. The line of cut is medial to the ethmoid sinus and the lateral one is between the outer edge of the superior and inferior orbital fissures. The use of cotton patties and thin brain spatula provide a protection to the fronto-basal dura as well as the periorbita covering the lacrimal gland (Fig. 1.2). The elevation of this flap will facilitate the extradural resection of the sphenoid wing and drilling of the anterior clinoid process. It will also help in identifying the orbito meningeal fold and the decompression of the superior orbital fissure, the optic canal, and the posterior orbit using a high-speed diamond burr.

The need for the double cut of the zygomatic arc is limited to the extended subtemporal approach proposed for surgical management of cavernous sinus lesions, complex basilar tip aneurysms, or upper clivus tumors as described by Dolenc and Hakuba. It does not warrant total skeletonization of the zygomatic arch and we advise to proceed with pre-platting rehearsal to achieve better alignment and good cosmetic results.

Recently, several authors tailored this approach and described less invasive variants that complement the pterional approach with the removal of the superior and lateral orbital rim but keeping the zygomatic arc intact.

1.2.3 Dolenc Approach and Kawase Approach

In the 1980s, Dolenc [24] introduced an innovative approach to treat complex paraclinoid aneurysms, cavernous sinus vascular lesions, and basilar tip aneurysms. It is a variant of FOZ approach, which provides the option of intradural or extradural approach to these lesions. Whereas Kawase [25, 26] in 1985 designed a subtemporal extradural access to the petrous apex and upper clivus to treat basilar A. aneurysms, Meckel's cave, and superior petroclival tumors (Fig. 1.3).

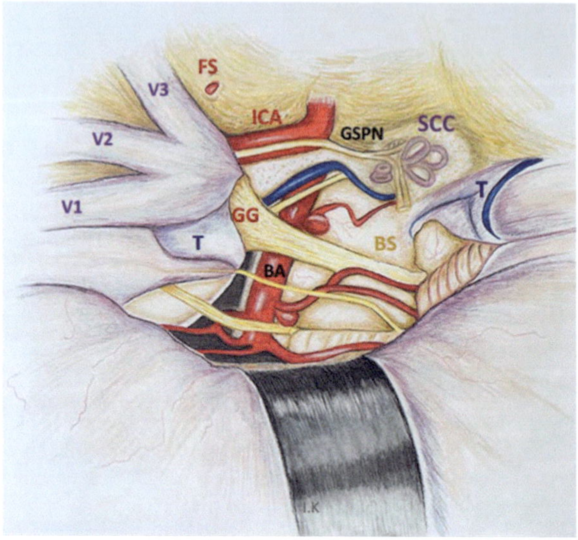

Fig. 1.3 Subtemporal extradural anterior petrosal transtentorial approach (Kawase). Artistic drawing illustrates exposure of the basilar artery and its branches aneurysms. Landmarks include GSPN/petrous carotid (ICA) lateral, arcuate eminence (SSC) posterior, Gasserian ganglion (GG) anterior, petrous ridge/tentorial edge "cut" (T) medial, (IAM) inferior

1.2.3.1 Intervention

Both approaches entail flattening of the lateral temporal fossa, obliteration of the foramen spinosum, and preserving the integrity of the greater and lesser superficial petrosal nerves (GSPN and LSPN) during the extradural exposure of the petrous carotid for proximal control while clipping of complex proximal paraclinoid aneurysms or proximal basilar A. aneurysms.

Furthermore, Dolenc's approach may weld with Kawase's approach as modified Dolenc-Kawase approach (MDK) to enhance such an exposure.

Recently, the rapid progress in neurovascular intervention supplants the regular use of these approaches and limits them to manage special complex or giant intracranial aneurysms [27].

1.3 Posterolateral Skull Base Approaches

Posterior circulation aneurysms represent 10% of all intracranial aneurysms and are primarily more centrally oriented. Their location, size, complexity, and confined regional anatomy may impose surgical challenges and dictate the selection of surgical approach. Pterional approach is a popular avenue to manage rostral basilar aneurysms, P1 and P1–P2 aneurysms, which represent 80% of posterior cerebral artery (PCA) aneurysms, whereas distal PCA aneurysms are amenable for surgery via a subtemporal approach for (posterior P2) or occipital interhemispheric transtentorial avenues for (P3). Treatment of most superior cerebellar artery (SCA) aneurysms entails neck clipping. Surgical approach options for management of its cisternal segment aneurysms are via pterional transsylvian, subtemporal transtentorial, or occipital transtentorial approaches. Basilar mid-trunk aneurysms are accessed via anterior or posterior petrosal presigmoid transtentorial combined approach. Vertebrobasilar aneurysms may require modified far-lateral or suboccipital trans-condylar approach. However, more lateral aneurysms of anterior inferior artery (AICA) and posterior inferior artery (PICA) aneurysms can be treated successfully via a simple lateral suboccipital or retrosigmoid approach for the former and a tailored far-lateral suboccipital trans-condylar approach or paramedian suboccipital approach for the latter.

1.3.1 Retrosigmoid Approach

The retrosigmoid approach provides a safe, versatile, multi-channel corridor to manage posterior circulation aneurysms or resect different types of tumor while maintaining the integrity of the surrounding neurovascular structures. It demands thorough knowledge of regional anatomy and expertise in microsurgical techniques. This approach represents an evolution from the unilateral suboccipital approach, first credited to Balance and Thomas Annandale [28] in 1894 and 1895 for removal of a vestibular schwannoma, popularized by Dandy in 1934 and eventually fine-tuned by others. The detailed cisternal and 3D-anatomy of the CPA are an important source of information to master the intervention, elegantly described by Yaşargil [29] and later by the comprehensive work of Rhoton [30].

1.3.1.1 Intervention

Placement of the patient into a semi-sitting or modified park bench position with 25° elevation of the upper trunk facilitates the venous outflow. Securing the head in a Mayfield head clamp with slight flexion and lateral rotation to the ipsilateral shoulder enhances visualization of the CPA and the tentorium. The intervention starts with a standard curvilinear incision 2–3 cm behind the postauricular sulcus, followed by incision of the soft tissue and exposure of the suboccipital region. A 4 × 4 cm craniotomy spans among three burr holes. One is over the asterion; a landmark corresponds to the underlying junction between the transverse sinus and sigmoid sinus junction. The second is along the same line about 4 cm medially and the third one is at the base of suboccipital region. Neuronavigation helps in planning this craniotomy and confirms the position of the lateral and sigmoid sinus in correlation with the standard practical method of drawing a virtual line from the zygomatic arch to the occipital protuberance as a reference to the course of the lateral sinus. The edge of the bony exposure should trace the posterior margin of the sigmoid sinus and the inferior margin of the transverse sinus. Dura opening starts with a

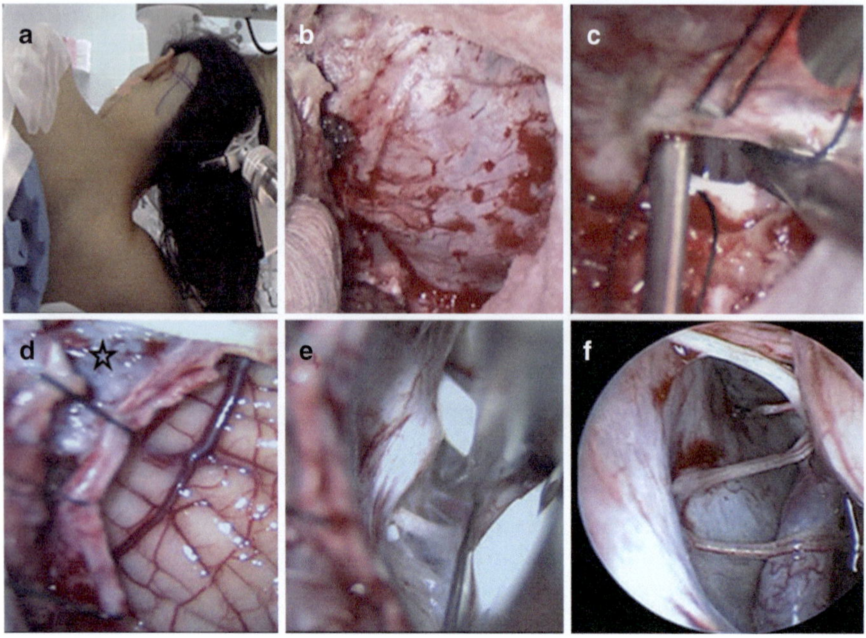

Fig. 1.4 Left retrosigmoid approach. (**a**) Modified park-bench position, easy curved incision, and localization of lateral and sigmoid sinuses. (**b**) Suboccipital lateral craniotomy extend to both lateral and sigmoid sinuses' edge. (**c**) Primary small basal dura incision to release CSF from the basal cistern "cisterna magna". (**d**) Y-shaped dura incision. Dura leaflets are reflect over the sinuses "dural sinus *". (**e**) Direct access to left CPA cisterns, showing 7 and 8 nerves complex entering the IAM and caudal cranial nerves. (**f**) Endoscopic view of the lower CPA with excellent visualization of the caudal cranial nerves over the vertebral A

small initial dural incision over the vicinity of the cisterna magna to allow for controlled egress of cerebrospinal fluid, which provides relaxation of the underlying cerebellum. Eventually, opening of the dura in Y-shaped forming superior and lateral leaflets that are reflected over the transverse and sigmoid sinuses leaves the medial part of the dura to cradle and cover the cerebellum and prevent its herniation (Fig. 1.4).

Microsurgical exposure starts with sharp incision of the upper CPA cistern, subarachnoidal dissection, and minimal retraction of the cerebellum. Identification of the internal auditory canal and maintaining the integrity of seven and eight cranial nerves complex, as well as the petrosal vein and the trigeminal nerve and special care of the sixth nerve in the depth. Evaluate the configuration of the aneurysm and its relationship to the parent vessel, surrounding neurovascular structures, with special attention to adjacent perforators and the brain stem. Judge the need for temporary clipping or the feasibility to apply a permanent clip safely after preselection of the size and type of the clip.

1.3.2 *Combined Presigmoid Retrolabyrinthine Petrosal Approach*

Hakuba described this approach in 1980; later refined and popularized by others [31–39], it provides a panoramic view to Meckel's cave, petroclival region, and anterior aspect of the brain stem and basilar artery.

1.3.2.1 Intervention

This intervention entails a combination of retrolabyrinthine presigmoid, retrosigmoid, and subtemporal avenues. An inverted J-shaped skin incision is fashioned from the zygoma arch at the pre-tragus curving up two fingerbreadths above the pinna and descending posterior and inferior behind the mastoid process, followed by release and reflection of the temporalis muscle inferiorly.

The bony exposure includes three steps (Fig. 1.5): step 1: Elevation of a temporal-suboccipital bone flap in one or two pieces using two bur holes spanned on both

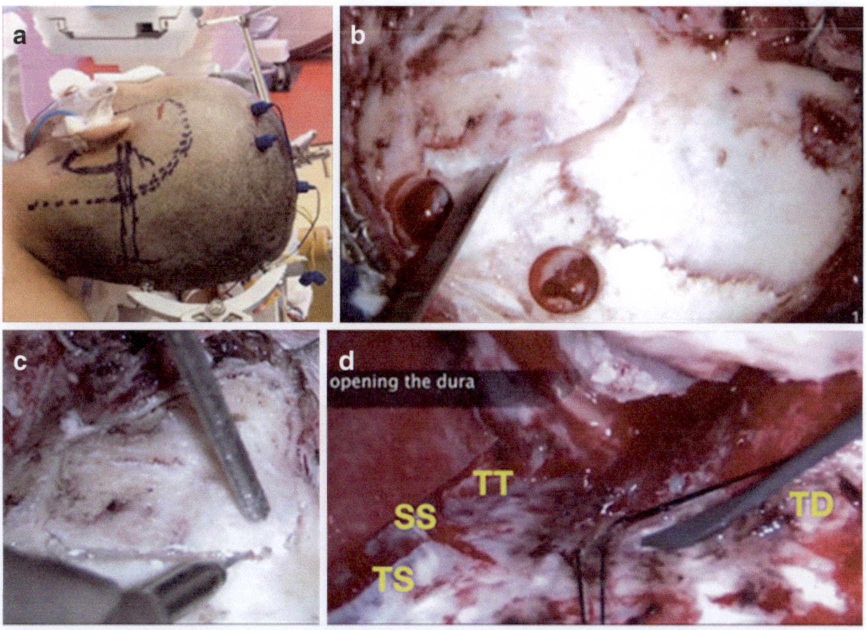

Fig. 1.5 Combined supra-infratentorial presigmoid retrolabrynthine approach. (**a**) Left park-bench position. Inverted J-shaped scalp incision with marking of the lateral sinus as shown. (**b**) Temporal suboccipital craniotomy in one or two pieces using 1–2 sets of burr-holes alongside the lateral sinus. (**c**) Complement boney exposure by elevation of a mastoid flap, drilling the air cells to skeletonize the sigmoid sinus. (**d**) Incision of the subtemporal and presigmoid dura "Trautman triangle" for double ligation of superior petrosal Vein. Transverse sinus (TS), Sphenoid sinus (SS), Trautman triangle dura (TT), Temporal dura (TD)

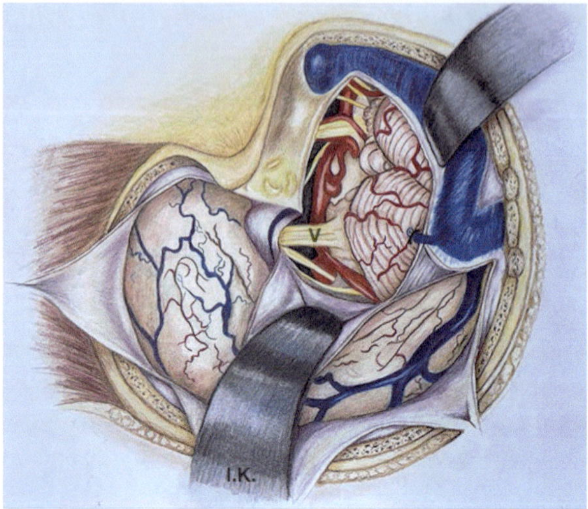

Fig. 1.6 Modified Hakuba approach. Artistic drawing illustrates the wide exposure of basilar artery system, anterior aspect of the brain stem, and cranial nerves III–XI and identifies an aneurysm at the origin of AICA with least retraction

sides of the transverse sinus just lateral to the asterion with special attention not to injure the lateral sinus or the vein of Labbé. Step 2: Performing a simple mastoidectomy by elevating a triangular mastoid cortical flap that is extended from the supramastoid ridge to the mastoid tip using a pediatric oscillating saw or B1 Midas Rex cuter. Drilling out the air cells of the antrum and exposing the presigmoid dura (Trautman triangle) and skeletonizing the sigmoid sinus down to the jugular bulb. The latter maneuver is crucial to allow maximal mobilization of the sigmoid sinus upon incising the tentorium. Special attention should be paid to preserve the integrity of the semicircular canals and the fallopian canal of the facial nerve. Step 3: Opening of the presigmoid and temporal-basal dura, followed by coagulation, double ligation, and cutting of the superior petrosal sinus. Eventually, incision of the tentorium is performed toward its free edge in parallel to the petrous ridge and posterior to the entry of the fourth nerve under the tent.

The merits of this approach rest on its direct multi-channel access to the CPA, Meckel's cave, ambient and prepontine cisterns, and petroclival region, providing a panoramic exposure of the anterior aspect of the brain stem, the basilar artery, and its proximal branches with least retraction of the cerebellum or brain stem. This approach is of a great value in management of several Vertebrobasilar system aneurysms. These include the P2–P3, proximal SCA, basilar tip and trunk, AICA, and some PICA aneurysms, especially the complex or giant ones (Fig. 1.6). This approach often entails significant bone drilling and increases the operative time and potential associated complications.

Recently, considering the major leap in the field of endovascular interventions and the hybrid use of endoscopic skull base surgery, we opt to restrict the indications for such a tedious approach to specific conditions. In particular, this refers to patients with giant petroclival skull base tumors with the aim of achieving more radical resection and a better long-term outcome as well as to treat difficult and special complex or giant vertebrobasilar aneurysms and the ones that failed neurovascular intervention.

1.3.3 Far-Lateral Approach and Extreme Lateral Inferior Trans-Condylar Approach (Elite)

These approaches provide direct access to remove tumors sited at the anterolateral aspect of the foramen magnum and the brain stem, or are used to manage aneurysms of the Vertebrobasilar junction and basilar trunk below the origin of AICA [40–45]. They agree with the general concept of skull base surgery by the removing of more bones in favor of better exposure and minimal cerebellar retraction.

1.3.3.1 Intervention

The author adopts the tailored far-lateral approach variant but performed in 3-quarter prone position [45], described as follows: Incision of the skin behind the ear in curvilineal fashion, about 2 cm posterior to the mastoid, followed by incision of the muscles and subperiosteal exposure of the suboccipital bone and the posterior lip of the foramen magna. Elevation of suboccipital bone flap using one burr hole. Enhancing the exposure by extending the bone removal laterally and resect the posterior rim of the foramen magnum up to the occipital condyle, C1 posterior arc and its ipsilateral transverse process using high-speed drill and a small rongeur (Fig. 1.7).

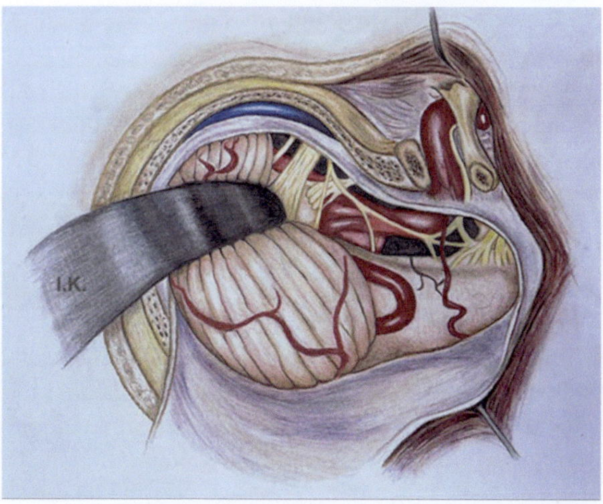

Fig. 1.7 Artistic drawing of far-lateral suboccipital approach right side in lateral or ¾ prone position. The bone exposure includes unilateral suboccipital craniotomy, the posterior lip of foramina magnum, and the C1 hemi-lamina. Exposure of extra and intradural segment of the vertebral artery (VA) for proximal control and surgical management of aneurysms at the Vertebrobasilar junction or PICA with tailored drilling of the occipital condyle and without transposition of the vertebral artery

Opening of the dura, after the exposure of the vertebral artery in the suboccipital triangle and trace it to its dura entrance. Sharp opening of the CPA cisterna and cisterna magna with possible section of the dentate ligament facilitate the exposure of regional neurovascular structure with minimal cerebellar retraction. These include Vertebrobasilar junction aneurysms, vertebral artery or PICA aneurysms.

Tailored drilling of the occipital condyle or the jugular tubercle may be deemed necessary in special cases of complex or giant aneurysms to improve their exposure and management. However, the protracted and tedious nature of the extreme far-lateral inferior trans-condylar approach (ELITE) variant with transposition of the vertebral artery and associated complication of instability has tempered its use [43]. This was also due to the rapid advancement in endovascular intervention as a popular minimally invasive alternative treatment option.

1.4 Recommended NS-Strategies for Management of Intracranial Aneurysms

Surgical indication and rehearsal of surgical intervention rest on proper evaluation of patients' clinical conditions and meticulous review of their images. Selection of the proper skull base approach is an important step in the surgical management of intracranial aneurysms. However, there is no substitute for judicious strategy and fine microsurgical dexterity. The latter warrants special training, experience, and profound knowledge of clip types and clipping methods.

The most popular clips are the MRI-compatible Yaşargil and Sugita titanium clips (crossed shaft alpha design resembling the first Greek letter alpha). They are available in different sizes and shapes including fenestrated clips to preserve intimate perforator or parent vessel during clipping. Other special clips include booster clip, t-bar fenestrated clip, and the Sundt graft clips for potential use in some cases of blister aneurysms or during catastrophic aneurysmal neck tears. Method of clipping is to be tailored to the shape, size, configuration, oscillatory stress index (OSI) and flow dynamic study, neck size and ratio, orientation, relation to adjacent perforators and parent vessel, and rupture site. These methods encompass variety of simple clipping, tandem clipping, interlocking clipping, pilot/tentative, staged or progressive clipping, and vessel reconstructive clipping.

Primary consideration for temporary clipping is a judgment call and as needed. However, in recent practice, it is reserved for cases of premature rupture and during treatment of complex and giant aneurysms [29]. Special attention is paid not to compromise a retrograde filling of other uninvolved innocent branches. The temporary clip should not be used in lieu of a permanent clip and its use should be timed out, not to exceed 5 minutes (or 10–15 min on and off), and under normotensive conditions. The Yaşargil temporary clip closing pressure shows 0.88–1.08 N (90–110 g) and for the permanent clip 1.47–1.96 N (150–180 g). Whereas for Sugita temporary clips closing pressure is 0.69 N (70 g) and for permanent clip ranges 1.27–1.47 (130–150 g) [46, 47].

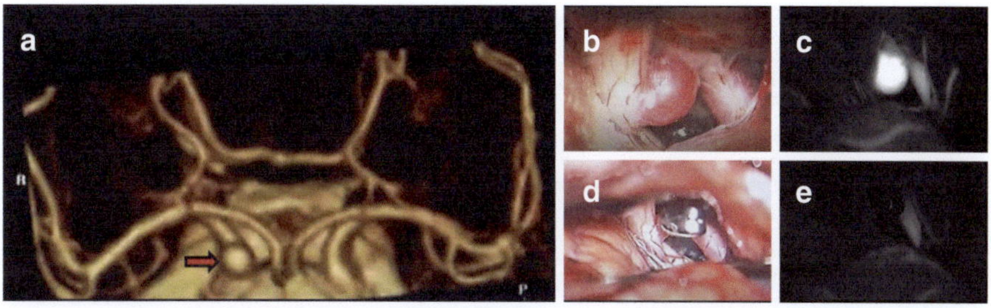

Fig. 1.8 (**a**) CT angiography depicting right ICA aneurysm "red arrow". (**b** + **c**) Intraoperative microscopic and ICG angiographic views of R. ICA' aneurysm "preclipping". (**d** + **e**) Intraoperative microscopic and ICG angiographic views confirm the complete obliteration of the ICA aneurysm post clipping with normal flow in the parent vessel. ("Courtesy G. Broggi")

The author's strategies consider the use of bipolar coagulation in some cases to shrink the neck of an aneurysm for better clipping or to treat blister aneurysm, rapping or entrapment of fusiform aneurysm, complemented with bypass procedure using vascular graft conduit or direct vascular anastomosis. The selection of bypass type should rely on the quantitative flow measurement. The innovative hybrid use of endoscopy, 3D ICG angiography, and quantitative flow measurement to check clip position and complete occlusion of the aneurysm while maintaining good vascular flow in the parent vessels and adjacent perforators or a good flow in the graft have added great value to the surgical outcome [48–50] (Fig. 1.8).

1.5 Conclusion

Most anterior circulation aneurysms are amenable to clipping via simple pterional approach using the concept of "subarachnoidal surgery" as coined by Yaşargil. However, some aneurysms may require a more intricate approach such as modified FOZ or Dolenc approach to have better exposure, proximal control or provide an adequate space to apply a temporary clip such as in some proximal ophthalmic/ICA aneurysms, paraclinoid aneurysms, and distal basilar aneurysms.

Posterior circulation aneurysms represent only 10–15% of all IAs but they are more difficult to manage. A simple suboccipital, retrosigmoid, or paramedian suboccipital approach may suffice for clipping most peripheral aneurysms of SCA, AICA, and PICA aneurysms. However, proximal branch' aneurysms, Vertebrobasilar junction and basilar trunk aneurysms demand advanced skull base exposures to pave the way for fine microsurgical techniques. These approaches include Kawase approach, combined petrosal or tailored far-lateral approach as described above. The same strategies may apply for giant anterior or posterior circulations intracranial aneurysms. The newly introduced innovative approach of transclival access is still in its infancy and demands more clinical and scientific validation.

Table 1.1 Proposed features of complex aneurysms [51, 52]

• Giant aneurysm (≥25 mm diameter)	• Broad neck aneurysm
• Calcification of the aneurysmal wall	• Intraluminal thrombus
• Wall structure (blister-like, dissecting)	• Vulnerable configuration (angioarchitecture)
• Location (difficult access)	• Parent artery/perforators (part of aneurysm)
• Embedding or adherent to neural structures	• Absence of collateral circulation
• Previous endovascular treatment	• Previously failed surgery

Nowadays, neurosurgeons' ingenuity and talent are taxed with more complex aneurysms, giant aneurysms, blister and small aneurysms, and aneurysms with hematoma, in addition to managing post-endovascular intervention failures [51, 52] (Table 1.1).

A good number of these lesions are not amenable to achieving a long-lasting and successful outcome with endovascular treatment option. On the other hand, elderly patients, presence of severe co-morbidities, vasospasm, calcification of the aneurysm neck, and unfavorable anatomy represent high-risk situations for surgery intervention. Recent innovation in endovascular treatment using pipeline or flow converter stents has proven helpful in treating a specific category of difficult aneurysms. Therefore, the important role of a joint vascular team should not be underestimated, with expertise of both disciplines contributing towards the evaluation and selection of the best treatment option for their patients to achieve rewarding outcomes.

References

1. Dott NM. Intracranial aneurysms cerebral arterio-radiography and surgical treatment. Edinb Med J. 1933;2:219–34.
2. Dandy WE. The surgical treatment of intracranial aneurysms of the internal carotid artery. Ann Surg. 1941;2:336–40. https://doi.org/10.1097/00000658-194109000-00003.
3. Norlen G, Olivecrona H. The treatment of aneurysms of the circle of Willis. J Neurosurg. 1953;10(4):404–15. https://doi.org/10.3171/jns.1953.10.4.0404. PMID: 13070065.
4. Drake CG. Bleeding aneurysms of the basilar artery. Direct surgical management in four cases. J Neurosurg. 1961;18:230–8.
5. Drake CG. The treatment of aneurysms of the posterior circulation. Clin Neurosurg. 1979;26:96–144.
6. Drake CG, Peerless SJ, Hernesniemi JA. Surgery of vertebrobasilar aneurysms—London, Ontario experience on 1767 patients. Vienna: Springer-Verlag Wien Publishers; 1995.
7. Krayenbuhl HA, Yaşargil MG, Flamm ES, Tew JM Jr. Microsurgical treatment of intracranial saccular aneurysms. J Neurosurg. 1972;2:678–86. https://doi.org/10.3171/jns.1972.37.6.0678.
8. Yaşargil MG, Antic J, Laciga R, Jain KK, Hodosh RM, Smith RD. Microsurgical pterional approach to aneurysms of the basilar bifurcation. Surg Neurol. 1976;2:83–91.
9. Sugita K, Kobayashi S, Takemae T, Tada T, Tanaka Y. Aneurysms of the basilar artery trunk. J Neurosurg. 1987;66:500–5. https://doi.org/10.3171/jns.1987.66.4.0500.
10. Heuer GJ, Dandy WE. A new hypophysis operation. Johns Hopkins Hosp Bull. 1918;29:154.

11. Dandy WE. Intracranial arterial aneurysms. New York: Hafner; 1944. Reprinted.
12. Kanaan IN. Trans-eyebrow mini-orbitozygomatic pterional approach for minimally invasive skull base surgery. Minim Invas Neurosurg. 2005;48(1):34–8.
13. Lan Q, Gong Z, Kang D, et al. Microsurgical experience with keyhole operations on intracranial aneurysms. Surg Neurol. 2006;66(Suppl 1):S2–9.
14. Fischer G, Stadie A, Reisch R, Hopf NJ, Fries G, Böcher-Schwarz H, et al. The keyhole concept in aneurysm surgery: results of the past 20 years. Oper Neurosurg. 2011;68:45–51. Back to cited text no. 1.
15. McArthur LL. An aseptic surgical access to the pituitary body and its neighborhood. JAMA. 1912;58:2009–11.
16. Frazer CH. An approach to the hypophysis through the anterior cranial fossa. Ann Surg. 1913;57(2):145–50.
17. Jane JA, Park TS, Pobereskin LH, et al. The supraorbital approach: technical note. Neurosurgery. 1982;11(4):537–42.
18. Pellerin P, Lesoin F, Dhellemmes P, et al. Usefulness of the orbitofrontomalar approach associated with bone reconstruction for frontotemporosphenoid meningiomas. Neurosurgery. 1984;15(5):715–8.
19. Hakuba A, Liu SS, Shuro N. The orbitozygomatic infratemporal approach: a new surgical technique. Surg Neurol. 1986;26(3):271–6.
20. Al-Mefty O. Supraorbital-pterional approach to skull base lesions. Neurosurgery. 1987;21:474–7.
21. Andaluz N, Keller JT, van Loveren HR, Zuccarello M. Anatomical and clinical study of the orbitopteri onal approach to anterior communicating artery aneu rysms. Neurosurgery. 2003;52(5):1140–9.
22. McDermott MW, Durity FA, Rootman J, et al. Combined frontotemporal- orbitozygomatic approach for tumors of the sphenoid wing and orbit. Neurosurgery. 1990;26(1):107–16.
23. Zabramski JM, Kiris T, Sankhla SK, Cabiol J, Spetzler RF. Orbitozygomatic craniotomy: technical note. J Neurosurg. 1998;89(2):336–41.
24. Dolenc VV. A combined epi-and subdural direct approach to carotidophthalmin artery aneurysms. J Neurosurg. 1985;62:667–72.
25. Kawase T, Toya S, Shiobara R, et al. Transpetrosal approach for aneurysms of the lower basilar artery. J Neurosurg. 1985;63:857–61.
26. Kawase T, Bertalanffy H, Otani M, et al. Surgical ap proaches for vertebrobasilar trunk aneurysms located in the midline. Acta Neurochir (Wien). 1996;138:402–10. https://doi.org/10.1007/BF01420302.
27. Mason AM, Michael Cawley C III, Barrow DL. Surgical management of intracranial aneurysms in the endovascular era: review article. Skull Base. 2011;21(4):233–42.
28. Ballance C. Some points in the surgery of the brain and its membranes. London: Macmillan; 1907.
29. Yaşargil MG. Microneurosurgery volume (1). New York: Thieme-Stratton; 1984. p. 25–53.
30. Rhoton AL. The cerebellopontine angle and posterior fossa cranial nerves by the retrosigmoid approach. Neurosurgery. 2000;47(Suppl_3):S93–S129.
31. Hakuba A, Nishimura S, Jang BJ. A combined retroauricular and preauricular transpetrosal-transtentorial approach to clivus meningiomas. Surg Neurol. 1988;30(2):108–16.
32. Samii M, Ammirati M. The combined supra-infratentorial pre-sigmoid sinus avenue to the petro-clival region. Surgical technique and clinical applications. Acta Neurochirur. 1988;95(1–2):6–12.
33. Giannotta SL, Maceri DR. Retrolabyrinthine transsigmoid approach to basilar trunk and vertebrobasilar artery junction aneurysms. J Neurosurg. 1988;69:461–6.
34. Fukushima T. Combined supra- and infra-parapetrosal approach for petroclival lesions. In: Sekhar LN, Janecka IP, editors. Surgery of cranial base tumors. New York: Raven Press; 1993. p. 661–9.
35. Spetzler RF, Daspit CP, Pappas CTE. The combined supra-and infratentorial approach for lesions of the petrous and clival regions; experience with 46 cases. J Neurosurg. 1992;76:588–99.

36. Couldwell WT, Fukushima T, Giannotta SL, et al. Petroclival meningiomas: surgical experience in 109 cases. J Neurosurg. 1996;84(1):20–8.
37. Seifert V. Direct surgery of basilar trunk and vertebrobasilar junction aneurysms via the combined trans petrosal approach. Neurol Med Chir (Tokyo). 1998;38(Suppl):86–92. https://doi.org/10.2176/nmc.38.suppl_86.
38. Wong R, Wong A, Stamates M, et al. Radiographic assessment of the presigmoid retrolabyrinthine approach. Surg Neurol Int. 2017;8:129.
39. Erkmen K, Pravdenkova S, Al-Mefty O. Surgical management of petroclival meningiomas: factors determining the choice of approach. Neurosurg Focus. 2005;19(2):E7.
40. Heros RC. Lateral suboccipital approach for vertebral and vertebrobasilar artery lesions. J Neurosurg. 1986;64:559–62.
41. Sen CN, Sekhar L. An extreme lateral approach to intradural lesions of the cervical spine and foramen magnum. Neurosurgery. 1990;27:197–294.
42. Sekhar LN, Kalia KK, Yonas H, Wright DC, Ching H. Cranial base approaches to intracranial aneurysms in the subarachnoid space. Neurosurgery. 1994;35:472–83.
43. Rhoton AL. The far-lateral approach and its transcondylar, supracondylar, and paracondylar extensions. Neurosurgery. 2000;47(Suppl):S195–209.
44. Hamilton MG, Spetzler RF. Surgical management of midbasilar and lower basilar aneurysms. In: Schmidek HH, editor. Operative neurosurgical techniques: indications, methods, and techniques. 4th ed. Philadelphia, PA: W.B. Saunders Company; 2000. p. 1247–60.
45. Nanda A, Vincent D, Vannemreddy PSS, Baskaya MK, Chanda A. Far-lateral approach to intradural lesions of the foramen magnum without resection of the occipital condyle. J Neurosurg. 2002;96:302–9.
46. Yaşargil Aneurysm Clip System Brochure [Internet]. Available from: https://www.aesculapusa.com/content/dam/aesculap-us/us/website/aesculap-inc/healthcareprofessionals/or-soultions/pdfs/DOC697-YASARAGIL%20Aneurysm%20Clip%20System%20Brochure-Rev%20H.pdf [Last cited on 2015 Feb 2].
47. Sugita2.pdf [Internet]. Available from: http://www.mizuhomedical.jp/sugita2.pdf [Last cited on 2015 Feb 2].
48. Imizu S, Kato Y, Sangli A, Oguri D, Sano H. Assessment of incomplete clipping of aneurysms intraoperatively by a near-infrared indocyanine green-video angiography (Niicg-Va) integrated microscope. Minim Invasive Neurosurg. 2008;51(4):199–203. https://doi.org/10.1055/s-2008-1080916. PMID: 186831099.
49. Nishiyama Y, Kinouchi H, Senbokuya N, Kato T, Kanemaru K, Yoshioka H, Horikoshi T. Endoscopic indocyanine green video angiography in aneurysm surgery: an innovative method for intraoperative assessment of blood flow in vasculature hidden from microscopic view case reports. J Neurosurg. 2012;117(2):302–8. https://doi.org/10.3171/2012.5.JNS112300. Epub 2012 Jun 8.
50. Yoshioka H, Kinouchi H. The roles of endoscope in aneurysmal surgery. Neurol Med Chir (Tokyo). 2015;55(6):469–78. https://doi.org/10.2176/nmc.ra.2014-0428. Published online 2015 Jun 2. PMCID: PMC4628198. PMID: 26041623.
51. Hanel RA, Spetzler RF. Surgical treatment of complex intracranial aneurysms. Neurosurgery. 2008;62(6 Suppl 3):1289–97; discussion 1297–1299.
52. Andaluz N, Zuccarello M. Treatment strategies for complex intracranial aneurysms: review of a 12-year experience at the University of Cincinnati. Skull Base. 2011;21(4):233–42. PMCID: PMC3312119, PMID: 22470266.

Chapter 2
Microsurgical Treatment of Deep and Eloquent AVMs

Phillip Cem Cezayirli, Hatice Türe, and Uğur Türe

Abbreviations

3D	Three dimensional
ACA	Anterior cerebral artery
AED	Antiepileptic drug
AP	Anteroposterior
ARUBA	A randomized controlled trial of unruptured brain AVMs
AVM	Arteriovenous malformation
CT	Computed tomography
CTA	Computed tomography angiography
DSA	Digital subtraction angiography
fMRI	Functional magnetic resonance imaging
ICA	Internal carotid artery
ICG	Indocyanine green
MCA	Middle cerebral artery
MRI	Magnetic resonance imaging

P. C. Cezayirli
Department of Neurosurgery, Yeditepe University School of Medicine, Istanbul, Turkey

Albert Einstein College of Medicine, Bronx, NY, USA

Montefiore Medical Center, Bronx, NY, USA
e-mail: pcezayir@montefiore.org

H. Türe
Department of Anesthesiology, Yeditepe University School of Medicine, Istanbul, Turkey

U. Türe (✉)
Department of Neurosurgery, Yeditepe University School of Medicine, Istanbul, Turkey

Y. Kato, A. Ansari (eds.), *Cerebrovascular Surgery*, Advances and Technical Standards in Neurosurgery 44, https://doi.org/10.1007/978-3-030-87649-4_2

mRS	Modified Rankin Scale
PCA	Posterior cerebral artery
SM	Spetzler–Martin

2.1 Introduction

The natural history of arteriovenous malformations (AVMs) varies based on their location and angio-architecture as well as the characteristics of the patient [1–5]. Unfortunately, there is no well-established grading system to predict the natural history of an individual AVM [4, 6–18]. Most authors cite general, prospective, or retrospective studies that provide low-level evidence of the natural history of AVMs but do not provide the natural history of an AVM in an individual patient. The ARUBA (A Randomized Controlled Trial of Unruptured Brain AVMs) trial was not designed to evaluate the natural history of AVMs based on angio-architectural or patient characteristics [6, 19–21]. Instead, this trial was designed to evaluate the benefit of medical management versus any treatment for unruptured AVMs, and the trial utilized the Spetzler–Martin (SM) grading system for AVMs to differentiate them [20, 22, 23]. The SM grading system is meant to be a guide to the surgical risks of microneurosurgical resection of an AVM and does not predict the natural history of the lesion nor the morbidity and mortality from different treatments [23–26].

AVMs can be in many locations throughout the central nervous system, including areas defined as "eloquent" according to the SM grading system [23]. These areas are termed eloquent because damage to them may cause noticeable morbidity in the patient when evaluated with relatively crude bedside examinations and outcome scales such as the Glasgow Outcome Scale or modified Rankin Scale (mRS) [23, 25, 27–29].

According to limited cases series and registries, deep AVMs have a natural history of a higher risk of hemorrhage, morbidity, and mortality [7, 17, 30–36]. The marginal benefits of treating deep AVMs or AVMs with deep venous drainage may be much greater than the marginal benefits of treating superficial AVMs with superficial drainage [7, 32, 36].

No randomized controlled trial compares different interventional treatment modalities directly, although many prospective and retrospective studies have been done to evaluate the different treatments of AVMs [4, 37, 38]. Microneurosurgical resection has the highest treatment success rates with similar overall morbidity and mortality when compared with endovascular embolization and radiosurgery as singular treatments [4, 18, 37, 39–47]. The promise of preoperative embolization is to decrease operative time and blood loss, and improve outcomes; however, the utility of preoperative embolization has been called into question in recent evaluations [48–59].

We aim to show that microneurosurgical resection of deep and eloquent AVMs can be done in a safe and effective manner to benefit the patient. Advances in preoperative and intraoperative tools have made this resection safer with good outcomes that beat the natural history of deep and eloquent AVMs. Importantly, deep AVMs can have a more worrisome natural history that should lower the threshold for treatment and, in our view, the natural history of an individual AVM for an individual patient is of utmost importance. Lastly, we do not believe that the term "eloquent" should be used to describe certain areas of the brain because this designation indicates that there are non-eloquent areas of the brain. Certainly, some areas of the brain have more obvious and striking effects if they are damaged; however, in the most common AVMs that have a compact nidus, there should be no intervening normal brain within the AVM. Therefore, any damage to surrounding brain tissue can and should be avoided when utilizing microneurosurgical techniques and adjuncts [2, 60].

2.2 Standards

2.2.1 Description

Deep and eloquent brain AVMs have come to be graded with the Spetzler–Martin system, as established in their seminal paper in 1986 [23], which was later simplified by Hamilton and Spetzler [28] and Spetzler and Ponce [61] and supplemented by other authors [23, 28, 61–63]. For surgical planning and decision making, we categorize AVMs based on the topographical and vascular terminology described by Yaşargil [1–3] and later modified by Valavanis and associates [1–3, 46] (Fig. 2.1). We do not alter our treatment decisions based on predictive systems of surgical outcome or eloquence and drainage patterns; instead, our decision to treat is based on concern over future hemorrhage and morbidity from the AVM in the individual

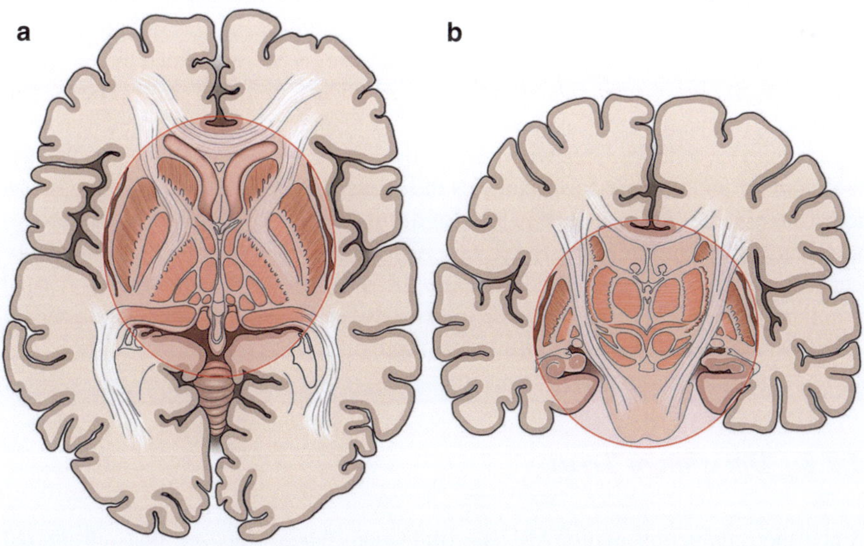

Fig. 2.1 Axial (**a**) and coronal (**b**) depictions of deep (or central) regions of the brain delineated by the darker, encircled regions. Convexity (or pallial) regions of the brain are outside of the encircled deep region. (Adapted from Yaşargil's Microneurosurgery, Volume IIIb [2])

patient. In particular, evidence of venous hypertension is one of our greatest indications for treatment. This may be indicated by cardiac output failure, papilledema, a venous varix, or venous dilation, stasis, or stenosis (especially stenosis of the deep venous system) [1–3, 64].

As described by Yaşargil and later modified by Valavanis, the arterial supply of an AVM may have both dominant and supplementary channels, which may be direct or indirect [1–3]. Understanding the specific variations of the arteries involved in an AVM is vital to surgical planning and ensuring a safe surgical resection. Specifically, differentiating and recognizing where and when an artery does (or does not) end in the nidus of an AVM is essential to ensuring safe and effective surgical resection.

The size of the nidus of an AVM has been classically based on anteroposterior and lateral angiographic images, but more recently magnetic resonance imaging (MRI) and 3D reconstructions have enabled more accurate and sensitive descriptions of AVM size [1–3]. We utilize Yaşargil's classification of AVM nidus size: micro (0.5–1.0 cm), small (1–2 cm), moderate (2–4 cm), large (4–6 cm), and giant (>6 cm), with a nidus that may be compact, multifocal, or diffuse [1–3].

The two main locations of lesions described by Yaşargil (and later modified by Valavanis) are the convexity (or pallial) AVMs and the central (or deep) AVMs [1–3]. The modification provided by Valavanis and Yaşargil helps in understanding the likely vascular supply and venous drainage patterns. We agree that diffuse (non-compact) AVMs with normal brain tissue intermingled between areas of the nidus are likely distinct entities with a different natural history and management [3, 65], as described and termed by Lasjaunius and associates as cerebral proliferative angiopathy [66], and we do not believe they are suitable candidates for microneurosurgical resection.

To clarify the term *diffuse*, there is the pseudo-diffuseness of an AVM from secondary perinidal angiogenesis (as described by Lawton and others), and there is the diffuse AVM with a different natural history (that Lasjaunius calls cerebral proliferative angiopathy) [1–3, 46, 61, 62, 65–69]. Pseudo-diffuse AVMs, as defined by Valavanis, are AVMs that have moderate or extensive secondary perinidal angiogenesis, and super-selective angiography is required to delineate the nidus from perinidal secondary changes [3, 46]. We agree with Lawton that AVMs with these secondary changes are more difficult to treat—especially as the changes increase; however, there seems to be inter-institutional variance in rates of diffuseness, and we believe these secondary changes require further study [61, 66]. AVMs with minimal or no perinidal angiogenesis allow the surgeon to differentiate the nidus from the surrounding normal brain; however, AVMs with moderate to extensive secondary perinidal angiogenesis, which Valavanis called pseudo-diffuse, are more difficult to treat [3, 46, 62, 66].

2.2.2 Decision to Treat

Since the completion of the ARUBA trial, many have proposed that unruptured AVMs should be medically managed; however, we believe the angio-architecture of the AVM and the characteristics of the patient dictate our decision to treat, not a poorly constructed randomized controlled trial [19, 20, 22]. The hallmarks of prior rupture include conspicuous hemorrhage when the patient presents acutely and as seen on computed tomography (CT), along with hemosiderin seen on MRI [70, 71]. Seizures, headaches, and neurological changes may be reasons for initial imaging in the outpatient setting, and the symptomatology or signs may correlate with the AVM [1–3]. Flow-related aneurysms indicate increased flow to the AVM, but there are mixed and inconclusive results as to whether a flow-related aneurysm correlates with a risk of AVM hemorrhage, but the aneurysm should be treated if the AVM itself will be left alone and watched [2–4, 7, 14, 72]. Venous hypertension, stasis, and outflow stenosis are our greatest indications to treat the AVM, but most patients with these venous changes have evidence of prior hemorrhage or signs and symptoms from the AVM; however, the evidence and classification of these venous changes are neither well established nor codified for deciding treatment [1–4, 7, 9, 10, 12, 13, 15, 29, 36, 44, 46, 73, 74].

For the past 30 years, the Spetzler–Martin grading system has defined AVMs based on venous drainage location, eloquent locations, and size; however, this system (and later iterations) does not predict the risk of hemorrhage or morbidity from the AVM itself but instead predicts the risk of microneurosurgical resection [24, 26, 75]. The venous drainage location does not affect our decision to treat, but it does help guide us for surgical planning. We do not differentiate our surgical decisions based on eloquent locations, but we do discuss the risks, benefits, and alternatives of resection with the patient based on the patient, the anatomical location of the AVM, and the AVM's angio-architecture. In particular, venous hypertension seen on preoperative imaging and/or the patient's signs and symptoms of venous hypertension are our greatest indication for treating a patient's AVM, in particular with occlusion of the straight sinus [1–3, 64].

2.2.3 *Microneurosurgical Technique*

The standard for resecting a brain AVM does not change based on the depth, venous drainage, size, or presumed eloquence. The microneurosurgical technique used to approach these lesions developed over the second half of the twentieth century [1, 2, 76–79]. Careful study of preoperative imaging and anatomical knowledge are vital for successful microneurosurgical resection of an AVM, which helps the surgeon understand the flow, arterial supply, and venous system. This understanding in turn helps with setting up the next steps of the procedure: the operative approach and patient positioning [1–3, 80],

When possible, we plan our operative approach so that the main venous drainage is deep rather than superficial, although this is often not feasible with convexity AVMs. Additionally, we plan our approach through a fissure, sulcus, or the least amount of brain [2]. We utilize a wide opening and craniotomy to maximize visualization of the AVM and surrounding anatomy [2]. After opening the dura (utilizing the Doppler and intraoperative ultrasound to avoid premature damage to the AVM), we perform indocyanine green (ICG) video-angiography before any further dissection, which allows us to evaluate the flow and direction of the observed vessels [1, 2, 81–85]. Our intraoperative view and understanding of the AVM and ICG video are compared to our expected view and the angio-architecture of the AVM based on preoperative studies and our anatomical and pathological knowledge of the disease. Prior to disrupting the AVM, we open sulci, fissures, and arachnoid around and adjacent to the AVM to identify important arterial and venous anatomy while allowing for egress of cerebrospinal fluid and brain relaxation [1, 2]. Once the important superficial anatomy has been exposed and identified, we compare what we see through the microscope to what we expected when looking at preoperative imaging and intraoperative ultrasound, which we find more accurate than neuronavigation [1–3, 83, 84]. To better understand the AVM, we repeat ICG video-angiography with or without the temporary placement of AVM or temporary aneurysm clips for temporary occlusion of suspected vessels. This maneuver allows us to better understand the AVM and its angio-architecture, except in small, simple AVMs (where it is not required). This technique can be repeated multiple times, especially for moderate, large, and complex AVMs [81, 82]. Additionally, the microvascular ultrasonic flow probe can be used with or without temporary clips to define the flow of the arterial and venous systems of the AVM throughout dissection and resection [83, 86].

We then work around the AVM in circumferential fashion, taking time to differentiate direct feeding vessels from indirect or transit arteries before coagulating any vessel [2]. When in doubt, we may place temporary AVM clips or temporary aneurysm clips for trial occlusions to look for AVM and cortical changes before coagulating and cutting a vessel. This maneuver may be coupled with intraoperative Doppler and/or ICG to better show the angio-architecture and flow dynamics of the AVM and potential changes [2, 81, 83]. Sacrifice of the primary draining vein is avoided until the end; however, supplementary venous elimination may be required to advance resection [2]. The primary draining vein and supplementary and adjacent veins may be differentiated based on preoperative study of the AVM along with intraoperative ultrasound and Doppler, the microvascular ultrasonic flow probe, and ICG video-angiography with or without the temporary placement of AVM clips [1–3, 81, 83–86].

Preferably, if we can first find a direct avenue to the deep arterial feeders, we then coagulate and disconnect these before coagulating the larger and superficial feeding vessels [60]. Moving circumferentially along the AVM, smaller vessels (less than 0.5 mm) may be encountered, in which case the use of bipolar cautery should be decreased to prevent bursting the small, friable artery [2]. The bipolars are kept clean and changed often throughout surgery to prevent sticking to the vessels during coagulation [2]. Non-stick bipolars are an excellent adjunct for AVM resection to prevent sticking to the small, friable vessels; however, these bipolars do not have the same weight and opening force as our normal bipolar set, so our use of the non-stick bipolars is limited because of their less familiar feel. Before coagulation of any artery, a few millimeters of the artery should be visible. This guideline has two primary benefits: the first is further identification of the target artery and the second is preventing the vessel from retracting deeper into the brain and re-bleeding [2]. To aid in exposing the vessel, the suction and/or a small cotton patty can be used to retract brain tissue from the exiting vessel. Alternatively, the previously exposed adjacent sulci and fissures may be used to better visualize the targeted artery [2]. In many cases, the temporary placement of AVM clips on larger vessels is necessary to stop nuisance bleeding, which is more likely near the corona radiata, internal capsule, ependyma, caudate, thalamus, and cerebellar peduncles. Wide dissection of normal brain should be avoided, however, as should the removal of an AVM piecemeal [2].

Once the arterial feeders are disconnected from the AVM nidus, the final draining vein should appear collapsible and darker in color [2]. Generally, additional feeding arteries are often found hidden by the main draining vein [2, 60]. At this stage, any continuing bleeding or a draining vein that is not dark or collapsible provide evidence that AVM feeders remain and should be identified, dissected, coagulated, and cut [2]. Before removing the AVM completely, ICG and Doppler are done to confirm that the arterial feeding arteries have been removed [81, 83]. Once the draining vein is coagulated and cut, the AVM can be removed. Subsequently, the operative bed is irrigated frequently and the blood pressure confirmed to be normal (not hypotensive) while we wait for the intraoperative angiogram to be done, which is usually at least 30 min after the AVM is removed. After the angiogram, we return to the microscope to evaluate the surgical bed; this is about 1 h after removal of the AVM.

The most difficult portion of the surgery is towards the end because of the presence of deep perforating arteries supplying the AVM. Lawton's cooperative study with the Helsinki group evaluated his supplementary grading system, which found that deep arterial supply affects outcome [2, 60, 64, 87]. The temporary placement of AVM clips or temporary aneurysm clips on feeding arteries is vital to prevent hemorrhage and/or identify sources of bleeding from these deep perforating arteries. We routinely apply these clips at different points throughout the case, but especially before coagulating the deep, small feeding vessels [2, 60]. For deep feeders emanating from the ventricle, it is best to enter the ventricle to identify the source arteries before coagulating these feeders [2]. When difficult-to-identify bleeding sources appear, adenosine can be given to pause cardiac activity to relieve bleeding, especially towards the end of surgery [88]. In some cases, we leave AVM or aneurysm clips on a feeding vessel postoperatively; unfortunately, as no titanium AVM clips exist, these clips cause significant artifact on postoperative MRIs.

Generally, the conduction of anesthesia for AVM resection follows the same recommendations for neuroanesthesia; however, some key points can be lifesaving for patients undergoing craniotomy. Volatile anesthetics and vasodilators can directly relax vascular smooth muscle and should be avoided. Thus, we use total intravenous anesthesia with propofol and remifentanil infusions [18]. Standard monitoring methods with four-lead electrocardiogram, peripheral oxygen saturation, both invasive and non-invasive arterial blood pressure, central venous pressure, and core temperature are utilized. However, the use of a continuous plethsymographic variability index, non-invasive hemoglobin measurement, or arterial pressure-based cardiac output monitoring may be used to manage fluid administration and follow-up transfusion trigger thresholds, given the potential for massive, rapid, and persistent blood loss [89]. Thromboelastometry of whole blood is useful for monitoring hemostasis capabilities throughout major vascular surgeries [90]. Monitoring the patient's intravascular volume status throughout the perioperative period is essential to understand the changes that occur before, during, and after major surgery. In our clinical practice, we restrict intravascular fluid infusions during cranial surgeries to between 0.5 and 1.0 mL/kg/h, which is supplemented as indicated when using invasive and non-invasive monitoring methods. Because AVMs are highly vascular lesions, the anesthesia team is ready to provide adenosine-induced transient asystole to aid with intraoperative hemostasis and prevent precarious situations during removal of the lesion [88].

Transfusion strategies should be planned preoperatively for patients with an AVM to allow for better timed and beneficial blood management. Packed red blood cells are primarily the red blood cells remaining after most of the plasma is removed from 1 unit of whole blood; thus, they do not contain platelets or clotting factors. Although fresh whole blood would be ideal, the amount of testing needed to screen the blood makes it largely impractical on a moment's notice. In clinical practice, blood donors can be prepared preoperatively, and early administration of fresh frozen plasma during expected major bleeding should be planned for as it can decrease coagulopathy and improve survival [91]. We give fresh frozen plasma before transfusing red blood cells, and we prefer giving fresh whole blood for major bleeding. Despite the sparse literature on transaxemic acid used in cranial surgeries, our anesthesia team administers it at the time of incision during major neurovascular surgeries, and they provide 24 h of postoperative dosing to minimize postoperative bleeding complications. To maintain hemodynamic stability, our anesthesia team wakes our patients up slowly and extubates them in the intensive care unit after major vascular surgeries. During the 24–48 h after surgery, the mean arterial blood pressure is kept within normal limits with the use of angiotensin-converting enzyme inhibitors (such as captopril) and calcium channel blockers (such as amlodipine). Most importantly, our anesthesia team screens, evaluates, and optimizes our patients weeks in advance, continues to manage them in the intensive care unit postoperatively, and works with our neurosurgery group as a single, cohesive team for the benefit of the patient.

Typically, we do not incorporate hypotension during or after AVM resection, although we do discuss the possible need for it with our anesthesia team before every AVM resection [2, 92–95]. Postoperative hemorrhage, stroke, or long-term deficits are indications that the nidus or involved vessels were misidentified, thereby damaging uninvolved brain regions [2]. The nidus of the AVM does not have function, nor do the end vessels of an AVM supply normal brain [1–3, 60, 96].

We do not routinely use pre- or postoperative embolization or radiation therapy for our patients; however, we do encounter and operate on previously embolized and radiated AVMs, which can make the surgery more difficult [2, 3, 49, 50, 59, 60, 97, 98]. In rare instances, we do request preoperative embolization of an AVM when there is a deep lenticulostriate or perforating arterial supply. Unfortunately, these perforating arterial feeders can rarely be embolized preoperatively [3, 59, 87].

2.3 Advances

Since the advent of microneurosurgical techniques, additional and beneficial advances have made the microneurosurgical resection of AVMs safer for our patients. Routinely, we utilize ICG video-angiography, microvascular Doppler, intraoperative ultrasound, a microvascular flow probe, preoperative advanced MRI techniques (including diffusion tensor imaging and functional MRI), preoperative angiography with 3D reconstructions, intraoperative angiography, postoperative MRI, and MRI and angiography at the 3-month follow-up.

Angiography allows for preoperative, intraoperative, and postoperative assessment of AVMs [1–3]. Newer and more advanced digital software for angiography allows for qualitative and quantitative assessment of flow dynamics and 3D reconstructions of the lesions [10, 74]. Computed tomography angiography (CTA) and newer dynamic CTA techniques allow assessment of the AVM along with its anatomic information beyond the vasculature [1–3, 37, 99, 100]. The advent of MRI has offered a different vantage point of the brain and vasculature compared to CT, CTA, and angiography; however, the most recent advances in MRI are advanced imaging such as diffusion tensor imaging and functional MRI (fMRI) to evaluate these so-called eloquent areas of the brain [1–3, 96, 101]. Quantitative evaluation of vascular flow assessment is possible with newer MRI techniques [11, 12]. Once the operative approach and plan are formulated with these advanced imaging techniques, the intraoperative adjuncts are available.

In 1979, Nornes and colleagues described the use of Doppler to assess cerebral hemodynamics intraoperatively for both aneurysms and AVMs [102]. In 1989, Rubin and associates described the intraoperative use of ultrasound with colored Doppler flow imaging for AVMs [103]. The quality of ultrasound and Doppler have increased significantly in the past 40 years and provide significant information to the surgeon to allow for safer and more effective surgeries (our experience with ultrasound and cottonoid placement has been accepted for publication) [83, 104, 105]. The microvascular ultrasonic flow probe allows for the quantitative assessment of individual vessel flow dynamics that are affected throughout the dissection and with temporary placement of micro-AVM clips or temporary aneurysm clips [83, 106]. Finally, intraoperative angiography allows us to evaluate our surgical resection of the AVM before closing the site and waking up the patient [2, 3]. The benefit of intraoperative angiography is the time added before and after the angiogram to re-evaluate the surgical bed.

In 2003, Raabe and colleagues illustrated the use of indocyanine green under video fluorescence to capture intraoperative vascular flow dynamics in a qualitative fashion [107]. Later, they incorporated this technique into a surgical microscope, allowing for intraoperative observation of vascular flow [107, 108]. In more recent years, more advanced software and algorithms have augmented visualization of this flow, overlying the direct visualization of the brain and vasculature in real-time and quantitative evaluation of flow dynamics intraoperatively [81–83, 85]. Unfortunately, there are limits to the number of times ICG can be given, and the depth of visualization of ICG is limited; however, newer techniques with ICG are being developed that allow a deeper view, along with endoscopic ICG use [107, 109–111]. The limitations of ICG video-angiography are the reason intraoperative angiography is essential for successful microsurgical resection.

Some authors have documented their use of preoperative or even postoperative embolization and/or radiosurgery for AVMs [30, 35, 48, 55, 57, 58, 112]. In our view, any patient with an AVM that should be treated should be viewed as a microsurgical candidate first [1–3]. Only for diffuse AVMs (from cerebral proliferative angiopathy) that are symptomatic do we suggest things such as staged embolization or radiosurgery [2, 3, 46, 61, 62, 65–69]. In the future, preoperative embolization may become more useful if lenticulostriate and deep perforating arteries feeding the AVM can be safely embolized preoperatively [2, 3, 46, 55, 59, 66, 87, 98].

2.4 Controversies

In 1986, the Spetzler–Martin grading system was first introduced and focused on larger AVM size, deep venous drainage, and the location of the AVM in eloquent brain as being the greatest risk factors for poor outcomes after microsurgical resection. The scale ranges from 1 to 5 with 5 being the highest risk for postoperative morbidity and mortality [23]. In later prospective and retrospective studies, the SM grading system has been validated by others, Many authors suggest that most AVMs of grades 1 or 2 can be treated safely with microneurosurgical resection with good outcomes, grade 3 should be evaluated on a case-by-case basis, and grades 4 and 5 should not be resected except in special circumstances [28, 63, 75].

In our view, the size of the AVM affects the length of the surgery more than the risks of the operation because of the increased amount of dissection required [2, 3]. In some instances, deep venous drainage makes the surgery easier than if the vein were draining superficially. This is because of the required surgical approach and the need to preserve the primary draining vein until the end of the AVM resection, especially in interhemispheric approaches, such as a cingulate AVM with drainage to the deep venous system [1, 2]. Additionally, deep venous drainage is a risk factor for future hemorrhage and worse morbidity and mortality from such hemorrhages [31–33].

The original 1986 Spetzler–Martin paper delineated eloquent regions of the brain as the following areas: motor, speech, and visual cortex (with their associated white matter pathways), the hypothalamus and thalamus, the internal capsule, the brain stem, the cerebellar peduncles, and deep cerebellar nuclei [23]. Left out of the areas denoted "eloquent" are the limbic and paralimbic areas (including the insula, mediobasal temporal region, and cingulate gyrus), the pallidum and striatum, and the entirety of the ventricular system [113]. The vasculature of AVMs may be more difficult in these non-eloquent regions because of their involvement with and proximity to deep perforating feeding vessels, for example, AVMs of the mediobasal temporal region and insula [1–3, 113]. More important is the separation of the brain into eloquent and non-eloquent regions, which we believe to be unwise.

In 1993, Itzhak Fried wrote a comment in the *Journal of Neurosurgery* about the use of the term "eloquence" and asked for a definition of non-eloquent cortex [114]. He pointed out that the inability to monitor an area at this point or grossly notice a change on a bedside exam does not mean the area is not eloquent [114]. As Fried reminded, large swaths of the frontal lobes, systematically destroyed in a frontal leucotomy, clearly are eloquent regions required for the intricate functions of the brain [114]. He pointed out that Charles Drake had been the greatest propagator of the term "eloquent" to identify certain areas of the brain [114]. Drake replied to Fried's comment in the same journal issue and provided the origin of the term "eloquent" as follows [114]. Wilder Penfield had been a visiting lecturer at Drake's institution in 1960 when Drake described Penfield's epilepsy surgery as eloquent [114]. Perhaps as an ode to Penfield, Drake transformed the use of eloquent from a description of a type of surgery to certain areas of the brain, with Drake referring to eloquent areas at least as early as 1965 in a paper on the treatment of aneurysms [115]. Drake formalized the use of eloquent areas of the brain, in regard to AVM surgery, in a 1979 paper on his experience with resection of AVMs [79]. Around the same time as Spetzler and Martin's 1986 paper, other scoring systems were published that similarly differentiated eloquent areas of the brain [25, 75, 116]. Of course, injury to regions of the brain with more obvious clinical changes may be more clearly seen on a bedside exam; however, these gross neurological exams and outcome scores do not consider more nuanced outcomes such as sexual function or higher-order functions that make humans distinct from other animals [117]. We believe the terms eloquent brain and non-eloquent or silent brain are dangerous: just because we cannot hear or see a change does not mean it is not there, just as not hearing a dog whistle does not mean it is silent. In our view, regardless of the location, size, and venous drainage location of an AVM, our decision to treat is based on the patient and the AVM angio-architecture, while our surgical approach is based on the AVM.

Much has been written about the ARUBA trial in the years after its publication, with some of the most outspoken critics coming from centers that were part of the trial [6, 21, 40, 43, 118–120]. Importantly, of the 1740 patients screened at the institutions involved in the ARUBA trial, only 226 were enrolled and randomized. Of the 18 patients undergoing microsurgical resection included in the trial of the 114 interventional-arm patients, only 5 had microsurgical resection alone. Thus the majority of morbidity in the intervention arm stemmed from singular treatment with endovascular or radiosurgery therapies or combination treatments [6, 21, 22, 40, 43, 118, 119, 121]. An additional issue with the trial, in our view, is the use of the Spetzler–Martin grading scale to differentiate between AVMs, when the SM scale was not designed to predict future hemorrhage, nor does it predict future hemorrhage in recent evaluations [23, 26]. Additionally, the SM scale was not designed to predict outcomes of non-microsurgical interventions and has not been found to do so [24, 122, 123]. The ARUBA trial was an opportunity to better understand the natural history of AVMs based on differences in patients and AVMs, but the opportunity was squandered [6, 20, 21]. Lastly, the term "unruptured" is relative to the timing and quality of the imaging: certainly, a 7 T MRI would find more signs of hemorrhage than a 1.5 T MRI [70, 71]. Our view regarding the treatment of AVMs is based on the patient and the AVM angio-architecture, not the subjective and ill-advised definition of ruptured status and eloquent brain.

We are not against the use of embolization for an AVM, but in our experience the embolization of superficial feeders is not helpful and changes the hemodynamics of the AVM [49–51, 59, 98]. In particular, "complete" embolization does not allow for coagulation and shrinking of the AVM, which makes the AVM firmer and more difficult to work around because millimeters are lost that could allow for better differentiation between the nidus and the brain [2, 3, 49, 59, 60]. Preoperative embolization of lenticulostriate, perforating, or ependymal vessels of the AVM would be helpful, but this is rarely possible and deemed a risky procedure [2, 3, 34, 35, 46, 49, 50, 55–59, 87, 98].

2.5 Illustrative Cases

2.5.1 Case 1

A 37-year-old right-handed female with a 4-year history of headache and generalized seizures came to our institution for treatment. She was taking one antiepileptic drug (AED). Her headache was progressive, but the seizures were well controlled.

Preoperative imaging with MRI revealed a left lateral, frontal, mixed gyral-sulcal convexity AVM, with a single compact nidus and a venous varix (Fig. 2.2) [1–3, 125]. This was a mixed gyral-sulcal insular fronto-opercular AVM with subcortical extension to the internal capsule and head of the caudate nucleus, along with ventricular extension to the frontal horn of the lateral ventricle. The location was within the inferior frontal gyrus, considered Broca's area between Brodmann areas 44 and 45. On fMRI, there was speech activation anterior and posterior to the AVM nidus, indicating this AVM was within Broca's speech area. The left lateral ventricular subependymal venous system appeared congested on the MRI. The angiogram showed M1–M5 involvement with the AVM's primary feeders from M1 lateral lenticulostriates and the superior trunk of M2. There was also a venous varix, tortuous deep venous drainage, and stenosis indicative of venous hypertension, but only minimal perinidal angiogenesis. Not shown on the angiogram was the presumed deep perforator anterior cerebral artery (ACA) supply to the AVM, including the recurrent artery of Heubner. The vascular steal from the primary middle cerebral artery (MCA) feeders concealed much of the deep perforator supply to the AVM [1–3, 80]. The AVM was large (4–6 cm) with a greatest diameter of 6 cm. This AVM had deep and superficial drainage. Under the Spetzler–Martin grading system, this lesion would be considered grade 4 because of the deep venous drainage, size between 3 and 6 cm, and eloquent location.

The AVM was resected through a left pterional approach. The pars opercularis was intact, the patient's headaches and seizures resolved, and there was no speech

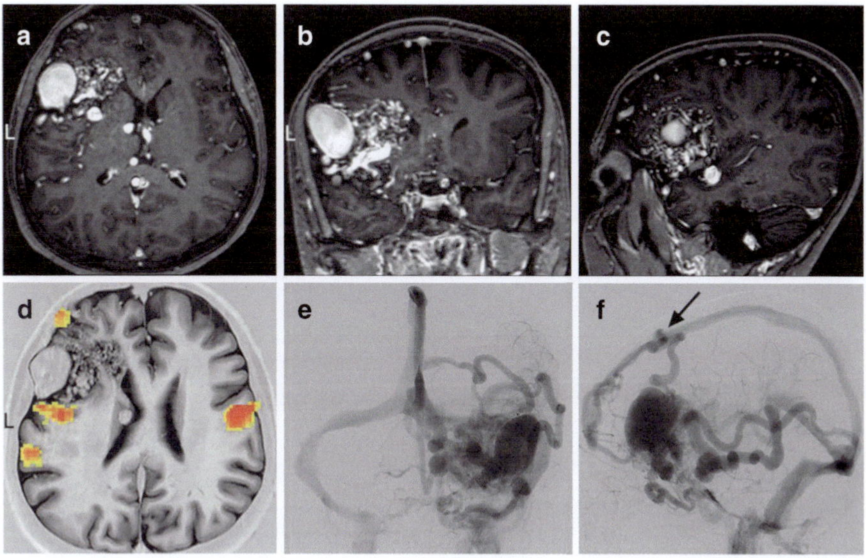

Fig. 2.2 Case 1: Preoperative T1-weighted MRI with contrast in axial (**a**), coronal (**b**), and sagittal (**c**) views show a large, mixed gyral-sulcal AVM of the left insular fronto-opercular region. There is subcortical extension deep to the head of the caudate nucleus and internal capsule, along with a ventricular extension to the frontal horn of the lateral ventricle. **Please note:** For axial and coronal MRIs and CTs, the senior author flips the image in the horizontal plane so that the left side of the brain (L) is on the left side of the image. fMRI in the axial view (**d**) indicates language activation anterior and posterior to the AVM nidus. Left ICA DSA in AP (**e**) and lateral (**f**) views: the arrow indicates venous stenosis leading to the superior sagittal sinus, with the angiogram showing M1–M5 MCA involvement with the AVM primary feeders from the M1 lateral lenticulostriate arteries and superior trunk of the M2 MCA [80, 124]. There is a venous varix with tortuous deep venous drainage and stenosis, indicating venous hypertension, but only minimal (or local) perinidal angiogenesis. The venous hypertrophy and varix are clearly visible on the DSA images (**e**, **f**). The angiogram does not show the presumed deep supply to the AVM from the ACA perforators, including the recurrent artery of Heubner. This is likely due to vascular steal from the primary feeders coming from the MCA [1–3]

difficulty (Figs. 2.3 and 2.4). In the early postoperative period, the patient had mild speech difficulties that resolved within 2 weeks, a status that was confirmed at the 3-month postoperative visit. The patient's preoperative mRS was 1, improving to 0 at the 3-month follow-up visit.

Not included in the Spetzler–Martin system is perinidal angiogenesis. The Lawton-Young supplemental grading system includes perinidal angiogenesis, which the authors term "diffuse," but there are varying rates of determination of these secondary effects between institutions [61, 62, 66, 69]. Super-selective angiography allows for better delineation between the nidal margins of the AVM and the secondary perinidal angiogenesis, and this tool should be part of any assessment of an AVM [3, 46, 69]. In this patient, although there was perinidal angiogenesis, it was subjectively minimal, which was more readily discernable in the operative view.

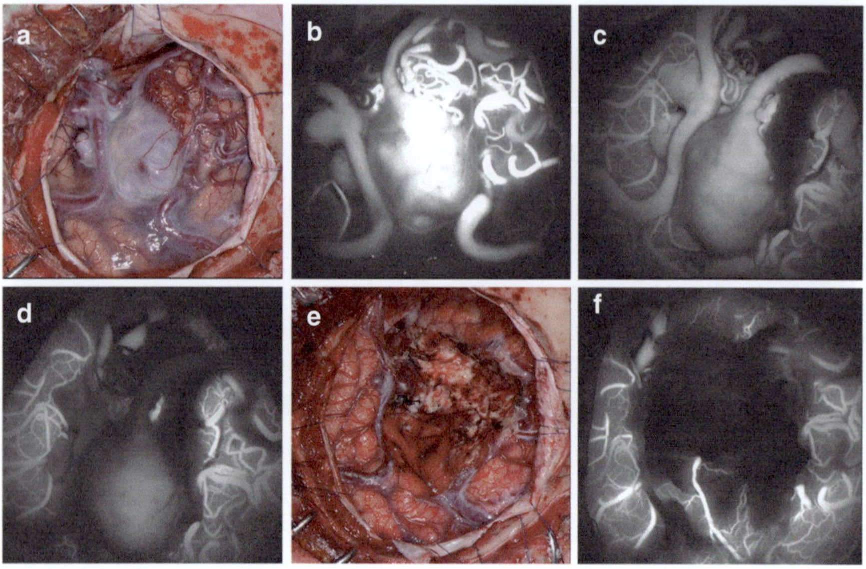

Fig. 2.3 Case 1 intraoperative images: The AVM before resection with the dura opened are depicted in a photograph (**a**) and corresponding ICG video-angiography (**b**). Early in the dissection of the AVM, ICG video-angiography (**c**) showed the initial superior plane around the AVM nidus. Later in dissection and coagulation of the AVM, additional ICG video-angiography (**d**) revealed diminished venous outflow from the AVM. Finally, after extirpation of the AVM, a photograph of the surgical bed (**e**) and ICG video-angiography (**f**) confirmed removal of the AVM

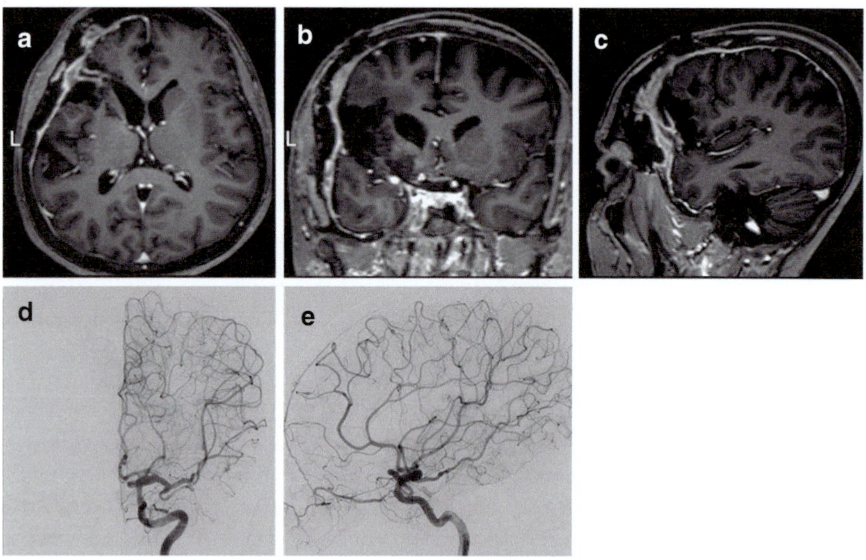

Fig. 2.4 Case 1: Postoperative T1-weighted MRI with contrast in axial (**a**), coronal (**b**), and sagittal (**c**) views shows complete resection of the AVM. (L) indicates the left side of the brain in axial and coronal views. Postoperative left ICA DSA in AP (**d**) and lateral (**e**) views shows filling of the normal vascular territories, loss of early venous drainage, and preservation of the lenticulostriate arteries

The authors of the Lawton-Young grading system had thought that a deep perforator supply to an AVM would affect outcomes; however, this was not found to be the case in their later paper, contrary to their prior publication [62, 66]. In 2019, Lawton collaborated on a follow-up study of the Lawton-Young grading system with the neurosurgery group in Helsinki, and they found that a deep perforator supply does affect outcomes [64]. We agree that a deep perforator supply makes the treatment of an AVM more difficult, but we agree with Yaşargil and others that venous hypertension and venous stenosis are indications to treat an AVM [2, 3, 64, 66, 87].

2.5.2 Case 2

A 27-year-old right-handed female with a recent history of sudden-onset headache, nausea, and vomiting was found to have an AVM at an outside hospital, 1 month prior to her surgery at our institution. The patient reported episodes occurring 4–5 times per year of a burning smell that others could not detect followed by 5–10 s of being able to hear others but not move, speak, or perceive her surroundings. These symptoms suggested limbic seizures without loss of consciousness. She was finally started on one AED once the lesion was found, but the episodes did not completely resolve. An outside institution recommended radiosurgery.

The MRI sequence revealed a right central (or deep), parenchymal limbic system AVM within the middle and posterior parahippocampal gyrus with ventricular extension, and without clear perinidal angiogenesis (Fig. 2.5). This right middle mediobasal temporal AVM had a single compact nidus, no venous varix, apparent venous hypertension, and hemorrhage on the posterior aspect. Angiography showed the arterial feeders to be the right inferior temporal branches from the P2 and P3 segments of the posterior cerebral artery (PCA) [80]. The AVM was small (1–2 cm), and 2 cm in greatest diameter. Venous drainage was to the temporal basal veins reaching to the galenic venous system with the appearance of venous stenosis leading to the galenic venous system. The angiogram did not seem to show perinidal angiogenesis and, if there were any, it was likely small and localized. Under the Spetzler–Martin grading system, this AVM would be considered grade 2 because of deep venous drainage, a size less than 3 cm, and its location not in an eloquent area.

The AVM was resected through the right-sided paramedian, supracerebellar, transtentorial (PST) approach with the patient in the semi-sitting position, along with a selective amygdalohippocampectomy to treat the seizures, a novel approach to an AVM in this location (Figs. 2.6 and 2.7) [127]. The presumed seizures resolved, and the patient could be taken off AEDs. Her vision remained intact postoperatively. The preoperative mRS of 1 improved to 0 by the 3-month follow-up visit.

Interestingly, the limbic system has been largely excluded from the delineated eloquent areas of the brain [113]. Beyond the fact that emotions and memories are important for our individual characteristics and should be considered eloquent, the vasculature and surrounding parenchyma make the mediobasal temporal region a

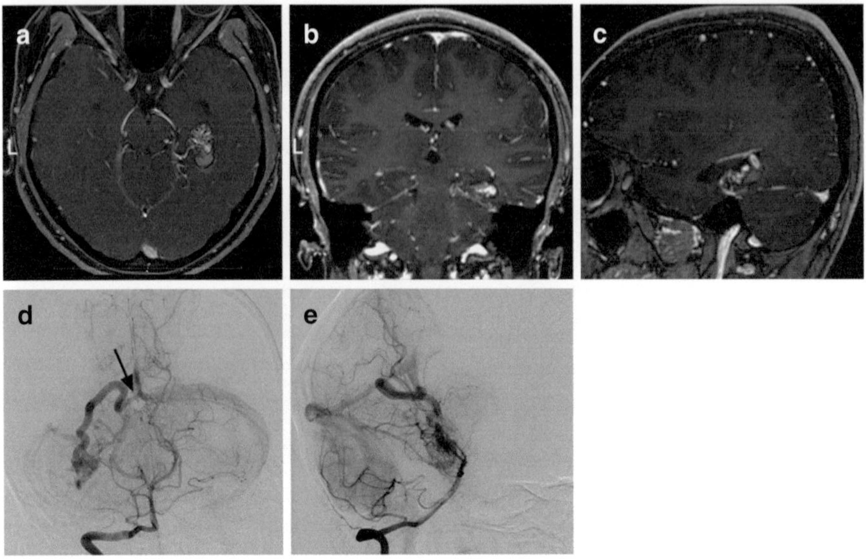

Fig. 2.5 Case 2: Preoperative T1-weighted MRI with contrast in axial (**a**), coronal (**b**), and sagittal (**c**) views shows a right middle mediobasal temporal AVM. On preoperative right vertebral artery DSA in AP (**d**) and lateral (**e**) views, the arrow indicates venous stenosis just proximal to the vein of Galen, just distal to the venous hypertrophy of the AVM. The arterial feeders are the right inferior temporal branches from the P2 and P3 segments of the PCA [80, 126]

difficult and dangerous area for resection of AVMs. This point is underappreciated and underweighted in the SM grading system.

2.5.3 Case 3

A 47-year-old right-handed male came to us with a recent onset of generalized tonic-clonic seizures emanating from where the AVM was found, with a subsequent focal seizure without loss of consciousness or generalization after starting to take AEDs. Before his referral to us, surgeons at an outside institution attempted embolization but stopped after completing only a small amount.

The preoperative MRI showed a right, mixed, deep, anterior insular AVM with both parenchymal and subarachnoid characteristics (Fig. 2.8) [1–3, 125]. Angiography outlined the arterial supply from the right M1 lateral lenticulostriates, the superior trunk of M2, and the recurrent artery of Heubner [80, 124]. Venous drainage was through the deep middle cerebral (sylvian) vein to the basal venous and subsequent galenic venous system, along with drainage to the superficial sylvian venous system. The AVM was 3 cm in greatest dimension, thus considered of moderate size (2–4 cm), making the lesion an SM grade 3 based on its deep venous drainage, non-eloquent location, and size between 3 and 6 cm.

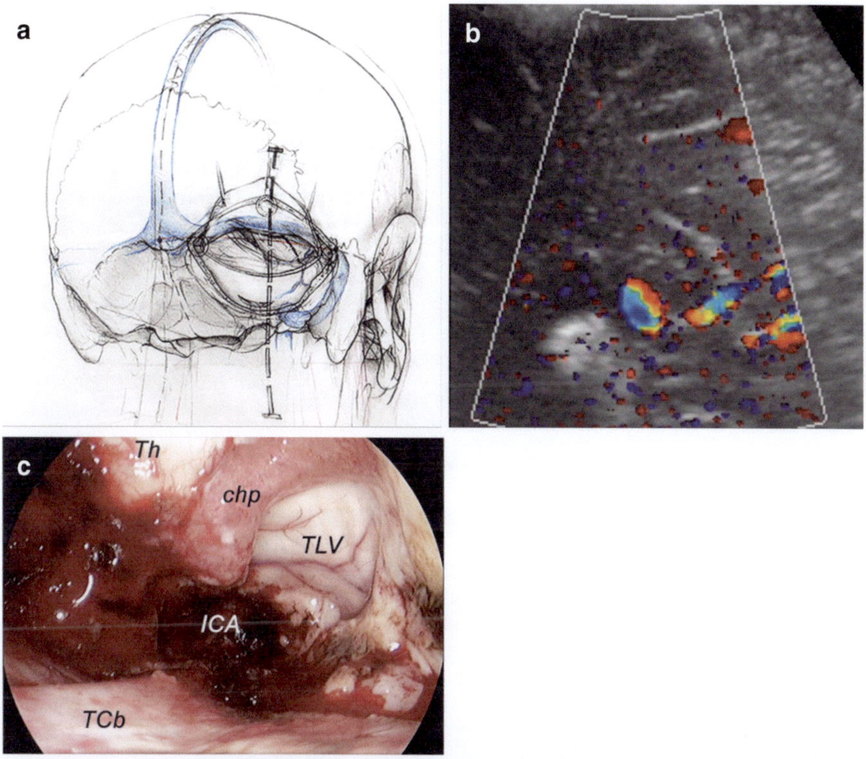

Fig. 2.6 Case 2: Illustration of the operative angle of view to the mediobasal temporal region via the right paramedian supracerebellar transtentorial approach with the patient in the semi-sitting position (**a**) [127]. Intraoperative ultrasound of the mediobasal temporal region and parts of the AVM nidus (**b**) are indicated with color-flow Doppler imaging of the ultrasound. An intraoperative endoscopic photograph taken after resection of the AVM and selective amygdalohippocampectomy (**c**) show the exposure of the choroid plexus (*chp*) of the right temporal horn of the lateral ventricle (*TLV*), the subpial view of the internal carotid artery (*ICA*), the right thalamus (*Th*), and the tentorium cerebelli (*TCb*) [80, 128]

The AVM was resected through a right pterional craniotomy via the trans-sylvian approach, with preservation of normal transit vessels including the lenticulostriates and the recurrent artery of Heubner (Figs. 2.9 and 2.10). The patient had a preoperative mRS of 1 that improved to 0 by the 3-month follow-up visit.

The insula is not included as an eloquent region of the brain, although many important emotions and visceral functions are affected by the insular region. If eloquence is differentiated by gross and clear functions at risk, then the adjacent basal ganglia and lenticulostriates that are often involved with insular lesions should be accounted for in predicting outcomes from surgery. Damage to those structures would lead to loud and clear deficits that could not be called silent.

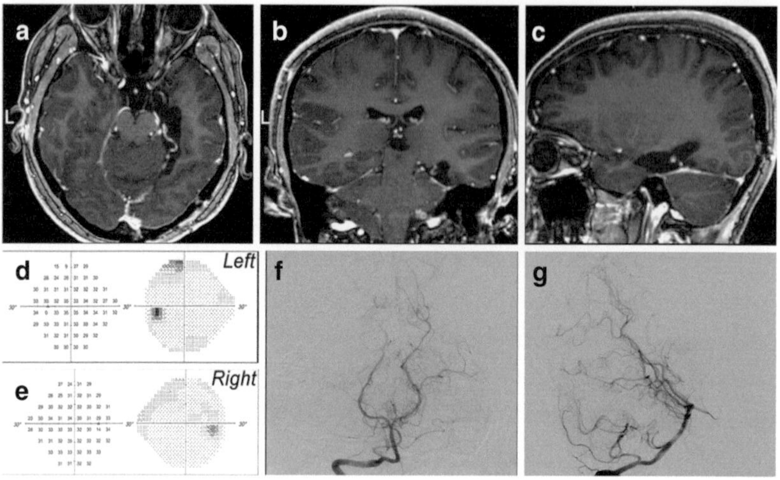

Fig. 2.7 Case 2: Postoperative T1-weighted MRI with contrast in axial (**a**), coronal (**b**), and sagittal (**c**) views shows removal of the AVM and amygdalohippocampectomy through the PST approach. Postoperative visual field testing of the left (**d**) and right (**e**) eyes illustrate the preservation of the visual fields through the PST approach to the mediobasal temporal region. Postoperative right vertebral DSA in AP (**f**) and lateral views (**g**) shows filling of the PCA and normal cerebral vasculature, along with loss of early venous filling

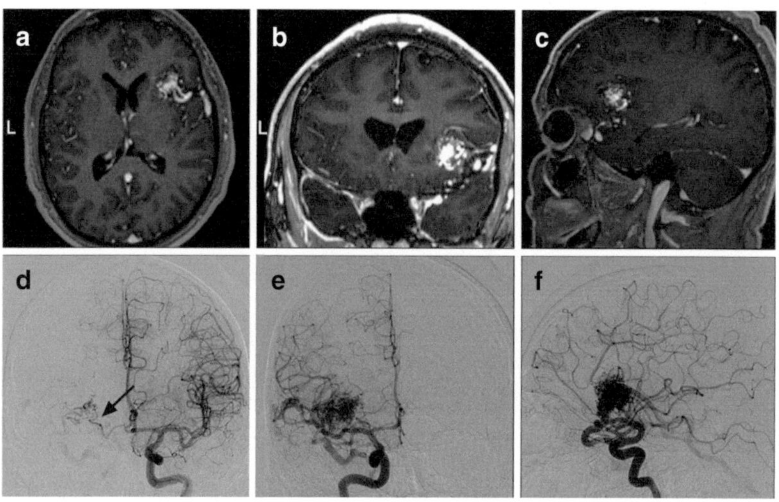

Fig. 2.8 Case 3: Preoperative T1-weighed MRI with contrast in axial (**a**), coronal (**b**), and sagittal (**c**) views shows a moderate-sized, mixed, deep AVM of the right anterior insular region. On the preoperative left ICA DSA in AP view (**d**), the arrow indicates the feeding vessel to the AVM from the recurrent artery of Heubner. Preoperative right ICA DSA in AP (**e**) and lateral (**f**) views illustrates the mostly compact nidus with early venous drainage to the Galenic venous system and arterial supply from the right M1 MCA lateral lenticulostriates, the superior trunk of the M2 MCA, and the recurrent artery of Heubner from the ACA

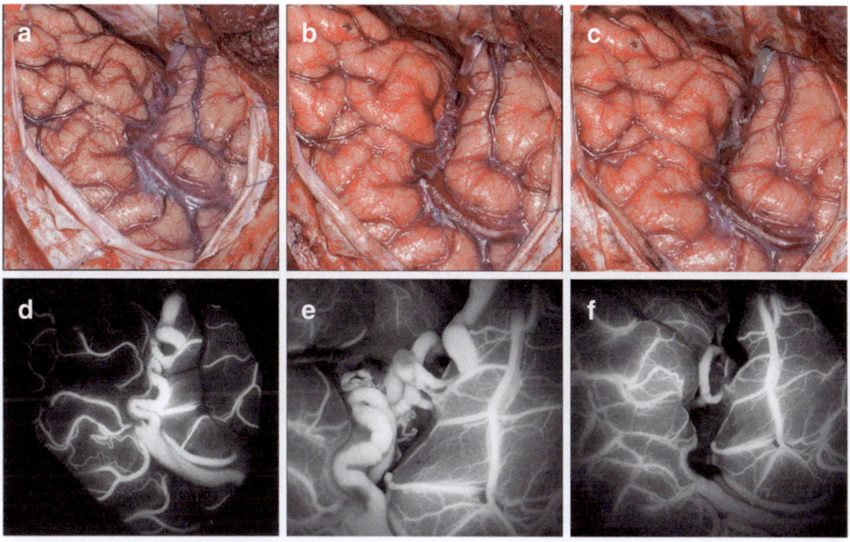

Fig. 2.9 Case 3: Intraoperative images: The photograph after dural opening prior to dissection around the AVM (**a**) is followed by an intraoperative photograph early in dissection after the sylvian fissure is split (**b**), and the final photograph (**c**) was taken after resection of the AVM. The corresponding ICG video-angiography pictures are after dural opening prior to dissection around the AVM (**d**), early in dissection after splitting the sylvian fissure (**e**), and the final ICG video-angiography picture after resection of the AVM (**f**), with (**d**), (**e**), and (**f**) corresponding to the photographs of (**a**), (**b**), and (**c**), respectively

2.5.4 Case 4

A 41-year-old right-handed female presented at our clinic with a history of right-sided numbness and focal motor seizures, with subsequent right-sided Todd's monoparesis of the arm and hand that resolved 2 h after seizures and which started 1 month before she came to us. She was started on one AED, which reduced the frequency of seizures. She had no gross neurological deficits on exam.

The MRI sequence revealed a left lateral convexity, middle post-central gyrus, gyral AVM with a compact nidus (Fig. 2.11). Angiography delineated the arterial supply from the distal branches of the MCA and ACA, specifically the paracentral artery from the ACA and the anterior parietal artery of the MCA [124, 126]. The AVM had superficial drainage through the ascending venous system to the superior sagittal sinus, with narrowing of the drainage before the entrance to the sinus. No perinidal angiogenesis was apparent on the MRI or angiogram; if it was present, then it was likely small and localized. The nidus of the AVM was 2.6 cm in greatest diameter, thus, a moderate size (2–4 cm). Under the Spetzler–Martin grading system, this AVM was grade 2 because of its size less than 3 cm, superficial drainage, and location in an eloquent area.

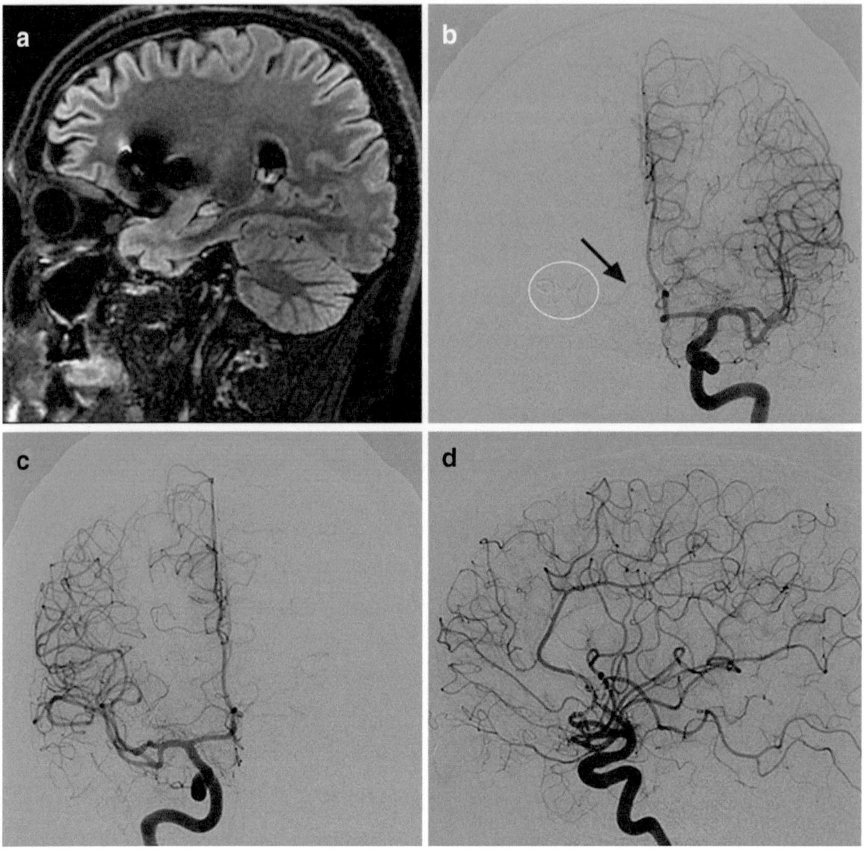

Fig. 2.10 Case 3: The postoperative T2-weighted MRI FLAIR in coronal view (**a**) has significant artifact from the three aneurysm clips on deep AVM feeding vessels from the lenticulostriate arteries and the recurrent artery of Heubner. This illustrates the need for titanium (or minimal artifact) AVM clips. The postoperative left ICA DSA in AP view (**b**) shows diminished pathologic shunting through the right recurrent artery of Heubner. The encircled region includes the shadow of the aneurysm clips at the distal end of the right recurrent artery of Heubner. The arrow points to the recurrent artery of Heubner with diminished pathologic shunting. Postoperative right ICA DSA in AP (**c**) and lateral (**d**) views after complete extirpation of the AVM shows preservation of the normal cerebral vasculature, including the transit lenticulostriate perforators

The AVM was resected through a left frontoparietal craniotomy (Figs. 2.12 and 2.13). Postoperatively, the patient had a mild right-sided monoparesis of the right hand and arm that resolved within 5 days. His AEDs were stopped at 1 year with complete resolution of the seizures. The preoperative mRS of 1 improved to 0 by the 3-month follow-up visit.

Even if located in an eloquent location, convexity AVMs with a compact nidus are easier to resect compared to deeper lesions. We believe the surgical risk for an eloquent convexity AVM is very low when treated microsurgically, even when larger than the lesion in this case.

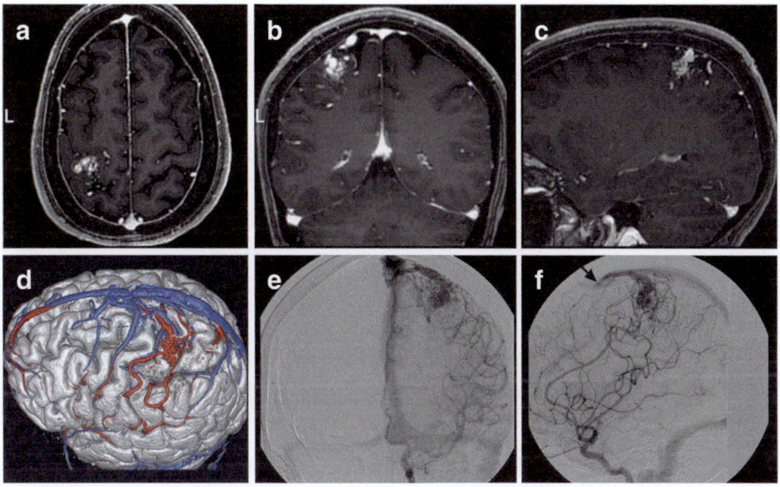

Fig. 2.11 Case 4: Preoperative T1-weighted MRI with contrast in axial (**a**), coronal (**b**), and sagittal (**c**) views show the left post-central gyrus AVM. The 3D reconstruction of preoperative imaging (**d**) delineates likely arterial flow in red and venous outflow in blue. Preoperative left ICA DSA in AP (**e**) and lateral (**f**) views: the arrow indicates venous stenosis (in **f**) just distal to the venous hypertrophy of the major draining vein prior to draining into the superior sagittal sinus. The branches are the paracentral artery from the distal ACA and the anterior parietal artery of the distal MCA [80, 124, 126]

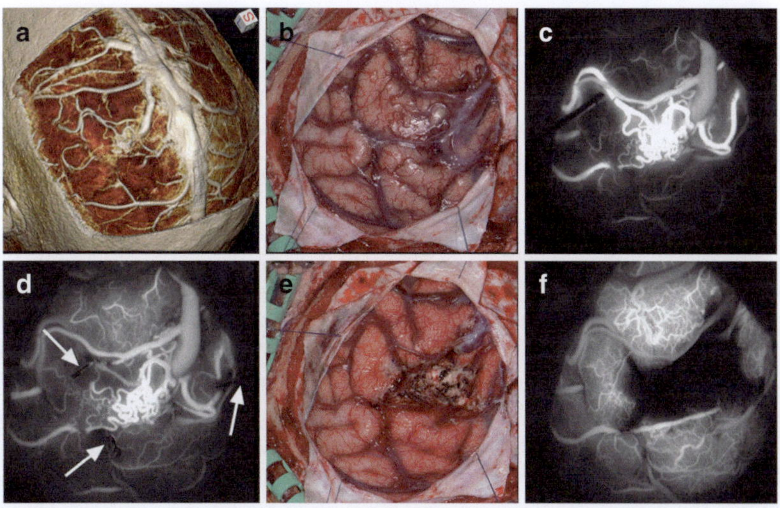

Fig. 2.12 Case 4: a reconstruction of preoperative imaging (**a**) shows the removal of scalp and bone layers to aid in operative planning [129]. A photograph after the craniotomy and opening of the dura, prior to dissection around the AVM (**b**), illustrates the largely hidden nidus of this gyral AVM. ICG video-angiography was performed (**c**) early in dissection around the AVM, after the sulci surrounding the AVM nidus were opened. An additional round of ICG video-angiography (**d**) with the placement of temporary aneurysm clips (arrows) aided in understanding the angio-architecture and flow of the AVM. The post-resection photograph (**e**) and ICG video-angiography (**f**) show complete removal of the AVM nidus

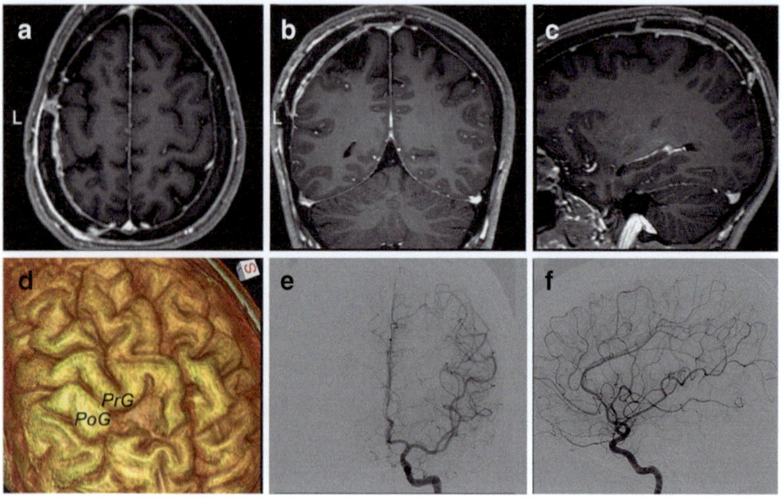

Fig. 2.13 Case 4: Postoperative T1-weighted MRI with contrast in axial (**a**), coronal (**b**), and sagittal (**c**) views after complete removal of the AVM nidus show the preservation of surrounding structures, including the pre-central gyrus. A 3D reconstruction of the postoperative imaging (**d**) illustrates the resection of the AVM nidus with preservation of surrounding eloquent regions of the brain, including the pre-central gyrus (*PrG*) and non-nidal post-central gyrus (*PoG*) [128]. The postoperative left ICA DSA in AP (**e**) and lateral views (**f**) shows preservation of the normal cerebral vasculature and loss of early venous drainage

2.5.5 Case 5

A 36-year-old right-handed male came to us with an 8-year history of shuffling and loss of strength in his left foot. Imaging done at that time showed a right paracentral AVM. He underwent gamma-knife treatment three separate times at an outside center. The second session was 6 months after the first (approximately 7 years prior to presenting at our clinic). The patient was started on a single AED at the time of the first gamma-knife treatment even though he had no clear seizure episodes before then. One year after the first gamma-knife treatment (6 months after the second), the patient began to have episodes of ascending numbness starting in his left foot, which were treated with a 1-week course of steroids. However, they intermittently occurred every 2–3 months thereafter. Two years prior to presentation in our clinic, he underwent a third gamma-knife treatment (5 years after the first therapy) due to incomplete resolution of the AVM on serial imaging. Over the year prior to presentation in our clinic, the patient progressively lost strength in his left arm and leg. He had a focal motor seizure with generalization 2 weeks before coming to us. On exam, he was hemiparetic on his left side, with a score of 2/5 in his left anterior tibial region and 3/5 in his left extensor hallicus longus.

An MRI sequence revealed a right convexity paracentral lobule (parasagittal dorsal frontal region) and pre-central gyrus AVM with a compact nidus. There were

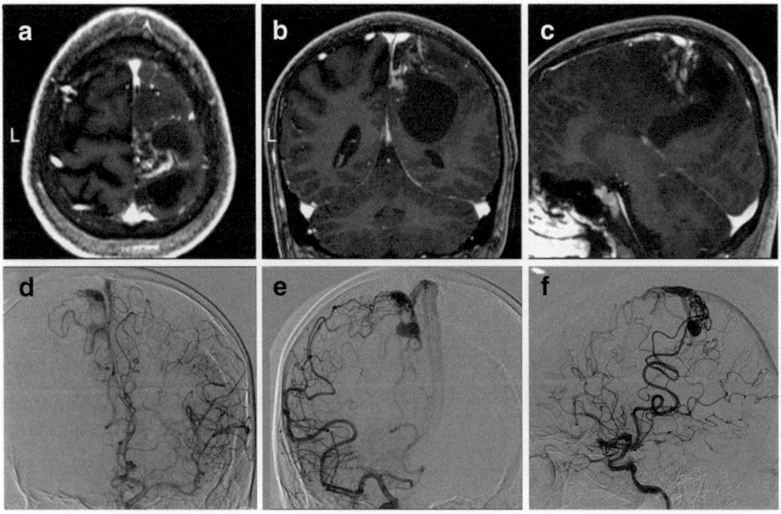

Fig. 2.14 Case 5: Preoperative T1-weighted MRI with contrast in axial (**a**), coronal (**b**), and sagittal (**c**) views of the right paracentral lobule and pre-central gyrus AVM shows cystic components with associated vasogenic edema lateral, anterior, posterior, and inferior to the AVM nidus. The preoperative left ICA DSA in AP view (**d**) reveals the distal ACA supply to the AVM from the right paracentral artery, which is not seen as clearly in the right ICA injection [80, 126, 130]. Preoperative right ICA DSA in AP (**e**) and lateral (**f**) views shows the distal MCA supply to the AVM from the central artery with venous dilation seen on the AP view [124]

also post-gamma-knife-induced cystic components straddling the AVM in the pre- and post-central regions (Fig. 2.14). The primary arterial supply to the AVM was from the distal ACA via the right paracentral artery and the MCA via the central artery. Superficial drainage was to the superior sagittal sinus, and deep venous drainage was to the pericallosal venous system to the galenic system. The AVM was moderate in size (2–4 cm) with the largest diameter of 4 cm. Under the Spetzler–Martin grading system, this AVM was considered grade 4 because it was larger than 3 cm, had superficial and deep drainage, and was in an eloquent location.

The AVM was resected via a right frontoparietal paramedian craniotomy (Figs. 2.15 and 2.16).

The patient improved postoperatively to have weakness only in the anterior tibial region of 3/5 strength, with complete resolution of weakness in the arm and proximal leg. The patient's preoperative mRS of 3 improved to 1 by the 3-month follow-up visit.

Radiosurgery is marketed as a minimally invasive procedure with minimal risks; however, radiosurgery has a 3-year latency period with AVMs and, during this time, there are changes to the angio-architecture and flow that can have poorly predicted effects on the AVM and surrounding tissue [4, 39, 97, 131]. Cysts, seizures, new deficits, and hemorrhage risk after radiosurgery are not predicted by the SM grading

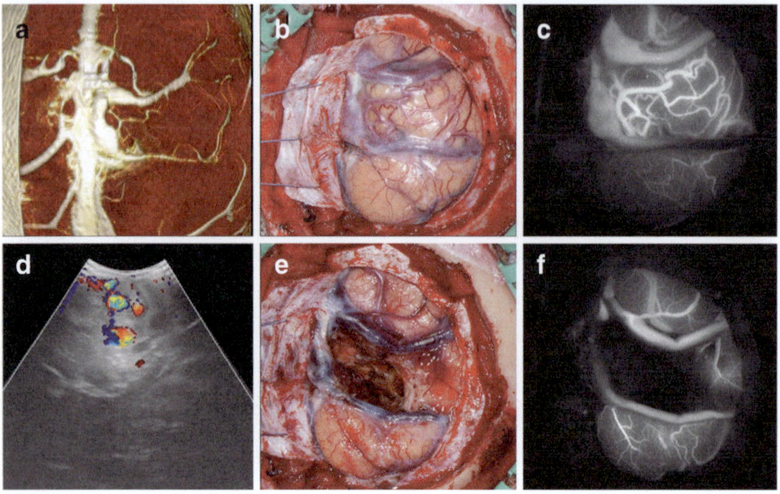

Fig. 2.15 Case 5: Preoperative 3D reconstruction for surgical planning (**a**) illustrates the venous structures bordering the AVM nidus. A photograph (**b**) and corresponding video-angiography (**c**) were taken after the craniotomy and durotomy but before resection of the AVM. The intraoperative ultrasound with color Doppler imaging reveals the AVM nidus and surrounding cyst (**d**). A post-resection photograph (**e**) and ICG video-angiography (**f**) after resection of the AVM show preservation of the adjacent sulcal veins draining into the superior sagittal sinus

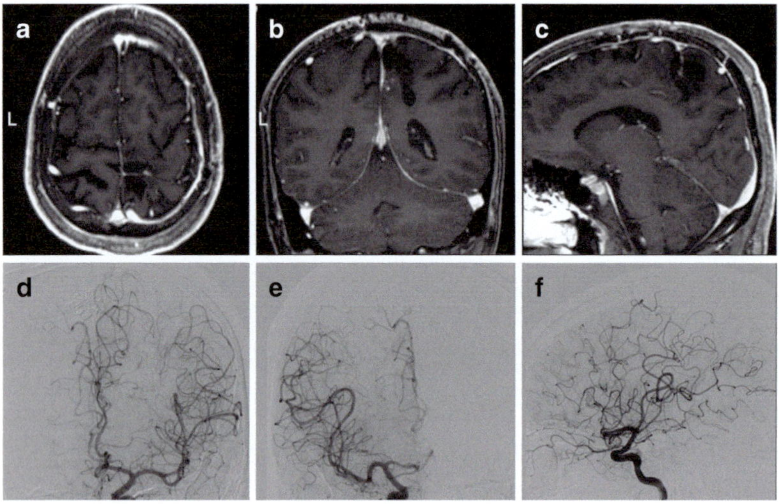

Fig. 2.16 Case 5: Postoperative T1-weighted MRI with contrast in axial (**a**), coronal (**b**), and sagittal (**c**) views after resection of the AVM show the resolution of mass effect and edema from the cyst. The postoperative left ICA DSA in AP view (**d**) highlights the loss of pathologic shunting to the AVM from the paracentral artery of the distal right ACA. The postoperative right ICA DSA in AP (**e**) and lateral views (**f**) illustrates preservation of the normal cerebral vasculature and loss of the pathologic early venous drainage

system and were not accounted for in the ARUBA trial [22–24, 120, 122, 131]. Most importantly, because only 18 microneurosurgical resections were included in the ARUBA trial, the vast majority of morbidity and mortality from treatment are from non-microneurosurgical interventions, such as endovascular and radiation therapy [6, 21, 121].

2.5.6 *Case 6*

A 38-year-old right-handed female presented at our clinic with intracerebral hemorrhage followed by partial embolization 1 year prior. She underwent partial embolization with coils and NBCA at an outside hospital at the time of her initial hemorrhage. She was taking one AED but had not had a clear history of any prior seizures. On exam, the patient was grossly intact.

The MRI sequence showed a left deep (or central) supero-posterior limbic, parenchymal AVM of the (callosocingular) parasplenial area with a compact nidus. It involved the splenium and cingulate isthmus, along with extension into the ventricle (Fig. 2.17). The arterial supply was from the distal segment of the pericallosal artery (the parietal internal inferior artery) of the A5 ACA branches, the posterior

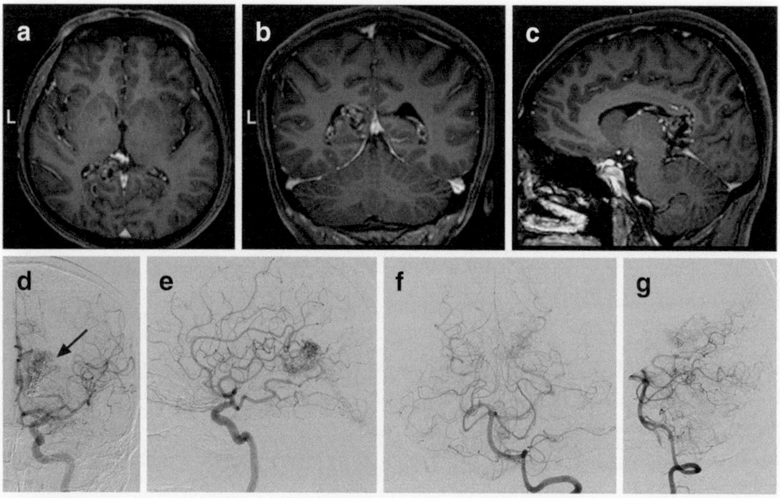

Fig. 2.17 Case 6: Preoperative T1-weighted MRI with contrast in axial (**a**), coronal (**b**), and sagittal (**c**) views show a left parasplenial callosocingular AVM. Preoperative left ICA DSA in AP (**d**) and lateral (**e**) views shows a distal ACA supply from the A5 segment of the pericallosal artery (the parietal internal inferior artery). The arrow (**d**) shows prior embolization material from an outside institution [80, 126, 130]. Preoperative left vertebral artery DSA in AP (**f**) and lateral (**g**) views illustrates the arterial supply to the AVM from the PCA via the medial posterior choroidal artery of the P2–P3 PCA, the posterior pericallosal artery of the P3 PCA, and the parieto-occipital artery of the P4 PCA [80, 126, 130]

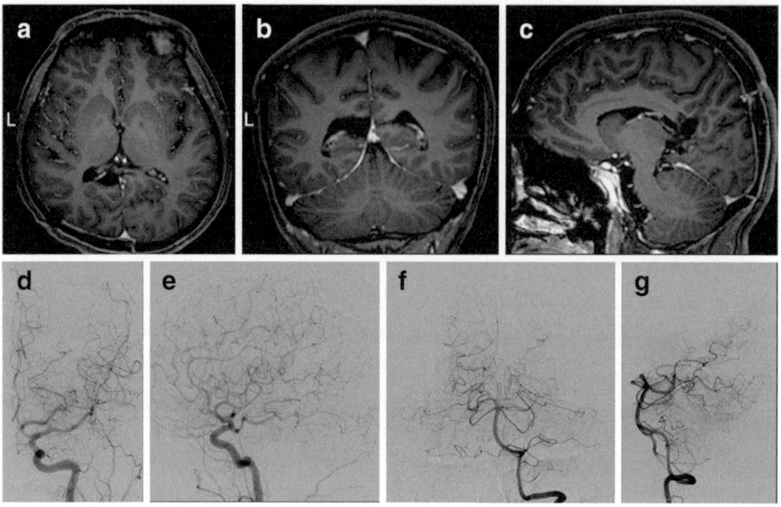

Fig. 2.18 Case 6: Postoperative T1-weighted MRI with contrast in axial (**a**), coronal (**b**), and sagittal (**c**) views was done after AVM resection. Postoperative left ICA DSA in AP (**d**) and lateral (**e**) views shows that most of the prior embolization material has been resected with the AVM. The postoperative left vertebral artery DSA in AP (**f**) and lateral (**g**) views reveals the loss of early venous drainage from the AVM with preservation of normal cerebral vasculature

pericallosal artery of P3, the medial posterior choroidal artery of P2–P3, and the parieto-occipital artery from P4 of the PCA [80, 126, 130]. The AVM had deep drainage to the galenic venous system, and was of moderate size (2–4 cm) measuring 2.5 cm in greatest diameter. Under the Spetzler–Martin grading system, this AVM was considered grade 2 because its size was less than 3 cm, it had deep drainage, and was located in a non-eloquent area.

A left-sided posterior interhemispheric approach was used for resection (Fig. 2.18). The patient's AEDs were stopped 1 year after surgery and she is asymptomatic, without speech or memory issues. Her preoperative mRS of 1 improved to 0 postoperatively.

The risks of parasplenial AVMs are underappreciated. These lesions are in a watershed zone with two arterial systems providing supply, are adjacent to the galenic venous system, are involved with the non-redundant splenium of the corpus callosum and the limbic system, and are near the visual pathways [2].

2.5.7 Case 7

A 41-year-old right-handed male presented to an outside institution with a left thalamic intracerebral hemorrhage and intraventricular hemorrhage. At initial presentation, he was comatose but recovered over the next week. He was treated with EVD and

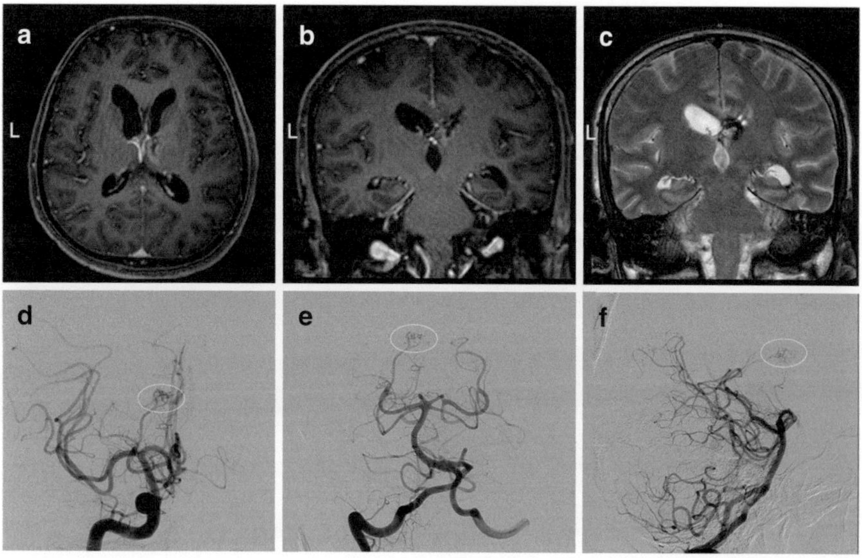

Fig. 2.19 Case 7: Preoperative T1-weighted MRI was done with contrast in axial (**a**) and coronal views (**b**), and T2-weighted MRI without contrast in the coronal view (**c**) of the right anterior thalamic AVM. Preoperative right ICA DSA in AP view (**d**) reveals the anterior choroidal arterial supply to the AVM. The right vertebral DSA in AP (**e**) and lateral (**f**) views shows the AVM with supply from the medial posterior choroidal artery of P2–P3 and thalamoperforators of P1 from the PCA [80, 126]

medical management. Upon discharge, the patient was hemiplegic but improved to mild right-sided hemiparesis by the time he was seen in our clinic 45 days later. He had been prescribed AEDs after his initial hemorrhage but had no clear history of seizures.

The MRIs showed a right central, parenchymal AVM of the anterior thalamus (within the superior, anterior thalamus of the striatocapsulothalamic subregion) with ventricular extension (Fig. 2.19) [1–3]. The feeding arteries were the anterior choroidal artery, the medial posterior choroidal artery of P2–P3, and thalamoperforators from P1 arteries of the PCA [1–3, 80]. The venous drainage was deep to the thalamostriate vein of the subependymal deep venous system. There was no venous hypertension or varix, and the lesion was small (1–2 cm) at 1.2 cm. This AVM was grade 3 on the Spetzler–Martin scale because of its eloquent location, small size, and deep venous drainage.

The AVM was resected through a right parasagittal frontal craniotomy via the anterior interhemispheric transcallosal approach (Figs. 2.20 and 2.21). On postoperative exam, the patient's weakness had resolved and the AEDs were stopped by 1 year postoperatively. The preoperative mRS of the patient was 2 and improved to 0 by the 3-month follow-up.

Although the thalamus is deemed an eloquent location and has deep venous drainage, these lesions can be safely resected when they face a ventricular or cisternal surface [104, 132]. Additionally, the prior hemorrhage helped create dissection

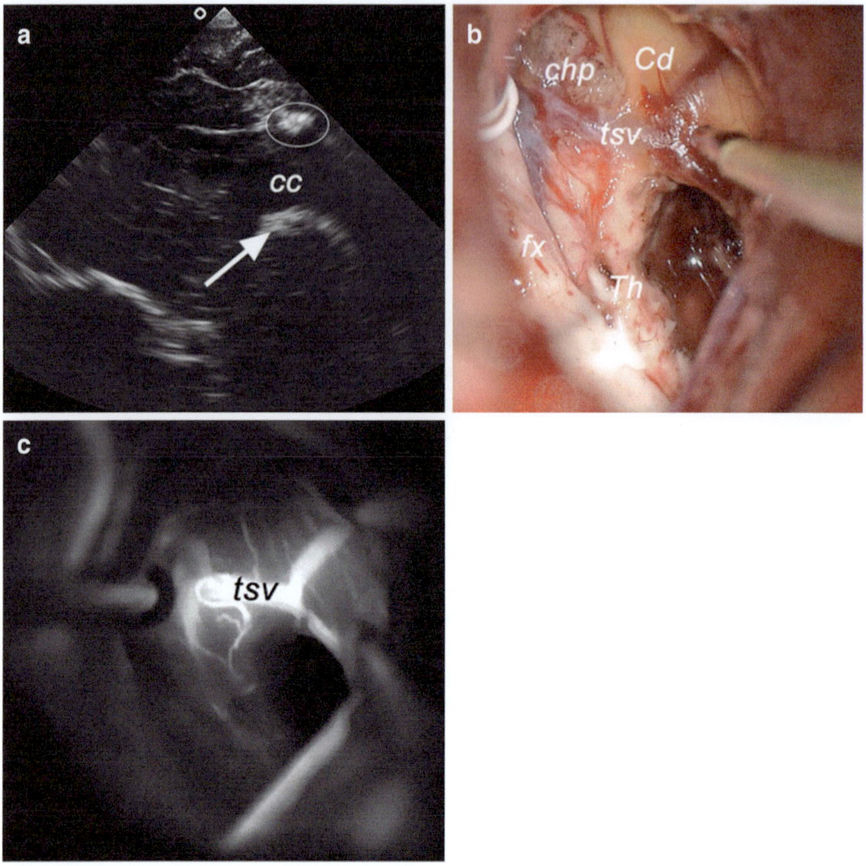

Fig. 2.20 Case 7: On intraoperative ultrasound (**a**) the arrow points to a cottonoid placed before the callosotomy to confirm the point of entry into the ventricle [104]. The encircled area within (**a**) indicates the cottonoid placed over the corpus callosum (cc). The arrow points to the underlying thalamic AVM. An intraoperative photograph taken after resection of the AVM (**b**) illustrates the surrounding fornix (*fx*), the perinidal thalamus (*Th*), the choroid plexus (*chp*), the caudate nucleus (*Cd*), and the thalamostriate vein (*tsv*). Corresponding ICG video-angiography (**c**) confirmed the preservation of the thalamostriate vein (*tsv*) [128]

planes around the AVM. Of utmost importance in these AVMs are differentiating the feeding supply from non-involved thalamoperforators and preserving the thalamostriate and internal cerebral veins.

2.6 Conclusion

Deep and eloquent AVMs can be safely resected to the benefit of the patient through microneurosurgical techniques and the use of advanced pre- and intraoperative tools. The extirpation of an AVM through microneurosurgical resection

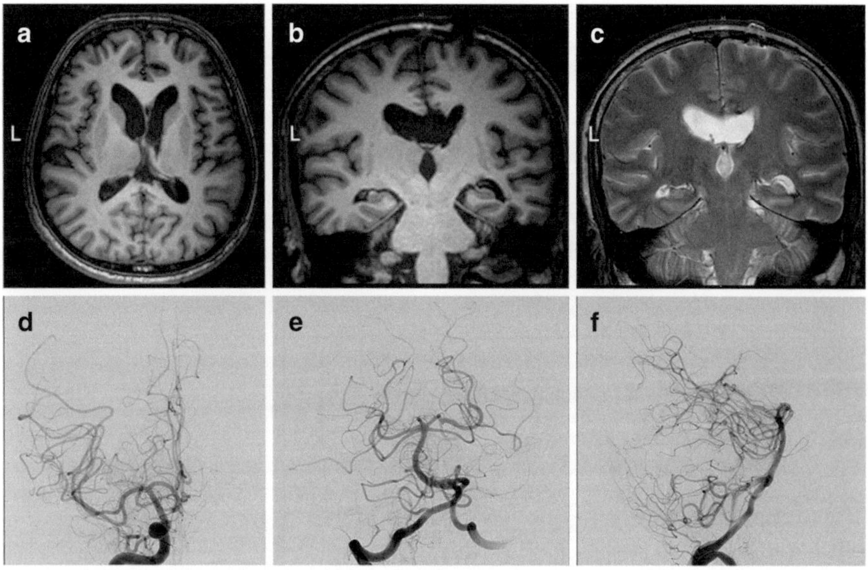

Fig. 2.21 Case 7: Postoperative T1-weighted MRI without contrast in axial (**a**) and coronal (**b**) views and postoperative T2-weighted MRI without contrast in the coronal view (**c**) were taken after complete removal of the AVM. Postoperative right ICA DSA in AP view (**d**) and right vertebral DSA in AP (**e**) and lateral (**f**) views show preservation of the normal cerebral vasculature, including the transit thalamoperforators from the P1 segment of the PCA [2, 80]

immediately removes the risk of future hemorrhage, neurological deterioration, and anxiety for the patient. The depth and function of brain tissue surrounding an AVM should be discussed with the patient when considering the risks, benefits, and alternatives to surgery; however, these AVMs can be safely resected and, in our minds, *should* be resected when the patient is at risk of future hemorrhage, morbidity, and mortality otherwise. Based on the patient's images, signs, and/or symptoms, the AVM should be treated if there is associated venous hypertension. Perinidal angiogenesis and deep perforating arteries make the treatment of an AVM more difficult; however, advanced techniques, improved imaging, and expert super-selective angiography help the surgeon for the benefit of the patient.

References

1. Yasargil MG. Microneurosurgery, volume IIIA: AVM of the brain, history, embryology, pathological considerations, hemodynamics, diagnostic studies, microsurgical anatomy. New York: Georg Thieme Verlag; 1987. https://medone.thieme.com.
2. Yasargil MG. Microneurosurgery, volume IIIB: AVM of the brain, clinical considerations, general and special operative techniques, surgical results, nonoperated cases, cavernous and venous angiomas, neuroanesthesia. New York: Georg Thieme Verlag; 1988.
3. Valavanis A, Yaşargil MG. The endovascular treatment of brain arteriovenous malformations. In: Cohadon F, Dolenc VV, Antunes JL, Nornes H, Pickard JD, Reulen H-J, et al., editors.

Advances and technical standards in neurosurgery, vol. 24. Vienna: Springer Vienna; 1998. p. 131–214. https://doi.org/10.1007/978-3-7091-6504-1_4.
4. Chen C-J, Ding D, Derdeyn CP, Lanzino G, Friedlander RM, Southerland AM, et al. Brain arteriovenous malformations: a review of natural history, pathobiology, and interventions. Neurology. 2020;95:917–27. http://www.ncbi.nlm.nih.gov/pubmed/33004601.
5. Locksley HB. Natural history of subarachnoid hemorrhage, intracranial aneurysms and arteriovenous malformations. Based on 6368 cases in the cooperative study. J Neurosurg. 1966;25:219–39. http://www.ncbi.nlm.nih.gov/pubmed/5911370.
6. Volovici V, Schouten JW, Vajkoczy P, Dammers R, Meling TR. Unruptured arteriovenous malformations. Stroke. 2021;52:1143–6. http://www.ncbi.nlm.nih.gov/pubmed/33494639.
7. Garzelli L, Shotar E, Blauwblomme T, Sourour N, Alias Q, Stricker S, et al. Risk factors for early brain AVM rupture: cohort study of pediatric and adult patients. Am J Neuroradiol. 2020;41:2358–63. http://www.ncbi.nlm.nih.gov/pubmed/33122204.
8. Ding D, Chen C-J, Starke RM, Kano H, Lee JYK, Mathieu D, et al. Risk of brain arteriovenous malformation hemorrhage before and after stereotactic radiosurgery. Stroke. 2019;50:1384–91. http://www.ncbi.nlm.nih.gov/pubmed/31043153.
9. Alqadi M, Brunozzi D, Linninger A, Amin-Hanjani S, Charbel FT, Alaraj A. Cerebral arteriovenous malformation venous stenosis is associated with hemodynamic changes at the draining vein-venous sinus junction. Med Hypotheses. 2019;123:86–8. http://www.ncbi.nlm.nih.gov/pubmed/30696602.
10. Lin TM, Yang HC, Lee CC, Wu HM, Hu YS, Luo CB, et al. Stasis index from hemodynamic analysis using quantitative DSA correlates with hemorrhage of supratentorial arteriovenous malformation: a cross-sectional study. J Neurosurg. 2019;132:1–9. http://www.ncbi.nlm.nih.gov/pubmed/31026828.
11. Brunozzi D, Hussein AE, Shakur SF, Linninger A, Hsu C-Y, Charbel FT, et al. Contrast time-density time on digital subtraction angiography correlates with cerebral arteriovenous malformation flow measured by quantitative magnetic resonance angiography, angioarchitecture, and hemorrhage. Neurosurgery. 2018;83:210–6. http://www.ncbi.nlm.nih.gov/pubmed/29106647.
12. Shakur SF, Valyi-Nagy T, Amin-Hanjani S, Ya'Qoub L, Aletich VA, Charbel FT, et al. Effects of nidus microarchitecture on cerebral arteriovenous malformation hemodynamics. J Clin Neurosci. 2016;26:70–4. http://www.sciencedirect.com/science/article/pii/S0967586815005354.
13. Abecassis IJ, Xu DS, Batjer HH, Bendok BR. Natural history of brain arteriovenous malformations: a systematic review. Neurosurg Focus. 2014;37:E7. http://www.ncbi.nlm.nih.gov/pubmed/25175445.
14. Gross BA, Du R. Natural history of cerebral arteriovenous malformations: a meta-analysis. J Neurosurg. 2013;118:437–43. http://www.ncbi.nlm.nih.gov/pubmed/23198804.
15. Lv X, Wu Z, Jiang C, Yang X, Li Y, Sun Y, et al. Angioarchitectural characteristics of brain arteriovenous malformations with and without hemorrhage. World Neurosurg. 2011;76:95–9. https://linkinghub.elsevier.com/retrieve/pii/S1878875011001173.
16. Stapf C, Mast H, Sciacca RR, Choi JH, Khaw AV, Connolly ES, et al. Predictors of hemorrhage in patients with untreated brain arteriovenous malformation. Neurology. 2006;66:1350–5. www.neurology.org.
17. Stefani MA, Porter PJ, TerBrugge KG, Montanera W, Willinsky RA, Wallace MC. Large and deep brain arteriovenous malformations are associated with risk of future hemorrhage. Stroke. 2002;33:1220–4. http://www.ncbi.nlm.nih.gov/pubmed/11988594.
18. Ogilvy CS, Stieg PE, Awad I, Brown RD, Kondziolka D, Rosenwasser R, et al. Recommendations for the management of intracranial arteriovenous malformations. Circulation. 2001;103:2644–57. http://www.ncbi.nlm.nih.gov/pubmed/11382737.
19. Mohr JP, Overbey JR, Von Kummer R, Stefani MA, Libman R, Stapf C, et al. Functional impairments for outcomes in a randomized trial of unruptured brain AVMs.

Neurology. 2017;89(14):1499–506. http://www.neurology.org/lookup/doi/10.1212/WNL.0000000000004532.
20. Mohr JP, Overbey JR, Hartmann A, von Kummer R, Al-Shahi Salman R, Kim H, et al. Medical management with interventional therapy versus medical management alone for unruptured brain arteriovenous malformations (ARUBA): final follow-up of a multicentre, non-blinded, randomised controlled trial. Lancet Neurol. 2020;19:573–81. www.thelancet.com/neurology.
21. Magro E, Gentric J-C, Darsaut TE, Ziegler D, Bojanowski MW, Raymond J. Responses to ARUBA: a systematic review and critical analysis for the design of future arteriovenous malformation trials. J Neurosurg. 2017;126:486–94. http://www.ncbi.nlm.nih.gov/pubmed/27128584.
22. Mohr JP, Parides MK, Stapf C, Moquete E, Moy CS, Overbey JR, et al. Medical management with or without interventional therapy for unruptured brain arteriovenous malformations (ARUBA): a multicentre, non-blinded, randomised trial. Lancet. 2014;383:614–21. http://www.ncbi.nlm.nih.gov/pubmed/24268105.
23. Spetzler RF, Martin NA. A proposed grading system for arteriovenous malformations. J Neurosurg. 1986;65:476–83. http://www.ncbi.nlm.nih.gov/pubmed/3760956.
24. Tayebi Meybodi A, Lawton MT. Modern radiosurgical and endovascular classification schemes for brain arteriovenous malformations. Neurosurg Rev. 2020;43:49–58. http://www.ncbi.nlm.nih.gov/pubmed/29728873.
25. Luessenhop AJ. AVM grading in assessing surgical risk. J Neurosurg. 1987;66:637–8. http://www.ncbi.nlm.nih.gov/pubmed/3559733.
26. Stefani MA, Sgarabotto Ribeiro D, Mohr JP. Grades of brain arteriovenous malformations and risk of hemorrhage and death. Ann Clin Transl Neurol. 2019;6:508–14. http://www.ncbi.nlm.nih.gov/pubmed/30911574.
27. van Swieten JC, Koudstaal PJ, Visser MC, Schouten HJ, van Gijn J. Interobserver agreement for the assessment of handicap in stroke patients. Stroke. 1988;19:604–7. http://www.ncbi.nlm.nih.gov/pubmed/3363593.
28. Hamilton MG, Spetzler RF. The prospective application of a grading system for arteriovenous malformations. Neurosurgery. 1994;34:2–7. https://academic.oup.com/neurosurgery/article/34/1/2/2857379.
29. Joint Writing Group of the Technology Assessment Committee American Society of Interventional and Therapeutic Neuroradiology; Joint Section on Cerebrovascular Neurosurgery a Section of the American Association of Neurological Surgeons and Congress of Neur, Atkinson RP, Awad IA, Batjer HH, Dowd CF, Furlan A, et al. Reporting terminology for brain arteriovenous malformation clinical and radiographic features for use in clinical trials. Stroke. 2001;32:1430–42. http://ahajournals.org.
30. Lawton MT, Hamilton MG, Spetzler RF. Multimodality treatment of deep arteriovenous malformations: thalamus, basal ganglia, and brain stem. Neurosurgery. 1995;37:29–36. http://www.ncbi.nlm.nih.gov/pubmed/8587687.
31. Tew JM, Lewis AI, Reichert KW. Management strategies and surgical techniques for deep-seated supratentorial arteriovenous malformations. Neurosurgery. 1995;36:1065–72. https://academic.oup.com/neurosurgery/article/36/6/1065/2757617.
32. de Oliveira E, Tedeschi H, Siqueira MG, Ono M, Rhoton AL. Arteriovenous malformations of the basal ganglia region: rationale for surgical management. Acta Neurochir (Wien). 1997;139:487–506. http://link.springer.com/10.1007/BF02750990.
33. Gross BA, Duckworth EAM, Getch CC, Bendok BR, Batjer HH. Challenging traditional beliefs: microsurgery for arteriovenous malformations of the basal ganglia and thalamus. Neurosurgery. 2008;63:393–410; discussion 410–1. http://www.ncbi.nlm.nih.gov/pubmed/18812951.
34. Potts MB, Young WL, Lawton MT. Deep arteriovenous malformations in the basal ganglia, thalamus, and insula. Neurosurgery. 2013;73:417–29. http://www.ncbi.nlm.nih.gov/pubmed/23728451.

35. Potts MB, Jahangiri A, Jen M, Sneed PK, McDermott MW, Gupta N, et al. Deep arteriovenous malformations in the basal ganglia, thalamus, and insula: multimodality management, patient selection, and results. World Neurosurg. 2014;82:386–94. http://www.ncbi.nlm.nih.gov/pubmed/24657255.
36. Laakso A, Dashti R, Juvela S, Isarakul P, Niemelä M, Hernesniemi J. Risk of hemorrhage in patients with untreated Spetzler-Martin grade IV and V arteriovenous malformations. Neurosurgery. 2011;68:372–8. http://www.ncbi.nlm.nih.gov/pubmed/21135742.
37. Kato Y, Dong V, Chaddad F, Takizawa K, Izumo T, Fukuda H, et al. Expert consensus on the management of brain arteriovenous malformations. Asian J Neurosurg. 2019;14:1074. http://www.ncbi.nlm.nih.gov/pubmed/31903343.
38. Zuurbier SM, Salman RAS. Interventions for treating brain arteriovenous malformations in adults. Cochrane Database Syst Rev. 2019:CD003436. http://www.ncbi.nlm.nih.gov/pubmed/31503327.
39. de Tribolet N. Radiosurgery of deep arteriovenous malformations. J Neurosurg. 2004;100:205–7. http://www.ncbi.nlm.nih.gov/pubmed/15086224.
40. Rutledge WC, Abla AA, Nelson J, Halbach VV, Kim H, Lawton MT. Treatment and outcomes of ARUBA-eligible patients with unruptured brain arteriovenous malformations at a single institution. Neurosurg Focus. 2014;37:E8. http://www.ncbi.nlm.nih.gov/pubmed/25175446.
41. Potts MB, Lau D, Abla AA, Kim H, Young WL, Lawton MT. Current surgical results with low-grade brain arteriovenous malformations. J Neurosurg. 2015;122:912–20. http://www.ncbi.nlm.nih.gov/pubmed/25658789.
42. Han PP, Ponce FA, Spetzler RF. Intention-to-treat analysis of Spetzler—Martin grades IV and V arteriovenous malformations: natural history and treatment paradigm. J Neurosurg. 2003;98:3–7. http://www.ncbi.nlm.nih.gov/pubmed/12546345.
43. Morgan MK, Davidson AS, Assaad NNA, Stoodley MA. Critical review of brain AVM surgery, surgical results and natural history in 2017. Acta Neurochir (Wien). 2017;159:1457–78. http://www.ncbi.nlm.nih.gov/pubmed/28555270.
44. Cenzato M, Boccardi E, Beghi E, Vajkoczy P, Szikora I, Motti E, et al. European consensus conference on unruptured brain AVMs treatment (supported by EANS, ESMINT, EGKS, and SINCH). Acta Neurochir (Wien). 2017;159:1059–64. http://www.ncbi.nlm.nih.gov/pubmed/28389875.
45. Pollock BE, Gorman DA, Brown PD. Radiosurgery for arteriovenous malformations of the basal ganglia, thalamus, and brainstem. J Neurosurg. 2004;100:210–4. http://www.ncbi.nlm.nih.gov/pubmed/15086226.
46. Valavanis A, Pangalu A, Tanaka M. Endovascular treatment of cerebral arteriovenous malformations with emphasis on the curative role of embolisation. Interv Neuroradiol. 2005;11:37–43. http://www.ncbi.nlm.nih.gov/pubmed/20584458.
47. Kano H, Kondziolka D, Flickinger JC, Yang H, Flannery TJ, Niranjan A, et al. Stereotactic radiosurgery for arteriovenous malformations, part 4: management of basal ganglia and thalamus arteriovenous malformations. J Neurosurg. 2012;116:33–43. http://www.ncbi.nlm.nih.gov/pubmed/22077451.
48. Catapano JS, Frisoli FA, Nguyen CL, Wilkinson DA, Majmundar N, Cole TS, et al. Spetzler-Martin grade III arteriovenous malformations: a multicenter propensity-adjusted analysis of the effects of preoperative embolization. Neurosurgery. 2021;88(5):996–1002. http://www.ncbi.nlm.nih.gov/pubmed/33427287.
49. Donzelli GF, Nelson J, McCoy D, McCulloch CE, Hetts SW, Amans MR, et al. The effect of preoperative embolization and flow dynamics on resection of brain arteriovenous malformations. J Neurosurg. 2020;132:1836–44. http://www.ncbi.nlm.nih.gov/pubmed/31100732.
50. Morgan MK, Davidson AS, Koustais S, Simons M, Ritson EA. The failure of preoperative ethylene-vinyl alcohol copolymer embolization to improve outcomes in arteriovenous malformation management: case series. J Neurosurg. 2013;118:969–77. http://www.ncbi.nlm.nih.gov/pubmed/23350776.

51. Henkes H, Gotwald TF, Brew S, Kaemmerer F, Miloslavski E, Kuehne D. Pressure measurements in arterial feeders of brain arteriovenous malformations before and after endovascular embolization. Neuroradiology. 2004;46:673–7. http://www.ncbi.nlm.nih.gov/pubmed/15205863.
52. Haw CS, TerBrugge K, Willinsky R, Tomlinson G. Complications of embolization of arteriovenous malformations of the brain. J Neurosurg. 2006;104:226–32. http://www.ncbi.nlm.nih.gov/pubmed/16509496.
53. Kim LJ, Albuquerque FC, Spetzler RF, McDougall CG. Postembolization neurological deficits in cerebral arteriovenous malformations: stratification by arteriovenous malformation grade. Neurosurgery. 2006;59:53–9; discussion 53–9. www.neurosurgery-online.com.
54. Rutledge C, Nelson J, Lu A, Nisson P, Jonzzon S, Winkler EA, et al. Cost determinants in management of brain arteriovenous malformations. Acta Neurochir (Wien). 2020;162:169–73. http://www.ncbi.nlm.nih.gov/pubmed/31760534.
55. Crowley RW, Ducruet AF, McDougall CG, Albuquerque FC. Endovascular advances for brain arteriovenous malformations. Neurosurgery. 2014;74:S74–82. http://www.ncbi.nlm.nih.gov/pubmed/24402496.
56. Baharvahdat H, Blanc R, Fahed R, Pooyan A, Mowla A, Escalard S, et al. Endovascular treatment as the main approach for Spetzler–Martin grade III brain arteriovenous malformations. J Neurointerv Surg. 2021;13(3):241–6. http://www.ncbi.nlm.nih.gov/pubmed/32989031.
57. Conger A, Kulwin C, Lawton M, Cohen-Gadol A. Endovascular and microsurgical treatment of cerebral arteriovenous malformations: current recommendations. Surg Neurol Int. 2015;6:39. http://www.ncbi.nlm.nih.gov/pubmed/25883831.
58. Crowley RW, Ducruet AF, Kalani MYS, Kim LJ, Albuquerque FC, McDougall CG. Neurological morbidity and mortality associated with the endovascular treatment of cerebral arteriovenous malformations before and during the Onyx era. J Neurosurg. 2015;122:1492–7. http://www.ncbi.nlm.nih.gov/pubmed/25816081.
59. Morgan MK, Heller GZ. The role of embolization before surgery for Spetzler-Ponce class B and C brain AVMs: a prospective cohort series. J Neurosurg Sci. 2018;62:429–36. http://www.ncbi.nlm.nih.gov/pubmed/29480692.
60. Hashimoto N. Microsurgery for cerebral arteriovenous malformations: a dissection technique and its theoretical implications. Neurosurgery. 2001;48:1278–81. https://academic.oup.com/neurosurgery/article/48/6/1278/3773532.
61. Kim H, Abla AA, Nelson J, McCulloch CE, Bervini D, Morgan MK, et al. Validation of the supplemented Spetzler-Martin grading system for brain arteriovenous malformations in a multicenter cohort of 1009 surgical patients. Neurosurgery. 2015;76:25–33. http://www.ncbi.nlm.nih.gov/pubmed/25251197.
62. Lawton MT, Kim H, McCulloch CE, Mikhak B, Young WL. A supplementary grading scale for selecting patients with brain arteriovenous malformations for surgery. Neurosurgery. 2010;66:702–13. http://www.ncbi.nlm.nih.gov/pubmed/20190666.
63. Spetzler RF, Ponce FA. A 3-tier classification of cerebral arteriovenous malformations. J Neurosurg. 2011;114:842–9. http://www.ncbi.nlm.nih.gov/pubmed/20932095.
64. Hafez A, Koroknay-Pál P, Oulasvirta E, Elseoud AA, Lawton MT, Niemelä M, et al. The application of the Novel Grading Scale (Lawton-Young Grading System) to predict the outcome of brain arteriovenous malformation. Neurosurgery. 2019;84:529–36. http://www.ncbi.nlm.nih.gov/pubmed/29733392.
65. Lasjaunias PL, Landrieu P, Rodesch G, Alvarez H, Ozanne A, Holmin S, et al. Cerebral proliferative angiopathy. Stroke. 2008;39:878–85. http://www.ncbi.nlm.nih.gov/pubmed/18239181.
66. Du R, Keyoung HM, Dowd CF, Young WL, Lawton MT. The effects of diffuseness and deep perforating artery supply on outcomes after microsurgical resection of brain arteriovenous malformations. Neurosurgery. 2007;60:638–46; discussion 646–8. http://www.ncbi.nlm.nih.gov/pubmed/17415200.

67. Chin LS, Raffel C, Gonzalez-Gomez I, Giannotta SL, McComb JG. Diffuse arteriovenous malformations: a clinical, radiological, and pathological description. Neurosurgery. 1992;31:863–8; discussion 868–9. http://www.ncbi.nlm.nih.gov/pubmed/1436409.
68. Fierstra J, Spieth S, Tran L, Conklin J, Tymianski M, ter Brugge KG, et al. Severely impaired cerebrovascular reserve in patients with cerebral proliferative angiopathy. J Neurosurg Pediatr. 2011;8:310–5. http://www.ncbi.nlm.nih.gov/pubmed/21882924.
69. Spears J, TerBrugge KG, Moosavian M, Montanera W, Willinsky RA, Wallace MC, et al. A discriminative prediction model of neurological outcome for patients undergoing surgery of brain arteriovenous malformations. Stroke. 2006;37:1457–64. http://www.ncbi.nlm.nih.gov/pubmed/16690897.
70. Abla AA, Nelson J, Kim H, Hess CP, Tihan T, Lawton MT. Silent arteriovenous malformation hemorrhage and the recognition of "unruptured" arteriovenous malformation patients who benefit from surgical intervention. Neurosurgery. 2015;76:592–600. http://www.ncbi.nlm.nih.gov/pubmed/25714514.
71. Chen X, Cooke DL, Saloner D, Nelson J, Su H, Lawton MT, et al. Higher flow is present in unruptured arteriovenous malformations with silent intralesional microhemorrhages. Stroke. 2017;48:2881–4. http://www.ncbi.nlm.nih.gov/pubmed/28855391.
72. Cunha e Sa MJ, Stein BM, Solomon RA, McCormick PC. The treatment of associated intracranial aneurysms and arteriovenous malformations. J Neurosurg. 1992;77:853–9. http://www.ncbi.nlm.nih.gov/pubmed/1432126.
73. da Costa L, Wallace MC, ter Brugge KG, O'Kelly C, Willinsky RA, Tymianski M. The natural history and predictive features of hemorrhage from brain arteriovenous malformations. Stroke. 2009;40:100–5. http://www.ncbi.nlm.nih.gov/pubmed/19008469.
74. Burkhardt J-K, Chen X, Winkler EA, Cooke DL, Kim H, Lawton MT. Delayed venous drainage in ruptured arteriovenous malformations based on quantitative color-coded digital subtraction angiography. World Neurosurg. 2017;104:619–27. http://www.ncbi.nlm.nih.gov/pubmed/28457930.
75. Grüter BE, Sun W, Fierstra J, Regli L, Germans MR. Systematic review of brain arteriovenous malformation grading systems evaluating microsurgical treatment recommendation. Neurosurg Rev. 2021. http://link.springer.com/10.1007/s10143-020-01464-3.
76. Sundt TM. Neurovascular microsurgery. World J Surg. 1979;3:53–65. http://www.ncbi.nlm.nih.gov/pubmed/483834.
77. Stein BM, Wolpert SM. Arteriovenous malformations of the brain. I: current concepts and treatment. Arch Neurol. 1980;37:1–5. https://jamanetwork.com/.
78. Stein BM, Wolpert SM. Arteriovenous malformations of the brain. II: current concepts and treatment. Arch Neurol. 1980;37:69–75. https://jamanetwork.com/.
79. Drake CG. Cerebral arteriovenous malformations: considerations for and experience with surgical treatment in 166 cases. Neurosurgery. 1979;26:145–208. https://academic.oup.com/neurosurgery/article/26/CN_suppl_1/145/4099519.
80. Rhoton AL. The cerebrum. Neurosurgery. 2007;61:37–118. http://www.ncbi.nlm.nih.gov/pubmed/18813175.
81. Foster CH, Morone PJ, Tomlinson SB, Cohen-Gadol AA. Application of indocyanine green during arteriovenous malformation surgery: evidence, techniques, and practical pearls. Front Surg. 2019;6:70. http://www.ncbi.nlm.nih.gov/pubmed/31921884.
82. Kato N, Prinz V, Dengler J, Vajkoczy P. Blood flow assessment of arteriovenous malformations using intraoperative indocyanine green videoangiography. Stroke Res Treat. 2019;2019:1–8. http://www.ncbi.nlm.nih.gov/pubmed/31007890.
83. Della Puppa A, Scienza R. Multimodal flow-assisted resection of brain AVMs. Acta Neurochir Suppl. 2016;123:141–5. http://www.ncbi.nlm.nih.gov/pubmed/27637641.
84. Walkden JS, Zador Z, Herwadkar A, Kamaly-Asl ID. Use of intraoperative Doppler ultrasound with neuronavigation to guide arteriovenous malformation resection: a pediatric case series. J Neurosurg Pediatr. 2015;15:291–300. http://www.ncbi.nlm.nih.gov/pubmed/25525933.

85. Kato Y, Yamada Y, Sadato A, Nouri M, Cherian I, Tanaka T, et al. Intraoperative anatomical and hemodynamic analysis of intracerebral arteriovenous malformations by semi-quantitative color-coded indocyanine green videoangiography. Asian J Neurosurg. 2017;12:638. http://www.ncbi.nlm.nih.gov/pubmed/29114275.
86. Amin-Hanjani S, Meglio G, Gatto R, Bauer A, Charbel FT. The utility of intraoperative blood flow measurement during aneurysm surgery using an ultrasonic perivascular flow probe. Oper Neurosurg. 2006;58:ONS-305–12. http://www.ncbi.nlm.nih.gov/pubmed/16582654.
87. Morgan MK, Drummond KJ, Grinnell V, Sorby W. Surgery for cerebral arteriovenous malformation: risks related to lenticulostriate arterial supply. J Neurosurg. 1997;86:801–5. http://www.ncbi.nlm.nih.gov/pubmed/9126895.
88. Luostarinen T, Takala RSK, Niemi TT, Katila AJ, Niemelä M, Hernesniemi J, et al. Adenosine-induced cardiac arrest during intraoperative cerebral aneurysm rupture. World Neurosurg. 2010;73:79–83. https://doi.org/10.1016/j.surneu.2009.06.018.
89. Cannesson M, Desebbe O, Rosamel P, Delannoy B, Robin J, Bastien O, et al. Pleth variability index to monitor the respiratory variations in the pulse oximeter plethysmographic waveform amplitude and predict fluid responsiveness in the operating theatre. Br J Anaesth. 2008;101:200–6. https://doi.org/10.1093/bja/aen133.
90. Marc Samama C, Thiry D, Elalamy I, Diaby M, Guillosson J-J, Kieffer E, et al. Perioperative activation of hemostasis in vascular surgery patients. Anesthesiology. 2001;94:74–8. http://www.ncbi.nlm.nih.gov/pubmed/11135724.
91. Snyder CW, Weinberg JA, McGwin G, Melton SM, George RL, Reiff DA, et al. The relationship of blood product ratio to mortality: survival benefit or survival bias? J Trauma Inj Infect Crit Care. 2009;66:358–64. http://www.ncbi.nlm.nih.gov/pubmed/19204508.
92. Spetzler RF, Wilson CB, Weinstein P, Mehdorn M, Townsend J, Telles D. Normal perfusion pressure breakthrough theory. Neurosurgery. 1978;25:651–72. https://academic.oup.com/neurosurgery/article/25/CN_suppl_1/651/4099752.
93. Young WL, Kader A, Prohovnik I, Ornstein E, Fleischer LH, Ostapkovich N, et al. Pressure autoregulation is intact after arteriovenous malformation resection. Neurosurgery. 1993;32:491–7. http://www.ncbi.nlm.nih.gov/pubmed/8474637.
94. Al-Rodhan NRF, Sundt TM, Piepgras DG, Nichols DA, Rßfenacht D, Stevens LN. Occlusive hyperemia: a theory for the hemodynamic complications following resection of intracerebral arteriovenous malformations. J Neurosurg. 1993;78:167–75. http://www.ncbi.nlm.nih.gov/pubmed/8421198.
95. Spetzler RF, Hargraves RW, McCormick PW, Zabramski JM, Flom RA, Zimmerman RS. Relationship of perfusion pressure and size to risk of hemorrhage from arteriovenous malformations. J Neurosurg. 1992;76:918–23. http://www.ncbi.nlm.nih.gov/pubmed/1588424.
96. Soldozy S, Akyeampong DK, Barquin DL, Norat P, Yağmurlu K, Sokolowski JD, et al. Systematic review of functional mapping and cortical reorganization in the setting of arteriovenous malformations, redefining anatomical eloquence. Front Surg. 2020;7:514247. http://www.ncbi.nlm.nih.gov/pubmed/33195382.
97. Ilyas A, Chen C-J, Ding D, Buell TJ, Raper DMS, Lee C-C, et al. Radiation-induced changes after stereotactic radiosurgery for brain arteriovenous malformations: a systematic review and meta-analysis. Neurosurgery. 2018;83:365–76. http://www.ncbi.nlm.nih.gov/pubmed/29040700.
98. Morgan MK, Zurin AAR, Harrington T, Little N. Changing role for preoperative embolisation in the management of arteriovenous malformations of the brain. J Clin Neurosci. 2000;7:527–30. http://www.ncbi.nlm.nih.gov/pubmed/11029234.
99. Bi WL, Brown PA, Abolfotoh M, Al-Mefty O, Mukundan S, Dunn IF. Utility of dynamic computed tomography angiography in the preoperative evaluation of skull base tumors. J Neurosurg. 2015;123:1–8. http://www.ncbi.nlm.nih.gov/pubmed/25839925.
100. Salomon EJ, Barfett J, Willems PWA, Geibprasert S, Bacigaluppi S, Krings T. Dynamic CT angiography and CT perfusion employing a 320-detector row CT: protocol and current

clinical applications. Klin Neuroradiol. 2009;19:187–96. http://www.ncbi.nlm.nih.gov/pubmed/19705072.
101. Conger A, Kulwin C, Lawton M, Cohen-Gadol A. Diagnosis and evaluation of intracranial arteriovenous malformations. Surg Neurol Int. 2015;6:76. http://www.ncbi.nlm.nih.gov/pubmed/25984390.
102. Nornes H, Grip A, Wikeby P. Intraoperative evaluation of cerebral hemodynamics using directional Doppler technique. J Neurosurg. 1979;50:145–51. http://www.ncbi.nlm.nih.gov/pubmed/430124.
103. Rubin JM, Hatfield MK, Chandler WF, Black KL, DiPietro MA. Intracerebral arteriovenous malformations: intraoperative color Doppler flow imaging. Radiology. 1989;170:219–22. http://www.ncbi.nlm.nih.gov/pubmed/2642343.
104. Serra C, Türe H, Yaltırık CK, Harput MV, Türe U. Microneurosurgical removal of thalamic lesions: surgical results and considerations from a large, single-surgeon consecutive series. J Neurosurg. 2020:1–11. https://thejns.org/view/journals/j-neurosurg/aop/article-10.3171-2020.6.JNS20524/article-10.3171-2020.6.JNS20524.xml.
105. Keleş A, Harput MV, Türe U. Microneurosurgical removal of a globus pallidus tumor with cottonoid-guided intraoperative ultrasonography: 2-dimensional operative video. Oper Neurosurg. 2020;19:E154. http://www.ncbi.nlm.nih.gov/pubmed/31768549.
106. Amin-Hanjani S, Charbel FT. Is extracranial-intracranial bypass surgery effective in certain patients? Neurosurg Clin N Am. 2008;19:477–87. https://doi.org/10.1016/j.nec.2008.07.009.
107. Raabe A, Beck J, Gerlach R, Zimmermann M, Seifert V. Near-infrared indocyanine green video angiography: a new method for intraoperative assessment of vascular flow. Neurosurgery. 2003;52:132–9; discussion 139. www.neurosurgery-online.com.
108. Raabe A, Beck J, Seifert V. Technique and image quality of intraoperative indocyanine green angiography during aneurysm surgery using surgical microscope integrated near-infrared video technology. Zentralbl Neurochir. 2005;66:1–6. http://www.ncbi.nlm.nih.gov/pubmed/15744621.
109. Nishiyama Y, Kinouchi H, Senbokuya N, Kato T, Kanemaru K, Yoshioka H, et al. Endoscopic indocyanine green video angiography in aneurysm surgery: an innovative method for intraoperative assessment of blood flow in vasculature hidden from microscopic view. J Neurosurg. 2012;117:302–8. http://www.ncbi.nlm.nih.gov/pubmed/22680246.
110. Cai Z, Zhu L, Wang M, Roe AW, Xi W, Qian J. NIR-II fluorescence microscopic imaging of cortical vasculature in non-human primates. Theranostics. 2020;10:4265–76. http://www.ncbi.nlm.nih.gov/pubmed/32226552.
111. Kamada K, Guger C, Takeuchi F. Multispectrum indocyanine green videography for visualizing brain vascular pathology. World Neurosurg. 2019;132:e545–53. https://doi.org/10.1016/j.wneu.2019.08.078.
112. Oermann EK, Ding D, Yen C-P, Starke RM, Bederson JB, Kondziolka D, et al. Effect of prior embolization on cerebral arteriovenous malformation radiosurgery outcomes. Neurosurgery. 2015;77:406–17. http://www.ncbi.nlm.nih.gov/pubmed/25875580.
113. Türe U, Kaya AH. Principles for managing cavernous malformations in eloquent locations. In: Rigamonti D, editor. Cavernous malformations of the nervous system. Cambridge: Cambridge University Press; 2011. p. 161–72. https://www.cambridge.org/core/product/identifier/9781139003636%23c76427-3076/type/book_part.
114. Fried I. The myth of eloquent cortex, or what is non-eloquent cortex? J Neurosurg. 1993;78:1009–10. http://www.ncbi.nlm.nih.gov/pubmed/8487065.
115. Drake CG. Surgical treatment of ruptured aneurysms of the basilar artery. J Neurosurg. 1965;23:457–73. http://www.ncbi.nlm.nih.gov/pubmed/5858437.
116. Shi Y, Chen X. A proposed scheme for grading intracranial arteriovenous malformations. J Neurosurg. 1986;65:484–9. http://www.ncbi.nlm.nih.gov/pubmed/3760957.
117. Lazar RM. Neuropsychological function and brain arteriovenous malformations: redefining eloquence as a risk for treatment. Neurosurg Focus. 2001;11:1–4. http://www.ncbi.nlm.nih.gov/pubmed/16466236.

118. Link TW, Winston G, Schwarz JT, Lin N, Patsalides A, Gobin P, et al. Treatment of unruptured brain arteriovenous malformations: a single-center experience of 86 patients and a critique of the a randomized trial of unruptured brain arteriovenous malformations (ARUBA) trial. World Neurosurg. 2018;120:e1156–62. http://www.ncbi.nlm.nih.gov/pubmed/30218805.
119. Cenzato M, Tartara F, D'Aliberti G, Bortolotti C, Cardinale F, Ligarotti G, et al. Unruptured versus ruptured AVMs: outcome analysis from a multicentric consecutive series of 545 surgically treated cases. World Neurosurg. 2018;110:e374–82. http://www.ncbi.nlm.nih.gov/pubmed/29155066.
120. Ding D, Starke RM, Kano H, Mathieu D, Huang P, Kondziolka D, et al. Radiosurgery for cerebral arteriovenous malformations in a randomized trial of unruptured brain arteriovenous malformations (ARUBA)-eligible patients. Stroke. 2016;47:342–9. http://www.ncbi.nlm.nih.gov/pubmed/26658441.
121. Schramm J, Schaller K, Esche J, Boström A. Microsurgery for cerebral arteriovenous malformations: subgroup outcomes in a consecutive series of 288 cases. J Neurosurg. 2017;126:1056–63. https://thejns.org/view/journals/j-neurosurg/126/4/article-p1056.xml.
122. Pollock BE, Storlie CB, Link MJ, Stafford SL, Garces YI, Foote RL. Comparative analysis of arteriovenous malformation grading scales in predicting outcomes after stereotactic radiosurgery. J Neurosurg. 2017;126:852–8. http://www.ncbi.nlm.nih.gov/pubmed/27058199.
123. Gupta R, Adeeb N, Moore JM, Motiei-Langroudi R, Griessenauer CJ, Patel AS, et al. Validity assessment of grading scales predicting complications from embolization of cerebral arteriovenous malformations. Clin Neurol Neurosurg. 2016;151:102–7. http://www.ncbi.nlm.nih.gov/pubmed/27821297.
124. Türe U, Yaşargil MG, Al-Mefty O, Yaşargil DCH. Arteries of the insula. J Neurosurg. 2000;92:676–87. http://www.ncbi.nlm.nih.gov/pubmed/10761659.
125. Türe U, Yaşargil DCH, Al-Mefty O, Yaşargil MG. Topographic anatomy of the insular region. J Neurosurg. 1999;90:720–33. http://www.ncbi.nlm.nih.gov/pubmed/10193618.
126. Huber P, Yasargil MG, Krayenbühl H. Cerebral angiography. 2nd ed. New York: Georg Thieme Verlag; 1982.
127. Türe U, Harput MV, Kaya AH, Baimedi P, Firat Z, Türe H, et al. The paramedian supracerebellar-transtentorial approach to the entire length of the mediobasal temporal region: an anatomical and clinical study. J Neurosurg. 2012;116:773–91. http://www.ncbi.nlm.nih.gov/pubmed/22264179.
128. Mai JK, Paxinos G, Voss T. Atlas of the human brain. 3rd ed. New York: Elsevier; 2008.
129. Harput MV, Gonzalez-Lopez P, Türe U. Three-dimensional reconstruction of the topographical cerebral surface anatomy for presurgical planning with free OsiriX software. Oper Neurosurg. 2014;10:426–35. http://www.ncbi.nlm.nih.gov/pubmed/24662508.
130. Türe U, Yaşargil MG, Krisht AF. The arteries of the corpus callosum: a microsurgical anatomic study. Neurosurgery. 1996;39:1075–84. http://www.ncbi.nlm.nih.gov/pubmed/8938760.
131. Kano H, Kondziolka D, Flickinger JC, Yang H, Flannery TJ, Awan NR, et al. Stereotactic radiosurgery for arteriovenous malformations, part 3: outcome predictors and risks after repeat radiosurgery. J Neurosurg. 2012;116:21–32. http://www.ncbi.nlm.nih.gov/pubmed/22077445.
132. Serra C, Türe U, Krayenbühl N, Şengül G, Yaşargil DCH, Yaşargil MG. Topographic classification of the thalamus surfaces related to microneurosurgery: a white matter fiber microdissection study. World Neurosurg. 2017;97:438–52. http://www.ncbi.nlm.nih.gov/pubmed/27725299.

Chapter 3
Posterior Circulation Aneurysms

Demi Dawkins, Sima Sayyahmelli, and Mustafa K. Baskaya

3.1 Introduction

Posterior circulations aneurysms can be defined as aneurysms involving the basilar artery, posterior cerebral artery (PCA), superior cerebellar artery (SCA), vertebral artery (VA), posterior interior cerebellar artery (PICA), or anterior inferior cerebellar artery (AICA). They most commonly occur at the basilar tip followed by PICA and SCA aneurysms [1]. These aneurysms account for approximately 10–15% of all intracranial aneurysms and can be saccular, non-saccular or dissecting pseudoaneurysms [2]. Posterior circulation aneurysms have a higher tendency to rupture and become symptomatic in comparison to anterior circulation aneurysms [3, 4].

Historically microsurgical management of these aneurysms has been challenging and is associated with higher morbidity and mortality rates in comparison to anterior circulation aneurysms due to the proximity to vital structures such as perforators and cranial nerves, the deep location of the vertebrobasilar system, and bony confinements of the skull base requiring more difficult surgical approaches in order to achieve adequate exposure. These technical difficulties have had a major influence on the increasing popularity and advancement of endovascular technology for management of these aneurysms [3, 5]. As a result, open surgical treatment of posterior circulation aneurysms has decreased as endovascular therapies have grown.

Current treatment modalities for aneurysms in these locations vary widely including microsurgical clipping, trapping with bypass, wrapping, and various endovascular methods such as coiling, balloon or stent-assisted coiling, flow diversion, and vessel sacrifice, among others. How we approach these posterior circulation aneurysms surgically depends on the location of the aneurysm. We can categorize these

D. Dawkins · S. Sayyahmelli · M. K. Baskaya (✉)
Department of Neurological Surgery, University of Wisconsin-Madison, Madison, WI, USA
e-mail: baskaya@neurosurgery.wisc.edu

Y. Kato, A. Ansari (eds.), *Cerebrovascular Surgery*, Advances and Technical Standards in Neurosurgery 44, https://doi.org/10.1007/978-3-030-87649-4_3

as upper complex (PCA, basilar tip, SCA), middle complex (basilar trunk, AICA), or lower complex (vertebrobasilar junction, PICA, VA). For the upper complex, the approaches can include the pterional craniotomy with or without orbitozygomatic or transcavernous (Dolenc) modifications, subtemporal craniotomy, or Kawase approach. For the middle complex, you can utilize the Kawase, transpetrosal, transoral, or retrosigmoid approaches. Finally, for the lower complex you can reach these aneurysms via far lateral transcondylar or midline versus lateral suboccipital approaches [2, 6]. Optimal treatment, whether open surgical or endovascular, should be tailored to each individual patient taking into consideration the location and morphology of the aneurysm as well as age, condition, and anatomy of the patient.

3.2 Basilar Tip Aneurysms

Basilar tip (apex or bifurcation) aneurysms make up about half of all posterior circulation aneurysms making it the most common location in this group and represents approximately 7% of all aneurysms [1]. In 1961, Charles Drake performed the first successful obliteration of a basilar tip aneurysm via a subtemporal approach [1, 7]. Yasargil then advanced the transsylvian approach pioneering its use in the treatment of basilar apex aneurysms [8, 9]. Today the two fundamental approaches for clipping basilar apex aneurysms include the pterional and subtemporal approaches. These surgical exposures can be modified with orbitozygomatic osteotomies, anterior or posterior clinoidectomy, and/or transcavernous dissections [10, 11]. Microsurgical treatment of these aneurysms can be particularly challenging due to the length of the operative corridor, presence of numerous perforators, and risk of cranial nerve palsies. These concerns contribute to the higher surgical morbidity associated with clipping of basilar tip aneurysms and therefore these aneurysms in this location are largely managed endovascularly at most centers. Still, there are circumstances where microsurgical techniques are relevant including cases of difficult catheter access (either due to vessel tortuosity, stenosis, or occlusion), broad based aneurysms in younger patients (especially in ruptured cases where stenting with dual antiplatelet therapy is relatively contraindicated), large or giant aneurysms where there is brainstem compression, or cases where a non-fetal P1 is intricately incorporated into the neck of the aneurysm [11]. These instances highlight the importance of maintaining an understanding of the technical nuances required to safely treat these aneurysms surgically.

3.2.1 Preoperative Considerations

The following factors should be considered when treating basilar apex aneurysms including (1) aneurysm size, projection, and relationship to perforators, (2) presence and/or size of the posterior communicating artery (PComA), (3) position of the

P1 in relation to the aneurysm neck, and (4) relationship of the basilar bifurcation to the dorsum sellae and posterior clinoid process.

Basilar bifurcation aneurysms can be anteriorly projecting which is most common, posteriorly projecting, superiorly projecting, or combinations of these directions. Posteriorly projecting aneurysms typically have the most involvement with the basilar tip and P1 perforators and make visualization of these perforators more difficult. The perforators which require adequate attention and preservation include the posterior thalamo-perforators arising from P1, peduncular and thalamo-geniculate perforators from P2, and the anterior thalamo-perforators from the PComA [11, 12]. These perforators can occasionally be identified on preoperative angiography depending on their size, but they must always be identified at the time of surgery in order to safely preserve them. High or low basilar bifurcations will also influence the course these perforators travel. Higher bifurcations typically result in the P1 perforators traveling in a downward trajectory which can make them easier to dissect from the aneurysm, in contrast to lower bifurcations where the perforators travel upward often resulting in them being adherent to the aneurysm dome [11, 13].

The location of the basilar artery bifurcation may be the most important factor in deciding the surgical approach of these aneurysms. Basilar tip aneurysms within 5 mm of the posterior clinoid process or dorsum sellae are typically suitable candidates for anterolateral approaches. If the basilar bifurcation is low riding (more than 1 cm below the level of the posterior clinoid), then the view may be poor from an anterolateral approach unless it is modified with a transcavernous dissection and/or drilling of the posterior clinoid [14, 15]. A lateral subtemporal approach may provide a more optimal trajectory in cases of low riding basilar tips especially with the addition of tentorial division. In contrast, with high riding basilar bifurcations a subtemporal approach will result in significant temporal lobe retraction and are typically better suited with anterolateral routes modified with an anterior clinoidectomy in order to widen the optico-carotid or carotid-oculomotor triangles and/or sectioning of non-fetal or hypoplastic PcomA in the perforator free segment to increase the mobilization of both the internal carotid artery (ICA) and optic nerve [2, 12, 16, 17].

Choosing the side of the approach is another important preoperative consideration. Most surgeons typically favor approaching from the nondominant right hemisphere if possible due to better toleration of temporal and frontal lobe retraction, especially when utilizing a subtemporal approach. Other factors, which may affect the choice of laterality, include the presence of hematoma, presence of additional aneurysms, or preexisting third nerve palsies or hemiparesis [12]. The relationship of the P1 to the neck of the aneurysm can also be a consideration. If one P1 is situated higher than the other in relationship to the neck of the aneurysm, approaching it from that side may be favorable in order to avoid placing it at risk since there is usually poor visualization of the contralateral P1 [12, 16]. Finally, if the left PCOMA is more hypoplastic, it may be considered approaching from the left side since for better visualization, it is a safer choice for ligation [11, 12].

3.2.2 Surgical Approaches: Anterolateral

The anterolateral approach to the basilar tip evolved after the subtemporal approach and typically involves the standard pterional craniotomy and transsylvian dissection which was popularized by Yasargil in 1976 [8]. This surgical approach was further advanced by Dolenc, who introduced the transcavernous dissection with anterior clinoidectomy, optic nerve unroofing, and removal of the posterior clinoid or dorsum sellae to further widen the operative corridor [18]. Orbitotomy or full orbitozygomatic osteotomies are typically considered based on the size of the aneurysm, presence of a high riding bifurcation, or the rupture status [11, 12, 16, 19]. In contrast to the subtemporal approach, the anterolateral trajectory results in less temporal lobe retraction, but the posterior perforating arteries can be difficult to visualize and the PComA depending on its size can obstruct the view of the basilar apex. Our preference unless there is a very low bifurcation is to perform a pterional craniotomy with transcavernous dissection and extradural clinoidectomy with distal dural ring excision in order to optimize the exposure and increase the ability to manipulate the ICA and optic nerve. The transcavernous dissection also results in less traction on the oculomotor nerve [20]. In cases of large or ruptured aneurysms, we will consider adding the cranio-orbital modification.

After the initial bony approach, the dura is opened along the Sylvian fissure and the Sylvian fissure is opened which allows for safe mobilization of the temporal lobe. Brain relaxation can be achieved by opening the lamina terminalis. At this stage the basilar bifurcation is blocked from view by the optic nerve and internal carotid artery (ICA) and therefore the appropriate triangle for aneurysm dissection must be selected. The three main corridors include the optico-carotid, carotid-oculomotor, and supracarotid triangles [12]. The optico-carotid triangle is typically narrow with very limited options for maneuvering the ICA and optic nerve even with anterior clinoidectomy and optic nerve unroofing. In cases of a high riding bifurcation it may provide a better window for visualization, but it is often inadequate on its own for safe clipping of aneurysms in this region. The supracarotid triangle is rarely used for treating basilar tip aneurysms because it is often limited in cases of a long supraclinoid ICA segment and it is obstructed by numerous perforating arteries arising from the ICA bifurcation. Therefore, carotid-oculomotor triangle is often the preferred corridor. It is the largest window and can be widened by medial retraction of the ICA towards its perforators and posterior mobilization of the temporal lobe [12]. In cases of low-lying basilar bifurcations, division of the tentorial edge taking care to preserve the trochlear nerve and posterior clinoidectomy can also be employed in order to achieve proximal control on the basilar artery.

The dissection to the aneurysm it typically initiated by following the origin of the PComA to where it joins the PCA. Lillequist's membrane is opened carefully in order to enter the interpeduncular cistern. At this point the decision can be made to either carefully mobilize the PcomA or to ligate it if it is hypoplastic and significantly obstructs the operative corridor. Typically, the PComA is divided in the perforator free segment close to the PCA. Next, proximal control is identified ideally proximal to the SCA origin, but above the distal basilar artery perforators [11, 12]. In cases low-lying basilar bifurcations proximal control on the basilar trunk can be difficult or impossible to safely achieve.

The arachnoid dissection is then continued to completely expose the basilar bifurcation including the neck of the aneurysm, bilateral P1 segments and SCAs, and the perforators. The contralateral P1 and SCA are typically better visualized by this anterolateral approach in contrast to the subtemporal approach. Anteriorly projecting aneurysms can obstruct the view of the contralateral P1 and SCA at this stage and posteriorly projecting aneurysms can displace perforators further posteriorly typically making these the most difficult aneurysms to safely clip. Potential clip trajectories are based on the orientations of the P1 segments and location of the perforators. Final dissection and clipping can be performed with or without temporary basilar artery occlusion depending on how much manipulation of the aneurysm neck and dome is required to visualize all of these vital structures. Often to fully visualize perforators arising from the contralateral side, temporary clipping is required in order to soften the aneurysm and allow for more aggressive manipulation of the dome. When temporary clipping is employed we standardly increase the FiO_2 to 100%, optimize the systemic blood pressure to maintain cerebral perfusion, and limit clipping to 3 min with at least 5 min of intermittent reperfusion time between clipping.

Clipping is usually carried out by using the contralateral P1 origin to determine the angle of the clip blades. It is also equally critical to ensure no perforators are inadvertently included in the clip tines. For wide necked aneurysms, atherosclerotic walls, or previously coiled aneurysms, clipping strategies can often include stacked or tandem clipping where fenestrated clips are employed to preserve either perforators or the ipsilateral P1 [11, 12]. After final clip application, it is our practice to confirm aneurysm obliteration as well as preservation of the parent vessels and perforators with indocyanine green (ICG) angiography and a micro-Doppler probe. We also typically puncture the dome of the aneurysm with a needle or shrink it with careful bipolar cautery as a final confirmation.

3.2.3 Surgical Approaches: Lateral

The subtemporal approach is a direct lateral exposure of the basilar apex and therefore it typically allows visualization along the long axis of the aneurysm, parallel to the P1 segments of the PCA which is the trajectory often ideal for visualizing clip blades. However, the dissection and visualization of the contralateral P1 can be difficult. This approach is typically reserved for low-lying and posteriorly projecting basilar tip aneurysms as it allows for optimal visualization of the posteriorly directed perforators [11]. This approach should also be considered when there are bilateral fetal or large PComA. Proximal control is typically easier to obtain and visualize with this route. This approach, however, does result in significant temporal lobe retraction which makes brain relaxation critical often with use of a lumbar or external ventricular drain for intraoperative cerebral spinal fluid (CSF) diversion [11]. This should be an important consideration when managing ruptured aneurysms where the brain is already swollen and friable.

Typically, a temporal craniotomy is performed flush with the floor of the middle fossa. After the dura is opened CSF can be drained from the perimesencephalic cistern. The trochlear nerve should be identified prior to opening the tentorial edge. The superior petrosal sinus will be ligated. For small aneurysms, this exposure is typically enough, but the corridor can be widened by opening the posterior cavernous sinus and drilling the medial petrous apex and posterior clinoid process [11]. Aneurysm and perforator dissection and clip application can then be carried out as detailed above.

3.2.4 Case Example

3.2.4.1 Case 1

A 72-year-old man presented with a traumatic left-sided posterior temporal lobe contusion (Fig. 3.1a) and was found to have two incidental unruptured aneurysms, an anterior communicating artery (AcomA) aneurysm and a posteriorly projecting basilar tip aneurysm (Fig. 3.1b–d). After recovery from the injury, the patient did not proceed with endovascular intervention due to concerns about compliance with dual antiplatelet therapy and the presence of a second aneurysm which was amenable to clipping. The decision was made to proceed with a right-sided pterional transsylvian, transcavernous approach with extradural anterior clinoidectomy, and optic nerve unroofing for concurrent microsurgical clipping of both aneurysms.

After successful clipping of the AcomA aneurysm, we then turned our attention to microsurgical clipping of the basilar tip aneurysm via a transcavernous approach. The posterior communicating artery (PcomA) was followed posteriorly to the interpeduncular cistern by dividing the membrane of Liliequist. The PcomA was then visualized joining the PCA (Fig. 3.1e). The basilar artery and bilateral SCA and PCA were clearly identified. To avoid traction injury to the oculomotor nerve, the small PcomA was coagulated and divided in the perforator free segment. The posteriorly projecting basilar tip aneurysm (Fig. 3.1f) was brought into view and was completely obliterated with two aneurysm clips (Fig. 3.1g). The postoperative course was uneventful and he made an excellent recovery without any cranial nerve palsy. CT angiogram and 3D CT angiogram confirmed complete obliteration of both aneurysms (Fig. 3.1h, i).

3.3 Posterior Inferior Cerebellar Artery (PICA) Aneurysms

PICA aneurysms are relatively rare but make up approximately 0.5–3% of all intracranial aneurysms [21]. They most often involve the proximal segment of the PICA (69%), but they can also involve the proximal VA (3%), distal VA (17%), or distal

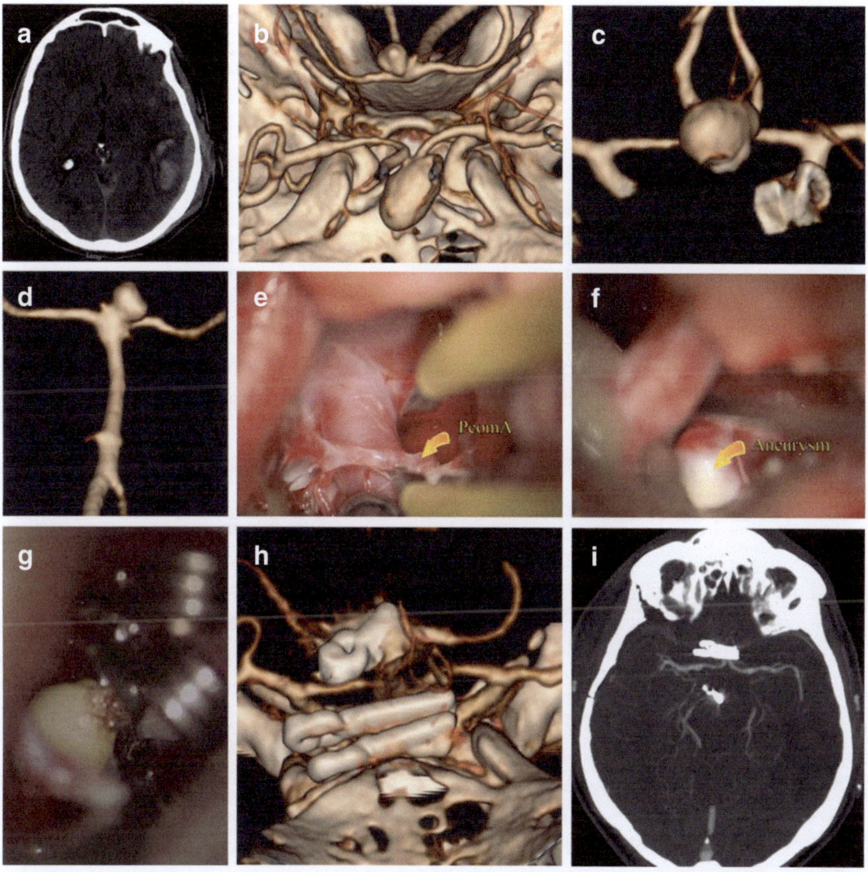

Fig. 3.1 (**a**) Head CT demonstrates initial traumatic left-sided posterior temporal lobe contusion. (**b**) 3D CT angiogram reconstruction shows two incidental unruptured aneurysms, (**c**) 12 mm AComA aneurysm and (**d**) 7 mm posteriorly projecting basilar tip aneurysm. (**e**) Intraoperative view showing the small PComA which was followed posteriorly until it joined PCA. (**f**) Intraoperative view showing the posteriorly projecting basilar tip aneurysm. (**g**) Intraoperative view showing complete obliteration of the aneurysm with two tandem clips. (**h**) Postoperative 3D CT angiogram and (**i**) axial CT angiogram confirm complete obliteration of both aneurysms

PICA (11%) [22]. They can be complex aneurysms to manage surgically due to their location at the skull base, close proximity to the lower cranial nerves, perforators, and brainstem, and highly variable courses of both the vertebral artery and PICA [1, 21]. Lower cranial nerve palsy or neuropraxia can occur even after minor manipulations and can be highly morbid resulting in dysphagia, dysarthria, or even airway compromise.

As with basilar tip aneurysms, there is continuous debate regarding clipping versus coiling of these aneurysms. The small nature of the PICA and the typically broad neck morphology of the aneurysms in this location favors clipping in many circumstances since the PICA will often times be at risk during coiling and stenting of these small vessels can occasionally result in sacrifice of the parent vessel due to in-stent stenosis or thrombosis. In general, older patients with significant medical co-morbidities and narrow-neck aneurysms may be more favorable for endovascular intervention.

3.3.1 Preoperative Considerations

Recognition of the many anatomical variants of the PICA, including a duplicated PICA, a unilateral or absent PICA, shared AICA-PICA trunk, VA termination in PICA, and extradural origins of PICA is critical [23]. The extradural variant can occur in up to 5–20% of cases and is the most important variant to recognize because it can place both the PICA and posterior spinal artery at risk during the initial extradural dissection of the V3 segment of the VA [23, 24]. As with basilar bifurcation aneurysms, understanding the bony skull base anatomy, in particular the C1 posterior arch (including the incompetent posterior arch variant), foramen magnum, and clivus, in relationship to the VA and PICA are important for preoperative planning.

There is a high incidence of non-saccular dissecting aneurysms in this location, which carry a high risk for both intraoperative bleeding and spontaneous rerupture [25, 26]. Due to the morphology of these aneurysms they are often not amenable to standard clipping or endovascular techniques and often require either open or endovascular parent vessel occlusion, trapping with bypass, wrapping, stent reconstruction, or flow diversion [27–29]. Dissecting aneurysms mainly involving the VA proximal to PICA are amenable treatment with proximal VA occlusion if the contralateral vertebral artery is adequate often confirmed by balloon test occlusion (BTO). Those dissecting aneurysms that involve the origin of PICA or that arise from PICA itself, often require microsurgical trapping with bypass or stent reconstruction. Distal PICA dissecting aneurysms can be treated with vessel sacrifice if absolutely necessary. This must be performed distal to the choroidal point which is the most superior point or apex of the PICA in the telovelotonsilar segment in order to ensure that the occlusion occurs distal to the origin of the PICA perforators supplying the dorsolateral medulla [30].

Bypass in this location should always be a consideration in cases of non-saccular dissecting aneurysms or aneurysms with large dysplastic morphologies in order to preserve the distal PICA territory and its perforators. Options can include in situ PICA-PICA side-to-side bypass, occipital-PICA end-to-side bypass, excision of distal aneurysms with end-to-end re-anastomosis, end-to-side reimplantation of the PICA into the proximal VA, and variations of these utilizing different interposition grafts including radial artery, saphenous vein, and others [31]. In general, it is our preference to preserve the parent vessel and its vascular territory when able.

3.3.2 Surgical Approaches

Selection of the approach for PICA aneurysms should take into consideration the segment of the PICA involved. For proximal PICA aneurysms (anterior medullary or lateral medullary segments), we typically prefer a far lateral or lateral suboccipital approach with or without condylectomy. For distal PICA aneurysms (tonsillomedullary, telovelotonsillar, or cortical segments), the midline suboccipital occipital approach is typically sufficient. In the rare cases of high riding PICA aneurysms where the PICA tonsillar loop comes to the level of the internal acoustic canal and cranial nerve 7 and 8 entry zones, we employ the retrosigmoid approach.

For surgical candidates, most PICA aneurysms require the use of the far lateral approach as first described by Heros [32]. When considering this approach, it is important to consider that drilling of more than one-third of the condyle can result in instability at the craniocervical junction. This limit intraoperatively can often be appreciated by reaching the condylar emissary vein. Only the minimal amount of condylar drilling should be performed that is needed for the exposure [6, 32, 33]. In cases of more distal PICA aneurysms (distal to the tonsillomedullary segment) midline or paramedian suboccipital approaches may be more appropriate [34]. This will require gentle lateral retraction of the tonsils or in cases of large aneurysms, unilateral subpial tonsillar resection can be performed.

For the far lateral approach the patient is positioned in the lateral park bench position with the head rotated and flexed towards the floor. We favor a hockey stick incision because it results in less muscle atrophy and neck pain, but linear or lazy "S" incisions can also be utilized for exposure. The lateral portion of the incision should extend up to the level of the superior nuchal line and turn inferolaterally towards the mastoid tip. This incision allows for harvesting of pericranium for duraplasty at the end of the case and a muscle cuff can also be left along the superior nuchal line for re-suspension of the suboccipital muscles during closure. The subperiosteal muscle dissection should extend down to the mastoid tip and digastric groove laterally and in the midline occurs in the avascular plane of the nuchal ligament to expose the foramen magnum as well as the posterior arch of C1 and the C2 spinous process and lamina.

We typically begin with a C1 hemilaminectomy and exposure of the V3 segment of the VA. The V3 segment can be located laterally in the sulcus arteriosus of C1 and can be easily identified and freed extradurally for early proximal control. A complex venous plexus typically surrounds the VA in this segment and can be a source of significant bleeding which can be managed with compression and irrigation. The lateral suboccipital craniotomy or craniectomy is then performed extending from the posterior border of the sigmoid sinus and superior nuchal line superiorly and the foramen magnum inferiorly. The lateral limit is the occipital condyle and medially it extends to the midline. The transcondylar drilling is variable and should be tailored to the extent needed for each individual case. The resection of the occipital condyle serves to widen the corridor to the ventral brainstem and can reduce retraction or manipulation of both the brainstem and cerebellum.

Once the dura is opened arachnoid dissection is carried out at the foramen magnum. Opening the arachnoid widely, especially around the lower cranial nerves is important in order to avoid traction injury or avulsion of these structures. The dentate ligament is often cut in order to facilitate a wider surgical corridor and allow more ventral visualization. Proximal control is then achieved intradurally from the V4 segment of the VA. Identification of PICA aneurysms can be achieved by either following the VA proximally or by identifying the tonsillar loop of PICA and tracing it back to its origin. The dissection windows are typically determined by the course of the lower cranial nerves and often the natural corridor is via the vagoaccesory triangle which provides access to the PICA origin [31]. Small perforator branches arising from the PICA are identified traveling medially to the medulla and must be preserved. The clipping strategy for most PICA aneurysms typically involves tandem clipping in order to reconstruct the neck and preserve the PICA origin which is typically incorporated into the neck of the aneurysm [31].

3.3.3 Case Examples

3.3.3.1 Case 2

A 34-year-old woman presented with Hunt and Hess (HH) grade 2, Fisher grade 3 subarachnoid hemorrhage (SAH) (Fig. 3.2a). DSA showed a ruptured complex, multilobed PICA aneurysm (Fig. 3.2b, c). She underwent a left-sided far lateral transcondylar skull base approach for microsurgical clipping of the PICA aneurysm using two tandem clips (Fig. 3.2e). Endovascular intervention was not pursued due to the complete

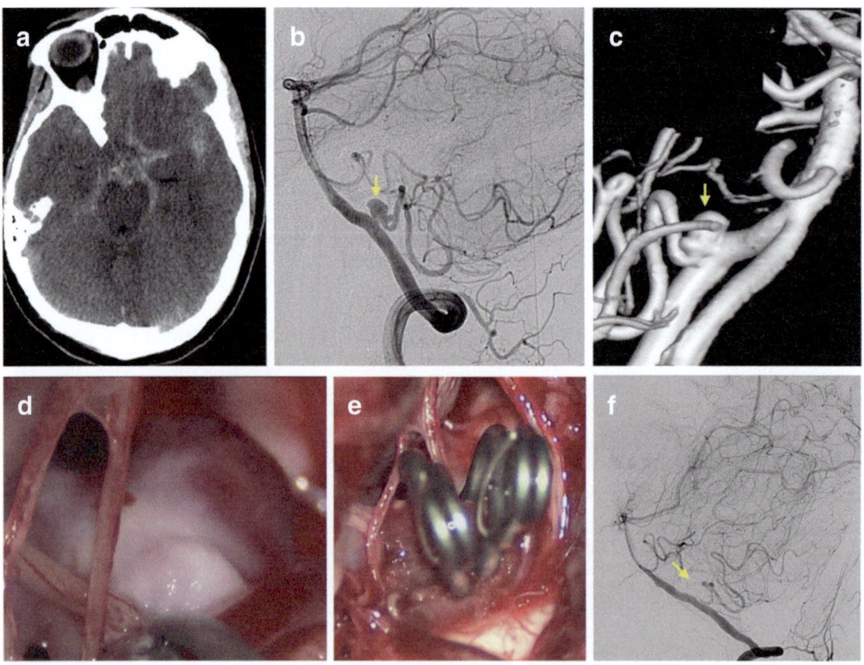

Fig. 3.2 (**a**) CT of the head shows Fisher grade 3 SAH most prominent in the left sylvian fissure and prepontine cisterns. (**b**) Lateral view DSA and (**c**) 3D-DSA show a 7 mm × 5 mm ruptured complex, multilobed PICA aneurysm (yellow arrow). (**d**) Intraoperative view shows complex multilobed PICA aneurysm. (**e**) Intraoperative view shows post-clipping configuration of the aneurysm. (**f**) Postoperative DSA shows complete obliteration of the aneurysm (yellow arrow)

incorporation of the large PICA branch into the neck of the aneurysm. Endovascular methods would have likely resulted in compromise of the PICA territory without stenting which would have been relatively contraindicated due to the need for dual antiplatelet therapy in the setting of SAH. Postoperative DSA showed complete obliteration of the aneurysm after an uneventful surgery and postoperative course (Fig. 3.2f).

3.3.3.2 Case 3

A 51-year-old man presented to the ED with headache, nausea, vomiting which rapidly progressed to the loss of consciousness and cardiac arrest (HH grade V). He underwent successful cardiopulmonary resuscitation and the head CT demonstrated substantial Fisher grade 3 SAH and hydrocephalus. An external ventricular drain (EVD) was placed (Fig. 3.3a) and DSA demonstrated a left-sided dissecting PICA aneurysm (Fig. 3.3b, c) which was not amenable to endovascular intervention without complete vessel sacrifice or use of dual antiplatelet therapy for stenting. The decision was made to proceed with bypass and trapping of the aneurysm. The possible options for revascularization included: (1) PICA-PICA bypass, which was not possible due to very high riding PICA loops which would have required significant resection of bilateral tonsils (Fig. 3.3d), (2) OA-PICA bypass, (3) V3-PICA bypass with RA interposition graft, and (4) V3-PICA bypass with SV interposition graft.

The patient underwent left-sided far lateral transcondylar skull base approach. Because of the body habitus of patient, the thick occipital bone (Fig. 3.3e, yellow dashed oval), and a very steep slope of the posterior fossa (Fig. 3.3f, yellow arrow), we extended the craniotomy supratentorial towards the nuchal line. There were several layers of complexity to this case. We were unable to identify an occipital artery during the dissection due to the body habitus of the patient. During the RA harvest, the plastic surgeon encountered in situ thrombosis of the RA towards the end of the dissection. Since the patient had a very sizable cephalic vein (CV) in the same field, we decided to harvest the CV for bypass (Fig. 3.3g). Bilateral PICA loops were high riding and we therefore had to perform a partial left tonsillar resection for complete exposure. We then performed a V3 to PICA bypass with CV interposition graft and with microsurgical trapping of the dissecting PICA aneurysm making sure to exclude any perforators (Fig. 3.3h–m). His hospital course was complicated by multiple treatments for severe vasospasm which was managed with balloon angioplasty and intra-arterial Verapamil. Postoperative DSA showed complete elimination of the aneurysm with a patent bypass (Fig. 3.3n–p). He made an excellent recovery with an mRS of 1 at 22-months follow-up.

3.3.3.3 Case 4

A 72-year-old woman with history of SAH due to a ruptured basilar tip aneurysm which was treated with coil embolization and required ventriculoperitoneal shunt placement for post-SAH hydrocephalus (Fig. 3.4a). She was lost to follow-up and subsequently presented to our hospital with HH grade 2, Fisher grade 4 SAH

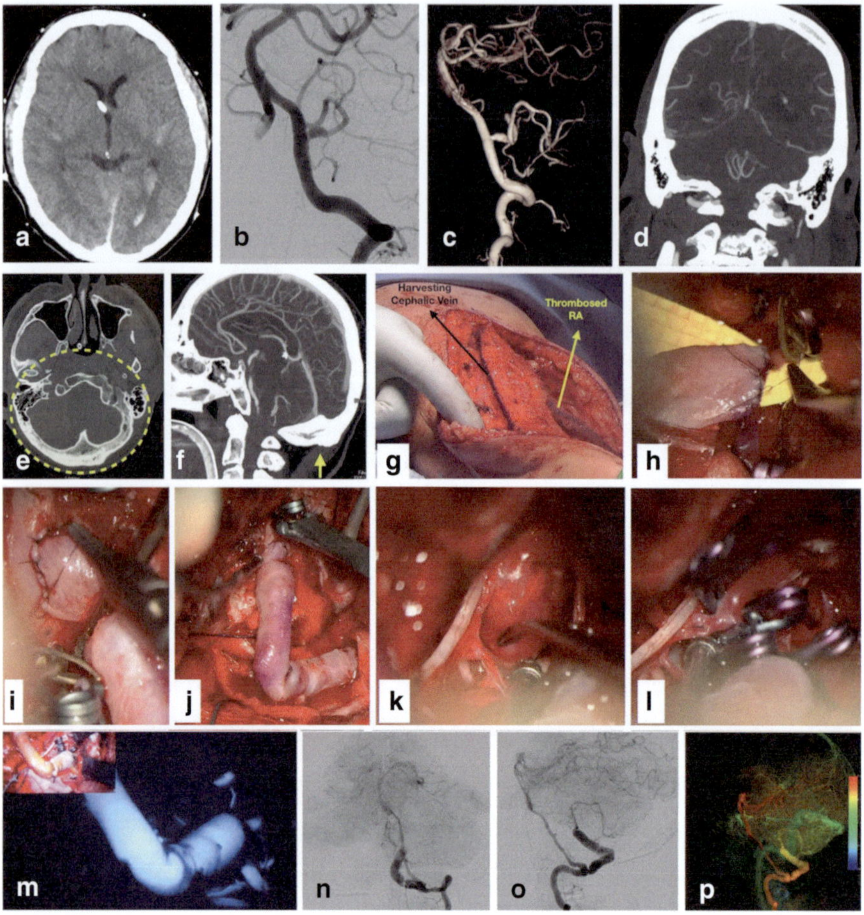

Fig. 3.3 (**a**) Head CT demonstrates substantial Fisher grade 3 SAH and ventriculostomy for hydrocephalus. (**b**) Lateral view DSA and (**c**) 3D-DSA show a left-sided dissecting PICA aneurysm. (**d**) Coronal section of the CT angiography shows very high riding PICAs. (**e**) Axial section of CT scan with bone window shows thick occipital bone (yellow dashed oval). (**f**) Sagittal section of CT angiography shows very steep slope posterior fossa (yellow arrow). (**g**) Intraoperative view of forearm during RA harvest with in situ thrombosis and the relative location of the harvested sizable CV. (**h**) Intraoperative view showing CV to PICA loop anastomosis, (**i**) intraoperative view showing V3 to CV anastomosis, (**j**) intraoperative view showing V3 to PICA bypass with CV interposition graft. (**k**) Intraoperative view showing dissecting PICA aneurysm. (**l**) Intraoperative view showing trapping of the dissecting PICA aneurysm, (**m**) intraoperative indocyanine green video angiography showing patent V3 to PICA bypass with CV interposition graft and trapping of the dissecting PICA aneurysm. (**n**) AP view DSA, (**o**) lateral view of DSA, and (**p**) perfusion study show complete trapping with a patent bypass

(Fig. 3.4b) from a ruptured left-sided distal tonsillomedullary segment PICA aneurysm (Fig. 3.4c, d). Due to multiple medical co-morbidities, we first considered endovascular treatment. Ultimately, the endovascular team deemed the aneurysm could

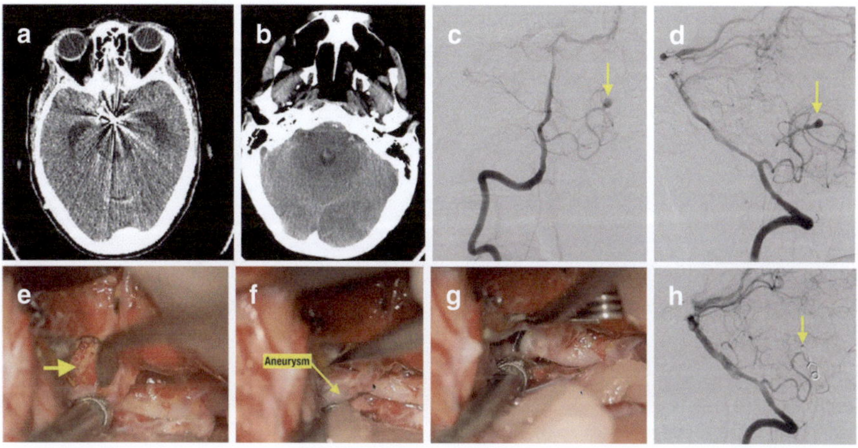

Fig. 3.4 (**a**) Axial head CT demonstrates the previously coiled basilar tip aneurysm. (**b**) Axial head CT without contrast shows Fisher 4 SAH. (**c, d**) AP and lateral view DSA confirm a ruptured left-sided 2–3 mm aneurysm of the tonsillomedullary segment of PICA (yellow arrow). (**e**) Intraoperative view showing hemosiderin staining which was the evidence of prior silent ruptures (yellow arrow). (**f**) Intraoperative view showing tonsillomedullary segment of PICA and the aneurysm (yellow arrow). (**g**) Intraoperative view showing successful clipping of the aneurysm. (**h**) Three-year follow-up DSA shows complete obliteration of the aneurysm and preservation of the parent vessel (yellow arrow)

not be treated without closing the parent artery. Therefore, the decision was made to proceed with a midline suboccipital craniotomy and microsurgical clipping of distal PICA aneurysm in order to preserve the distal PICA territory. Intraoperatively we encountered hemosiderin staining which was consistent with evidence of prior silent ruptures in the region (Fig. 3.4e). We then separated the tonsils with careful arachnoid dissection and identified the tonsillomedullary segment of PICA along with the aneurysm (Fig. 3.4f). Neuronavigation can also be employed if needed to locate the aneurysm. Successful reconstruction of the neck of the aneurysm with a single clip was performed (Fig. 3.4g). The surgery and postoperative course were uneventful and she made an excellent recovery. Three-year follow-up DSA showed complete obliteration of the aneurysm with preservation of the small distal PICA branch (Fig. 3.4h).

3.4 Vertebrobasilar Junction Aneurysms

Dandy was the first to describe his surgical exposure of a VA aneurysm in 1921 [35]. Since that time aneurysms in this location continue to present a challenge to cerebrovascular neurosurgeons due to the close relationship with both the lower cranial nerves and brainstem perforators. These aneurysms also have the added complexity that they are typically large with dysplastic morphologies and they involve exposure of bilateral VAs and the proximal basilar artery from a limited field of view which requires comfort with the variable anatomy of this region as well as modifications of the available skull base exposures of this region.

3.4.1 Preoperative Considerations

The anatomy of the VBJ is highly variable and therefore no single surgical approach can be routinely applied to aneurysms in these locations, therefore, treatment considerations must be tailored to each individual patient and the characteristics of their pathology. The basilar artery is formed by the joining of both intradural VAs in 80% of cases. Most often the left VA is dominant (80%), but these anatomical variants must be studied on preoperative imaging [36, 37]. In 5–10% of cases, the nondominant VA will continue alone and terminate as the PICA without joining the contralateral VA [37]. Additionally, the presence and size of the PcomA and the contralateral vertebral artery is also important, especially when considering collateral supply in the setting of possible VA sacrifice. The anatomy which also must be considered is the relationship of the VBJ to the clivus anteriorly, brainstem posteriorly, and petrous bone laterally as well as the course of the perforators arising from the VA, PICA, AICA, and proximal BA [37, 38]. Selecting the side of the approach is also important, especially when the VBJ is positioned in the midline. Factors to consider include the VA dominance, course of the occipital artery (OA), and projection of the aneurysm. In general most surgeons choose to approach the aneurysms from the side it shows laterality or where early proximal control can be easily achieved [37].

Cerebrovascular bypass should be considered preoperatively at least as a salvage plan in almost all VBJ aneurysms and at times it is needed as a first line treatment option. Preoperative angiography should include adequate imaging of the external carotid artery (ECA) to evaluate for potential donors including the caliber of the vessels and its geographical relationship to potential recipients. There are several donor vessel options for posterior circulation bypass including the superficial temporal artery (STA), radial artery (RA), saphenous vein (SV), and the OA. These is also consideration of in situ bypass with side-to-side PICA-PICA anastomosis among others. The OA is typically the most commonly used graft in posterior circulation revascularization due to its proximity to numerous recipient vessels in the posterior fossa. The suboccipital segment can be identified as it extends from the occipital groove to the superior nuchal line [37].

3.4.2 Surgical Approaches

Several skull base approaches can be considered when managing aneurysms of the VBJ. Working medial to lateral these can include, transclival, lateral suboccipital, transpetrosal, and far lateral transcondylar approaches. These approaches will all offer adequate exposure of the VBJ with increasing bony removal resulting in a wider corridor with less manipulation of brainstem structures. Often, the lateral suboccipital approach is adequate for most straightforward and small aneurysms of the VBJ, but it requires more lateral extension with transcondylar drilling and C1 laminectomy for larger or more complex aneurysms not only to achieve adequate exposure but also in consideration of achieving earlier and safe proximal control [32, 37].

The far lateral transcondylar approach is our preference for aneurysms in this location and is carried out as described earlier in the surgical approach to PICA aneurysms. Once the dura is opened, wide arachnoid dissection allows for better visualization of the deeper structures, less inadvertent retraction of the lower cranial nerves, and results in the release of CSF for brain relaxation. The dentate ligament is also cut if better access to the ventral medulla is necessary. The dissection then involves following the ipsilateral VA as it pierces the dura and then travels to join the contralateral VA to form the basilar artery. This early exposure of bilateral VAs and the proximal basilar artery provides both proximal and distal control prior to identification and dissection of the aneurysm. Ideally, a complete exposure should include the proximal basilar artery, bilateral VAs, the ipsilateral PICA origin, the ipsilateral AICA origin, perforators, cranial nerves 7 and 8, as well as the lower cranial nerves. Visualization of all of these structures will allow for safe clipping of these aneurysms utilizing the standard microsurgical techniques.

3.4.3 Case Example

3.4.3.1 Case 5

A 54-year-old man presented with progressive headaches, dizziness, and ataxia. CT angiogram demonstrated a giant saccular aneurysm of the vertebrobasilar junction resulting in brainstem compression (Fig. 3.5a). Two attempts at endovascular embolization were unsuccessful secondary to occlusive vasospasm of the VA. He was transferred to our hospital and underwent coil occlusion of right VA to decrease blood flow into the aneurysm since flow diverting stents were not being used at the time of his presentation. Eight-months following coiling, he developed progressive quadriparesis and lower cranial nerve dysfunction. CT angiogram at that time demonstrated interval growth of the VBJ aneurysm (Fig. 3.5b). Oblique and 3D DSA confirmed growth of aneurysm following coil occlusion of right VA (Fig. 3.5c, d).

The decision was made to proceed with a left-sided far lateral transcondylar skull base approach and microsurgical clipping of the complex giant VBJ aneurysm. Clip reconstruction was possible since the aneurysm did not involve 360° of the VA. We employed hypothermic circulatory arrest in order to decompress and soften the large aneurysm to allow for better manipulation of the dome. After 32 min of circulatory arrest, the aneurysm was completely obliterated and the neck was reconstructed with 12 aneurysm clips (Fig. 3.5e, f). Optimally circulatory arrest should

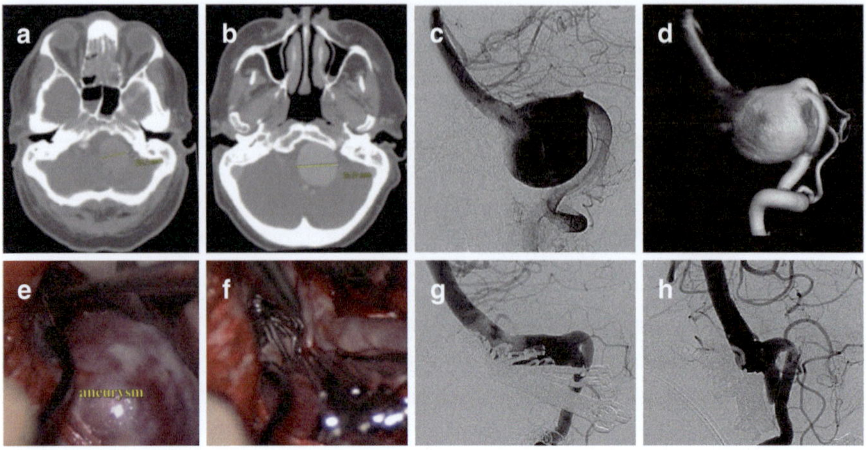

Fig. 3.5 (**a**) CT angiogram demonstrates a giant (2.5 cm) saccular aneurysm of the vertebrobasilar junction. (**b**) CT angiogram shows interval growth of the vertebrobasilar junction aneurysm 8-months after coil occlusion of right vertebral artery. (**c**) Oblique view DSA and (**d**) 3D DSA confirm the growth of aneurysm following coil occlusion of right vertebral artery. (**e**) Intraoperative view showing giant vertebrobasilar junction aneurysm. (**f**) Intraoperative view showing complete obliteration of the aneurysm with 12 aneurysm clips under 32 min of circulatory arrest. (**g**) Lateral view of DSA and (**h**) AP view DSA confirm complete obliteration of the aneurysm and the stump of the occluded right vertebral artery

not surpass 40 min. The surgery and postoperative course were uneventful and he tolerated the surgery and circulatory arrest well. Postoperative DSA confirmed complete obliteration of the aneurysm (Fig. 3.5g, h).

3.5 Aneurysms of the Basilar Trunk

Basilar trunk aneurysms are rare lesions and are defined as aneurysms located between the VBJ and SCA origins. This can include SCA aneurysms, AICA aneurysms, or aneurysms arising from large perforators of the basilar trunk. The majority of aneurysms in this location arise from the proximal SCA. The origin and size of the aneurysm is what dictates the approach taking into consideration the bony structures that often impede trajectories to reach this region. Surgical approaches to mid-basilar trunk are made difficult due to limitations from the clivus, distance below the posterior clinoid, and the interference of the petrous bone. Occasionally, approaching aneurysms in these locations may require one of the several variations of transpetrosal approaches, but transoral, Kawase, or retrosigmoid approaches can also be considered. The complexity of the approaches required to treat these aneurysms which is why endovascular treatment is has become more favorable at most institutions if it is technically feasible [39]. However, SCA aneurysms that are not amendable to endovascular treatment can be more favorable to microsurgical clipping than other basilar trunk aneurysms due to their accessibility and typically they are not as involved with the posterior thalamo-perforators which arise more distally at the basilar bifurcation.

SCA aneurysms or aneurysms of the distal basilar trunk can often be exposed and treated in a similar manner to basilar tip aneurysms either via a pterional approach modified with an extradural clinoidectomy, transcavernous dissection, and posterior clinoidectomy for more proximal aneurysms [14, 40, 41]. Alternatively, subtemporal approaches with division of the tentorium with or without anterior petrosectomy can be utilized and is often preferred in more proximal pathology [33, 41]. Again, the relationship of the basilar bifurcation to the posterior clinoid or dorsum sella is an important consideration in determining the appropriate surgical corridor. As described for the basilar bifurcation dissection the PComA is usually followed from its origin on the ICA to the PCA, and the PCA and SCA are identified in their standard positions on either side of the oculomotor nerve. Proximal control is achieved proximal to the SCA origin but distal to the basilar trunk perforators. Standard clipping strategies are then able to be employed.

3.6 Non-saccular Aneurysms of the Posterior Circulation

Gideon H. Wells described the first non-saccular posterior circulation aneurysms in 1922 [42]. Presently, posterior circulation non-saccular aneurysms continue to present challenges in treatment due to their involvement of brainstem perforators, extensive involvement in long segments of the vertebrobasilar system, and the absence of a discrete neck. Standard techniques including microsurgical clipping or endovascular coiling cannot typically be employed with these aneurysms. Although relatively uncommon with an incidence of less than 1%, their natural history can be associated with significant morbidity and mortality due to compression of the brainstem and cranial nerves, obstructive hydrocephalus, ischemic stroke from atheroembolism of partially thrombosed or calcified aneurysms, or rarely hemorrhage [3, 43, 44]. The natural history of these aneurysms is variable with a mortality rate reported up to 30% [43].

Non-saccular aneurysms of the posterior circulation have been subtyped by morphology in the literature as fusiform, dolichoectatic, or transitional [43, 45]. The fusiform subtype is defined as dilation of the vertebral or basilar artery >1.5 times normal, dolichoectatic subtype is the same amount of dilation, but involving the entire basilar artery, vertebral artery, or vertebrobasilar system, and transitional is the same amount of dilation with a superimposed further dilation of a part the disease segment [43]. In a longitudinal study of 159 patients with non-saccular vertebrobasilar aneurysms, Flemming et al. demonstrated that transitional and fusiform subtype aneurysms were more likely to be symptomatic with dolichoectatic aneurysms typically being asymptomatic. The only independent factor predicting aneurysm ruptured was the transitional morphology. Their cohort also showed a 6.7% per year risk of recurrent infarcts in patients who initially presented with stroke during 10-years follow-up. The most common cause of death in their study was stroke [43, 46]. Bhogal et al. suggested early treatment of asymptomatic, large fusiform, and transitional aneurysms due to their tendency to become symptomatic while preferring conservative management of dolichoectatic aneurysms with serial imaging with or without antiplatelet therapy as they typically have a more benign course [43].

Due to the high morbidity associated with the natural history of these aneurysms, treatment options have been sought after, but typically involves complex or high-risk procedures including trapping with or without bypass, endovascular or surgical sacrifice of a vertebral artery in order to reduce flow into the aneurysmal segment, or more recently flow diverting stents. Conservative or medical management with either antiplatelet therapy or anticoagulation has also been considered to reduce the incidence of thrombotic or atheroembolic ischemic strokes but thus far has demonstrated limited influence on long-term outcomes [27]. The success of surgical interventions has been limited due to the location at the skull base adding complexity to open surgical treatment and difficulty preserving brainstem perforators contributes to morbidity and mortality in both open and endovascular approaches [44, 47].

Surgical treatment of these aneurysms can be thought of as inducing flow reduction (vessel sacrifice) or flow reversal (bypass). The success of these interventions is based largely on the collateral supply from the posterior communicating artery. When a large posterior communicating artery is not present, bypass surgery should be favored over vessel sacrifice. The most common revascularization procedure for this pathology is the STA to SCA or PCA bypass with trapping of the diseased aneurysmal segment. Mortality rates with bypass have been reported as high as 45–62% [47, 48]. Flow reduction can be performed with dominant vertebral artery occlusion either by open surgical ligation or endovascular occlusion. This technique is most successful when disease is confined to the vertebral artery without involvement of the basilar artery [43]. Bilateral vertebral artery occlusion has also been attempted in extreme cases where patients are already presenting in poor clinical condition with limited treatment options, but again the presence of a large posterior communicating artery is the main predictor of a successful outcome [43].

Endovascular flow diversion for treatment of non-saccular posterior circulation aneurysms has been aggressively sought after because it allows for reconstruction of diseased segments and preservation of flow to the posterior circulation; however, at this time it does remain an off-label use of these devices. Additionally, coverage of critical brainstem perforators with flow diverting stents does not always resulted in preservation of flow through these small branches. Use of flow diverting stents requires the use of dual antiplatelet therapy which contributes to the reported high rates of hemorrhagic complications [49, 50]. Flow diversion also results in delayed or limited improvement in the symptoms related to mass effect from these aneurysms including brainstem compression, cranial neuropathies, and hydrocephalus. Endovascular treatments have recently shown promise as the technology has advanced in this specialty, but initial the popularity of flow diversion in the posterior circulation has ebbed and flowed as high complication rates have been reported in the literature [49].

Szikora et al. claimed that flow diverters seemed to be a supreme treatment option for large partially thrombosed non-saccular vertebrobasilar aneurysms [51]. But in 2012, a report from a single-center by Siddiqui et al. debated the efficacy of flow diverters for these challenging aneurysms based on a mortalities in 4 of 7 patients in their small series [49]. As techniques, devices and their applications have evolved the earlier reported high morbidity and mortality rates associated with posterior circulation flow diversion has improved. These improvements have been credited to better patient selection and indications, avoidance of flow diversion in partially thrombosed fusiform holobasilar aneurysms due to risk of occluding of critical pontine perforators, and limiting the number of overlapping devices to reduce risk of perforator occlusion [43, 52]. Also, the addition of coiling to flow diversion has led to less stent prolapse and reduced hemorrhagic complications, therefore contributing to better outcomes [3, 43, 52]. The difficulty with these cases continues to be indications for treatment and timing of intervention. Ultimately, the ideal indications and treatment modality have not been completely elucidated for this pathology, but recent reports would suggest that flow diversion shows promise when clinically indicated.

3.7 Endovascular Therapy for Posterior Circulation Aneurysms

The biggest advancements in the treatment of posterior circulation aneurysms in recent decades have been regarding endovascular intervention. With the improvements in technology and devices, more and more aneurysms are becoming suitable candidates for safe endovascular embolization. In addition to conventional primary coil embolization, the addition of newer devices including balloons for neck remodeling, stents, flow diverters, liquid embolics, and more recently Woven EndoBridge (WEB) devices for wide neck aneurysms have increased the spectrum of aneurysms amenable to endovascular treatment [53]. Due to the technical difficulty in treating these aneurysms surgically including risk to perforators and cranial nerves and complex skull base approaches requiring advanced technical skill, endovascular therapy has largely become the modality of choice for treating posterior circulation aneurysms at many centers.

Despite the safety and efficacy of endovascular embolization, there has been debate regarding its durability, mainly regarding higher rates of recurrence and higher rates of re-hemorrhage after coiling in comparison to clipping [54–58]. The biggest argument against endovascular treatment of all aneurysms is that coiling fails to reach the same standards of long-term complete aneurysm obliteration when compared with surgical clipping. Several trials and case series have documented the lower complete occlusion rates in embolization in comparison to clipping [55, 59]. This higher residual and recurrence rate often results in the need for multiple retreatments which compounds the periprocedural complications [3].

The widely debated International Subarachnoid Aneurysm Trial (ISAT) helped further advance the popularity and favoritism of endovascular therapy especially in cases of ruptured aneurysms when their results demonstrated the coiling group had lower risk of disability at 1 year in comparison to patients undergoing open surgical clipping. However, their data also reported the rate of technical failure during the procedure and long-term risk of re-bleeding was higher with coiling than clipping. It should also be noted that posterior circulation aneurysms were significantly under-represented in this trial (>97% were anterior circulation) [56]. The Cerebral Aneurysm Rerupture After Treatment (CARAT) study reported on a multicenter collaboration of 1001 patients treated with coil embolization or surgical clipping of ruptured intracranial aneurysms with a mean follow-up of 4 years. The authors concluded that the risk of re-hemorrhage tended to be greater after coil embolization (3.4%) than after surgical clipping (1.3%), but this did not reach statistical significance ($P = 0.09$). They also determined the degree of occlusion with the initial intervention is a strong predictor for re-hemorrhage in patients with SAH which supports the importance of complete occlusion of aneurysms, especially in cases of rupture [60].

In a study by Bohnstedt et al. to compare endovascular versus microsurgical treatment for basilar tip aneurysms, cranial nerve deficit, and hemiparesis were more common in the microsurgical group but aneurysm remnants were more common in endovascular group which was reduced with the addition of stenting. They concluded microsurgical treatment still has an important role in the selected basilar tip aneurysms to avoid re-treatment [61]. In terms of the clinical outcomes of oculomotor nerve palsies associated with microsurgical clipping of basilar apex aneurysms, the series of 103 aneurysms reported by Basma et al. demonstrated that an immediate postoperative oculomotor nerve palsy was seen in all of their patients but 32% of patients demonstrated complete recovery at the time of discharge and at 1 year only 3% of patients had a persistent third nerve palsy which only consisted of diplopia corrected with prism glasses [20].

Dissecting aneurysms of the posterior circulation represent a unique challenge due to their high bleed risk and their shape and morphology not being amenable to standard surgical or endovascular approaches. As discussed previously, these aneurysms are not often not amenable to primary clip reconstruction of the neck and therefore numerous endovascular strategies have evolved over the years. Endovascular methods such as the open surgical approaches include both vessel-sacrificing and vessel-preserving strategies. These can include parent vessel occlusion with coils or embolic material, stent placement, or flow diversion [50, 62–64]. Flow diversion is an encouraging endovascular option with a higher occlusion rate and a lower complication rate in comparison to other endovascular techniques in management of dissecting aneurysms [3]. Flow diverters can cause perforator infarcts or delayed rupture due to the use of dual antiplatelet therapy and therefore have not been popular for the use in the treatment of posterior circulation aneurysms amenable to other treatment modalities [52].

Overall, surgical versus endovascular treatment of posterior circulation aneurysms continue to be a controversial topic in cerebrovascular neurosurgery. At most centers, endovascular therapy is usually favored for most aneurysms in this territory but rational decision making should be tailored to each case instead of blanket statements being made regarding the treatment of these aneurysms. At our center, multidisciplinary assessments including surgeons capable of both endovascular and microsurgical treatments of these aneurysms are employed to guide the treatment strategies. As advancements in both fields are made, this will continue to be a topic for debate. Anatomy and individual patients will dictate the correct approach and therefore proficiency in the microsurgical techniques required to treat these aneurysms will continue to be both relevant and important.

References

1. Pia H. Classification of vertebro-basilar aneurysrns. Acta Neurochir. 1979;47:3–30.
2. Winn HR. Vascular. In: Youmans neurological surgery. 6th ed. Amsterdam: Elsevier; 2011.
3. Adeeb N, Ogilvy C, Griessenauer C, Thomas A. Expanding the indications for flow diversion: treatment of posterior circulation aneurysms. Neurosurgery. 2020;86(Suppl 1):76–84.
4. Bender M, Colby G, Jiang B, et al. Flow diversion of posterior circulation cerebral aneurysms: a single-institution series of 59 cases. Neurosurgery. 2019;84(1):206–16.
5. Tjahjadi M, Serrone J, Hernesniemi J. Should we still consider clips for basilar apex aneurysms? A critical appraisal of the literature. Surg Neurol Int. 2018;9:44.
6. Lawton MT, editor. Seven aneurysms: tenets and techniques for clipping. Thieme; 2011.
7. Drake C. Bleeding aneurysms of the basilar artery: direct surgical management in four cases. J Neurosurg. 1961;18(2):230–8.
8. Yasargil M, Laciga R, Jain K, Hodosh R, Smith R. Microsurgical pterional approach to aneurysms of the basilar bifurcation. Surg Neurol. 1976;6(2):83–91.
9. Yasargil M. Microneurosurgery. New York: Thieme Medical; 1984.
10. Bendok BR, Getch CC, Parkinson R, O'shaughnessy B, Batjer H. Extended lateral transsylvian approach for basilar bifurcation aneurysms. Neurosurgery. 2004;10(1):174–8.
11. Abecassis J, Shetty R, Sekhar L. Surgical treatment of basilar tip aneurysms. In: Massoud T, Kirollos R, Hacein-Bey L, editors. Basilar artery. New York: Nova Science; 2019. p. 435–48.
12. Lawton M. Basilar artery birfucation aneurysms. In: Seven aneurysms: tenets and techniques for clipping. New York: Thieme Medical; 2011.
13. Spetzler RF, Kalani YM, Nakaji P. Surgical therapies for basilar artery aneurysms. In: Spetzler R, Nakaji P, editors. Neurovascular surgery. 2nd ed. New York: Thieme Medical; 2015. p. 623–34.
14. Krisht AF, Kadri PAS. Surgical clipping of complex basilar apex aneurysms: a strategy for successful outcome using the pretemporal transzygomatic transcavernous approach. Neurosurgery. 2005;56(4 Suppl):15–8. https://doi.org/10.1227/01.NEU.0000156785.63530.4E.
15. Drake CG. Further experience with surgical treatment of aneurysm of the basilar artery. J Neurosurg. 1968;29(4):372–92. https://doi.org/10.3171/jns.1968.29.4.0372.
16. Batjer H. Aneurysms of distal basilar artery, the pterional approach. In: Samson D, editor. Intracranial aneurysms surgery: techniques. Bath: Future Publishing; 1990.
17. Youssef AS, Abdel Aziz K, Kim E-Y, Keller J, Zuccarello M, van Loveren H. The carotid-oculomotor window in exposure of upper basilar artery aneurysms: a cadaveric morphometric study. Neurosurgery. 2004;54(5):1181–9.
18. Dolenc S, Sustersic J, Skrbec M, Morina A. A transcavernous-transsellar approach to basilar tip aneurysms. Br J Neurosurg. 1987;1(2):251–9.
19. Drake CG. Treatment of aneurysms of the basilar artery. J Neurosurg. 1968;29:436–46.
20. Basma J, Ryttlefors M, Latini F, Pravdenkova S, Krisht A. Mobilization of the transcavernous oculomotor nerve during basilar aneurysm surgery: biomechanical bases for better outcome. Neurosurgery. 2014;10(1):106–14. https://doi.org/10.1227/NEU.0000000000000027.

21. Sejkorová A, Petr O, Mulino M, et al. Management of posterior inferior cerebellar artery aneurysms: what factors play the most important role in outcome? Acta Neurochir. 2017;159(3):549–58. https://doi.org/10.1007/s00701-016-3058-z.
22. Drake C. The treatment of aneurysms of the posterior circulation. Clin Neurosurg. 1979;26:96–144.
23. Seckin H, Ozkan A, Bauer A, Baskaya MK. Microsurgical anatomy of the posterior spinal artery via far-lateral transcondylar approach. J Neurosurg Spine. 2009;10(3):228–33.
24. Wang X, Tang G, Li M. Bilateral extradural posterior inferior cerebellar artery origins where vertebral artery ascends between transverse foramina of C-2 and C-1, with simultaneous right double origin PICA: rare case report and literature review. World Neurosurg. 2019;125:234–9. https://doi.org/10.1016/j.wneu.2019.01.233.
25. Yamaura A, Watanabe Y, Saeki N. Dissecting aneurysms of the intracranial vertebral artery. J Neurosurg. 1990;72(2):183–8.
26. Kawaguchi S, Sakaki T, Tsunoda S, et al. Management of dissecting aneurysms of the posterior circulation. Acta Neurochir. 1994;131(1–2):26–31.
27. Steinberg GK, Drake C, Peerless S. Deliberate basilar or vertebral artery occlusion in the treatment of intracranial aneurysms. Immediate results and long-term outcome in 201 patients. J Neurosurg. 1993;79(2):161–73.
28. Fukasawa I, Sasaki H, Nukui H. Surgical treatment for ruptured vertebral artery dissecting aneurysms. Neurol Med Chir (Tokyo). 1998;38(Suppl):104–6.
29. Yamada K, Hayakawa T, Ushio Y, et al. Therapeutic occlusion of the vertebral artery for unclippable vertebral aneurysm: relationship between site of occlusion and clinical outcome. Neurosurgery. 1984;15(6):834–8.
30. Lewis SB, Chang DJ, Peace DA, LaFrentz PJ, Day AL. Distal posterior inferior cerebellar artery aneurysms: clinical features and management. J Neurosurg. 2002;97:756–66.
31. Lawton MT. Posterior inferior cerebellar artery aneurysms. In: Conerly K, editor. Seven aneurysms: tenets and techniques for clipping. New York: Thieme Medical; 2011. p. 193–215.
32. Heros RC. Lateral suboccipital approach for vertebral and vertebrobasilar artery lesions. J Neurosurg. 1986;64(4):559–62. https://doi.org/10.3171/jns.1986.64.4.0559.
33. Samson D. Intracranial aneurysm surgery: techniques. Bath: Futura Publishing; 1990.
34. Ogilvy C, Quinones-Hinojosa A. Surgical treatment of vertebral and posterior inferior cerebellar artery aneurysms. Neurosurg Clin N Am. 1998;9(4):851–60.
35. Kretzer RM, Coon AL, Tamargo RJ, Walter E. Dandy's contributions to vascular neurosurgery: historical vignette. J Neurosurg. 2010;112(6):1182–91. https://doi.org/10.3171/2009.7.JNS09737.
36. Songur A, Gonul Y, Ozen O, et al. Variations in the intracranial vertebrobasilar system. Surg Radiol Anat. 2008;30:257–64.
37. Dogan I, Baskaya MK. Vertebrobasilar junction aneurysms: microsurgical treatment. In: Massoud TF, Kirollos R, Hacein-Bey L, editors. Basilar artery. New York: Nova Science; 2019. p. 519–34.
38. Grand W, Budny J, Gibbons K, Sternau L, Hopkins L. Microvascular surgical anatomy of the vertebrobasilar junction. Neurosurgery. 1997;40:1219–25.
39. Van Rooij W, Sluzewski M, Menovsky T, Wijnalda D. Coiling of saccular basilar trunk aneurysms. Neuroradiology. 2003;45(1):19–21.
40. Hakuba A, Nishimura S. The orbitozygomatic infratemporal approach: a new surgical technique. Surg Neurol. 1986;26(3):271–6.
41. Russin J, Spetzler R. Microsurgical management of aneurysms of the posterior cerebral, superior cerebellar, and anterior inferior cerebellar arteries. In: Spetzler R, Kalani M, Nakaji P, editors. Neurovascular surgery. New York: Thieme Medical; 2015.
42. Wells HG. Intracranial aneurysm of the vertebral artery. Arch Neurol Psychiatr. 1922;7(3):311–20.
43. Bhogal P, Perez M, Ganslandt O, Bazner H, Henkes H, Fischer S. Treatment of posterior circulation non-saccular aneurysms with flow diverters: a single-center experience and review of 56 patients. J Neurointerv Surg. 2017;9(5):471–81.

44. Church EW, Bigder MG, Sussman ES, et al. Treatment of posterior circulation fusiform aneurysms. J Neurosurg. 2020:1–7. https://doi.org/10.3171/2020.4.jns192838.
45. Flemming K, Wiebers D, Brown R Jr, Al E. The natural history of radiographically defined vertebrobasilar nonsaccular intracranial aneurysms. Cerebrovasc Dis. 2005;20:270–9.
46. Flemming K, Wiebers D, Brown R Jr, et al. The natural history of radiographically defined vertebrobasilar nonsaccular intracranial aneurysms. Cerebrovasc Dis. 2005;20(4):270.
47. Lawton MT, Abla AA, Rutledge WC, et al. Bypass surgery for the treatment of dolichoectatic basilar trunk aneurysms: a work in progress. Neurosurgery. 2016;79(1):83–99. https://doi.org/10.1227/NEU.0000000000001175.
48. Kalani MYS, Zabramski JM, Nakaji P, Spetzler RF. Bypass and flow reduction for complex basilar and vertebrobasilar junction aneurysms. Neurosurgery. 2013;72(5):763–75. https://doi.org/10.1227/NEU.0b013e3182870703.
49. Siddiqui A, Abla A, Kan P, et al. Panacea or problem: flow diverters in the treatment of symptomatic large or giant fusiform vertebrobasilar aneurysms. J Neurosurg. 2012;116(6):1258–66.
50. Coert BA, Chang SD, Do HM, Marks MP, Steinberg GK. Surgical and endovascular management of symptomatic posterior circulation fusiform aneurysms. J Neurosurg. 2007;106(5):855–65. https://doi.org/10.3171/jns.2007.106.5.855.
51. Szikora I, Turanyi E, Marosfoi M. Evolution of flow-diverter endothelialization and thrombus organization in giant fusiform aneurysms after flow diversion: a histopathologic study. Am J Neuroradiol. 2015;36(9):1716–20.
52. Natarajan S, Sonig A, Rai A, Carpenter J, Levy E, Siddiqui A. The safety of pipeline flow diversion in fusiform vertebrobasilar aneurysms: a consecutive case series with longer-term follow-up from a single US center. J Neurosurg. 2016;125(1):111–9.
53. Goyal N, Hoit D, Dinitto J, et al. How to WEB: a practical review of methodology for the use of the Woven EndoBridge. J Neurointerv Surg. 2020;12(5):512–20. https://doi.org/10.1136/neurintsurg-2019-015506.
54. Graves V, Strother C, Duff T, Perl J. Early treatment of ruptured aneurysms with Guglielmi detachable coils: effect on subsequent bleeding. Neurosurgery. 1995;37(4):640–7.
55. Vinuela F, Duckwiler G, Mawad M. Guglielmi detachable coil embolization of acute intracranial aneurysm: perioperative anatomical and clinical outcome in 403 patients. J Neurosurg. 1997;86(3):475–82.
56. Molyneux A, et al. International subarachnoid aneurysms trial (ISAT) of neurosurgical clipping versus endovascular coiling in 2143 patients with ruptured intracranial aneurysms: a randomised trial. Lancet. 2005;366(9488):809–17.
57. Raymond J, Roy D, Bojanowski M, Moumdjian R, L'Esperance G. Endovascular treatment of acutely ruptured and unruptured aneurysms of the basilar bifurcation. J Neurosurg. 1997;86(2):211–9.
58. Klein G, Szolar D, Leber K, Karaic R, Hausegger K. Basilar tip aneurysm: endovascular treatment with Guglielmi detachable coils--midterm results. Radiology. 1997;205(1):191–6.
59. Zubillaga FA, Guglielmi G, Vinuela F, Duckwiler GR. Endovascular occlusion of intracranial aneurysms with electrically detachable coils: correlation of aneurysm neck size and treatment results. AJNR Am J Neuroradiol. 1994;15(5):815–20.
60. Johnston SC, Dowd CF, Higashida RT, Lawton MT, Duckwiler GR, Gress DR. Predictors of rehemorrhage after treatment of ruptured intracranial aneurysms: the Cerebral Aneurysm Rerupture After Treatment (CARAT) study. Stroke. 2008;39(1):120–5. https://doi.org/10.1161/STROKEAHA.107.495747.
61. Bohnstedt B, Ziemba-Davis M, Sethia R, et al. Comparison of endovascular and microsurgical management of 208 basilar apex aneurysms. J Neurosurg. 2017;127(6):1342–52.
62. Aymard A, Gobin Y, Hodes J, et al. Endovascular occlusion of vertebral arteries in the treatment of unclippable vertebrobasilar aneurysms. J Neurosurg. 1991;74(3):393–8.
63. Halbach V, Higashida R, Dowd C, et al. Endovascular treatment of vertebral artery dissections and pseudoaneurysms. J Neurosurg. 1993;79(2):183–91.
64. Albuquerque F, Fiorella D, Han P, Al E. Endovascular management of intracranial vertebral artery dissecting aneurysms. Neurosurg Focus. 2005;18(2):E3.

Chapter 4
Ischemic Stroke Revascularization

Naoki Otani and Atsuo Yoshino

4.1 Standard Surgical Strategies and Techniques

4.1.1 Indications

Surgical indications are based on symptomatic (transient ischemic attack [TIA] or minor stroke) internal carotid artery (ICA) or middle cerebral artery (MCA) occlusive disease with misery perfusion demonstrated by quantitative single photon emission computed tomography (SPECT) study in the chronic phase at least 3 months after the final ischemic attack. Surgery should be limited to patients with a mismatch between the extent of decreased cerebral blood flow (CBF) and completed cerebral infarction. Patients with dependent activities of daily living caused by extensive cerebral infarction should be excluded.

4.1.2 Surgical Strategies

1. Preoperative medical treatment
   Dehydration should be avoided and antiplatelet medications should be continued to prevent recurrence of ischemic attack. Administration of multiple antiplatelet agents should be reduced to a single agent. Antiplatelet medications should be continued and hyperosmotic colloid infusion started intravenously 1 week before operation. However, administration of two or more antiplatelet agents should be

N. Otani · A. Yoshino (✉)
Division of Neurosurgery, Department of Neurological Surgery, Nihon University School of Medicine, Itabashi-ku, Tokyo, Japan
e-mail: otani.naoki@nihon-u.ac.jp

Y. Kato, A. Ansari (eds.), *Cerebrovascular Surgery*, Advances and Technical Standards in Neurosurgery 44, https://doi.org/10.1007/978-3-030-87649-4_4

given in the presence of continuing TIA. Any anticoagulant medication should be stopped at once and replaced by heparin continuous drip infusion.

2. Preoperative radiological evaluation
Cardiac health and the presence of ischemic heart disease and/or carotid stenosis is evaluated. Three-dimensional computed tomography angiography (3D-CTA) and/or digital subtraction angiography are mandatory to determine the surgical strategy (Fig. 4.1a). Quantitative SPECT should be performed to assess the vascular reserve to establish the surgical indication. Stage II area requires improved CBF because of decreased vascular reserve capacity, and indicates that bypass surgery could be justified (Fig. 4.1b).
3. Intraoperative anesthesia management
Information sharing with anesthesiology is essential, so blood pressure is maintained over 120 mmHg during general anesthesia to avoid unexpected induced hypotension caused by dehydration, and intravascular CO_2 level should be maintained around 40–45 mmHg under precise ventilation control.
4. Positioning
Just after induction of general anesthesia, the target recipient M4 arteries and superficial temporal artery (STA) should be marked on the cranial bone (Fig. 4.1c, d). Surgical decisions are based on the extent of craniotomy, tracing of the STA, and skin incision based on the findings of preoperative 3D-CTA (Fig. 4.1f). The head is secured by three-point fixation positioning, so that the craniotomy site is at the highest point of the upper body to prevent cerebrospinal fluid leakage (Fig. 4.1e). Shoulder pillows should be inserted to reduce the extensive strain on the neck especially in elderly patients.
5. STA harvesting
The following are our microsurgical tips for successful bypass surgery. The STA is prepared using the ultrasonic scalpel instrument (Harmonic Scalpel®; Ethicon Endo-Surgery, Cincinnati, OH) (Fig. 4.2a). Fricative heat of the supersonic irradiation induces protein denaturation, so the STA can be dissected with complete hemostasis [1]. Side branches can also be transected without injury to the main trunk, then the STA is elevated using vessel tape, and protein coagulation is achieved in 2 or 3 s (Fig. 4.2b). The frontal branch of the STA is also dissected (Fig. 4.2c), the main trunk is skeletonized quickly and safely, and dissection continued from the undersurface. This instrument allows faster and safer harvesting of the STA or radial artery (RA).
6. Craniotomy and preparation of anastomosis
The craniotomy is performed under the supratemporal line (Fig. 4.3a). Just before dural opening, indocyanine green (ICG) angiography is performed to confirm the location of the recipient superficial cerebral artery over the dura (Fig. 4.3b), and to trace the superficial cerebral artery (Fig. 4.3c, d), which helps to minimize extension of the dural opening (Fig. 4.3e) [2]. Trimming of the STA is easily performed using a needle (Fig. 4.4a, b). After cutting the end of the STA, direct marking using a skin marking pen is usually performed to clarify the vascular edge of the anastomosis layer (Fig. 4.4c). Direct marking of the vascular wall of the recipient artery is also useful (Fig. 4.4d–f). This method can con-

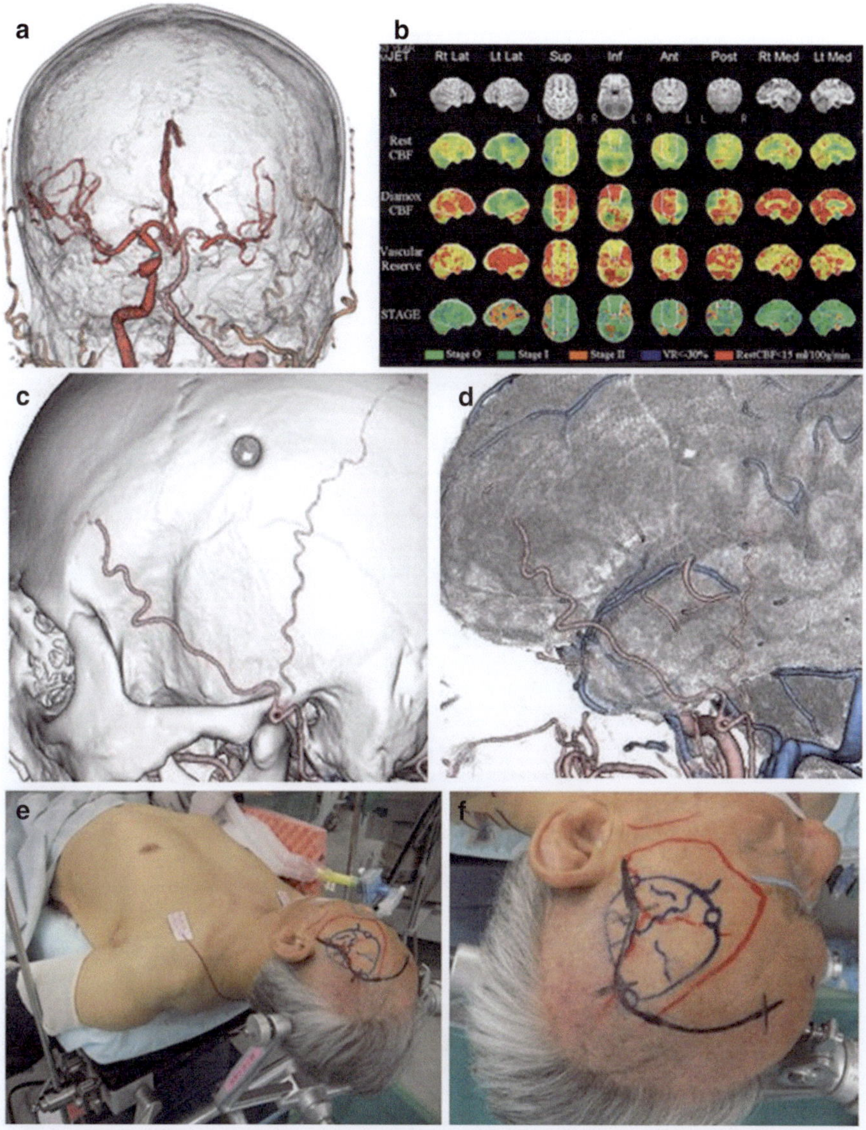

Fig. 4.1 Three-dimensional computed tomography angiography (3D-CTA) (**a**) and quantitative single photon emission computed tomography (**b**) should be performed to establish the surgical indication preoperatively. The superficial temporal artery (STA) (**c**) and targeted M4 (**d**) were superimposed based on the 3D-CTA data. The head was fixed and positioned so the craniotomy site is at the highest point of the upper body to prevent cerebrospinal fluid leakage (**e**). Extent of craniotomy, tracing of the STA, and skin incision were marked on the skin (**f**)

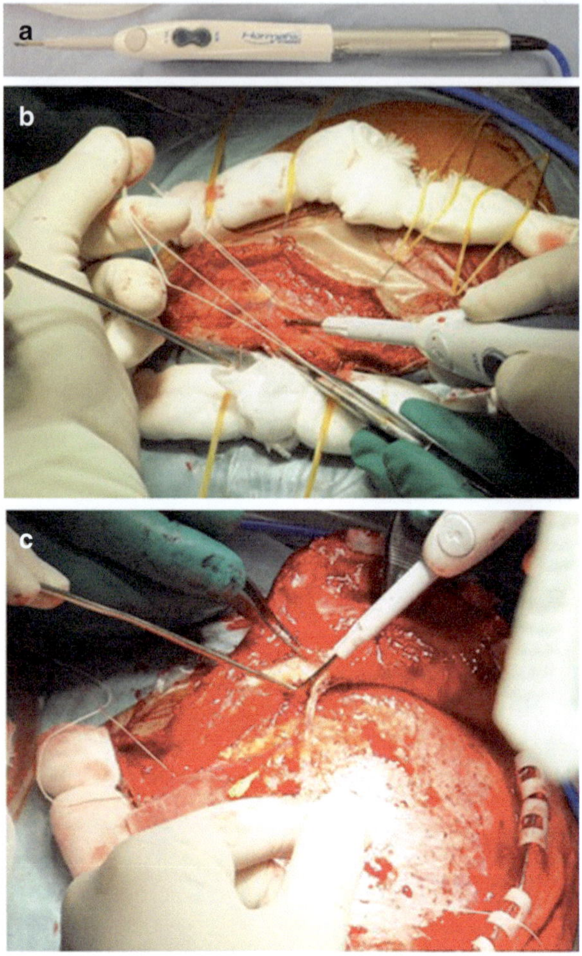

Fig. 4.2 Parietal branch (**b**) and frontal branch of the STA (**c**) were harvested using the Harmonic Scalpel (**a**)

firm only the outer vessel walls for anastomosis. Care should be taken to make the operative field broad, to avoid anastomosis at the border site of the craniotomy, and to maintain semi-wet condition and complete hemostasis.

7. Anastomosis
   Arteriotomy of the recipient artery should adopt the fish mouth type (Fig. 4.5a). Straight incision is desirable for recipient artery with small diameter of less than 1 mm. The length of the arteriotomy of the recipient artery is adjusted to about 3.0 mm with a scaled rubber sheet. Various anastomotic techniques can be performed including continuous, running, and intermittent suturing railroad methods (Fig. 4.5b). In particular, the anastomosis should be cross linked with manipulation of the microscope. After anastomosis, vessel patency is usually confirmed using Doppler sonography and ICG video-angiography (Fig. 4.5c, d). Finally, complete hemostasis and arachnoid plasty are performed to prevent chronic subdural hematoma.

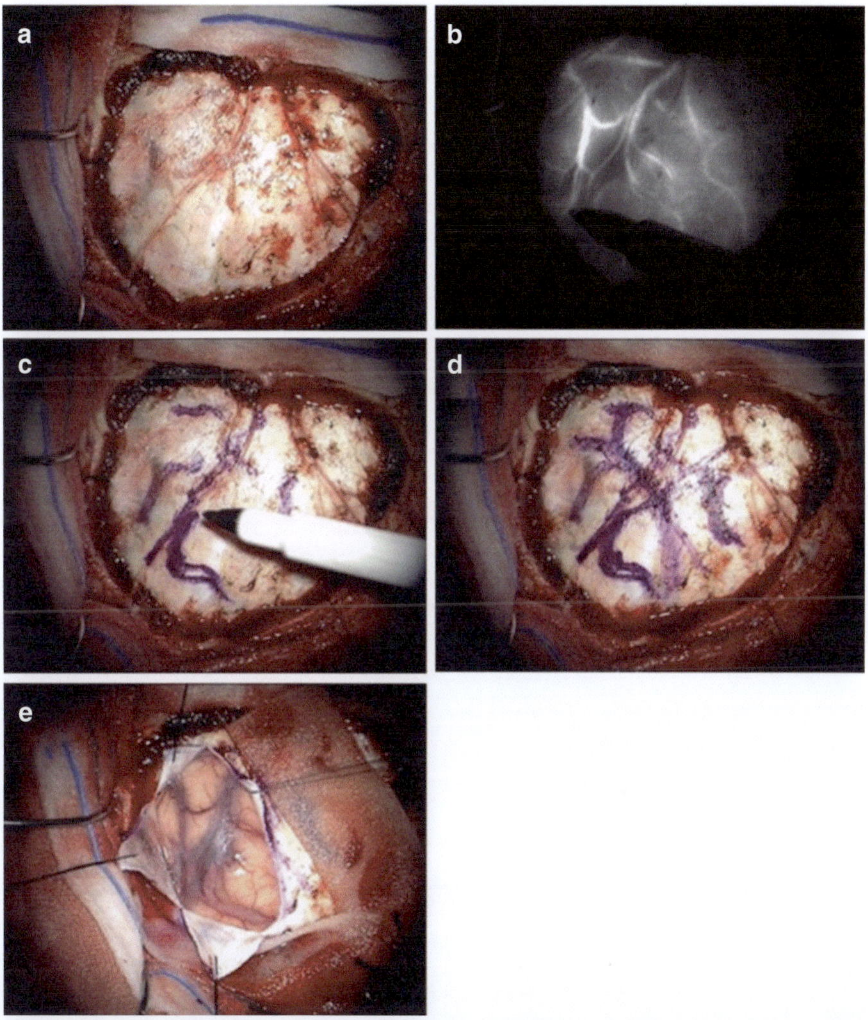

Fig. 4.3 Extradural indocyanine green tracing was performed for precise and safe dural incision (**a**–**e**)

8. Skin closure and postoperative concerns including wound problems
   STA flow patency must be monitored using the Doppler blood flow meter until the subcutaneous suture is completed, because the STA patency is sometimes obstructed at the edge of the cranial bone and/or temporal muscles. We recommend skin closure just above the STA using nylon sutures to avoid injury to the STA. After the operation, blood pressure control should achieve normo-tension to avoid hypervascular syndrome. Medical treatment can be started for prevention of chronic subdural hematoma such as administration of tranexamic acid [3] and/or herbal Kampo medicine Goreisan [4]. Many patients who require bypass

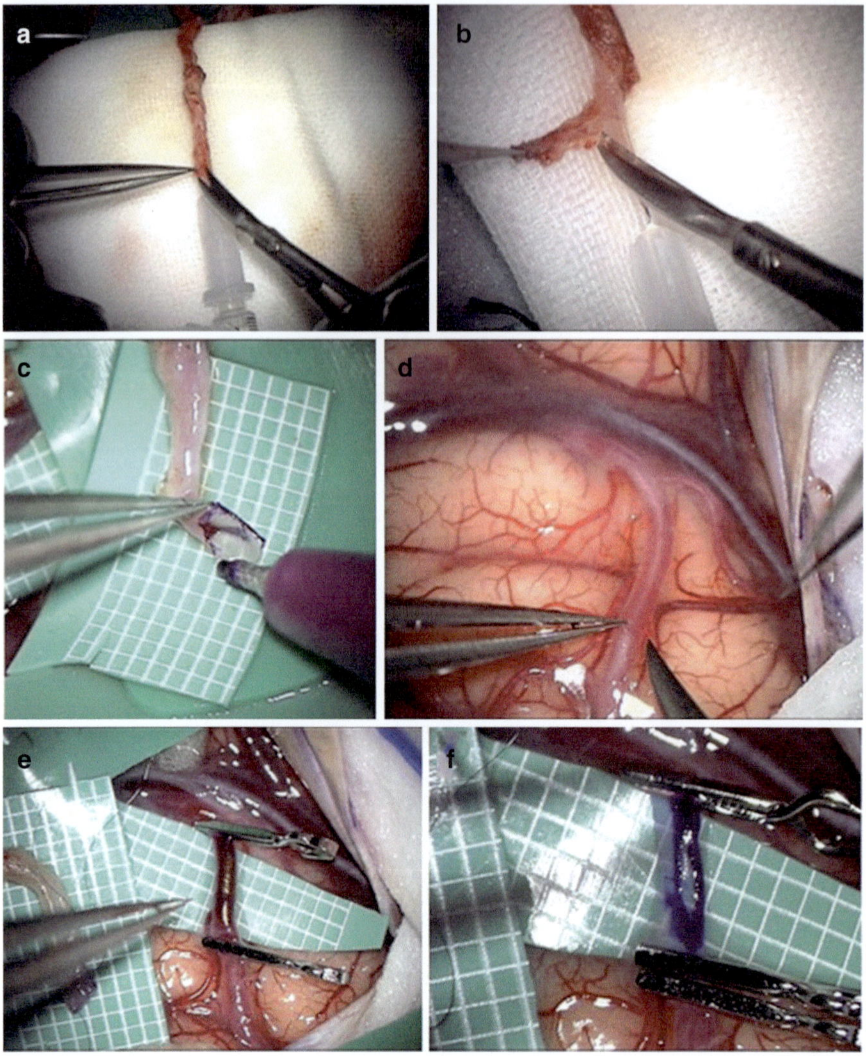

Fig. 4.4 Trimming of the STA is easily performed using a needle (**a**, **b**). Direct marking of the donor STA (**c**) and the recipient M4 artery (**d**–**f**) can help to clarify the vascular edge for the anastomosis

surgery have several risk factors such as diabetes and/or atherosclerosis. Furthermore, the STA is peeled off and sacrificed, so wound problems are possible after bypass surgery. Hyperbaric oxygen (HBO) therapy, which is useful to treat skin disorders, can be recommended in the early stage of wound problems. The period of HBO therapy depends on the severity of the skin problems after surgery [5].

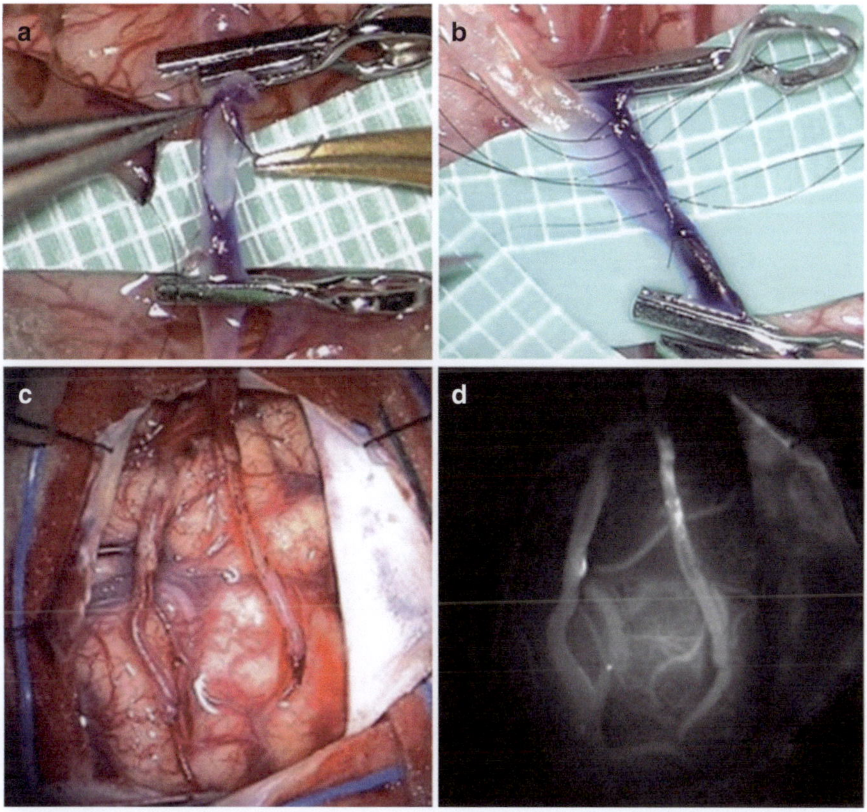

Fig. 4.5 Stay suture (**a**) and suture methods (**b**). Indocyanine green video-angiography was used to confirm the vascular patency after anastomosis (**c**, **d**)

4.2 Advanced Surgical Strategies and Techniques

4.2.1 Occipital Artery (OA)-Posterior Inferior Cerebellar Artery (PICA), STA-Superior Cerebellar Artery (SCA), STA-Posterior Cerebral Artery (PCA) Bypass for Posterior Circulation Ischemia

OA-PICA bypass is performed in the three-quarter prone position (Fig. 4.6a). The ipsilateral mastoid process becomes the highest point in the operating field. The inverted U-shaped skin incision is begun in the cervical midline over the C4 process (Fig. 4.6c), and further extended to the cervical region if condylectomy is required. The OA is routinely secured, and the suboccipital muscles are peeled away layer by

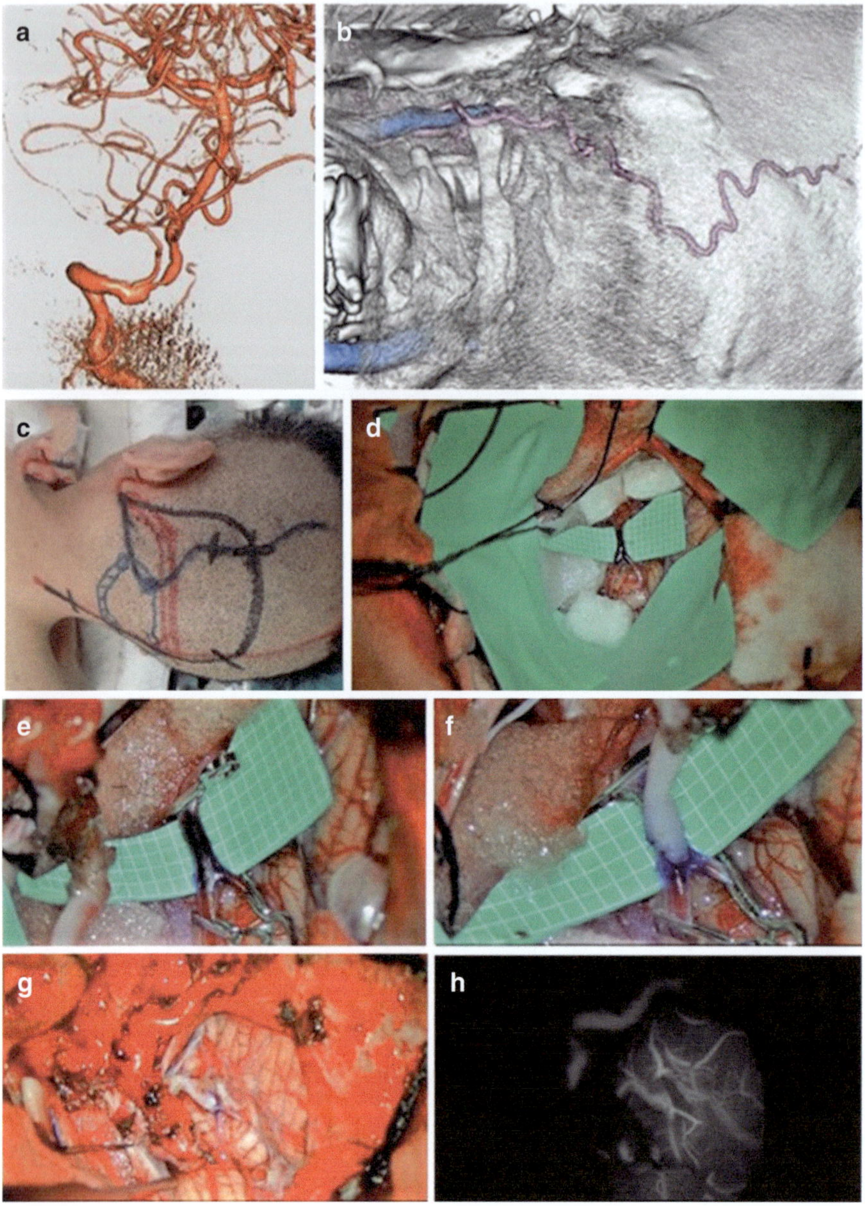

Fig. 4.6 Occipital artery (OA)-posterior inferior cerebellar artery (PICA) bypass for symptomatic vertebral artery stenosis (**a**). Running course of the OA was superimposed using the 3D-CTA data (**b**). Transcondylar fossa approach allows a shallow surgical field for anastomosis of the OA to the recipient PICA, the caudal loop of the PICA (**c**–**g**). Finally, vascular patency was confirmed using indocyanine green video-angiography (**h**)

layer (Fig. 4.6b). The suboccipital craniotomy is extended unilaterally from the foramen magnum in the midline, and then back around the foramen magnum. The supracondylar area of the suboccipital bone is removed (far lateral approach), and the sigmoid-magnum triangle is sufficiently removed, the condylar emissary vein is cauterized, and the condylar fossa is fully exposed and removed (transcondylar fossa approach). A semicircular dural incision is made from the cervical dura to the lateral edge of the craniotomy. The vertebral artery is secured intradurally. The inferior cranial nerve is secured and the caudal loop of the PICA is identified (Fig. 4.6d). OA-PICA bypass is then performed (Fig. 4.6e–h).

STA-SCA or STA-PCA bypass is performed using the subtemporal approach. Cutting of the cerebellar tent can be helpful to expose the SCA, and the minitranspetrosal approach is used to access the PCA, which requires exposure of the partial presigmoid dura around the superior petrosal sinus, to achieve a wide operative field.

4.2.2 Bonnet Bypass for Unilateral Common Carotid Artery (CCA) Occlusion

No effective surgical procedure is available for CCA occlusion, because the blood flow of the ipsilateral STA is often less efficient in the presence of CCA occlusion. The first Bonnet bypass using a saphenous vein (SV) graft was described in 1980, in which the blood flow of the SV graft was 20–50 mL/min, or enough to supply the circulation area, and the harvested SV graft can be longer than the RA [6]. On the other hand, the SV graft can be easily twisted and occluded by the tension of the skin flap. Therefore, the optimal method is to form a gutter in the skull to hold the vein graft which is fixed using a mini-plate to prevent such complications (Fig. 4.7) [7].

4.2.3 Reverse Bypass Using a Naturally Formed "Bonnet" STA for Symptomatic CCA Occlusion

Hemodynamic cerebral ischemia results in the development of ischemic symptoms after CCA occlusion, so "bonnet" bypass using an RA or SV graft is usually considered. However, if a spontaneously formed "bonnet" STA with sufficient retrograde blood flow from the contralateral STA is available, a so-called "reversed" arterial bypass should be considered (Fig. 4.8), because this surgical procedure can be performed both safely and less invasively [8].

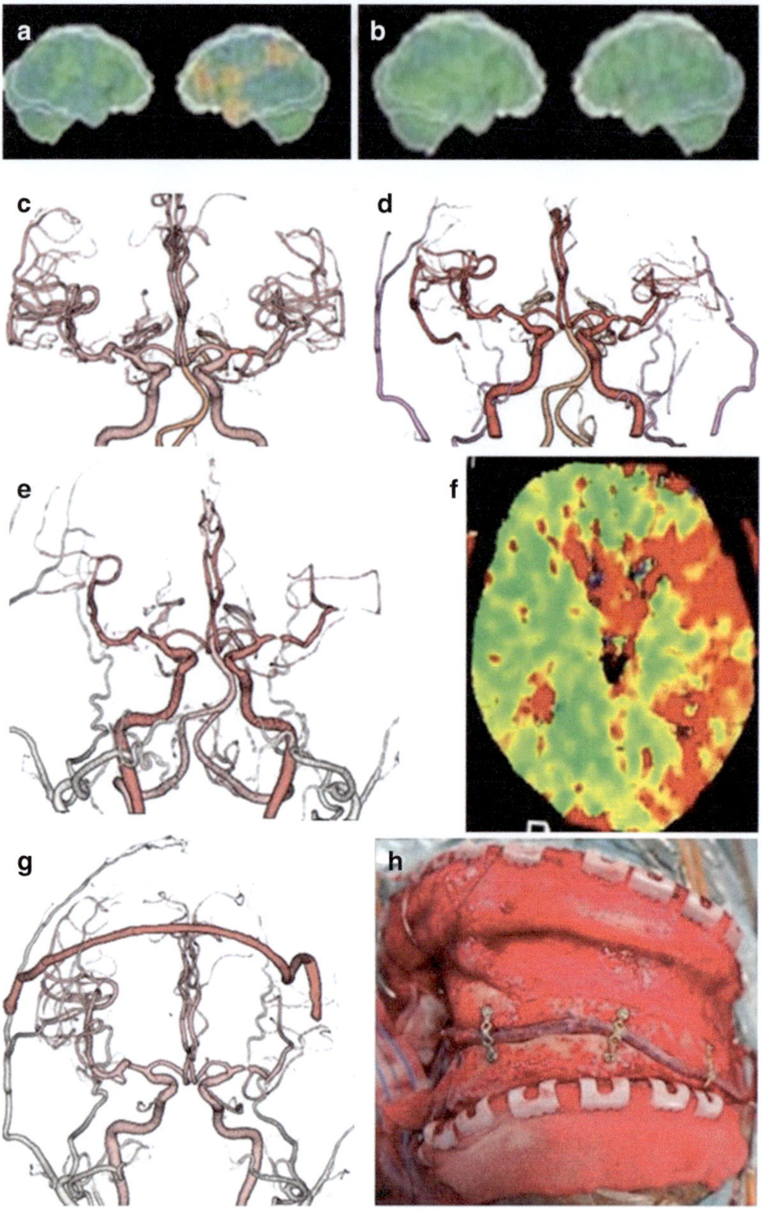

Fig. 4.7 Bonnet bypass for unilateral common carotid artery occlusion. The patient suffered multiple transient ischemic attack symptoms caused by vascular reserve disorder (**a**) due to left M1 severe stenosis (**c**), and underwent left STA-middle cerebral artery (MCA) bypass (**d**) with improved vascular reserve dysfunction (**b**). Five years later, the left STA donor artery was obstructed (**e**), and vascular reserve disorder and recurrent symptoms occurred (**f**). Bonnet bypass was performed using a saphenous vein (SV) graft (**g**). SV graft can be easily twisted and occluded by the tension of the skin flap, so we formed a gutter in the skull to hold the vein graft which was fixed using a mini-plate to prevent such complications (**h**)

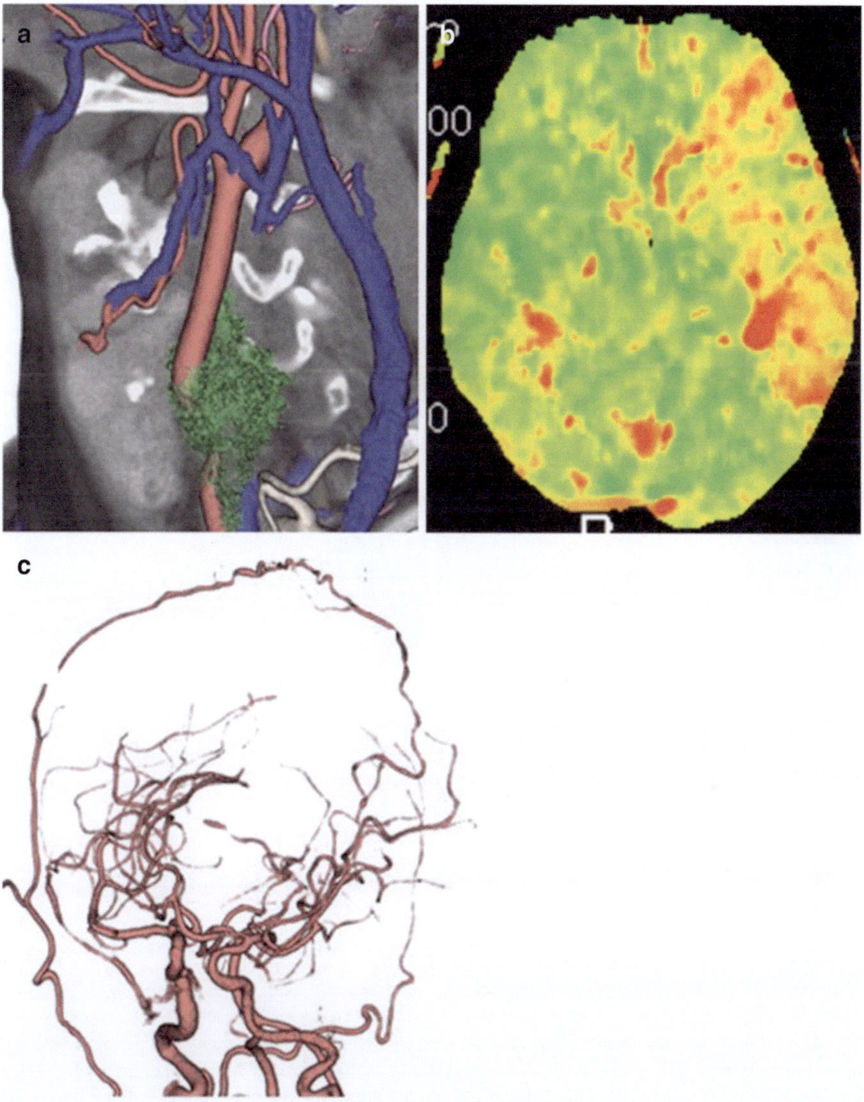

Fig. 4.8 "Reverse" bypass using a naturally formed bonnet STA (**c**) for symptomatic common carotid artery occlusion (**b**) caused by thyroid tumor (**a**)

4.2.4 Absence of Donor Artery Such as the STA

Ischemia of the MCA territory with absent and/or hypoplastic STA may require RA graft for anastomosis from the proximal STA trunk around the zygomatic arch to the M3/M4 segment (Fig. 4.9). Ischemia of the anterior cerebral artery territory may be treated by RA graft for bypass surgery from the proximal STA trunk to the A3/A4 segment [9, 10].

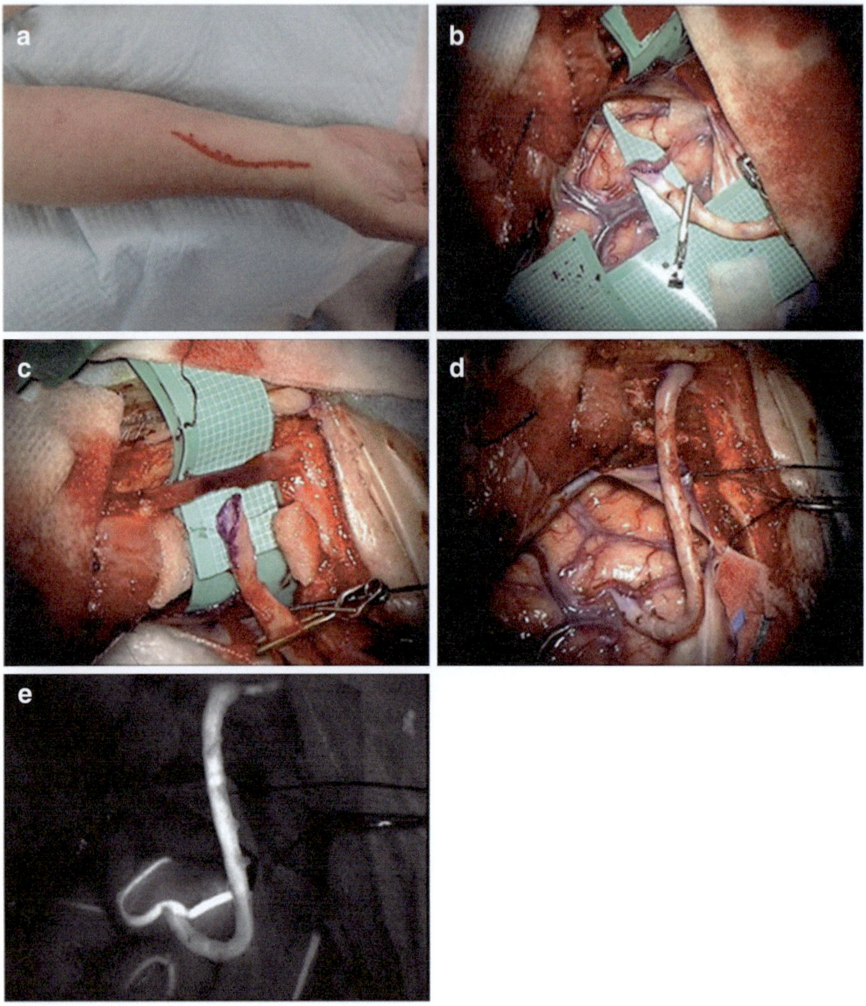

Fig. 4.9 STA absent as a donor artery. Radial artery (RA) graft (**a**) can be used for bypass surgery from the proximal STA trunk around the zygomatic arch (**c**) to the M3/M4 segment (**b**). After M4-RA-STA proximal bypass (**d**), indocyanine green angiography confirmed vascular patency (**e**)

4.2.5 Multiple Stenotic Lesions

Bilateral ICA stenosis and/or occlusion (Fig. 4.10a, c), similar to moyamoya disease, requires that blood pressure is maintained over 120 mmHg to avoid unexpected hypotension caused by dehydration, and intravascular CO_2 level is maintained around 40–45 mmHg by precise ventilation control during general anesthesia. Care is required at three-point fixation to not injure the STA in the contralateral side in case of second operation (Fig. 4.10b). After unilateral bypass surgery, the vascular reserve of the opposite side may also improve (Fig. 4.10d).

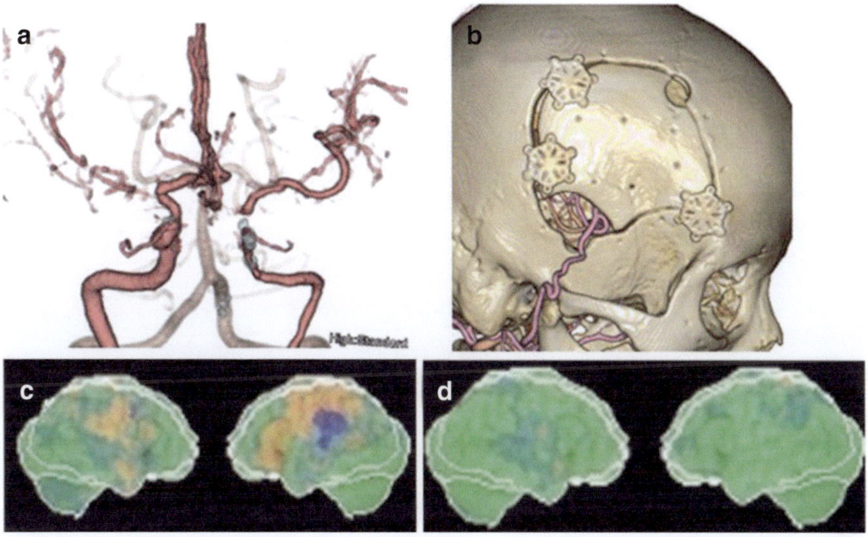

Fig. 4.10 Bilateral internal carotid artery stenosis with vascular reserve dysfunction (**a**, **c**). After unilateral bypass surgery (**b**), the contralateral side also had improved vascular reserve (**d**)

Tandem stenotic lesions with coexisting carotid artery stenosis and intracranial ICA and/or M1 stenosis require preferential treatment of lesions close to the heart side as a basic concept. The STA as a donor artery can be the cause of low flow in the anastomotic vessels with stenosis of the origin of the external carotid artery (ECA). Percutaneous transluminal angioplasty and/or stent may be effective to enlarge the stenosis of the origin of the ECA. In this case, ECA calcification was very severe, so we performed carotid endarterectomy simultaneously with double bypass surgery (Fig. 4.11).

4.3 Controversies

4.3.1 Surgical Indications

The extracranial-intracranial (EC-IC) bypass study failed to confirm the effectiveness for preventing cerebral ischemia in patients with atherosclerotic arterial disease in the ICA and MCA in 1985 [11]. Review of ongoing trials and research registers and reference lists of relevant articles concluded that EC/IC bypass surgery were neither superior nor inferior to only medical care in 2010 [12]. However, the surgical indications for revascularization based on cerebrovascular reserve dysfunction was not considered. Recently, the Carotid Occlusion Surgery Study failed to show benefit for the surgical group with respect to ipsilateral stroke recurrence at 2 years after treatment, despite improved cerebral hemodynamics and excellent

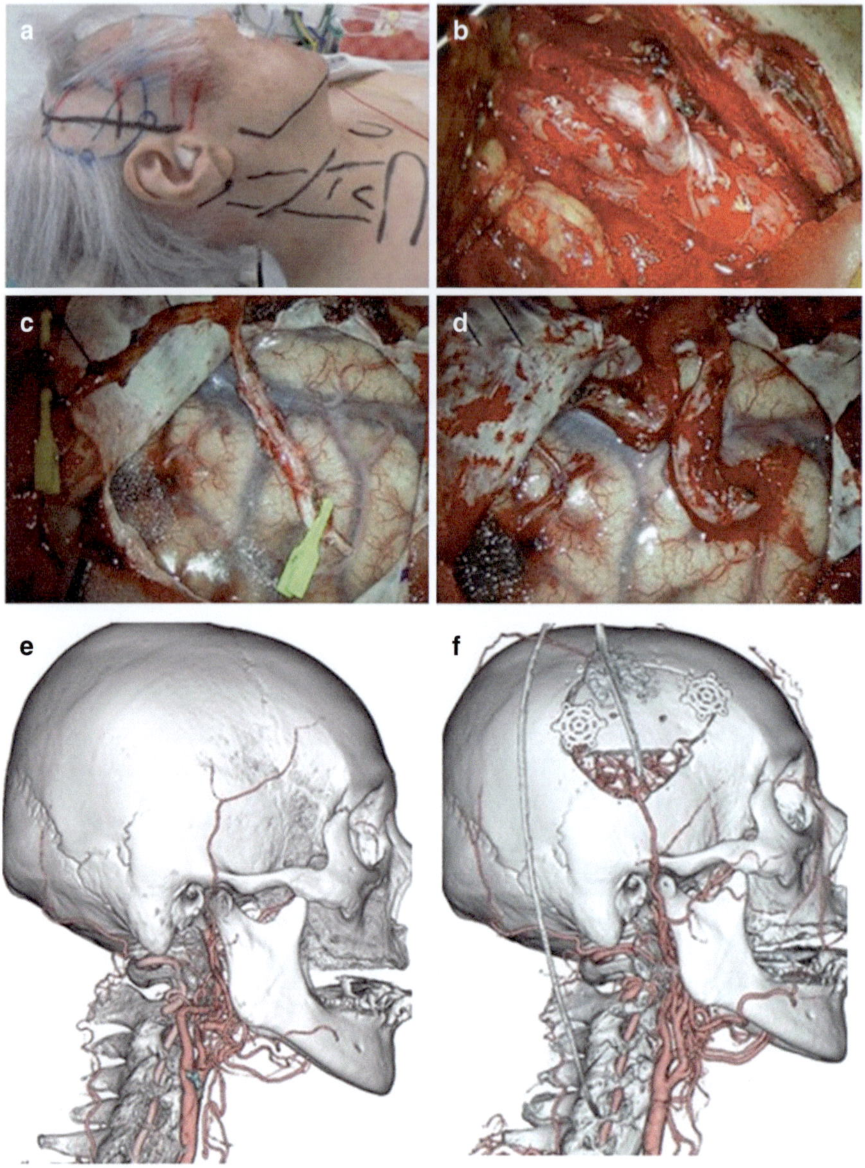

Fig. 4.11 Severe stenosis and calcification of the origin of the external carotid artery (**e**). Combined carotid endarterectomy (**a**, **b**) and STA-MCA double bypass (**c**, **d**) were simultaneously performed (**f**)

bypass graft patency rates [13]. However, the recurrence rate of cerebral infarction with medical treatment was low, and the extensive perioperative complications in the bypass treatment group probably led to the lack of advantage for bypass surgery [13, 14]. On the other hand, the recurrence rate of cerebral infarction was lower in the bypass surgery group than in the medical treatment group [15–17]. In these series, EC-IC bypass has proven to be significantly effective in patients with symptomatic MCA (or/and) ICA stenotic (or occlusive) disease with misery perfusion (stage II) area on positron emission tomography or SPECT. The surgical technique and strategies must be refined to indicate bypass surgery for more strict surgery indications as well as continue to reduce complications as much as possible.

4.3.2 Acute Phase (Emergency) Bypass

Intravenous tissue plasminogen activator (t-PA) therapy for acute cerebral infarction is effective as a standard treatment, but the recanalization rate remains at 30–40% [18]. Recently, mechanical thrombectomy using retrieval stents was found to be effective in a large multicenter comparative study [19–22]. The outcome after 3 months was better in the stent treatment group than in the t-PA treatment group, with no difference in complication rate and mortality rate. A comparative study of several devices found improved surgical results and fewer complications. However, the recanalization rate remained at only about 80%. Therefore, no gold standard therapy is available for technically difficult cases or treatment inappropriate cases outside the time limit for endovascular treatment.

Revascularization techniques may be effective against impairment of cerebrovascular reserve capacity [23–25]. Hemodynamic brain disorder may be avoided with the improvement of CBF reserve capacity after bypass surgery, so bypass surgery will be effective for hemodynamic cerebral infarction manifesting as progressive symptoms in the acute phase.

Thrombus retrieval therapy using a stent retriever was effective for acute cerebral infarction in three randomized controlled trials [19–21]. Therefore, the American Heart Association/American Stroke Association guidelines indicate intravascular treatment using a stent retriever for acute cerebral infarction under the following conditions: independent in daily life before onset, ineffective intravenous therapy using recombinant t-PA, occlusive disease of the ICA to M1 of the MCA, National Institutes of Health Stroke Scale >6 or higher moderate disorder, no extensive infarct area with Alberta Stroke Program Early Computed Tomography Score >6 points, and within 6.0 h of onset [22]. However, no therapeutic guidelines have been established for cases that do not satisfy these conditions, especially for 6 h or more after onset of symptoms, or if mechanical thrombectomy was ineffective. Emergency EC-IC bypass may be effective for non-cardiac cerebral artery occlusive disease [26, 27] (Fig. 4.12).

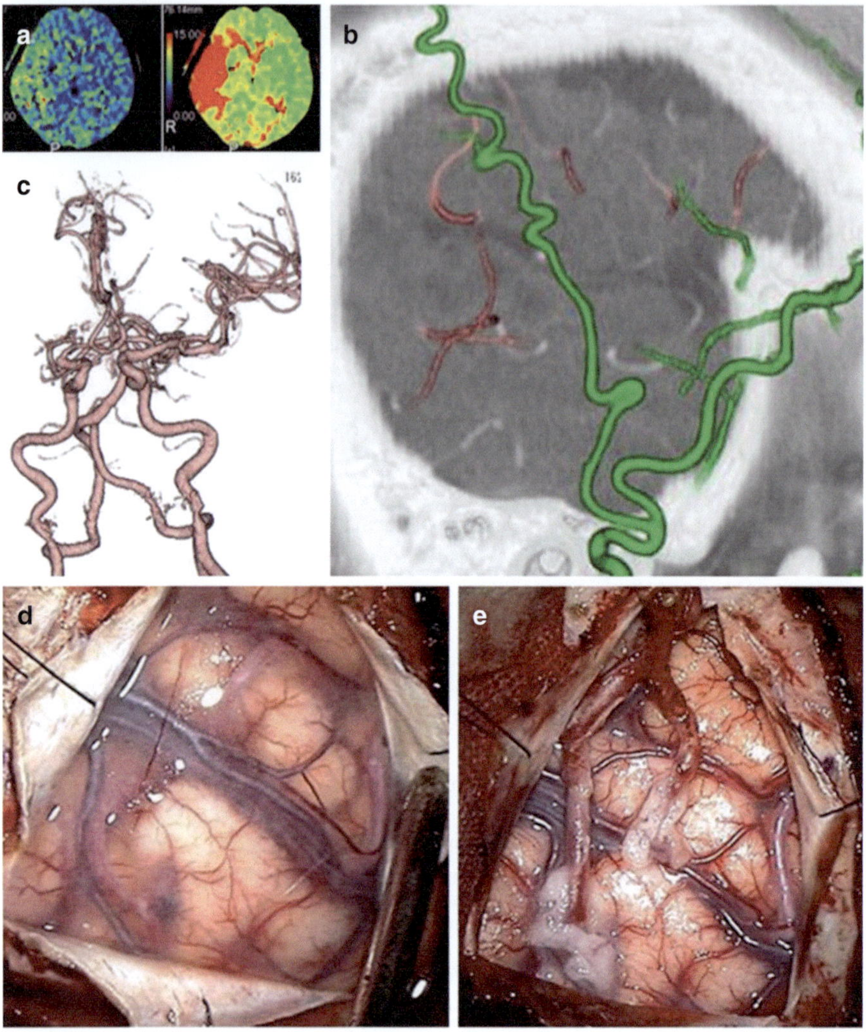

Fig. 4.12 Intravenous tissue plasminogen activator therapy for acute cerebral infarction failed to improve right M1 obstruction (**c**) with vascular reserve disturbance (**a**), so emergent bypass was performed (**b**, **d**, **e**)

References

1. Wada K, Nawashiro H, Arimoto H, Ohkawa H, Ono K, Takahara T. Usefulness of an ultrasonic scalpel to harvest and skeletonize the superficial temporal artery for extracranial-intracranial bypass surgery. Neurosurgery. 2009;65(6 Suppl):141–7; discussion 147-8
2. Otani N, Wada K, Toyooka T, Takeuchi S, Tomiyama A, Mori K. Usefulness of dural surface tracing of the cortical vessels with indocyanine green videoangiography just prior to dural opening for various cerebrovascular diseases. Surg Neurol Int. 2017;8:201.

3. Kageyama H, Toyooka T, Tsuzuki N, Oka K. Nonsurgical treatment of chronic subdural hematoma with tranexamic acid. J Neurosurg. 2013;119(2):332–7.
4. Yasunaga H. Effect of Japanese herbal Kampo medicine Goreisan on reoperation rates after burr-hole surgery for chronic subdural hematoma: analysis of a national inpatient database. Evid Based Complement Alternat Med. 2015;2015:817616. https://doi.org/10.1155/2015/817616.
5. Larsson A, Engström M, Uusijärvi J, Kihlström L, Lind F, Mathiesen T. Hyperbaric oxygen treatment of postoperative neurosurgical infections. Neurosurgery. 2002;50(2):287–95; discussion 295–6
6. Spetzler RF, Roski RA, Rhodes RS, Modic MT. The "bonnet bypass". Case report. J Neurosurg. 1980;53(5):707–9.
7. Matsumoto T, Otani N, Wada K, Ohtsuka Y, Fujii T, Yoshiura T, Kumagai K, Fujii K, Toyooka T, Mori K. Surgical strategies and technical tips for bonnet bypass using a saphenous vein graft for common carotid artery occlusion: a report of three cases and review of the literature. Surg Cerebral Stroke. 2017;45(5):409–13. [Japanese]
8. Otani N, Wada K, Sakakibara F, Nagatani K, Takeuchi S, Tomura S, Osada H, Mizokami D, Yamashita T, Shiotani A, Mori K. "Reverse" bypass using a naturally formed "bonnet" superficial temporal artery in symptomatic common carotid artery occlusion: a case report. Neurol Med Chir (Tokyo). 2014;54(10):851–3.
9. Otani N, Wada K, Toyooka T, Takeuchi S, Tomiyama A, Mori K. Surgical strategies for ruptured complex aneurysms using skull base technique and revascularization surgeries. Asian J Neurosurg. 2018;13(4):1165–70.
10. Wada K, Otani N, Toyooka T, Takeuchi S, Tomiyama A, Mori K. Superficial temporal artery to anterior cerebral artery hemi-bonnet bypass using radial artery graft for prevention of complications after surgical treatment of partially thrombosed large/giant anterior cerebral artery aneurysm. J Stroke Cerebrovasc Dis. 2018;27(12):3505–10.
11. EC/IC Bypass Study Group. Failure of extracranial-intracranial arterial bypass to reduce the risk of ischemic stroke. Results of an international randomized trial. N Engl J Med. 1985;313(19):1191–200.
12. Fluri F, Engelter S, Lyrer P. Extracranial-intracranial arterial bypass surgery for occlusive carotid artery disease. Cochrane Database Syst Rev. 2010;2010(2):CD005953.
13. Powers WJ, Clarke WR, Grubb RL Jr, Videen TO, Adams HP Jr, Derdeyn CP, Investigators COSS. Extracranial-intracranial bypass surgery for stroke prevention in hemodynamic cerebral ischemia: the Carotid Occlusion Surgery Study randomized trial. JAMA. 2011;306(18):1983–92.
14. Reynolds MR, Grubb RL Jr, Clarke WR, Powers WJ, Zipfel GJ, Adams HP Jr, Derdeyn CP, Carotid Occlusion Surgery Study Investigators. Investigating the mechanisms of perioperative ischemic stroke in the Carotid Occlusion Surgery Study. J Neurosurg. 2013;119(4):988–95.
15. JET Study Group. Japanese EC-IC Bypass Trial (JET Study). Study design and interim analysis. Surg Cerebral Stroke. 2002;30(2):97–100. [Japanese]
16. Sandow N, von Weitzel-Mudersbach P, Rosenbaum S, König S, Buchert R, Mehl SR, Garbe A, Vajkoczy P. Extra-intracranial standard bypass in the elderly: perioperative risk, bypass patency and outcome. Cerebrovasc Dis. 2013;36(3):228–35.
17. Muroi C, Khan N, Bellut D, Fujioka M, Yonekawa Y. Extracranial-intracranial bypass in atherosclerotic cerebrovascular disease: report of a single centre experience. Br J Neurosurg. 2011;25(3):357–62.
18. Bhatia R, Hill MD, Shobha N, Menon B, Bal S, Kochar P, Watson T, Goyal M, Demchuk AM. Low rates of acute recanalization with intravenous recombinant tissue plasminogen activator in ischemic stroke: real-world experience and a call for action. Stroke. 2010;41(10):2254–8.
19. Berkhemer OA, Fransen PS, Beumer D, van den Berg LA, Lingsma HF, Yoo AJ, Schonewille WJ, Vos JA, Nederkoorn PJ, Wermer MJ, van Walderveen MA, Staals J, Hofmeijer J, van Oostayen JA, Hofmeijer J, Boiten J, Brouwer PA, Emmer BJ, de Bruijn SF, van Dijk LC, Kappelle LJ, Lo RH, van Dijk EJ, de Vries J, de Kort PL, van Rooij WJ, van den Berg JS, van Hasselt BA, Aerden LA, Dallinga RJ, Visser MC, Bot JC, Vroomen PC, Eshghi O, Schreuder TH, Heijboer RJ, Keizer K, Tielbeek AV, den Hertog HM, Gerrits DG, van den Berg-Vos

RM, Karas GB, Steyerberg EW, Flach HZ, Marquering HA, Sprengers ME, Jenniskens SF, Beenen LF, van den Berg R, Koudstaal PJ, van Zwam WH, Roos YB, van der Lugt A, van Oostenbrugge RJ, Majoie CB, Dippel DW, MR CLEAN Investigators. A randomized trial of intraarterial treatment for acute ischemic stroke. N Engl J Med. 2015;372(1):11–20. Erratum in: N Engl J Med. 2015;372(4):394

20. Goyal M, Demchuk AM, Menon BK, Eesa M, Rempel JL, Thornton J, Roy D, Jovin TG, Willinsky RA, Sapkota BL, Dowlatshahi D, Frei DF, Kamal NR, Montanera WJ, Poppe AY, Ryckborst KJ, Silver FL, Shuaib A, Tampieri D, Williams D, Bang OY, Baxter BW, Burns PA, Choe H, Heo JH, Holmstedt CA, Jankowitz B, Kelly M, Linares G, Mandzia JL, Shankar J, Sohn SI, Swartz RH, Barber PA, Coutts SB, Smith EE, Morrish WF, Weill A, Subramaniam S, Mitha AP, Wong JH, Lowerison MW, Sajobi TT, Hill MD, ESCAPE Trial Investigators. Randomized assessment of rapid endovascular treatment of ischemic stroke. N Engl J Med. 2015;372(11):1019–30.
21. Campbell BC, Mitchell PJ, Kleinig TJ, Dewey HM, Churilov L, Yassi N, Yan B, Dowling RJ, Parsons MW, Oxley TJ, Wu TY, Brooks M, Simpson MA, Miteff F, Levi CR, Krause M, Harrington TJ, Faulder KC, Steinfort BS, Priglinger M, Ang T, Scroop R, Barber PA, McGuinness B, Wijeratne T, Phan TG, Chong W, Chandra RV, Bladin CF, Badve M, Rice H, de Villiers L, Ma H, Desmond PM, Donnan GA, Davis SM, EXTEND-IA Investigators. Endovascular therapy for ischemic stroke with perfusion-imaging selection. N Engl J Med. 2015;372(11):1009–18.
22. Powers WJ, Derdeyn CP, Biller J, Coffey CS, Hoh BL, Jauch EC, Johnston KC, Johnston SC, Khalessi AA, Kidwell CS, Meschia JF, Ovbiagele B, Yavagal DR, American Heart Association Stroke Council. 2015 American Heart Association/American Stroke Association focused update of the 2013 guidelines for the early management of patients with acute ischemic stroke regarding endovascular treatment: A guideline for healthcare professionals from the American Heart Association/American Stroke Association. Stroke. 2015;46(10):3020–35.
23. Chou CW, Chang JH, Lin SZ, Cho DY, Cheng YW, Chen CC. Extracranial-intracranial (EC-IC) bypass of symptomatic middle cerebral artery (MCA) total occlusion for haemodynamic impairment patients. Br J Neurosurg. 2012;26(6):823–6.
24. Low SW, Teo K, Lwin S, Yeo LL, Paliwal PR, Ahmad A, Sinha AK, Teoh HL, Wong LY, Chong VF, Seet RC, Chan BP, Yeo TT, Chou N, Sharma VK. Improvement in cerebral hemodynamic parameters and outcomes after superficial temporal artery-middle cerebral artery bypass in patients with severe stenoocclusive disease of the intracranial internal carotid or middle cerebral arteries. J Neurosurg. 2015;123(3):662–9.
25. Schmiedek P, Piepgras A, Leinsinger G, Kirsch CM, Einhüpl K. Improvement of cerebrovascular reserve capacity by EC-IC arterial bypass surgery in patients with ICA occlusion and hemodynamic cerebral ischemia. J Neurosurg. 1994;81(2):236–44.
26. Horiuchi T, Nitta J, Ishizaka S, Kanaya K, Yanagawa T, Hongo K. Emergency EC-IC bypass for symptomatic atherosclerotic ischemic stroke. Neurosurg Rev. 2013;36(4):559–64; discussion 564-5
27. Nussbaum ES, Janjua TM, Defillo A, Lowary JL, Nussbaum LA. Emergency extracranial-intracranial bypass surgery for acute ischemic stroke. J Neurosurg. 2010;112(3):666–73.

Chapter 5
Hemorrhagic Stroke: Endoscopic Aspiration

Alberto Feletti and Alessandro Fiorindi

5.1 Introduction

Hemorrhagic stroke is due to bleeding of a ruptured vessel into the brain. It can be subdivided into intracerebral hemorrhage (ICH), intraventricular hemorrhage (IVH), and subarachnoid hemorrhage (SAH). As hemorrhage can rapidly expand, causing consciousness impairment and neurological deficits, progression of hemorrhagic stroke is often associated with severe morbidity and high mortality [1]. Hypertension and cerebral amyloid angiopathy are the most common causes of ICH, while the usual causes of spontaneous SAH are ruptured aneurysms, arteriovenous malformations, vasculitis, arterial dissection, and dural sinus thrombosis. IVH can be divided into primary or secondary. Primary IVH originates from intraventricular sources or lesions in contact with the ventricular walls and is limited to the ventricular system. Secondary IVH derives from an intraparenchymal or subarachnoid hemorrhage which extend into the ventricular system at a later time. About 30% of IVHs are primary and 70% are secondary [2, 3].

ICH and IVH are devastating diseases with a high social impact. ICH causes 10–15% of first-ever strokes, with a 30-day mortality rate of 35–52% and only 20% of survivors expected to have full functional recovery after 6 months [4, 5]. Overall

Supplementary Information The online version contains supplementary material available at (https://doi.org/10.1007/978-3-030-87649-4_5).

A. Feletti (✉)
Department of Neurosciences, Biomedicine, and Movement Sciences, Institute of Neurosurgery, University of Verona, Verona, Italy
e-mail: alberto.feletti@univr.it

A. Fiorindi
Unit of Neurosurgery, Spedali Civili, University of Brescia, Brescia, Italy

Y. Kato, A. Ansari (eds.), *Cerebrovascular Surgery*, Advances and Technical Standards in Neurosurgery 44, https://doi.org/10.1007/978-3-030-87649-4_5

incidence of spontaneous ICH worldwide is 24.6 per 100,000 persons-years [6]. IVH can complicate SAH and ICH in 15 and 40% of patients, respectively [7]. It has been shown that >20 mL of intraventricular blood is associated with poor prognosis [8, 9]. The mortality rate of IVH is as high as 42.6–83.3% [7].

Besides the primary bleed, the hemorrhage continues to cause brain tissue damages not only because of mass effect, but also due to the activation of the coagulation cascade and hemoglobin breakdown, with consequent excitotoxic edema and progressive neurotoxicity [10]. Actually, it has been shown that the coagulation cascade is involved in brain edema that develops adjacent to a brain hemorrhage [11]. Therefore, reduction of the hemorrhage volume can be necessary to diminish secondary burden and improve outcomes of the patients.

Although historically the accepted treatments for hemorrhagic stroke have included conservative medical treatment and craniotomy with surgical evacuation, endoscopic treatment has been gaining consensus in the last years, particularly for ICH and IVH. This chapter will focus on ICH and IVH, as such hemorrhages can be potentially treated with endoscopic techniques.

5.2 Intracerebral Hemorrhage

5.2.1 Standards

Nowadays the standards of care in case of ICH are mainly based on medical treatment, reserving surgery only if the volume of hemorrhage is life-threatening or if hydrocephalus occurs. Of course, the cause of hemorrhage must be investigated and eventually treated. In any case the control of intracranial pressure (ICP) must be secured. Although there is a general consensus about the fact that conservative treatment is preferable if ICP is under control, the treatment modality of hemorrhage itself when ICP increases is debated.

5.2.1.1 Case Illustration 1

A 73-year-old female patient was admitted for headache and right hemiparesis. CT scan revealed a left ICH (Fig. 5.1a). Her medical history included chronic atrial fibrillation, hypertension, obstructive sleep apnea syndrome, gastric reflux disease, and chronic obstructive pulmonary disease. The patient was on warfarin therapy (INR at admittance: 2.53). She was initially treated conservatively. Four hours later, due to neurological deterioration, a new CT scan was performed, with evidence of increased ICH volume (Fig. 5.1b). The patient underwent craniotomy and microsurgical removal of ICH (Fig. 5.1c).

Craniotomy and Microsurgical Removal: Two multicenter clinical trials have studied the role of surgery in ICH. The International **S**urgical **T**rial in **I**ntra**C**erebral **H**aemorrhage (STICH) compared early surgery versus initial conservative

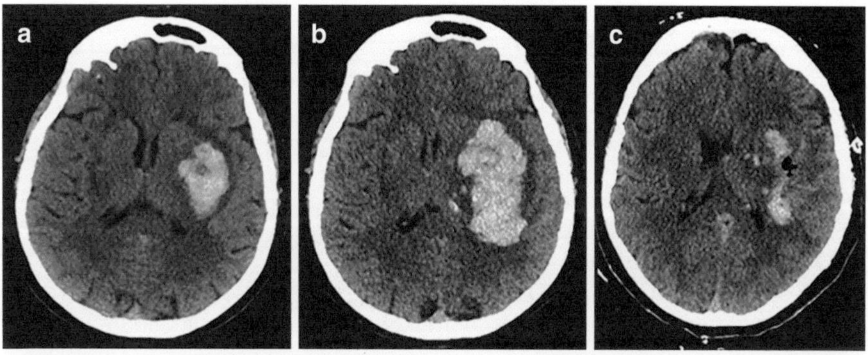

Fig. 5.1 Case Illustration 1. (**a**) CT scan showing a left ICH. (**b**) Second CT scan 4 h after the first one, showing the increased ICH volume. (**c**) CT scan after craniotomy and evacuation of ICH

treatment in patients with spontaneous supratentorial ICH [12]. This trial found no difference in mortality rates between groups. Another trial, STICH II, was designed with a more homogeneous population of patients to assess whether early surgery could improve outcomes in conscious patients with a superficial ICH and without IVH [13]. However, the STICH II trial also failed to demonstrate substantial improvement in patient outcome and mortality with surgery. Nonetheless, STICH II results are debated because surgery could be done in any fashion, without any distinction between open craniotomy and minimally invasive techniques. Overall, STICH I and STICH II trials have failed to show evidence of clinical benefit from an open surgical approach. Potentially, these discouraging results could be due to iatrogenic injury.

Fibrinolytic Therapy: The use of fibrinolytic agents in addition to minimally invasive surgery (MIS) has been investigated by some trials. Wang et al. compared conservative management in 182 patients with CT-guided craniopuncture with aspiration followed by the administration of a urokinase solution over 3–5 days in 195 patients [14]. At 90-day follow-up, the interventional group showed better functional outcomes (64% vs. 40.9%; $p < 0.01$), but no differences in mortality rates were noted. Similarly, Sun et al. compared craniotomy and craniopuncture followed by urokinase infusion in 304 patients [15]. Although the latter group had better outcomes, there were no significant differences on neurological function and mortality rates on follow-up.

The **M**inimally **I**nvasive **S**urgery and **rt**PA for **I**ntracerebral Hemorrhage **E**vacuation (MISTIE) trial was a multicentric phase II RCT designed to assess the safety and efficacy of alteplase combined with MIS for the treatment of supratentorial ICH, compared to the best medical standard of care [16]. The authors showed a significant reduction of ICH volume in the alteplase group (57% vs. 5% reduction; $p < 0.0001$). No difference in 7- to 30-day mortality was observed between the two cohorts. The MISTIE III trial, a multicentric phase III RCT, was then designed to assess morbidity and mortality associated with the same surgical technique [17]. Data demonstrated that a residual hemorrhage volume less than 15 mL was significantly associated with favorable functional outcome, except for cases with moderate to large

ICH. At 1-year follow-up, the alteplase cohort showed a decreased mortality compared to the medical treatment group ($p \leq 0.037$). However, the trial failed to show improvement of functional outcome compared with the medically treated arm.

5.2.2 *Advances*

5.2.2.1 Case Illustration 2

A 67-year-old lady was admitted to our emergency room for sudden loss of consciousness with left hemiplegia. A CT scan revealed the presence of a large right parietal intraparenchymal hemorrhage with mass effect (Fig. 5.2a). No vascular malformations were detected at angio-CT. Being the patient in poor but not desperate conditions (E1M4Vt), and also considering the absence of major comorbidities, surgery was urgently performed. The hemorrhage was approached with a rigid endoscope through an enlarged burr hole (Fig. 5.2b). An immediate post-operative CT scan showed a good evacuation of the hematoma without complications (Fig. 5.2c).

Rigid Endoscopy: The use of an endoscope to treat cerebral hemorrhage is not new. In 1985 Auer et al. described for the first time a novel endoscopic technique to remove intracerebral hemorrhages, with or without involvement of the ventricular system, using a rigid endoscope [18]. Their randomized study, including 100 patients affected by spontaneous supratentorial ICH, showed that 6-month mortality rate was significantly lower in the surgical cohort, compared to conventional medical management. This benefit appeared limited to patients <60 years old and to subcortical ICH, and improvement of functional outcome after surgery was not proved. Many new developments in medicine commonly pass through three stages. First, it is ridiculed. Second, it is violently opposed. Third, it is accepted as being self-evident [19]. Auer's technique did not have a different fate. Initially it was received without enthusiasm, and later it was criticized because apparently not easily reproducible. Therefore, this technique was almost abandoned, with only a few exceptions in the beginning of the XXI century, almost 15 years after Auer's report [20–23]. More recently, endoscopic removal of intraparenchymal hemorrhage has been re-proposed as a minimally invasive and effective way to manage this kind of patients [24–26]. Endoscopic hematoma removal of supratentorial intracerebral hemorrhage has also been performed under local anesthesia, with reduction of operative time compared to craniotomy [27]. A meta-analysis by Xia et al. showed a lower mortality rate in patients undergoing minimally invasive surgery, compared to craniotomy (OR: 0.76; 95% CI 0.60–0.97) [25]. Moreover, the minimally invasive surgery group showed a statistically significant decrease in rebleeding compared to the medically treated cohort (OR: 0.42; 95% CI 0.19–0.95). Similarly, in their meta-analysis Tang et al. reported lower mortality rate and reduction of rebleeding in patients treated with minimally invasive surgery compared to those treated with craniotomy or conservative therapy [24]. A recent meta-analysis showed that

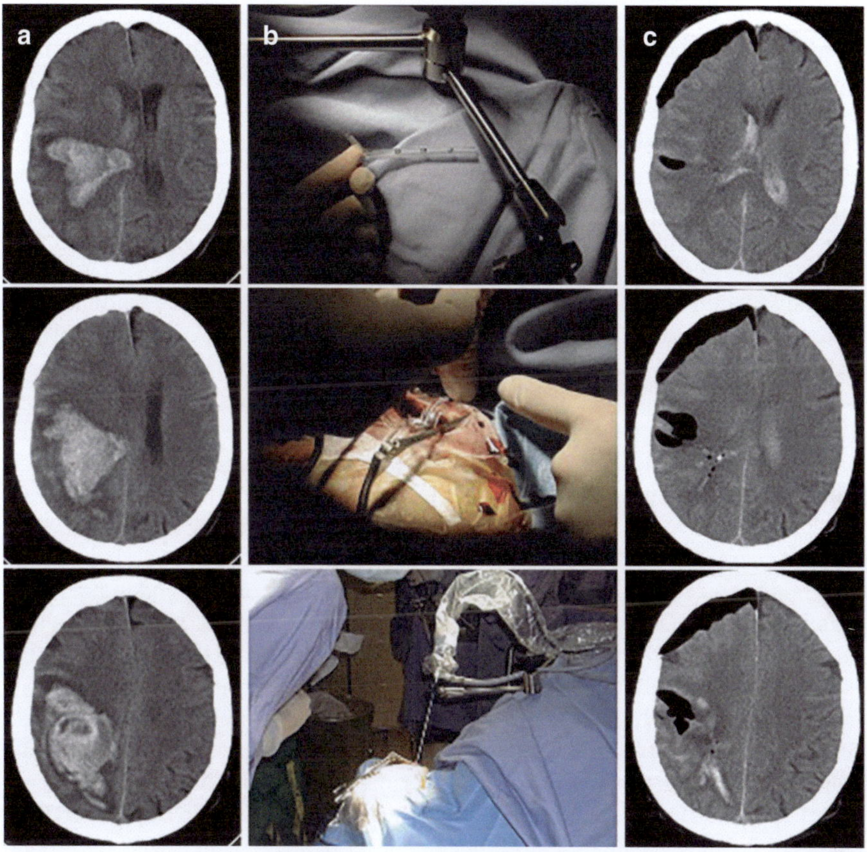

Fig. 5.2 Case Illustration 2. (**a**) CT scan revealing the presence of a large right parietal ICH with mass effect. (**b**) Surgical endoscopic aspiration of ICH. A transparent tubular retractor was used (*top panel*). The retractor was inserted into the hematoma through an enlarged burr hole (*middle panel*), and a rigid endoscope was introduced through the retractor into the hematoma (*bottom panel*). (**c**) An immediate post-operative CT scan showed a good evacuation of the hematoma

neuroendoscopic surgery for supratentorial hypertensive ICH has lower complications, but no superior advantages in morbidity rates compared to craniotomy [26].

In the recent years, new additional tools and techniques for ICH evacuation have been introduced, as BrainPath/Myriad (NICO, Indianapolis, Indiana, USA) and the Apollo (first generation)/Artemis (second generation) Systems (Penumbra, Alameda, California, USA). The Nico BrainPath is a minimally invasive tubular retractor consisting of a transparent sheath and an obturator, designed to reduce iatrogenic damage when reaching the ICH. It is introduced through a small craniotomy and a dural opening large enough to allow the advancement of the device into the clot under neuronavigation. The obturator is then removed, and ICH can be removed with assistance of either microscopic/exoscopic or endoscopic visualization, eventually with the aid of the Myriad handpiece, a device that can help to remove dense ICH by cutting, suction, and blunt dissection. Similar transparent tubular retractors are also available, including the Vycor Viewsite, which has an oval shape [28]. Prybylowski et al. retrospectively reviewed all 11 patients who underwent BrainPath endport-assisted microsurgical evacuation of ICH. They reported a median reduction in ICH volume of 87%, a median reduction in midline shift of 38%, a 90-day functional independence rate (mRS 0-2) of 36%, and an ICH-related mortality rate of 36% [29]. Bauer et al. prospectively collected data on 18 patients who underwent BrainPath evacuation of ICH. They reported a mean ICH volume reduction of 95.7% (±5.8%; $p < 0.001$), no hemorrhagic recurrences, an increase in the mean GCS of 5 ± 2.3, and a mortality rate of 5.6% in the first 30 days [30]. More recently, Labib et al. performed a multicentric study including 39 patients who were operated with BrainPath-assisted evacuation of ICH [31]. They reported clot reduction between 50 and 89% in 72% of patients, with statistically significant improvement of the median GCS (median post-operative GCS of 14). At follow-up, mRS score was ≤2 in 52% of patients, with no mortalities.

The Apollo/Artemis is an aspiration/irrigation device which includes a vibrational element with unclogging function. It can be inserted into the working channel of a rigid endoscope, allowing the removal of ICH under constant endoscopic visualization through a burr hole or a mini-craniotomy. Fiorella et al. reported a significant ICH volume reduction in the three patients operated with the device [32]. Tan et al. treated eight patients, and they reported a significant reduction in ICH volume [33]. A larger study by Goyal et al. compared 18 patients treated with the Apollo device and 54 patients who underwent standard medical treatment [34]. The authors found that the surgical group showed lower median residual ICH volume (15 vs. 40 cm^3; $p < 0.001$) and reduced in-hospital mortality (28% vs. 56%; $p = 0.041$). A multicentric study by Spiotta et al., including 29 patients treated with the Apollo system, demonstrated a mean reduction in ICH volume of 54.1% ± 39.1% ($p < 0.001$), and a mortality rate of 13.8% [35]. Kellner et al. proposed a novel neuroendoscopic technique called **S**tereotactic **ICH** **U**nderwater **B**lood **A**spiration (SCUBA), which is performed in two phases [36]. Initially, an introducer sheath is inserted into the distal part of the hematoma and along its main axis, under neuronavigation assistance. The hematoma is aspirated with the Apollo device under neuroendoscopic vision. After clearing all visible clots, the cavity is passively infused with normal saline through a side port while the second side port also remains fully open to prevent pressurization of the cavity. In this way, the cavity can be fully explored under endoscopic visualization and bleeding sources can be identified and eventually cauterized. The authors reported a significant decrease in mean ICH volume, with an average evacuation of 88.2%.

Griessenauer et al. compared patients treated with the Apollo device and BrainPath including 5 patients per group, and they showed no overall differences in ICH volume evacuation between the two methods [37].

The **I**ntraoperative Stereotactic **C**omputed Tomography-Guided **E**ndoscopic **S**urgery (ICES) trial was designed to test the hypothesis that intraoperative computerized tomographic image-guided endoscopic surgery is safe and effective to remove ICH [38]. Twenty patients (14 surgical and 4 medical) were included with primary ICH of >20 mL volume within 48 h of ICH onset, and outcomes were evaluated at 6 and 12 months. Surgery was successfully completed in all cases, with immediate reduction of hemorrhagic volume by 68 ± 21.6%. One surgically related bleed was reported, but no mortality. Neurological outcome at 180 and 365 days was better (mRS 0-3) in the surgical group compared to the medical group (42.9 and vs. 23.7%; $p = 0.19$).

5.3 Intraventricular Hemorrhage

5.3.1 Standards

Similar to ICH, also in the case of IVH the standards of care are mainly based on medical treatment, reserving surgery only if the hemorrhage causes hydrocephalus. However, besides increased ICP, other deleterious effects of intraventricular blood are a threaten to the patient. Some studies suggested that direct mass effect of the IVH can potentially reduce cerebral blood flow [39] and that the mass effect of clots distending the ventricle walls is the most important mechanism responsible for hemorrhagic ventricular dilatation [40]. Others indicated extensive damage to the ependymal and subependymal layers caused by blood clots themselves, due to direct mass effect and also to inflammatory response [41, 42].

IVH has been identified as an independent prognostic factor of poor outcome and has been associated with a 78% risk of death if no specific treatment is adopted [9, 43, 44]. In cases of ICH, the additional presence of IVH significantly increases the risk of death compared to ICH alone (51.2% vs. 19.5%) [45]. Moreover, IVH at presentation has been associated with only a 20% rate of favorable outcome [46]. In cases of IVH secondary to SAH the risk of death is higher if patients are not treated with EVD, compared to those undergoing EVD (84% vs. 67%) [45]. This evidence supports the rationale of fast and extensive IVH removal.

Several grading scales have been suggested to estimate IVH severity and to predict outcome. Graeb et al. were the first to identify the correlation between the amount of intraventricular blood and outcome and proposed a grading score from 0 to 12 points, which is currently the most commonly used grading system to classify the severity of IVH [47]. The score results from summing a maximum of 2 points each for third and fourth ventricle and 4 points for each lateral ventricle. Subsequently, the LeRoux score and the IVH Score were developed to offer a more objective method to quantify the amount of intraventricular blood and predict the functional outcome [48, 49].

5.3.1.1 Case Illustration 3

A 51-year-old man was urgently admitted to hospital after the onset of acute headache and vomiting, with left hemiparesis. A head CT scan showed a right thalamic hemorrhage with tetraventricular extension (Fig. 5.3a). A right EVD was initially placed (Fig. 5.3b). Two days later, as the EVD was not properly draining and the patient's neurological status was worsening, a second EVD was placed in the left lateral ventricle (Fig. 5.3c). A CT scan performed 11 days after admission confirmed blood wash out from the fourth ventricle, with residual clots in the lateral and third ventricles (Fig. 5.3d). Because of communicating hydrocephalus, a VP-shunt was subsequently placed.

External Ventricular Drainage: EVD represents the most common procedure in cases of IVH and is recognized as a level B class of evidence [50]. It can be used as a rescue maneuver in emergency setting to control ICP. Secondarily, it is an outflow

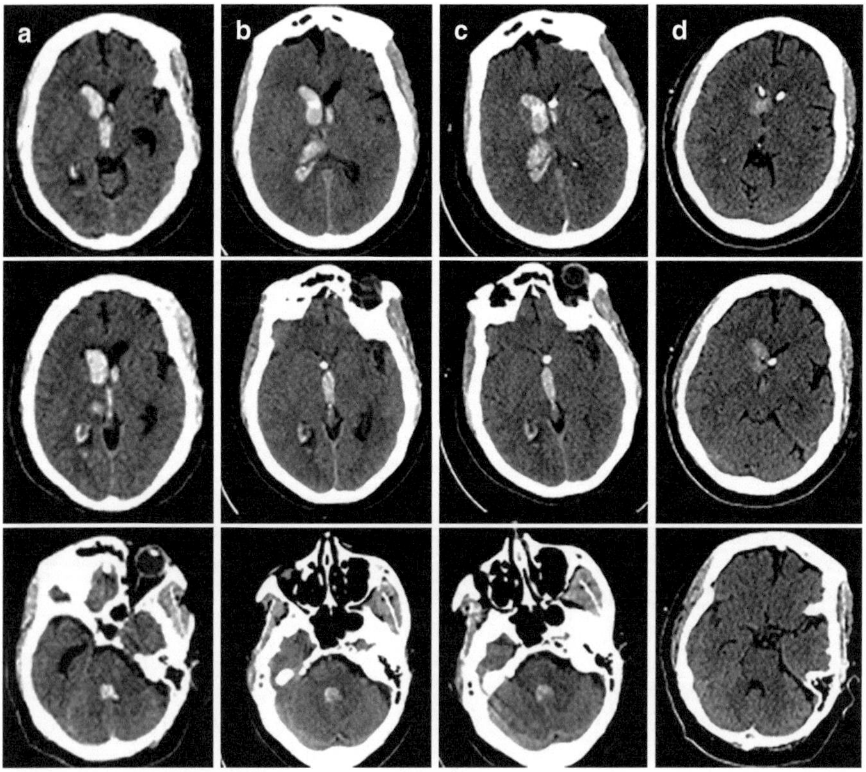

Fig. 5.3 Case Illustration 3. (**a**) CT scan showing a right thalamic hemorrhage with tetraventricular extension. (**b**) A right EVD was initially placed. (**c**) A contralateral EVD was placed in the left lateral ventricle, as the first EVD was not draining any more. (**d**) A CT scan performed 11 days after admission confirmed blood wash out from the fourth ventricle, with residual clots in the lateral and third ventricles

way for blood, as soon as clots are degraded and lysed. However, it is often necessary to place EVD bilaterally in these cases, and nevertheless EVD frequently becomes obstructed by coagulated blood. Studies of serial CT scans seemed to suggest that IVH usually disappears over a period of 2–3 weeks after the hemorrhage [51]. Conversely, postmortem examinations revealed that intraventricular blood persists for months after a hemorrhage [52]. Although intraventricular hematoma can become isodense to CSF over time, giving the false impression that IVH has resolved, the fibrinolytic system of CSF is limited, and blood may remain in the ventricles for months after hemorrhage, contributing to the patient's poor clinical status [52]. Consequently, EVD needs to be left in place for a long time before a satisfactory wash out is obtained. Moreover, it has been shown that EVD alone is often not effective in improving the poor prognosis in patients with IVH [52, 53].

Craniotomy and Microsurgical Removal: Craniotomy has also been proposed as a method to remove IVH in a fast way and under direct microscopic vision, through a frontal corticectomy [54], with a trans-corpus callosum route [55, 56], or through a posterior fossa approach to the fourth ventricle [57]. Some authors suggested a high occipital transcortical approach, pointing out that the entire region of the lateral ventricle, including the inferior horn, corpus, and posterior horn can be set free of blood clots in a single operative field [58]. Although good results have been reported in single-center series, there are no studies comparing mortality rates and functional outcomes between craniotomy and other less invasive techniques. Moreover, it is quite difficult to get rid of blood clots from the third and the fourth ventricles using this approach.

5.3.1.2 Case Illustration 4

A 16-year-old boy was admitted with GCS 3 after a traumatic brain injury. A head CT scan revealed an IVH (Fig. 5.4a), and a right EVD was placed (Fig. 5.4b). One day later, the EVD was not functioning. Intrathecal 10,000 IU u-PA were administered twice per day, and the patency of the EVD was restored. Two days later, CT scan confirmed the initial lysis of blood clots (Fig. 5.4c). A CT scan 8 days after admission (7 days after the first u-PA administration) confirmed the progressive clots lysis, although blood residues were still present (Fig. 5.4d). Twenty-five days after admission, a CT scan confirmed the complete resorption of IVH (Fig. 5.4e). The patient underwent VP-shunt due to communicating hydrocephalus.

Fibrinolytic Therapy: Clinicians have started administration of fibrinolytic agents directly into the ventricular system with the aim to keep the EVD patent and to expedite the resolution of IVH. The use of fibrinolysis in a patient affected by an intracranial bleeding can be at first seen as a paradox. However, before the initiation of fibrinolytic therapy, the hemorrhagic episode is usually over, eventual conditions predisposing to a worsening of the hemorrhage (coagulopathy and elevated blood pressure) have been corrected, and any source of bleeding (ruptured aneurysm or AVM) has been controlled by surgical or endovascular means [59]. Nevertheless, the risk of rebleeding due to fibrinolytic therapy cannot be excluded [41, 60].

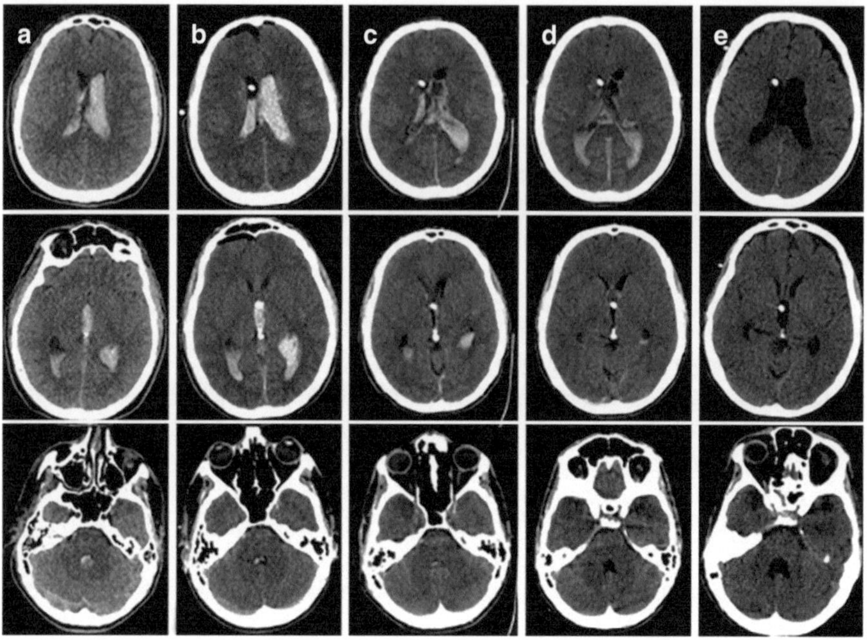

Fig. 5.4 Case Illustration 4. (**a**) CT scan showing a post-traumatic IVH. (**b**) A right EVD was placed. (**c**) CT scan performed 2 days after the beginning of intraventricular fibrinolytic therapy shows the initial lysis of blood clots. (**d**) A CT scan 7 days after the first administration of fibrinolytic agent confirms the progressive clots lysis, although blood residues are still present. (**e**) CT scan 25 days after admission confirming the complete resorption of IVH

After the first published reports [61, 62], several studies confirmed that the direct administration of fibrinolytic agents into the ventricular system can speed up the dissolution of IVH [45, 63–65]. Recombinant tissue plasminogen activator (t-PA/alteplase) and urokinase plasminogen activator (u-PA) are the most commonly used fibrinolytic agents. Usually intermittent boluses administration is adopted, although continuous infusion has also been proposed for u-PA. It takes at least 2–3 days to get some evident results with t-PA, as confirmed by CT scans [41], and a bit longer with u-PA. In any case, beneficial effects on ICP, ventricular size, and mortality have been documented in large series and meta-analyses, while different effect sizes are generated when different functional outcome tools are used [66]. In the **C**lot **L**ysis: **E**valuating **A**ccelerated **R**esolution of IVH III (CLEAR III) trial, patients with ICH $\leq$30 cm^3 with associated IVH were randomized into two groups (placebo and intrathecal recombinant t-PA 1 mg every 8 h through an EVD [67]). The trial proved that mortality at 180 days was significantly lower in the t-PA group, and in a subgroup of patients with IVH volumes >20cm^3 functional outcomes were better. Although clinical studies of fibrinolytic therapy for IVH have found a 30–35% reduction in mortality, they failed to prove an improved neurologic outcome for the survivors. Nevertheless, intrathecal fibrinolytic therapy can have some complications, as rebleeding, hemorrhage along the EVD, meningitis, and ventriculitis [41, 59, 60, 62, 68, 69].

5.3.2 *Advances*

5.3.2.1 Case Illustration 5

A 74-year-old male without a significant medical history suffered headache with nausea and vomiting during a hypertensive crisis. After admission, he underwent head CT scan that documented a spontaneous ICH, presumably originated from the head of the right caudate nucleus and opened into the ventricle, leading to tetraventricular inundation (Fig. 5.5a). Head CT-angiogram was negative for vascular malformations. In order to avoid prolonged necessity of bilateral EVD, he underwent immediate endoscopic treatment with fiberscope. Attention was particularly focused on cleaning the aqueduct and the fourth ventricle to rapidly reestablish the physiological CSF dynamics. There were no complications during the procedure and the patient slowly improved his neurological condition. Post-operative head CT scan confirmed the satisfactory cleaning of the third and fourth ventricles, and the unblocking of the aqueduct of Sylvius (Fig. 5.5b). The patient was discharged to the rehabilitation department and freed from external ventricular drainage 10 days after the procedure.

Flexible and Rigid Endoscopy: After the initial report by Auer, other surgeons' experience revealed that there is a significant difference between the hard and dense intracerebral hemorrhage and the gelatinous, fragile clots of early intraventricular hemorrhages [70–74]. This evidence, along with the technical improvement of optics and instrumentation, and the need for less invasive methods to remove the

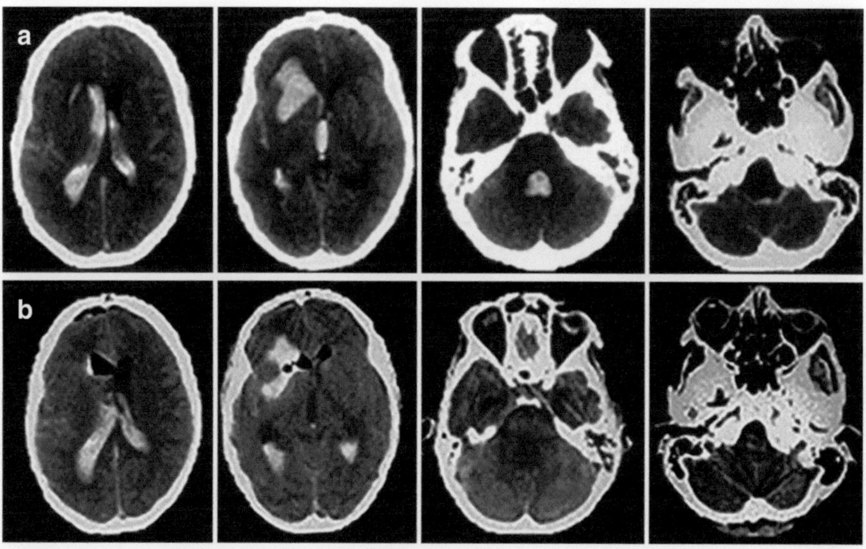

Fig. 5.5 Case Illustration 5. (**a**) CT scan showing IVH due to a spontaneous ICH at the level of the right caudate nucleus. (**b**) Post-operative head CT scan after IVH aspiration with flexible scope, confirming the satisfactory cleaning of the third and fourth ventricles, and the unblocking of the aqueduct of Sylvius

hemorrhagic mass and decrease intracranial pressure in these patients, prompted neurosurgeons to try again the endoscopic approach, which became more and more accepted [7, 75, 76]. Actually, massive IVH requires aggressive and fast management not just to reduce ICP. It has been reported that the occurrence of IVH significantly increases the risk of death from ICH or cerebellar hemorrhage [77–79], and also the risk of delayed cerebral ischemia after SAH [80].

Endoscopic removal of IVH can be performed with two different instruments: a rigid scope or a flexible scope. Initially, only the rigid scope was used to clear the ventricles from blood clots, and promising results were reported in terms of volume of removed IVH and safety [7, 20, 23, 81]. In some cases, an ETV was also performed, in order to resolve the obstructive hydrocephalus due to the blockade of the cerebral aqueduct and fourth ventricle, which cannot be explored with rigid instruments [20, 82]. A biportal approach is usually adopted to remove blood clots from both lateral ventricles [20, 82–84].

Chen et al. compared endoscopic surgery with rigid scope and EVD for the treatment of 48 patients with IVH, and they found that endoscopic surgery was associated with shorter ICU stay and with lower shunt-dependent hydrocephalus [85]. A similar study including 42 patients confirmed that endoscopic surgery allows for a higher hematoma clearance rate, fewer complications, and better outcomes [86]. Other studies focused on endoscopic irrigation in cases of neonatal IVH reporting lower shunt rates and fewer complications such as infections and development of multiloculated hydrocephalus, compared to conventional temporary CSF diversion [87, 88]. Ding et al. studied the combination of endoscopic hematoma evacuation and intraventricular lavage and reported improved hematoma clearance rate and good outcomes [89].

With the development of steerable scopes, which can nicely adapt to the complex and irregular geometry of the ventricular system, it was possible to extend the exploration to all ventricular cavities, with the chance of aspirating blood clots even from the fourth ventricle. Kamikawa et al. were the first to use a flexible scope in patients affected by IVH [21]. In their series of four neonates, the scope was used to observe the ventricles, perform ETV, coagulate eventual bleeding sources and choroid plexus, and relieve hydrocephalus by simple irrigation. However, Longatti et al. introduced a more extensive use of flexible scope to actively aspirate blood clots from all ventricles, obtaining the complete restoration of the ventricular system patency [72, 73, 90]. The technique requires a precoronal, paramedian curved skin incision of about 3 cm at the side of the lateral ventricle with the largest amount of blood, and the burr hole should not be too lateral than 1.5–2 cm from the midline in order to obtain a direction towards the cerebral aqueduct as straight as possible [91, 92]. A semirigid 14-French peel-away introducer catheter is used to cannulate the lateral ventricle. Although several types of steerable scopes are available, only those with an external diameter up to 4 mm should be used for this procedure, as larger sizes would not allow a safe navigation of the cerebral aqueduct (Fig. 5.6). The flexible scope is used with a free-hand technique. Initially, the vision is severely impaired because the tip of the scope is dipped in blood clots. Although this can be worrisome and frustrating, intermittent irrigation with Ringer lactate and aspiration

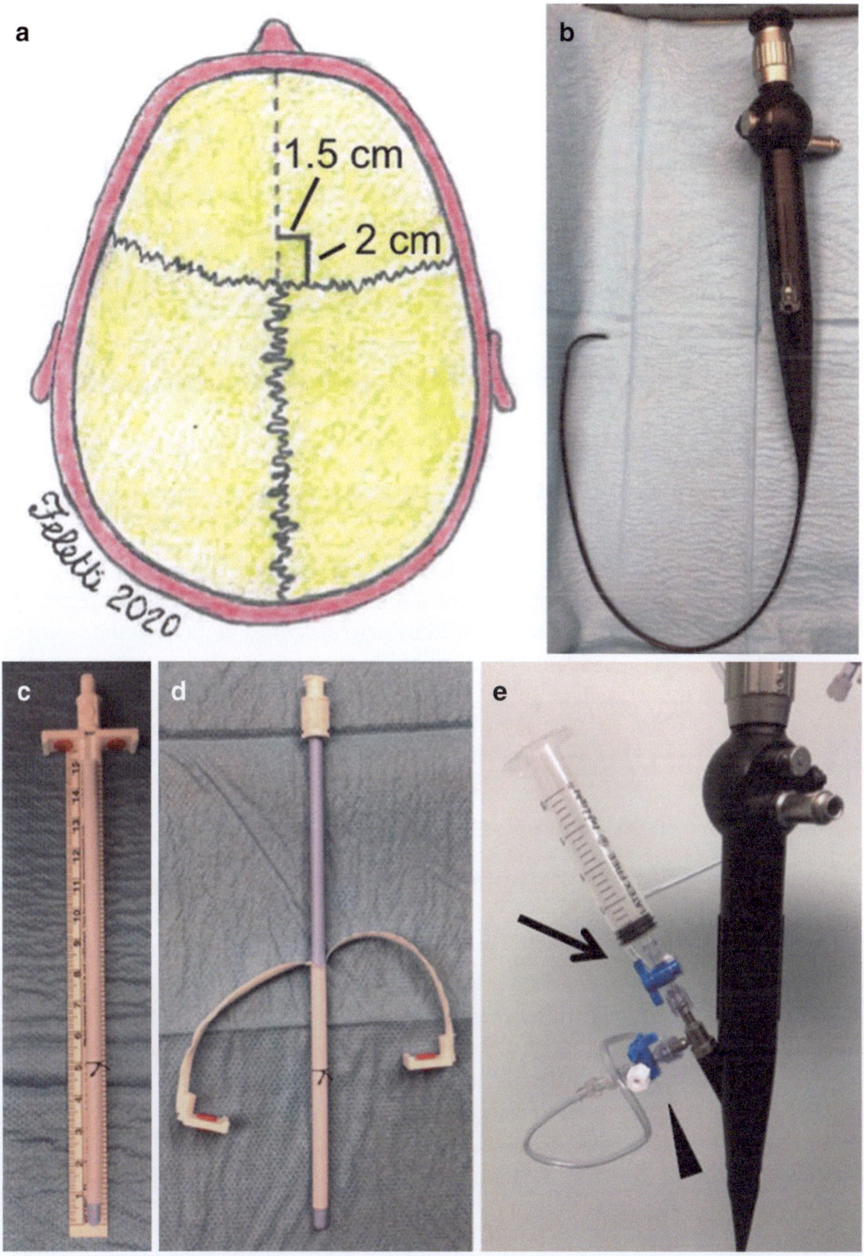

Fig. 5.6 (**a**) The precoronal burr hole should be placed at about 1.5 cm from the midline. (**b**) Flexible endoscope (Karl Storz, Tuttlingen, Germany). (**c**) The peel-away length is marked using a stitch placed at about 5 cm from the tip. (**d**) After cannulation of the ventricle, the peel-away is opened and the mandrel removed. (**e**) A 20-mL syringe (*arrow*) and a catheter (*arrowhead*) are connected to the outer ends of the scope for aspiration and irrigation, respectively (Feletti et al., How I do it: flexible endoscopic aspiration of intraventricular hemorrhage. Acta Neurochir 2020, 162:3141–3146. Published with permission)

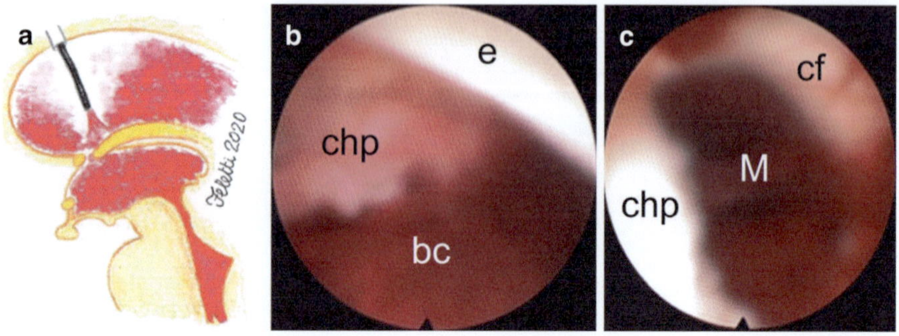

Fig. 5.7 Clots aspiration from the lateral ventricle. (**a**) Artist's illustration showing the tip of the endoscope in the lateral ventricle. (**b**) The tip of the scope is directed backwards: after the initial aspiration of blood clots (*bc*), the choroid plexus (*chp*) and the ependyma (*e*) of the floor and lateral wall of the right lateral ventricle are unveiled. (**c**) Directing the tip of the scope anteriorly, the choroid plexus (*chp*) leads to the foramen of Monro (*M*), contoured by the column of the fornix (*cf*) and still obstructed by clots (Feletti et al., How I do it: flexible endoscopic aspiration of intraventricular hemorrhage. Acta Neurochir 2020, 162:3141–3146. Published with permission)

using an external 20 mL syringe connected to the outer end of the scope, grants the breaking of the clots, that can be removed by active aspiration through the working channel of the scope. Care must be taken by the second operator to promptly stop aspiration when the whitish color of the ependymal layer is seen on the screen, and to alternate irrigations to clear the field and improve the vision. Usually, the first anatomic landmark to be exposed is the choroid plexus, which can be followed forwards until the foramen of Monro is identified (Fig. 5.7, Video 5.1). A standard septostomy can be performed in order to partially remove blood clots from the contralateral ventricle. Advancing the scope into the third ventricle, the same maneuvers (aspiration and irrigation) unveil the mammillary bodies and tuber cinereum. After the anterior third ventricle is cleared, the tip of the scope is bent backwards, and clots are aspirated from the posterior third ventricle. In this way, the posterior and habenular commissures, the roof of the third ventricle, and the adytum of the cerebral aqueduct are uncovered (Fig. 5.8). In expert hands, the aqueduct can be safely crossed, and clots can be removed from the fourth ventricle, restoring the patency of the foramina of Luschka and Magendie (Fig. 5.9, Video 5.2). The peel-away diameter is larger than that of the scope, allowing free CSF outflow during irrigation, without any risk of acute iatrogenic hydrocephalus and ICP increase. However, this is not the case when exploring the fourth ventricle, as the scope occupies the entire diameter of the cerebral aqueduct. Therefore, aspiration and irrigation must be carefully balanced in this region, to avoid local hypertension and bradycardia. After eventual active sources of bleeding have been ruled out, an EVD is left in place to monitor ICP and drain CSF, if needed. EVD is usually kept open at about 10–15 cm from the tragus and can generally be weaned off over the following 2–3 days.

This technique can be immediately performed after coiling, in those cases when IVH is caused by a ruptured aneurysm [93]. Safety and good outcomes obtained

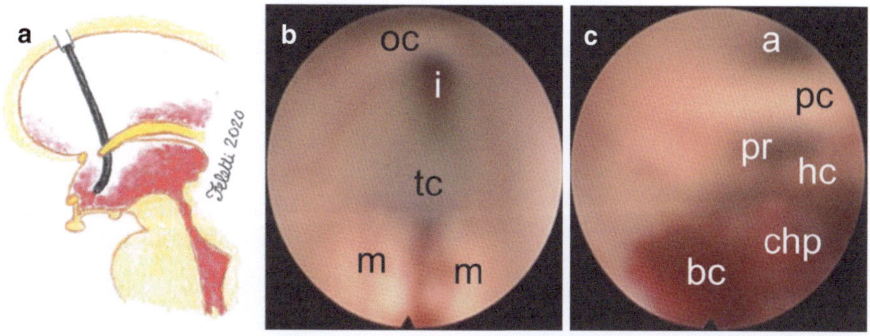

Fig. 5.8 Clots aspiration from the third ventricle. (**a**) Artist's illustration showing the direction of the endoscope through the foramen of Monro into the third ventricle. (**b**) Appearance of the anterior third ventricle after clots aspiration: mammillary bodies (*m*) and tuber cinereum (*tc*) are usually the first anatomical landmarks that can be seen, followed by the infundibulum (*i*) and the optic chiasm (*oc*). (**c**) Residual blood clots (*bc*) in the posterior third ventricle. The choroid plexus on the roof of the third ventricle, the habenular commissure (*hc*), the pineal recess (*pr*), the posterior commissure (*pc*), and the adytum of the cerebral aqueduct (*a*) are visible (Feletti et al., How I do it: flexible endoscopic aspiration of intraventricular hemorrhage. Acta Neurochir 2020, 162:3141–3146. Published with permission)

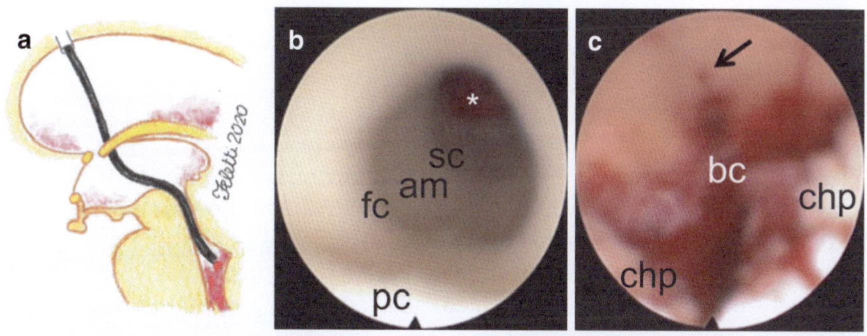

Fig. 5.9 Clots aspiration from the fourth ventricle. (**a**) Artist's illustration showing the transaqueductal navigation of the fourth ventricle. (**b**) Closer inspection of the cerebral aqueduct reveals the first constriction, the ampulla (*am*), the second constriction (*sc*), and blood clot hampering the egressus of the cerebral aqueduct (*asterisk*). (**c**) The inferior triangle of the fourth ventricle: after blood aspiration, the choroid plexus (*chp*) on the roof of the ventricle and the canalis centralis medullaris at the calamus scriptorius (*black arrow*) are now visible. Blood clots (*bc*) are still obstructing the foramen of Magendie (Feletti et al., How I do it: flexible endoscopic aspiration of intraventricular hemorrhage. Acta Neurochir 2020, 162:3141–3146. Published with permission)

with this technique have been confirmed by different groups [71]. It has been shown that flexible endoscopic aspiration of IVH plus EVD reduces shunting rates by 34%, when compared with external drainage alone [94]. Endoscopy should be performed in the first 48 h after the hemorrhagic event, otherwise the blood clots can get stiff and harder to be aspirated [91]. For this reason, delayed endoscopic IVH removal is often incomplete and may not prevent communicating hydrocephalus [95]. A similar procedure, with a flexible scope introduced from the fourth ventricle up to the third ventricle, has been also described in cases of patients operated in the prone position with a microsurgical technique, with the aim of aspirating eventual blood clots that might wedge into the cerebral aqueduct and the third ventricle and potentially cause acute hydrocephalus during the post-operative course [96].

5.3.3 Controversies Discussion

ICH and IVH associated with impaired neurological status have always been a challenge for neurosurgeons, due to their deep location or extension. Craniotomy has traditionally been adopted to reduce the mass effect and to save the patient's life. However, the discouraging results in terms of functional outcome have prompted neurosurgeons to find different treatment strategies, which could not only be effective to decrease ICP, but also not harmful to the surrounding brain structures. In the last years, new MIS techniques tried to overcome the evident limits of conventional surgery by developing safer and more effective methods to remove hematomas. Despite several studies and meta-analyses, the best method to treat ICH and IVH is still controversial.

5.3.3.1 ICH

The MISTIE II trial proved the technical feasibility of a catheter-based pharmacological therapy of ICH. However, the MISTIE III trial failed to show improvement of functional outcome compared to the standard medical therapy. For this reason, thrombolytic therapy for ICH is still debated, especially after the introduction of minimally invasive mechanical methods that offer the possibility to safely and effectively remove the hematoma in a single and relatively fast procedure, with immediate ICP control. Such techniques proved to be very efficient in reducing clot volume and mortality, but the benefit on functional outcome is not clear yet, as only small multicenter series are available. Similarly, it is still not clear if a specific device is better than others to remove ICH with a minimally invasive technique. Three ongoing trials will hopefully help to find answers to these questions. The **E**arly Mi**N**imally Invasive **R**emoval of **ICH** trial (ENRICH trial) is a multicenter, randomized, adaptive clinical trial comparing standard medical management to early surgical hematoma evacuation (less than 24 h) using minimally invasive parafascicular surgery (MIPS) with NICO BrainPath. The INVEST trial is a randomized, controlled trial to investigate the safety and efficacy of image-guided minimally invasive endoscopic surgery with Apollo, compared to the best medical management for supratentorial ICH. The MIND trial is a prospective, multicenter study evaluating minimally invasive hematoma evacuation with the Artemis device, and comparing it with the best medical management. In any case, specific studies should also clarify how to choose the best entry point on the cerebral cortex and the optimal trajectory. Although the shorter distance between the cortex and hematoma is often selected, a frontal access to avoid relevant white matter fascicles and a direction along the major extension of the hematoma appear nowadays more reasonable.

It is likely that the trend in the treatment of ICH will progressively move towards endoscopic MIS, if the ongoing trials will show good results not only in terms of reduced mortality, but also in terms of better functional outcome, compared to the best medical treatment. The possibility for the new generations of neurosurgeons to be more exposed and trained on endoscopy can potentially facilitate the shift to MIS in the management of ICH.

5.3.3.2 IVH

IVH management is probably even more controversial than ICH. The traditional EVD is a very simple and fast maneuver, and therefore it is still the most commonly performed treatment in such cases, despite its evident limits. The infusion of fibrinolytic agents through EVD is still debated. It can speed up the process of clots lysis and IVH resolution, but it takes several days to act, and it can potentially increase the risk of hemorrhage, ventriculitis, and meningitis.

The recent results with endoscopic aspiration of IVH are very promising, as this technique can remove the blood mass effect immediately, facilitating ICP control and reducing EVD obstructions and replacements. It has been shown that endoscopy can also potentially reduce shunt-dependency of these patients. Nevertheless, this benefit must be confirmed by larger studies, and is probably dependent on the primary cause of IVH and timing of surgery. Moreover, endoscopy in IVHs, where vision is severely impaired by blood, requires practice and training, especially if a flexible endoscope, with the aim of cleaning also the fourth ventricle, is used. The side where to place the burr hole is also debated. Although the lateral ventricle with less blood would be easier to cannulate and navigate, it is preferable to choose the side with the highest amount of blood, in order to have more chances to remove most of the IVH in the lateral ventricle. In cases of tetraventricular hemorrhage, some authors suggested a biportal approach to clear both lateral ventricles. Others proposed a single burr hole, and a septostomy to access the opposite lateral ventricle, in order to have just one intraparenchymal route. Anyway, in our experience, restoration of CSF circulation, i.e. cleaning of third and fourth ventricles, appears to have a greater impact on outcome, particularly on reducing shunt-dependency, than total removal of blood in the lateral ventricles.

Endoscopy for IVH is questioned by someone because of the alleged risk of rebleeding during the procedure, and because of the potentially troublesome hemostasis. However, this risk can be significantly reduced in the preoperative stage. After CT scan, patients should undergo an angio-CT scan or a digital subtraction angiography (DSA) to rule out obvious causes of the hemorrhage, and eventually treat any vascular malformation before endoscopic aspiration of IVH. Identification and correction of coagulation disorders in the preoperative setting, and maintenance of mean arterial blood pressure below 110 mmHg during endoscopy are also required.

The best endoscope to remove IVH is also controversial. Rigid scopes surely provide a better quality of vision compared to flexible scopes. However, they can reach only the lateral and the third ventricles, without any possibility to explore the cerebral aqueduct and the fourth ventricle. It has been demonstrated that hemorrhagic dilation of the fourth ventricle is a significant outcome predictor [53, 97]. For this reason, the removal of blood clots from the fourth ventricle seems very important to obtain better outcomes, although randomized trials are lacking about this topic. Flexible scopes appear to be the only way to completely and directly remove blood from the entire ventricular system, even from the cerebral aqueduct and the fourth ventricle. Flexible instruments also better adapt to the anatomy of the ventricular system, and for this reason, according to some authors, they minimize the risk of iatrogenic damage. The alleged better outcomes, less risk of damages to the brain structures, and reduced shunt-dependency with flexible scopes are still debated and require further and larger studies.

References

1. Chen S, Zeng L, Hu Z. Progressing haemorrhagic stroke: categories, causes, mechanisms and managements. J Neurol. 2014;261(11):2061–78.
2. Angelopoulos M, Gupta SR, Azat KB. Primary intraventricular hemorrhage in adults: clinical features, risk factors, and outcome. Surg Neurol. 1995;44(5):433–6; discussion 437
3. Rosen DS, Macdonald RL, Huo D, Goldenberg FD, Novakovic RL, Frank JI, et al. Intraventricular hemorrhage from ruptured aneurysm: clinical characteristics, complications, and outcomes in a large, prospective, multicenter study population. J Neurosurg. 2007;107(2):261–5.
4. Broderick J, Connolly S, Feldmann E, Hanley D, Kase C, Krieger D, et al. Guidelines for the management of spontaneous intracerebral hemorrhage in adults: 2007 update: a guideline from the American Heart Association/American Stroke Association Stroke Council, High Blood Pressure Research Council, and the Quality of Care and Outcomes in Research Interdisciplinary Working Group. Stroke. 2007;38(6):2001–23.
5. Caceres JA, Goldstein JN. Intracranial hemorrhage. Emerg Med Clin North Am. 2012;30(3):771–94.
6. van Asch CJ, Luitse MJ, Rinkel GJ, van der Tweel I, Algra A, Klijn CJ. Incidence, case fatality, and functional outcome of intracerebral haemorrhage over time, according to age, sex, and ethnic origin: a systematic review and meta-analysis. Lancet Neurol. 2010;9(2): 167–76.
7. Zhang Z, Li X, Liu Y, Shao Y, Xu S, Yang Y. Application of neuroendoscopy in the treatment of intraventricular hemorrhage. Cerebrovasc Dis. 2007;24(1):91–6.
8. de Weerd AW. The prognosis of intraventricular hemorrhage. J Neurol. 1979;222(1):46–51.
9. Tuhrim S, Horowitz DR, Sacher M, Godbold JH. Volume of ventricular blood is an important determinant of outcome in supratentorial intracerebral hemorrhage. Crit Care Med. 1999;27(3):617–21.
10. Lee KR, Kawai N, Kim S, Sagher O, Hoff JT. Mechanisms of edema formation after intracerebral hemorrhage: effects of thrombin on cerebral blood flow, blood-brain barrier permeability, and cell survival in a rat model. J Neurosurg. 1997;86(2):272–8.

11. Lee KR, Betz AL, Kim S, Keep RF, Hoff JT. The role of the coagulation cascade in brain edema formation after intracerebral hemorrhage. Acta Neurochir. 1996;138(4):396–400; discussion 400-401
12. Mendelow AD, Gregson BA, Fernandes HM, Murray GD, Teasdale GM, Hope DT, et al. Early surgery versus initial conservative treatment in patients with spontaneous supratentorial intracerebral haematomas in the International Surgical Trial in Intracerebral Haemorrhage (STICH): a randomised trial. Lancet. 2005;365(9457):387–97.
13. Mendelow AD, Gregson BA, Rowan EN, Murray GD, Gholkar A, Mitchell PM, et al. Early surgery versus initial conservative treatment in patients with spontaneous supratentorial lobar intracerebral haematomas (STICH II): a randomised trial. Lancet. 2013;382(9890):397–408.
14. Wang W-Z, Jiang B, Liu H-M, Li D, Lu C-Z, Zhao Y-D, et al. Minimally invasive craniopuncture therapy vs. conservative treatment for spontaneous intracerebral hemorrhage: results from a randomized clinical trial in China. Int J Stroke. 2009;4(1):11–6.
15. Sun H, Liu H, Li D, Liu L, Yang J, Wang W. An effective treatment for cerebral hemorrhage: minimally invasive craniopuncture combined with urokinase infusion therapy. Neurol Res. 2010;32(4):371–7.
16. Hanley DF, Thompson RE, Muschelli J, Rosenblum M, McBee N, Lane K, et al. Safety and efficacy of minimally invasive surgery plus alteplase in intracerebral haemorrhage evacuation (MISTIE): a randomised, controlled, open-label, phase 2 trial. Lancet Neurol. 2016;15(12):1228–37.
17. Hanley DF, Thompson RE, Rosenblum M, Yenokyan G, Lane K, McBee N, et al. Efficacy and safety of minimally invasive surgery with thrombolysis in intracerebral haemorrhage evacuation (MISTIE III): a randomised, controlled, open-label, blinded endpoint phase 3 trial. Lancet. 2019;393(10175):1021–32.
18. Auer LM, Ascher PW, Heppner F, Ladurner G, Boné G, Lechner H, et al. Does acute endoscopic evacuation improve the outcome of patients with spontaneous intracerebral hemorrhage? Eur Neurol. 1985;24(4):254–61.
19. Grotenhuis A. If it can be done, it should be done,…or not? Acta Neurochir. 2016;158(4):649–53.
20. Horváth Z, Veto F, Balás I, Kövér F, Dóczi T. Biportal endoscopic removal of a primary intraventricular hematoma: case report. Minim Invasive Neurosurg. 2000;43(1):4–8.
21. Kamikawa S, Inui A, Kobayashi N, Tamaki N, Yamadori T. Intraventricular hemorrhage in neonates: endoscopic findings and treatment by the use of our newly developed Yamadori-type 8 ventriculoscope. Minim Invasive Neurosurg. 2001;44(2):74–8.
22. Nakano T, Ohkuma H, Ebina K, Suzuki S. Neuroendoscopic surgery for intracerebral haemorrhage—comparison with traditional therapies. Minim Invasive Neurosurg. 2003;46(5):278–83.
23. Oka K, Go Y, Yamamoto M, Kumate S, Tomonaga M. Experience with an ultrasonic aspirator in neuroendoscopy. Minim Invasive Neurosurg. 1999;42(1):32–4.
24. Tang Y, Yin F, Fu D, Gao X, Lv Z, Li X. Efficacy and safety of minimal invasive surgery treatment in hypertensive intracerebral hemorrhage: a systematic review and meta-analysis. BMC Neurol. 2018;18(1):136.
25. Xia Z, Wu X, Li J, Liu Z, Chen F, Zhang L, et al. Minimally invasive surgery is superior to conventional craniotomy in patients with spontaneous supratentorial intracerebral hemorrhage: a systematic review and meta-analysis. World Neurosurg. 2018;115:266–73.
26. Zhao X-H, Zhang S-Z, Feng J, Li Z-Z, Ma Z-L. Efficacy of neuroendoscopic surgery versus craniotomy for supratentorial hypertensive intracerebral hemorrhage: a meta-analysis of randomized controlled trials. Brain Behav. 2019;9(12):e01471.
27. Katsuki M, Kakizawa Y, Nishikawa A, Yamamoto Y, Uchiyama T. Endoscopic hematoma removal of supratentorial intracerebral hemorrhage under local anesthesia reduces operative time compared to craniotomy. Sci Rep. 2020;10(1):10389.
28. White T, Chakraborty S, Lall R, Fanous AA, Boockvar J, Langer DJ. Frameless stereotactic insertion of viewsite brain access system with microscope-mounted tracking device for resection of deep brain lesions: technical report. Cureus. 2017;9(2):e1012.

29. Przybylowski CJ, Ding D, Starke RM, Webster Crowley R, Liu KC. Endoport-assisted surgery for the management of spontaneous intracerebral hemorrhage. J Clin Neurosci. 2015;22(11):1727–32.
30. Bauer AM, Rasmussen PA, Bain MD. Initial single-center technical experience with the BrainPath system for acute intracerebral hemorrhage evacuation. Oper Neurosurg (Hagerstown). 2017;13(1):69–76.
31. Labib MA, Shah M, Kassam AB, Young R, Zucker L, Maioriello A, et al. The safety and feasibility of image-guided BrainPath-mediated transsulcul hematoma evacuation: a multicenter study. Neurosurgery. 2017;80(4):515–24.
32. Fiorella D, Gutman F, Woo H, Arthur A, Aranguren R, Davis R. Minimally invasive evacuation of parenchymal and ventricular hemorrhage using the Apollo system with simultaneous neuronavigation, neuroendoscopy and active monitoring with cone beam CT. J Neurointerv Surg. 2015;7(10):752–7.
33. Tan LA, Lopes DK, Munoz LF, Shah Y, Bhabad S, Jhaveri M, et al. Minimally invasive evacuation of intraventricular hemorrhage with the Apollo vibration/suction device. J Clin Neurosci. 2016;27:53–8.
34. Goyal N, Tsivgoulis G, Malhotra K, Katsanos AH, Pandhi A, Alsherbini KA, et al. Minimally invasive endoscopic hematoma evacuation vs best medical management for spontaneous basal-ganglia intracerebral hemorrhage. J Neurointerv Surg. 2019;11(6):579–83.
35. Spiotta AM, Fiorella D, Vargas J, Khalessi A, Hoit D, Arthur A, et al. Initial multicenter technical experience with the Apollo device for minimally invasive intracerebral hematoma evacuation. Neurosurgery. 2015;11(Suppl 2):243–51; discussion 251
36. Kellner CP, Chartrain AG, Nistal DA, Scaggiante J, Hom D, Ghatan S, et al. The Stereotactic Intracerebral Hemorrhage Underwater Blood Aspiration (SCUBA) technique for minimally invasive endoscopic intracerebral hemorrhage evacuation. J Neurointerv Surg. 2018;10(8):771–6.
37. Griessenauer C, Medin C, Goren O, Schirmer CM. Image-guided, minimally invasive evacuation of intracerebral hematoma: a matched cohort study comparing the endoscopic and tubular exoscopic systems. Cureus. 2018;10(11):e3569.
38. Vespa P, Hanley D, Betz J, Hoffer A, Engh J, Carter R, et al. ICES (intraoperative stereotactic computed tomography-guided endoscopic surgery) for brain hemorrhage: a multicenter randomized controlled trial. Stroke. 2016;47(11):2749–55.
39. Mayer SL, Kessler DB, Van Hurtum RL, et al. Effect of intraventricular blood on global cortical perfusion in acute intracerebral hemorrhage: a single photon emission computed tomographic study (abstract). Ann Neurol. 1995;38:228.
40. Mayfrank L, Kissler J, Raoofi R, Delsing P, Weis J, Küker W, et al. Ventricular dilatation in experimental intraventricular hemorrhage in pigs: characterization of cerebrospinal fluid dynamics and the effects of fibrinolytic treatment. Stroke. 1997;28(1):141–8.
41. Andrews CO, Engelhard HH. Fibrinolytic therapy in intraventricular hemorrhage. Ann Pharmacother. 2001;35(11):1435–48.
42. Pang D, Sclabassi RJ, Horton JA. Lysis of intraventricular blood clot with urokinase in a canine model: part 3. Effects of intraventricular urokinase on clot lysis and posthemorrhagic hydrocephalus. Neurosurgery. 1986;19(4):553–72.
43. Hanley DF. Intraventricular hemorrhage: severity factor and treatment target in spontaneous intracerebral hemorrhage. Stroke. 2009;40(4):1533–8.
44. Nieuwkamp DJ, de Gans K, Rinkel GJ, Algra A. Treatment and outcome of severe intraventricular extension in patients with subarachnoid or intracerebral hemorrhage: a systematic review of the literature. J Neurol. 2000;247(2):117–21.
45. Gaberel T, Magheru C, Emery E. Management of non-traumatic intraventricular hemorrhage. Neurosurg Rev. 2012;35(4):485–94; discussion 494-495
46. Steiner T, Diringer MN, Schneider D, Mayer SA, Begtrup K, Broderick J, et al. Dynamics of intraventricular hemorrhage in patients with spontaneous intracerebral hemorrhage: risk

factors, clinical impact, and effect of hemostatic therapy with recombinant activated factor VII. Neurosurgery. 2006;59(4):767–73; discussion 773-774
47. Graeb DA, Robertson WD, Lapointe JS, Nugent RA, Harrison PB. Computed tomographic diagnosis of intraventricular hemorrhage. Etiology and prognosis. Radiology. 1982;143(1):91–6.
48. Hallevi H, Dar NS, Barreto AD, Morales MM, Martin-Schild S, Abraham AT, et al. The IVH score: a novel tool for estimating intraventricular hemorrhage volume: clinical and research implications. Crit Care Med. 2009;37(3):969–74, e1
49. LeRoux PD, Haglund MM, Newell DW, Grady MS, Winn HR. Intraventricular hemorrhage in blunt head trauma: an analysis of 43 cases. Neurosurgery. 1992;31(4):678–84; discussion 684-685
50. Morgenstern LB, Hemphill JC, Anderson C, Becker K, Broderick JP, Connolly ES, et al. Guidelines for the management of spontaneous intracerebral hemorrhage: a guideline for healthcare professionals from the American Heart Association/American Stroke Association. Stroke. 2010;41(9):2108–29.
51. Bakshi R, Kamran S, Kinkel PR, Bates VE, Mechtler LL, Janardhan V, et al. Fluid-attenuated inversion-recovery MR imaging in acute and subacute cerebral intraventricular hemorrhage. AJNR Am J Neuroradiol. 1999;20(4):629–36.
52. Yamamoto Y, Waga S. Persistent intraventricular hematoma following ruptured aneurysm. Surg Neurol. 1982;17(4):301–3.
53. Shapiro SA, Campbell RL, Scully T. Hemorrhagic dilation of the fourth ventricle: an ominous predictor. J Neurosurg. 1994;80(5):805–9.
54. Shimoda M, Oda S, Shibata M, Tominaga J, Kittaka M, Tsugane R. Results of early surgical evacuation of packed intraventricular hemorrhage from aneurysm rupture in patients with poor-grade subarachnoid hemorrhage. J Neurosurg. 1999;91(3):408–14.
55. Holtzman RN, Brust JC, Ainyette IG, Bowers PP, Tikofsky RS, Lliguin HM, et al. Acute ventricular hemorrhage in adults with hydrocephalus managed by corpus callosotomy and fenestration of the septum pellucidum. Report of three cases. J Neurosurg. 2001;95(1):111–5.
56. Wang K-C, Lee J-E, Chen C-L, Tseng S-H, Kao M-C, Chen J-C. Interhemispheric transcorpus callosal approach in the treatment of ventricular hemorrhage with obstructive hydrocephalus. Surg Neurol. 2006;66(Suppl 2):S52–9; discussion S59
57. Lagares A, Putman CM, Ogilvy CS. Posterior fossa decompression and clot evacuation for fourth ventricle hemorrhage after aneurysmal rupture: case report. Neurosurgery. 2001;49(1):208–11.
58. Onoda K, Kurozumi K, Tsuchimoto S, Satoh T. Experience with the high occipital transcortical approach in the treatment of intraventricular hemorrhage. Report of two cases. J Neurosurg. 2001;94(2):315–7.
59. Engelhard HH, Andrews CO, Slavin KV, Charbel FT. Current management of intraventricular hemorrhage. Surg Neurol. 2003;60(1):15–21; discussion 21-22
60. Schwarz S, Schwab S, Steiner HH, Hacke W. Secondary hemorrhage after intraventricular fibrinolysis: a cautionary note: a report of two cases. Neurosurgery. 1998;42(3):659–62; discussion 662-663
61. Findlay JM, Weir BK, Stollery DE. Lysis of intraventricular hematoma with tissue plasminogen activator. Case report. J Neurosurg. 1991;74(5):803–7.
62. Shen PH, Matsuoka Y, Kawajiri K, Kanai M, Hoda K, Yamamoto S, et al. Treatment of intraventricular hemorrhage using urokinase. Neurol Med Chir (Tokyo). 1990;30(5):329–33.
63. Khan NR, Tsivgoulis G, Lee SL, Jones GM, Green CS, Katsanos AH, et al. Fibrinolysis for intraventricular hemorrhage: an updated meta-analysis and systematic review of the literature. Stroke. 2014;45(9):2662–9.
64. Litrico S, Almairac F, Gaberel T, Ramakrishna R, Fontaine D, Sedat J, et al. Intraventricular fibrinolysis for severe aneurysmal intraventricular hemorrhage: a randomized controlled trial and meta-analysis. Neurosurg Rev. 2013;36(4):523–30; discussion 530-531

65. Starnoni D, Oddo M, Maduri R, Messerer M, Daniel RT. Thrombolysis for non-traumatic intra-ventricular hemorrhage in adults: a critical reappraisal. Minerva Anestesiol. 2017;83(9):982–93.
66. Baker AD, Rivera Perla KM, Yu Z, Dlugash R, Avadhani R, Mould WA, et al. Fibrinolytic for treatment of intraventricular hemorrhage: a meta-analysis and systematic review. Int J Stroke. 2018;13(1):11–23.
67. Ziai WC, Tuhrim S, Lane K, McBee N, Lees K, Dawson J, et al. A multicenter, randomized, double-blinded, placebo-controlled phase III study of Clot Lysis Evaluation of Accelerated Resolution of Intraventricular Hemorrhage (CLEAR III). Int J Stroke. 2014;9(4):536–42.
68. Coplin WM, Vinas FC, Agris JM, Buciuc R, Michael DB, Diaz FG, et al. A cohort study of the safety and feasibility of intraventricular urokinase for nonaneurysmal spontaneous intraventricular hemorrhage. Stroke. 1998;29(8):1573–9.
69. Whitelaw A, Saliba E, Fellman V, Mowinckel MC, Acolet D, Marlow N. Phase I study of intraventricular recombinant tissue plasminogen activator for treatment of posthaemorrhagic hydrocephalus. Arch Dis Child Fetal Neonatal Ed. 1996;75(1):F20–6.
70. Bhattathiri PS, Gregson B, KSM P, Mendelow AD, STICH Investigators. Intraventricular hemorrhage and hydrocephalus after spontaneous intracerebral hemorrhage: results from the STICH trial. Acta Neurochir Suppl. 2006;96:65–8.
71. Hamada H, Hayashi N, Kurimoto M, Umemura K, Nagai S, Kurosaki K, et al. Neuroendoscopic removal of intraventricular hemorrhage combined with hydrocephalus. Minim Invasive Neurosurg. 2008;51(6):345–9.
72. Longatti PL, Martinuzzi A, Fiorindi A, Maistrello L, Carteri A. Neuroendoscopic management of intraventricular hemorrhage. Stroke. 2004;35(2):e35–8.
73. Longatti P, Fiorindi A, Martinuzzi A. Neuroendoscopic aspiration of hematocephalus totalis: technical note. Neurosurgery. 2005;57(4 Suppl):E409; discussion E409
74. Kiymaz N, Demir O, Cirak B. Is external ventricular drainage useful in primary intraventricular hemorrhages? Adv Ther. 2005;22(5):447–52.
75. Nagasaka T, Tsugeno M, Ikeda H, Okamoto T, Inao S, Wakabayashi T. Early recovery and better evacuation rate in neuroendoscopic surgery for spontaneous intracerebral hemorrhage using a multifunctional cannula: preliminary study in comparison with craniotomy. J Stroke Cerebrovasc Dis. 2011;20(3):208–13.
76. Nakagawa T, Suga S, Mayanagi K, Akaji K, Inamasu J, Kawase T, et al. Predicting the overall management outcome in patients with a subarachnoid hemorrhage accompanied by a massive intracerebral or full-packed intraventricular hemorrhage: a 15-year retrospective study. Surg Neurol. 2005;63(4):329–34; discussion 334-335
77. el Chami B, Milan C, Giroud M, Sautreaux JL, Faivre J. Intracerebral hemorrhage survival: French register data. Neurol Res. 2000;22(8):791–6.
78. Karnik R, Valentin A, Ammerer HP, Hochfelner A, Donath P, Slany J. Outcome in patients with intracerebral hemorrhage: predictors of survival. Wien Klin Wochenschr. 2000;112(4):169–73.
79. St Louis EK, Wijdicks EF, Li H. Predicting neurologic deterioration in patients with cerebellar hematomas. Neurology. 1998;51(5):1364–9.
80. Claassen J, Bernardini GL, Kreiter K, Bates J, Du YE, Copeland D, et al. Effect of cisternal and ventricular blood on risk of delayed cerebral ischemia after subarachnoid hemorrhage: the Fisher scale revisited. Stroke. 2001;32(9):2012–20.
81. Nomura S, Ishihara H, Yoneda H, Shirao S, Shinoyama M, Suzuki M. Neuroendoscopic evacuation of intraventricular hematoma associated with thalamic hemorrhage to shorten the duration of external ventricular drainage. Surg Neurol Int. 2010;1:43.
82. Yadav YR, Mukerji G, Shenoy R, Basoor A, Jain G, Nelson A. Endoscopic management of hypertensive intraventricular haemorrhage with obstructive hydrocephalus. BMC Neurol. 2007;7:1.
83. Idris Z, Raj J, Abdullah JM. Early experience in endoscopic management of massive intraventricular hemorrhage with literature review. Asian J Neurosurg. 2014;9(3):124–9.

84. Nishikawa T, Ueba T, Kajiwara M, Iwata R, Yamashita K. Combined treatment of ruptured aneurysm accompanied by intraventricular hemorrhage; neuroendoscopy and coiling: case report. Minim Invasive Neurosurg. 2008;51(6):354–7.
85. Chen C-C, Liu C-L, Tung Y-N, Lee H-C, Chuang H-C, Lin S-Z, et al. Endoscopic surgery for intraventricular hemorrhage (IVH) caused by thalamic hemorrhage: comparisons of endoscopic surgery and external ventricular drainage (EVD) surgery. World Neurosurg. 2011;75(2):264–8.
86. Song P, Duan F-L, Cai Q, Wu J-L, Chen X-B, Wang Y, et al. Endoscopic surgery versus external ventricular drainage surgery for severe intraventricular hemorrhage. Curr Med Sci. 2018;38(5):880–7.
87. Etus V, Kahilogullari G, Karabagli H, Unlu A. Early endoscopic ventricular irrigation for the treatment of neonatal Posthemorrhagic hydrocephalus: a feasible treatment option or not? A multicenter study. Turk Neurosurg. 2018;28(1):137–41.
88. Schulz M, Bührer C, Pohl-Schickinger A, Haberl H, Thomale U-W. Neuroendoscopic lavage for the treatment of intraventricular hemorrhage and hydrocephalus in neonates. J Neurosurg Pediatr. 2014;13(6):626–35.
89. Ding H-T, Han Y, Sun D-K, Nie Q-M. Efficacy and safety profile of neuroendoscopic hematoma evacuation combined with intraventricular lavage in severe intraventricular hemorrhage patients. Brain Behav. 2020;10(9):e01756.
90. Longatti P, Basaldella L. Endoscopic management of intracerebral hemorrhage. World Neurosurg. 2013;79(2 Suppl):S17.e1–7.
91. Feletti A, Basaldella L, Fiorindi A. How I do it: flexible endoscopic aspiration of intraventricular hemorrhage. Acta Neurochir. 2020;162(12):3141–6.
92. Luca B, Alessandro F, Alberto F, Pierluigi L. Intraventricular hemorrhage. In: Torres-Corzo JG, Rangel-Castilla L, Nakaji P, editors. Neuroendoscopic surgery. New York: Thieme. p. 169–79.
93. Longatti P, Fiorindi A, Di Paola F, Curtolo S, Basaldella L, Martinuzzi A. Coiling and neuroendoscopy: a new perspective in the treatment of intraventricular haemorrhages due to bleeding aneurysms. J Neurol Neurosurg Psychiatry. 2006;77(12):1354–8.
94. Basaldella L, Marton E, Fiorindi A, Scarpa B, Badreddine H, Longatti P. External ventricular drainage alone versus endoscopic surgery for severe intraventricular hemorrhage: a comparative retrospective analysis on outcome and shunt dependency. Neurosurg Focus. 2012;32(4):E4.
95. Nishikawa T, Takehira N, Matsumoto A, Kanemoto M, Kang Y, Waga S. Delayed endoscopic intraventricular hemorrhage (IVH) removal and endoscopic third ventriculostomy may not prevent consecutive communicating hydrocephalus if IVH removal was insufficient. Minim Invasive Neurosurg. 2007;50(4):209–11.
96. Feletti A, Stanzani R, Alicandri-Ciufelli M, Giliberto G, Martinoni M, Pavesi G. Neuroendoscopic aspiration of blood clots in the cerebral aqueduct and third ventricle during posterior fossa surgery in the prone position. Oper Neurosurg (Hagerstown). 2019;17(2):143–8.
97. Hughes JD, Puffer R, Rabinstein AA. Risk factors for hydrocephalus requiring external ventricular drainage in patients with intraventricular hemorrhage. J Neurosurg. 2015;123(6):1439–46.

Chapter 6
Functional Outcomes of Microsurgical Resection for Cavernous Malformations of the Brainstem

Ken-ichiro Kikuta, Makoto Isozaki, Yoshifumi Higashino, Toshiaki Kodera, Hidetaka Arishima, Ken Matsuda, Takahiro Yamauchi, Shinsuke Yamada, Ayumi Akazawa, Masamune Kidoguchi, Hideto Umeda, Yu Tsukinowa, and Ryota Hagiwara

6.1 Introduction

Cavernous malformations of the brainstem (CMB) involve 8–16% of the cavernous malformations in the central nervous system [1, 2]. Multistage hemorrhage within sinusoidal structures of CMB leads to expansion into a mulberry-like multi-lobular mass [3, 4]. The mass effect of CMB easily causes focal neurological deterioration, since a number of cranial nerve nuclei and long tracts are densely situated in the brainstem [5]. Recent technical innovation in neuroimaging, intraoperative electrophysiological monitoring, and image-guided navigation systems have allowed for safer and more accurate surgical resection of CMB than before [6–11]. In this chapter, we have discussed and retrospectively examined the functional outcomes of surgery for CMB in our institution.

6.2 Surgical Indication, Approach, and Resection

Patients with hemorrhagic onset, with progressive neurological symptoms, and with CMB extending very close to the pial or ependymal layer were indicated to surgical resection. Thirty-three surgical procedures were performed in 25 patients. Patients

K.-i. Kikuta (✉) · M. Isozaki · Y. Higashino · T. Kodera · H. Arishima · K. Matsuda
T. Yamauchi · S. Yamada · A. Akazawa · M. Kidoguchi · H. Umeda · Y. Tsukinowa
R. Hagiwara
Department of Neurosurgery, Division of Medicine, Faculty of Medical Sciences, University of Fukui, Fukui, Japan
e-mail: kikuta@u-fukui.ac.jp

Y. Kato, A. Ansari (eds.), *Cerebrovascular Surgery*, Advances and Technical Standards in Neurosurgery 44, https://doi.org/10.1007/978-3-030-87649-4_6

without hemorrhagic onset and no neurological symptoms or without CMB not extending to the pial or ependymal layer were excluded from surgical indication. The safe entry point on the brainstem was determined as the point at which the pial or ependymal layer between the CMB and subarachnoid space or ventricle was the thinnest. Free software "No-kan" for ipad or iphone (https://brain-3dcg.org) can also clearly provide geometrical information about neural tract, cranial nerve fibers, cranial nerve nuclei, and safe entry zone on the brainstem. The optimal operative trajectory was determined as the arrow line connecting the safe entry point and the center of the CMB.

Surgery was performed around 1 month after the date of latest hemorrhagic episode because hematoma got easily evacuated by suction at that time. Dorsal midbrain CMBs were resected through unilateral superior and inferior colliculus by using occipital transtentorial approach. Ventral midbrain CMBs were resected through the cerebral peduncle between corticospinal tract (CST) and the origin of oculomotor nerve by using pterional or orbitozygomatic approach. Most pontine CMBs were resected through unilateral supra-facial triangle on the floor of the fourth ventricle by using telovelar approach. Some of the lateral pontine CMBs were resected through lateral pontine surface between origins of facial and glossopharyngeal nerve by using lateral suboccipital craniotomy. Some ventral pontine CMBs were resected through lateral pontine surface between origins of trigeminal and vestibulocochlear nerve by using posterior transpetrosal approach. Medullary CMBs were resected through the dorsal medulla around the olive or through the dorsal midline medulla just caudal to the obex by using midline suboccipital craniotomy. Evacuation of hematoma through 5–10 mm incision on the safe entry point, decompression of CMB, meticulous dissection of the capsule, and en bloc resection was the common surgical procedure.

6.3 Judgment of Complete Resection

As previously reported, we evaluated surgeries for CMB as follows: preoperative magnetic resonance imaging (MRI) demonstrated that the lesion was a homogeneous hyperintense mass, and the surgery was defined as complete resection or incomplete resection based on intraoperative findings. When preoperative MRI study revealed other findings, complete resection was determined according to whether postoperative MRI study in the postoperative chronic stage within 2 months after surgery demonstrated lesions distinct from the peripheral hemosiderin rim [12].

6.4 Our Experience

Twenty-five consecutive patients with CMB surgically treated at the University of Fukui Hospital between 2006 and 2021. There were 11 men and 14 women, with ages ranging from 13 to 61 years (mean ± SD = 37 ± 12 years). All patients had a single CMB presenting with one or more clinical hemorrhagic episodes. Neurological functions, namely motor, sensory, cerebellar, and cranial nerve functions, were evaluated on admission and at discharge. Modified Rankin Scale (mRS) scores were evaluated before surgery, 1 month after surgery, and at the final follow-up.

Univariable analysis was performed using a paired t-test, chi-square test, or Mann–Whitney *U*-test. Multivariable analysis was performed using linear regression analysis with significant clinical factors at univariate analysis. All statistical analyses were performed using JMP 15.2.0 (SAS Institute Inc.) and the free software R (https://cran.r-project.org/), with an error probability of less than 0.05 considered significant. The number of previous hemorrhages ranged from 1 to 5 (mean ± SD = 2.7 ± 1.0). The lesion size ranged from 10 to 30 mm (mean ± SD = 21 ± 8 mm). The location of malformation was the medulla in seven patients, dorsal pons in ten patients, lateral pons in seven patients, and ventral pons in one patient. The average of the mRS scores on admission and mRS scores at the final follow-up was 2.9 points and 1.7 points, respectively. The mRS scores at the final follow-up were significantly lower than the mRS scores on admission ($p = 0.0025$, paired *t*-test) (Table 6.1).

6.5 Results of 33 Operations

Two patients underwent three operations while two other patients underwent two operations due to recurrent hemorrhage after incomplete resection. Two patients underwent two surgeries due to residual lesions. A total of 33 surgeries were performed in 25 patients. The surgical approach used was the midline suboccipital approach in 20 operations, the lateral suboccipital approach in four operations, the presignmoid approach in four operations, the subtemporal approach in three operations, the pterional approach in one operation, and the occipital transtentorial approach in one operation. Deterioration of mRS scores after surgery was observed in eight patients. The average of the preoperative mRS score and mRS score at 1 month after operation was 3.1 points and 2.9 points, respectively. There was no statistical difference between preoperative mRS and mRS at 1 month after surgery ($p = 0.4138$, paired *t*-test) (Table 6.2). Logistic regression analysis showed that favorable outcomes (mRS score at the final follow-up ranging from 0 to 2) were significantly related to the size of the lesion ($p = 0.0448$), preoperative mRS scores ($p = 0.0338$), and mRS scores at 1 month after surgery ($p = 0.0107$). Multivariable analysis indicated that mRS scores at 1 month after surgery were the most significant factors related to favorable outcomes ($p = 0.00005$). (Table 6.2).

6.6 Recurrent Hemorrhage During Follow-up

The duration between the date of the final operation and the date of the final follow-up, or between the date of the final operation and the date of recurrent hemorrhage, ranged from 1 to 190 months (mean ± SD = 71 ± 58 months, median = 59 months).

Table 6.1 Characteristics of the 25 patients

Case No.	Age	Sex	mRS on admission	No. of previous hemorrhage	Location of CMB	Size (mm)	mRS at final) Follow-up
1	31	M	4	1	Medulla	15	1
2	35	F	2	4	Medulla	20	2
3	52	F	5	2	Medulla	30	0
4	13	M	5	1	Medulla	20	0
5	35	F	2	3	Medulla	15	0
6	29	F	2	1	Dorsal pons	15	2
7	38	F	4	3	Dorsal pons	30	5
8	61	M	2	3	Dorsal pons	25	0
9	33	F	1	3	Dorsal pons	20	1
10	37	F	3	2	Lateral pons	30	4
11	57	M	3	3	Ventral midbrain	20	3
12	48	M	5	4	Lateral midbrain	10	5
13	26	M	1	2	Lateral midbrain	15	1
14	40	F	4	3	Dorsal pons	30	1
15	29	F	4	4	Dorsal pons	40	1
16	42	M	3	2	Lateral pons	10	1
17	56	F	5	5	Lateral pons	30	2
18	28	M	1	4	Lateral pons	10	1
19	36	M	1	2	Medulla	10	1
20	28	M	2	3	Dorsal pons	30	3
21	39	F	4	3	Lateral pons	15	2
22	51	F	2	3	Dorsal pons	21	1
23	15	M	1	2	Dorsal pons	15	0
24	24	F	1	2	Dorsal pons	20	2
25	44	F	5	3	Medulla	30	3

Table demonstrating the age, sex, mRS scores on admission, number of previous hemorrhages, localization and size of the lesion, and mRS scores at the final follow-up *M* male, *F* female, *C* complete resection, *I* incomplete resection

Among the 33 operations, complete resection was achieved in 24 operations, while 9 operations were judged as incomplete. Recurrent hemorrhage occurred after seven operations, while six occurred after incomplete resections. The frequency of recurrent hemorrhage was significantly higher after incomplete resection than after complete resection ($p = 0.0002$). The mRS scores at the final follow-up after incomplete resection (2.9 ± 1.1) were significantly higher than those after complete resection (1.6 ± 1.3) ($p = 0.01$) (Table 6.2).

Table 6.2 Results of the 33 operations

Operation No.	Case No.	Preop mRS score	Size (mm)	Location	Surgical approach	Complete resection	mRS Score I mo. postop	Postop deterioration of mRS	Recurrent hemorrhage	Duration of follow-up after final op (mos)
1	1	4	15	Medulla	Midline suboccipital	C	3	0	0	156
2	2	2	20	Medulla	Midline suboccipital	C	2	1	1	162
3	3	5	30	Medulla	Midline suboccipital	C	2	0	0	111
4	4	5	20	Medulla	Midline suboccipital	C	2	0	0	65
s	5	2	15	Medulla	Midline suboccipital	C	1	0	0	82
6	6	2	15	Dorsal pons	Midline suboccipital	C	2	0	0	190
7		4	30	Dorsal pons	Midline suboccipital	I	4	0	1	19
8	7	4	30	Dorsal pons	Midline suboccipital	I	4	0	1	22
9		5	30	Dorsal pons	Midline suboccipital	C	5	0	0	152
10	8	2	25	Dorsal pons	Midline suboccipital	C	2	0	0	177
11	9	1	20	Dorsal pons	Midline suboccipital	C	1	0	0	15
12		3	30	Lateral pons	Lateral suboccipital	I	5	1	1	1
13	10	3	30	Lateral pons	Lateral suboccipital	I	5	1	1	1
14		3	30	Lateral pons	Lateral suboccipital	C	5	1	0	143
15	11	3	15	Ventral midbrain	Subtemporal	I	3	0	1	33
16		3	20	Ventral midbrain	Pterional	C	3	0	0	118
17	12	5	10	Lateral midbrain	Subtemporal	I	5	0	1	129

(continued)

Table 6.2 (continued)

Operation No.	Case No.	Preop mRS score	Size (mm)	Location	Surgical approach	Complete resection	mRS Score I mo. postop	Postop deterioration of mRS	Recurrent hemorrhage	Duration of follow-up after final op (mos)
18		5	10	Lateral midbrain	Subtemperal	I	5	0	0	115
19	13	1	15	Lateral midbrain	Occipital transtentorial	C	2	1	0	16
20	14	4	30	Dorsal pons	Midline suboccipital	C	3	0	0	70
21	15	4	40	Dorsal pons	Midline suboccipital	C	3	0	0	63
22	16	3	30	Lateral pons	Midline suboccipital	I	2	0	0	2
23		3	10	Lateral pons	Presigmoid	C	2	0	0	59
24	17	5	30	Lateral pons	Presigmoid	C	3	0	0	2
25		5	30	Lateral pons	Presigmoid	C	3	0	0	50
26	18	1	10	Lateral pons	Presigmoid	C	3	0	0	39
27	19	1	10	Medulla	Midline suboccipital	C	1	0	0	37
28	20	2	30	Dorsal pons	Midline suboccipital	C	2	0	0	33
29	21	4	15	Lateral pons	Lateral suboccipital	C	3	0	0	120
30	22	2	21	Dorsal pons	Midline suboccipital	C	3	1	0	108
31	23	1	15	Dorsal pons	Midline suboccipital	C	1	0	0	30
32	24	1	20	Dorsal pons	Midline suboccipital	I	2	1	0	26
33	25	5	30	Medulla	Midline suboccipital	C	5	1	0	8

Table demonstrating mRS scores on admission, size and localization of the lesion, operative approach, resection rate, mRS scores at 1 month after surgery, postoperative deterioration of mRS scores, subsequent recurrent hemorrhage, and duration of follow-up after the last operation (*C* complete resection, *I* incomplete resection)

6.7 Recovery of Neurological Symptoms

Before performing the 33 operations, motor weakness, sensory disturbance, and cerebellar ataxia were observed in 19, 21, and 18 patients, respectively. At the final follow-up, motor weakness, sensory disturbance, and cerebellar ataxia improved in 6, 8, and 18 patients, respectively. Improvements in sensory disturbances and cerebellar ataxia were significantly more frequent. A variety of cranial nerve symptoms were also observed before surgery, as shown in Table 6.3. Improvement of trigeminal nerve and lower cranial nerve symptoms was significantly more frequent (Table 6.3).

6.8 Representative Cases

6.8.1 Case 1

A 39-year-old woman with CMB in the lateral pons experienced three hemorrhages, which caused cerebellar ataxia and right facial palsy (Fig. 6.1a). Since the pial layer of the middle cerebellar peduncle was the thinnest, we performed surgical resection through lateral suboccipital craniotomy and electrophysiological monitoring of the facial nerve, lower cranial nerves, hypoglossal nerve, auditory evoked potential

Table 6.3 Table demonstrating the preoperative symptoms of motor, sensory, cerebellar, and cranial nerve function and any postoperative changes

	Preoperative symptoms	Postoperative changes				Postop. Improvement
		Improvement	Worsening	Unchanged	Newly	*p* value
Motor weakness	19	6	3	10	0	0.3299
Sensory disturbance	21	8	2	11	0	0.0075*
Cerebellar symptoms	18	10	2	6	1	0.0015*
Cranial nerve symptoms						
Oculomotor	3	0	2	1	3	0.4226
Trochlear	2	0	0	2	1	N.E.
Trigeminal	9	5	3	1	0	0.0509*
Abducence	16	7	2	7	1	0.09616
Facial	21	8	6	7	1	0.8007
Vestibulocochlear	10	5	1	4	1	0.1039
Lower cranial nerves	9	6	1	2	0	0.0593*
Hypoglossal	1	1	0	0	1	N.E.

(ABR), and motor evoked potential (MEP) (Fig. 6.1b). A 5-mm pial incision was made on the lateral pons between the vestibulocochlear nerve and glossopharyngeal nerve (Fig. 6.1c). The CMB was dissected and removed entirely (Fig. 6.1d, e). Postoperative MRI showed complete resection of the CMB (Fig. 6.1f). All symptoms disappeared after surgery.

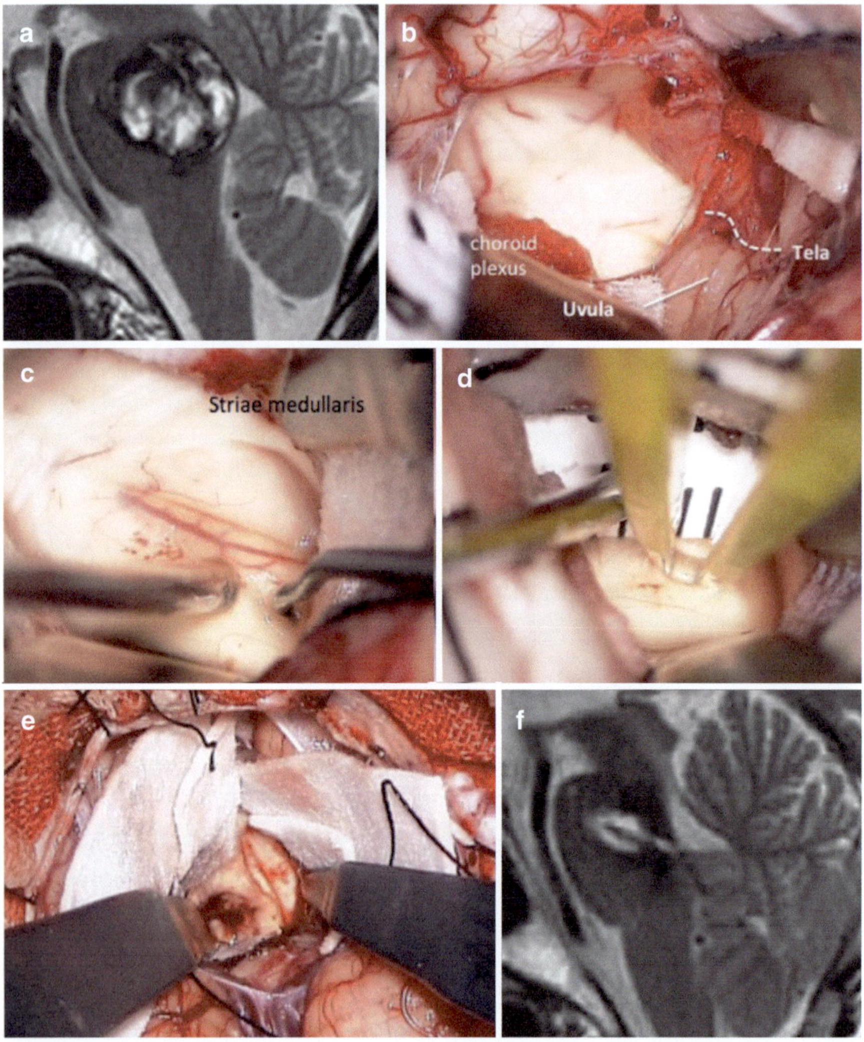

Fig. 6.1 A 39-year-old female with CMB in the lateral pons. (**a**) Preoperative MRI (T2*-weighted image, axial), (**b**) surgery through lateral suboccipital craniotomy, (**c**) 5 mm-long pial incision on the lateral pons between the vestibulocochlear nerve and the glossopharyngeal nerve, (**d**) Entire dissection of CMB, (**e**) Complete resection of CMB, (**f**) Postoperative MRI (T2*-weighted image, axial)

6.8.2 Case 2

A 51-year-old woman with CMB in the dorsal pons experienced three hemorrhages in 2 months, which caused left hemiparesis, left paresthesia, cerebellar ataxia, diplopia, right facial numbness, and right facial palsy (Fig. 6.2a). Since the ependymal layer of the floor of the fourth ventricle was the thinnest, we performed surgical resection through midline suboccipital craniotomy and telovelar approach under electrophysiological monitoring of the abducens nerve, facial nerve, auditory evoked potential (ABR), and sensory evoked potential (SEP) (Fig. 6.2b). After identification of the facial colliculus and the nucleus of the facial nerve by electrical stimulation (Fig. 6.2c), an ependymal incision of 5 mm was made at the right suprafacial triangle (Fig. 6.2d). The CMB was dissected and removed entirely (Fig. 6.2e). Postoperative MRI revealed complete resection of the CMB (Fig. 6.2f). All symptoms disappeared without paresthesia, which was limited to the left forearm.

6.9 Discussion

In our series, the mRS scores at the final follow-up were significantly lower than the mRS scores on admission. The functional outcome of CMB surgery was found to be generally feasible. Favorable outcome at the final follow-up was significantly related to the size of the lesion, preoperative mRS scores, and mRS scores at 1 month after surgery; the mRS score at 1 month after surgery was the most significant factor related to a favorable outcome. Chen LH et al. reported excellent results in 38 consecutive patients receiving CMB surgery under intraoperative neuronavigation and neurophysiological monitoring. Complete resection was achieved in 37 patients, and 94% of the patients showed favorable outcomes. Intraoperative neuronavigation and neurophysiological monitoring seemed to prevent postoperative deterioration, thus leading to favorable outcomes [11]. They also reported newly developing cranial nerve injury in 13, motor weakness in 3, and sensory disturbance in 6 patients. In our series, eight patients had newly developed cranial nerve injury and one patient had cerebellar symptoms. There were no new symptoms of motor weakness or sensory disturbances. Moreover, our study showed that preoperative sensory disturbance, cerebellar ataxia, trigeminal nerve symptoms, and lower cranial nerve symptoms showed significant recovery. Compared to those symptoms, motor weakness, diplopia, and facial nerve palsy seemed to be more difficult to recover.

There were only three patients with midbrain CMB in our series, and oculomotor palsy and abducens were residual in all patients. Tsuji Y et al. reported that the time interval between the onset of symptoms and surgery, age over 40 years, size of CMB over 18 mm, and poor mRS scores at admission are important predictors for persistent oculomotor palsy after surgery of midbrain CMB [13]. de Oliveira JG et al. reported the supracerebellar infratentorial approach to be an alternative approach

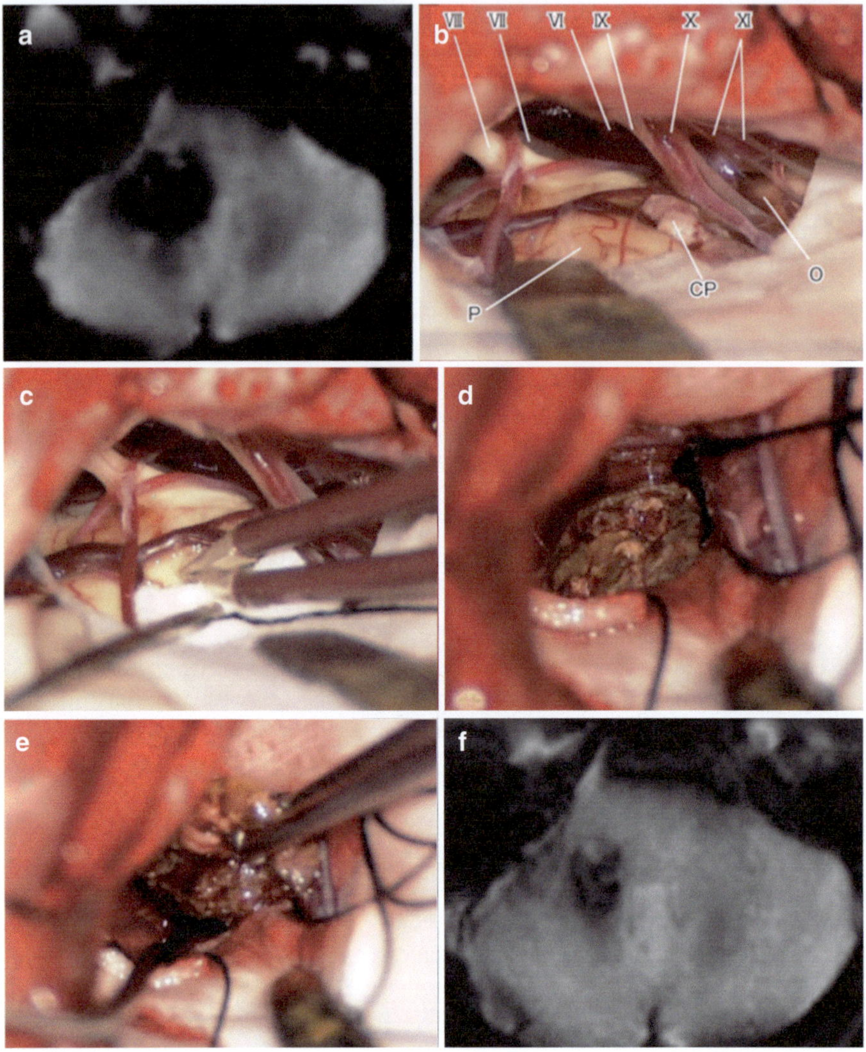

Fig. 6.2 A 51-year-old female with CMB in the dorsal pons. (**a**) Preoperative MRI (T2-weighted image, sagittal), (**b**) Telovelar approach under midline suboccipital craniotomy, (**c**) Electrical stimulation of the right facial nerve, (**d**) 5 mm-long incision of the floor of the fourth ventricle, (**e**) Entire dissection and complete resection of CMB, (**f**) Postoperative MRI (T2-weighted image, sagittal)

for midbrain CMB since it can provide the same or a better outcome in 88% of the patients [14].

Thirteen patients with pontine CMB were operated through the midline suboccipital approach, while eight patients underwent the lateral approach. There was no significant recurrence of postoperative abducens and facial nerve function with the two approaches. However, Bertalanffy et al. recommended the lateral approach when pontine CMB can be operated by either the medial or lateral approach, as the lateral approach is linked to significantly fewer occurrences of postoperative abducens and facial nerve palsies [15].

In our series, complete resection was achieved in 24 operations, while nine operations were incomplete. Recurrent hemorrhage was significantly more common in incomplete resection and was related to significantly higher mRS scores at the final follow-up. As CMB surgery usually involves a small entrance on the pial or ependymal surface, surgeons should attain mass reduction by evacuation of the hematoma first, and then aim to keep the margin of the capsule with meticulous hemostasis and manipulation. As long as surgeons operate on CMB using these principles, complete resection can be achieved in most cases.

6.10 Conclusions

Favorable outcomes of CMB surgery might be related to the achievement of complete resection and mRS at 1 month after surgery. Preoperative sensory, cerebellar, trigeminal nerve, and lower cranial nerve symptoms significantly improve after surgery.

References

1. Porter RW, Detwiler PW, Spetzler RF, Lawton MT, Baskin JJ, Derksen PT, Zabramski JM. Cavernous malformations of the brainstem: experience with 100 patients. J Neurosurg. 1999;90(1):50–8. https://doi.org/10.3171/jns.1999.90.1.0050.
2. Samii M, Eghbal R, Carvalho GA, Matthies C. Surgical management of brainstem cavernomas. J Neurosurg. 2001;95(5):825–32. https://doi.org/10.3171/jns.2001.95.5.0825.
3. Russel DS, Rubinstein LJ. Tumors and hematomas of the blood vessels. In: Russel DS, Rubinstein LJ, editors. The pathology of tumors of the nervous system. London: Arnold; 1959. p. 72–92.
4. Zabramski JM, Henn JS, Coons S. Pathology of cerebral vascular malformations. Neurosurg Clin N Am. 1999;10(3):395–410.
5. Zabramski JM, Wascher TM, Spetzler RF, Johnson B, Golfinos J, Drayer BP, Brown B, Rigamonti D, Brown G. The natural history of familial cavernous malformations: results of an ongoing study. J Neurosurg. 1994;80(3):422–32. https://doi.org/10.3171/jns.1994.80.3.0422.
6. Eisner W, Schmid UD, Reulen HJ, Oeckler R, Olteanu-Nerbe V, Gall C, Kothbauer K. The mapping and continuous monitoring of the intrinsic motor nuclei during brain stem surgery. Neurosurgery. 1995;37(2):255–65. https://doi.org/10.1227/00006123-199508000-00010.
7. Bertalanffy H, Tissira N, Krayenbühl N, Bozinov O, Sarnthein J. Inter- and intrapatient variability of facial nerve response areas in the floor of the fourth ventricle. Neurosurgery. 2011;68(1 Suppl Operative):23–31.; ; discussion 31. https://doi.org/10.1227/NEU.0b013e31820781fb.
8. Sarnthein J, Bozinov O, Melone AG, Bertalanffy H. Motor-evoked potentials (MEP) during brainstem surgery to preserve corticospinal function. Acta Neurochir. 2011;153(9):1753–9. https://doi.org/10.1007/s00701-011-1065-7. Epub 2011 Jun 10

9. Fritschi JA, Reulen HJ, Spetzler RF, Zabramski JM. Cavernous malformations of the brain stem. A review of 139 cases. Acta Neurochir. 1994;130(1–4):35–46. https://doi.org/10.1007/BF01405501.
10. Sandalcioglu IE, Wiedemayer H, Secer S, Asgari S, Stolke D. Surgical removal of brain stem cavernous malformations: surgical indications, technical considerations, and results. J Neurol Neurosurg Psychiatry. 2002;72(3):351–5. https://doi.org/10.1136/jnnp.72.3.351.
11. Chen LH, Zhang HT, Chen L, Liu LX, Xu RX. Minimally invasive resection of brainstem cavernous malformations: surgical approaches and clinical experiences with 38 patients. Clin Neurol Neurosurg. 2014;116:72–9. https://doi.org/10.1016/j.clineuro.2013.10.012. Epub 2013 Oct 31
12. Kikuta K, Nozaki K, Takahashi JA, Miyamoto S, Kikuchi H, Hashimoto N. Postoperative evaluation of microsurgical resection for cavernous malformations of the brainstem. J Neurosurg. 2004;101(4):607–12. https://doi.org/10.3171/jns.2004.101.4.0607.
13. Tsuji Y, Kar S, Bertalanffy H. Microsurgical management of midbrain cavernous malformations: predictors of outcome and lesion classification in 72 patients. Oper Neurosurg (Hagerstown). 2019;17(6):562–72. https://doi.org/10.1093/ons/opz026.
14. de Oliveira JG, Lekovic GP, Safavi-Abbasi S, Reis CV, Hanel RA, Porter RW, Preul MC, Spetzler RF. Supracerebellar infratentorial approach to cavernous malformations of the brainstem: surgical variants and clinical experience with 45 patients. Neurosurgery. 2010;66(2):389–99. https://doi.org/10.1227/01.NEU.0000363702.67016.5D.
15. Bertalanffy H, Ichimura S, Kar S, Tsuji Y, Huang C. Optimal access route for pontine cavernous malformation resection with preservation of abducens and facial nerve function. J Neurosurg. 2020:1–10. https://doi.org/10.3171/2020.7.JNS201023.

Chapter 7
Giant Aneurysm Management

Jianping Song and Ying Mao

7.1 Introduction

Giant intracranial aneurysms (GIAs) are classically defined as aneurysms larger than 25 mm in diameter [1, 2]. These rare intracranial events usually cause hemorrhage, mass effects, or thromboembolism and have a poor prognosis due to their complexity [1, 3–10]. Untreatable GIAs have an 80% risk of severe disability or even death within 5 years [11]. In prospective natural history studies, patients with unruptured, untreated giant aneurysms had a 5-year cumulative hemorrhage rate of 40–50% [12]. These aneurysms are among the most challenging lesions faced by neurosurgeons [13].

GIAs are complex, and they may have wide necks, intraluminal thrombi, perforators, and atherosclerotic/calcified walls. The morphology of GIAs can be saccular, fusiform, serpentine, or dolichoectatic, resulting in various hemodynamic changes and disease courses [1, 2, 10, 14–20]. Although clipping is still the gold standard in intracranial aneurysm treatment by vascular neurosurgeons, the complex nature of GIAs typically makes simple clipping impossible and requires more creative reconstructive or remodeling clipping techniques [1, 21–23]. Unfortunately, the number

J. Song · Y. Mao (✉)
Department of Neurosurgery, Huashan Hospital, Shanghai Medical College, Fudan University, Shanghai, China

Neurosurgical Institute of Fudan University, Shanghai, China

Shanghai Clinical Medical Center of Neurosurgery, Shanghai, China

National Center for Neurological Disorders, Shanghai, China
e-mail: maoying@fudan.edu.cn

Y. Kato, A. Ansari (eds.), *Cerebrovascular Surgery*, Advances and Technical Standards in Neurosurgery 44, https://doi.org/10.1007/978-3-030-87649-4_7

of neurosurgeons who have gained sufficient experience to master the skills required to treat GIAs is shrinking in the era of fast-growing endovascular treatment techniques [24, 25].

Revolutionary flow diverters have led to a paradigm shift in the treatment of GIAs from microsurgery to endovascular treatment, which now dominates the treatment of cavernous sinus (CS) segment and paraclinoidal internal carotid artery (ICA) aneurysms. The off-label use of flow diverters also showed a potential advantage in GIAs located beyond the ICA [13, 25–31]. However, the relatively low complete occlusion rate (≈75% at 6 months), higher recurrence possibility (>10%), potential requirement for lifetime anticoagulation medication, and unpredictable or even fatal complications (overall complication rate ≈10–15%), such as delayed/nonaneurysmal intraparenchymal hemorrhage, perforator occlusion, stroke, in-stent stenosis, and rerupture from endovascular flow diversion treatment, cannot be neglected [13, 21, 25, 26, 28–30, 32–35]. The techniques of the endovascular treatment of GIAs are beyond the scope of this chapter. However, if a previous endovascular therapy fails to occlude a GIA, more vascular neurosurgeons are required for additional surgery [24, 36].

Bypass surgery is still the last resort of vascular neurosurgeons to treat complex GIAs, regardless of the GIA morphology or previous treatment status [8, 23, 37–39]. This state-of-the-art bypass surgery now requires more innovation, creativity, and scientific and clinical evidence to push its boundary to achieve efficient and optimal bypass strategy selection [24]. Therefore, this chapter mainly discusses the standards, advances, and controversies in bypass surgery for GIAs.

7.2 Standards of Treatments

7.2.1 The Classification of Bypass Techniques

From our point of view, there are three primary bypass techniques utilized clinically: extracranial-intracranial (EC-IC) bypass, intracranial-intracranial (IC-IC) bypass, and combined bypass.

EC-IC bypass is the pioneering work of revascularization in the history of microneurosurgery [40]. A large armamentarium of EC-IC bypass strategies has been developed and refined over the past decades and widely adopted by neurosurgeons. EC-IC bypass can mainly be classified as high-flow, intermediate-flow, and low-flow bypass by the different flow rates provided through the donor or graft [41]. Flow matching, either overt or implicit, is a crucial consideration in bypass surgery related to the GIA location, demand in the revascularized territory, and donor caliber [42]. The flow rates in the ICA have been reported to be approximately 200 mL/min, 50–75 mL/min in the proximal middle cerebral artery (MCA), 20 mL/min in the distal MCA, 40 mL/min in the anterior cerebral artery (ACA), 28–33 mL/min in the posterior cerebral artery (PCA), 13 mL/min in the posterior inferior cerebellar artery (PICA), and 10 mL/min in the superior cerebellar artery [42–44]. We

Table 7.1 EC-IC bypass classification by different flow rates and common techniques

Classification	Flow rate (mL/min)	Common techniques
Low-flow	10–40	STA-MCA (usually M4); STA-PCA; OA-PICA
Intermediate-flow	40–100	STA-RA/GSV-MCA (M2 or M3); STA-RA/GSV-ACA; STA-RA/GSV-PCA
High-flow	100–200	ECA-RA/GSV-MCA (M2 or M3)

ECA external cerebral artery, *GSV* great saphenous vein, MCA middle cerebral artery, OA occipital artery, PCA posterior cerebral artery, RA radial artery, STA superficial temporal artery

summarized the most common EC-IC bypass techniques in Table 7.1. The flow rate in low-flow bypass offered by distal STA donors has been variably measured at 10–40 mL/min [42, 45]. Therefore, STA double branch bypass is sometimes performed to increase blood supply if possible. The occipital artery (OA) is also considered an alternative donor for low-flow bypass [46, 47]. Both have the capacity to dilate and increase flow over time (Case 3 [48, 49]). Unlike low-flow bypass, a graft is needed in intermediate-flow and high-flow EC-IC bypass. For intermediate bypass, the STA trunk is the most convenient donor, having a flow rate of approximately 40–100 mL/min [50, 51], and the internal maxillary artery (IMA) provides a similar flow rate of approximately 70–90 mL/min [42, 52, 53]. The donor in high-flow bypass is usually the external carotid artery (ECA). For the graft, the radial artery (RA) and great saphenous vein (GSV) are two primary sources, having flow rates of approximately 100 mL/min and 150 mL/min, respectively [42, 54]. The direction of the valvula venosa should not be neglected when using the GSV as a graft. However, the authors preferred using the RA as the graft artery, considering the significant caliber mismatch and higher GSV stenosis rate. The spasm issue during RA harvesting could be treated by the pressure distension technique [55, 56]. Due to the nature of EC-IC bypass, end-to-side anastomosis is the primary technique for revascularization [40, 42, 45, 50, 51].

Compared with EC-IC bypass, intracranial-intracranial (IC-IC) bypass used to be a challenging technique. Mostly, IC-IC bypass utilizes two vessels close to each other as donors and recipients. Therefore, there is little concern about the mismatch of blood flow and vessel caliber. IC-IC bypass can be classified into four types to meet revascularization requirements in various situations: in situ bypass, reimplantation, reanastomosis, and IC-IC bypass with an interpositional graft (Table 7.2). The technical barriers of IC-IC bypass have been gradually removed with the development of skull base approaches and fine surgical instruments [42, 57]. The authors preferred in situ bypass whenever possible. Among the IC-IC bypasses, side-to-side in situ bypass may have the potential advantage of best flow augmentation to the recipient territory due to the seamless hemodynamics achieved by the parallel donor and recipient vessels and larger stoma than end-to-side or end-to-end anastomosis [42, 57, 58].

The combination of different EC-IC and/or IC-IC bypasses has also been introduced for treating GIAs, especially for GIAs with direct branches or perforators originating from their sac that cannot be sacrificed without sequelae (Case 4). This

Table 7.2 Four IC-IC bypass techniques and examples

Techniques	Anastomosis technique	Examples
Reanastomosis	End-to-end	MCA (M1-M3)-MCA (M1-M3), PCA (P2)-PCA (P3), ACA-ACA, PICA-PICA
Reimplantation	End-to-side	PICA (P1)-VA (V4), MCA (M2)-MCA (M2), MCA (M3)-MCA (M3), ACA (A4)-ACA (A4)
In situ bypass	Side-to-side	MCA (M2)-MCA (M2), MCA (M3)-MCA (M3), PCA (P2)-SCA (S1), ACA (A4)-ACA (A4)
Bypass with an interpositional graft	End-to-end or end-to-side	ACA (A2)-RA-ACA (A4), ACA(A1)-RA-MCA (M2), MCA (M1)-RA-MCA (M2), VA (V3)-RA-PICA (P3)[a]

[a]Mostly classified as an IC-IC bypass, although V3 is the extracranial segment of the vertebral artery (VA)

kind of GIA requires comprehensive hemodynamic evaluation and maximal surgeon creativity. Tailored revascularization methods should be designed for each case [10, 38, 39, 56, 59–61].

7.2.2 *The Common Hemodynamic Assessment Technique*

1. *Balloon occlusion test (BOT)*

   GIAs may exhibit very different hemodynamics among different individuals, even at the same location. Therefore, a careful assessment of each case is required before and during treatment to develop the surgical strategy. The need for bypass surgery can be evaluated by temporary occlusion of the parent artery to determine the tolerance of its temporary or even permanent sacrifice. However, currently, there is not a single well-accepted standard. The most commonly used technique was the BOT (mostly 30 min) +/− pressure drop test [46, 62–68], which provides valuable information about the adequacy of collateral flow across the circle of Willis by angiography evaluation and neurological function examination. Other radiological assessments, including single-photon emission computed tomography (SPECT), positron emission tomography (PET), computed tomography perfusion imaging (CTP), and xenon-enhanced CT (xenon-CT), can be combined for a more accurate evaluation of the cerebrovascular reserve capacity [62–65, 68–77]. A modernized digital subtraction angiography (DSA) system is equipped with an advanced algorithm for angiography perfusion analysis [64, 70]. Complications arise from BOT itself in 0–8.3% of cases [78]. Nevertheless, BOT is a near-standard hemodynamic evaluation tool for complex ICA aneurysms and is well acknowledged in the neurosurgical community [46, 62–68]. BOT can also be applied in MCA or vertebrobasilar artery GIAs if a bypass is planned [79–83].
2. *Indocyanine Green Video Angiography (ICGVA) and Microvascular Doppler Ultrasonography (MDU)*

ICGVA and MDU are the two most commonly used noninvasive intraoperative flow evaluation modalities. ICGVA is the ideal alternative procedure for intracranial aneurysm surgery other than DSA. ICGVA can be applied to inspect aneurysm remnants, parent arteries, and perforators intraoperatively, with an 86–100% accordance rate compared to postoperative DSA [84–95]. In most cases, the discordance rate was considered insignificant. Aneurysm remnants are the main reason for most repositioned cases [84, 89, 94]. MDU is also an effective method to evaluate blood flow intraoperatively and is notable because it is inexpensive, noninvasive, and easy to learn. The strengths of MDU are speed and high availability, making it easy to apply even in primary hospitals. The reported sensitivity of MDU in aneurysm surgeries was 98–100% [96–101]. However, MDU application is easily affected by the detection angle and depth, and it is difficult to detect the back of the aneurysm [99, 102].

In addition, ICGVA-based techniques, such as flash fluorescence (direct and indirect), delayed fluorescence, or initial fluorescence, can provide quick, precise, reliable localization of an appropriate recipient artery for bypass when revascularization is needed [103, 104].

3. *Intraoperative Neurophysiologic Monitoring (IONM)*

   Motor evoked potentials (MEPs) and somatosensory evoked potentials (SSEPs) are the most widely used IONM methods in intracranial aneurysm surgery. SSEPs primarily evaluate the sensory system, but false positive and negative predictive values are high when evaluating the motor system. MEP monitoring, including transcranial and direct types, uses electrical stimulations targeted at the primary motor cortex to produce depolarized action potentials recorded along corticospinal tracts [81, 105–110]. Although there are no randomized, blinded, or prospective clinical studies on this subject, MEPs seem to be more sensitive than SEPs for warning of insufficient blood flow. MEPs can detect subcortical ischemia or infarction during the operation in less than 1 min, especially pure motor deficits caused by perforating arteries or large branches [81, 105–109]. Hence, MEPs may be a more sensitive method than SEPs for advanced warning of cerebral ischemia during GIA surgery [109]. Based on an MEP amplitude decrement of >50% (Stage 1, Case 4) or loss (Stage 2), a 2-stage warning criterion of MEP changes was advocated. The stage 1 warning was more sensitive to radiologic abnormalities, whereas the stage 2 warning better predicted motor status decline. Both wave loss and > 50% amplitude decrement of MEP monitoring showed good predictive value when used as part of a 2-stage warning criterion [81, 110].

7.2.3 Bypass Strategy for GIAs Located at Different Locations

GIAs mostly occur in the anterior circulations. For ICA GIAs, patients who did not tolerate the 30-minute BOT underwent ICA sacrifice (proximal occlusion) and high-flow ECA-RA-MCA flow-replacement bypass. For the patients who passed the 30-min BOT without developing neurologic deficits, additional capillary phase analysis and CTP scan were applied. If less than a 0.5-s delay during the capillary phase in the ipsilateral hemisphere on contralateral ICA angiography was detected, as well as no manifestations of hypoperfusion on CTP, the patients were likely to tolerate direct ICA sacrifice without EC-IC bypass. Otherwise, an STA-RA-MCA flow-replacement bypass combined with ICA sacrifice was considered (Case 1). GIA trapping was performed if retrograde filling of the aneurysm was detected during BOT or after ICA sacrifice (Fig. 7.1) [68, 109].

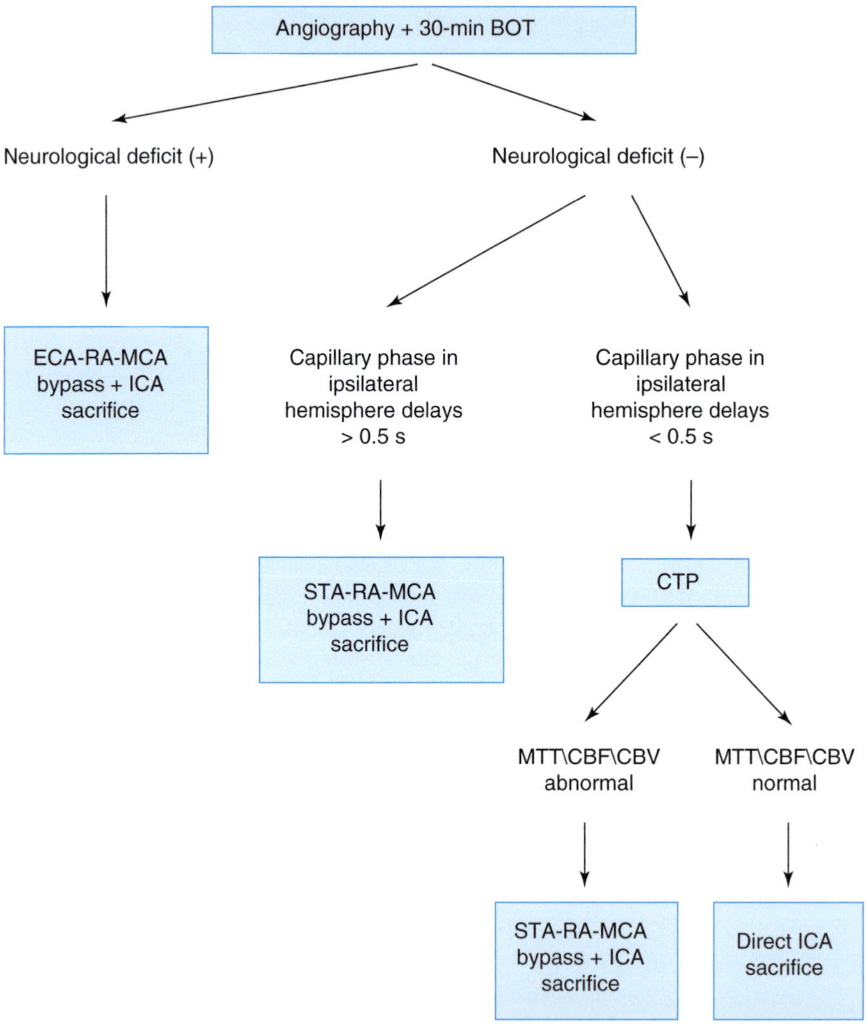

Fig. 7.1 Management algorithm for complex ICA aneurysms (Reproduced from: Zhu W, Tian Y, Zhou L, Song D, Xu B, Mao Y. Treatment Strategies for Complex Internal Carotid Artery (ICA) Aneurysms: Direct ICA Sacrifice or Combined with Extracranial-to-Intracranial Bypass. World Neurosurg. 2011; 75(3–4): 476–84)

For MCA GIAs, the surgical strategy was determined by angioarchitecture, and IONM is an essential safeguard for MCA GIA procedures. M1 aneurysms involving important perforating branches, such as lenticulostriate arteries (LSAs), usually cannot be clipped directly. In a patient with a positive BOT in the M1 segment, ECA-RA-MCA or STA-RA-MCA flow-reversal bypass can be combined with ipsilateral ICA occlusion (proximal trapping). The gradual intraaneurysm blood flow decrement is beneficial for promoting ischemic tolerance in the LSA supply areas and collateral LSA circulation. Early thrombosis development in the GIAs and the gradual intraaneurysm blood flow decrement will also lead to complete thrombosis of the M1 GIAs in most cases (Case 2) [61]. IC-IC in situ bypass and intermediate-flow EC-IC bypass (STA-RA-M3) with aneurysm trapping can be used to treat M2 segment (including M2 bifurcation) GIAs. Direct trapping of the aneurysmal parent arteries (except the central artery or the artery of the angular gyrus) can be performed in most GIAs beyond the M3 segment, and bypass can be performed under IONM guidance if necessary (Fig. 7.2) [61, 111]. A protective STA-MCA bypass can be applied if more prolonged temporary parent artery occlusion is needed for reconstructive clipping in particular MCA GIA cases [5].

Most anterior communicating artery (AcomA) aneurysms can be clipped directly or reconstructively. A tailored approach needs to be designed on a case-by-case basis for ACA GIAs. Bypass surgery is mainly applied in cases where A2 occlusion is required. EC-IC bypass can be performed with relatively easy access [112]. However, side-to-side A2-A2 or A3-A3 anastomoses are the primary techniques in most cases [113–115].

Posterior circulation GIAs are much rarer than anterior circulation GIAs. To date, there is no well-established bypass strategy for posterior circulation GIAs. Bypass surgery applied for posterior circulation GIA treatment includes EC-IC (mostly OA-PICA or STA-PCA bypass) and IC-IC bypass (such as PICA-PICA and PCA-SCA side-to-side bypass, PICA-VA reimplantation). A high degree of surgical skills is required for these procedures because the operating sites of the posterior circulation aneurysm are close to important tissues and the operating space is limited. Among GIAs, the basilar trunk GIA, which is usually fusiform or dolichoectatic, poses a unique, complicated entity for surgical treatment due to its deep location, nonsaccular morphology, and brainstem perforator involvement [11, 19, 116]. Bypass surgery combined with proximal or distal occlusion is the primary treatment modality, followed by active anticoagulant therapy to prevent acute thrombosis formation, which can result in unwanted perforator occlusion. Several reports have described bypass techniques using the PCA as the recipient, such as OA-PCA, STA-PCA, ECA-RA-PCA, or MCA-PCA, based on a case-by-case analysis. The surgical outcome is still unsatisfactory, with surgical and final mortality rates of 50% to 60%, respectively [11, 19, 116, 117].

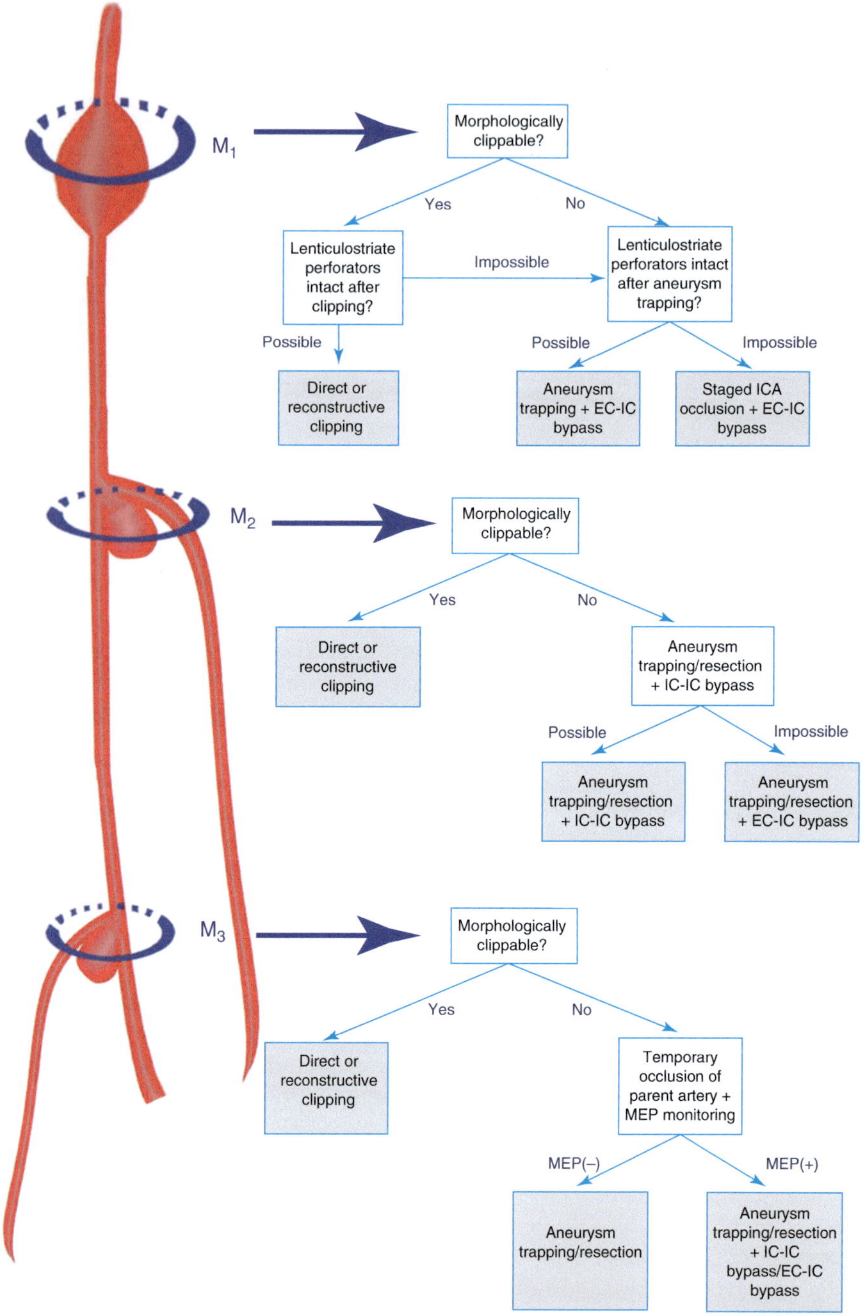

Fig. 7.2 The algorithm of our surgical strategies for treating complex MCA aneurysms (Reproduced from: Zhu W, Liu P, Tian Y, Gu Y, Xu B, Chen L, Zhou L, Mao Y. Complex middle cerebral artery aneurysms: a new classification based on the angioarchitecture and surgical strategies. Acta Neurochir. 2013; 155(8): 1481–91)

7.3 Case Illustration

Case 1 A 58-year-old man was admitted with a 3-month history of headache. Head MRI revealed multiple, partially thrombosed, giant aneurysms on both sides of the parasellar region (Fig. 7.3a). Cerebral DSA revealed a partially thrombosed GIA arising from the right intracavernous ICA. The left ICA occluded spontaneously, so the left ICA aneurysm was thrombosed completely (Fig. 7.3b, c). The blood supply to both hemispheres was mainly from the right ICA. Therefore, a bilateral STA-RA-MCA bypass was planned before occluding the right ICA. The patient initially underwent a left STA-RA-M2 bypass. Two weeks later, a right STA-RA-M2 bypass was performed, followed by prolonged cervical ICA occlusion (Fig. 7.3d–i). After completely occluding the right ICA, cerebral DSA confirmed that the graft was patent on both sides, but a slight narrowing of the left RA graft had caused the left MCA to be filled by the left STA through the RA graft and the right STA through the AComA (Fig. 7.3j–n). The patient showed no significant postoperative neurologic signs except for slight right oculomotor nerve palsy, which resolved entirely 3 months later.

Case 2
A 56-year-old man presented with a headache and aphasia that had persisted for 3 h. A CT scan in a local hospital showed a giant lesion in the left frontal lobe. After the lesion had been diagnosed as a giant unruptured and thrombotic MCA aneurysm, it was partially coiled (Fig. 7.4a, b). The patient was then transferred to our department. DSA revealed a giant serpentine aneurysm originating from the M1 segment, and direct clipping or further endovascular treatment was impossible (Fig. 7.4c–e). Furthermore, sacrifice of the LSA perforators would have been unavoidable if we had trapped the aneurysm. Therefore, a left STA-RA-M3 bypass followed by a staged left cervical ICA occlusion was performed; the ICA was finally occluded after 7 days (Fig. 7.4f, g). Postoperative DSA demonstrated that the aneurysm was completely obliterated, the ICA was sacrificed, and a bypass graft from the STA supplied the MCA territory (Fig. 7.4h, k). The patient did not present with any neurological deficits at the 3-month and 2-year follow-up appointments.

Case 3
A 58-year-old female underwent left STA-MCA double bypass 18 years ago due to transient cerebral ischemia and headache. At that time, DSA revealed a giant left serpentine aneurysm (Fig. 7.5a, b). During the surgery, a sizeable frontotemporal craniotomy was performed, and both frontal and parietal branches of the STA were harvested. Postoperative DSA showed the disappearance of the aneurysm and patent bypasses. Therefore, we did not perform an additional proximal occlusion by coiling. The patient recovered well without neurological deficits. The 2-year follow-up revealed a small recurrence at the proximal end of the aneurysm (Fig. 7.5c, d). The patient experienced several transient ischemic syndromes and was treated conservatively. Although the STA frontal branch-MCA bypass degenerated, the yearly follow-up DSA showed a dilated STA parietal branch-MCA bypass and reduced

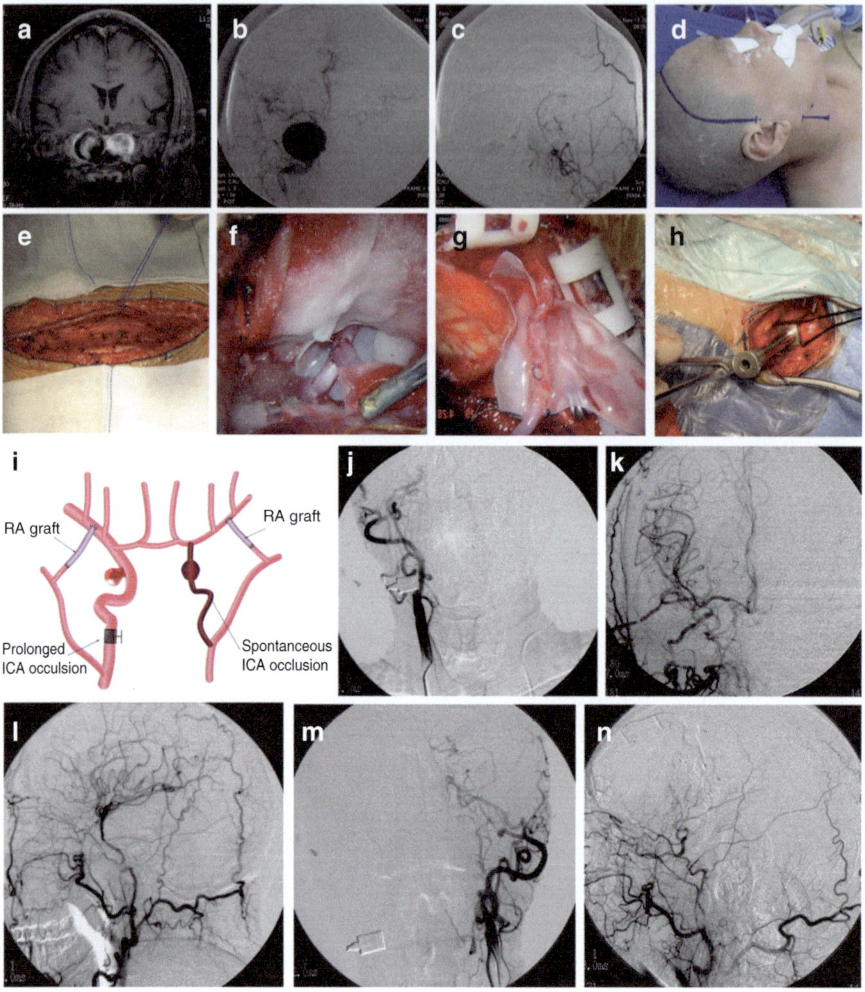

Fig. 7.3 (**a**) MRI depicted a mass lesion on the bilateral parasellar regions, indicating partially thrombosed giant aneurysms. (**b**, **c**) Cerebral DSA revealed a right ICA GIA (**b**) and spontaneous occlusion of the left ICA (**c**). (**d**) Skin incisions. (**e**) Patient position for RA graft harvesting procedure. (**f**) RA-MCA end-to-side anastomosis. (**g**) RA-STA end-to-end anastomosis. (**h**) Prolonged ICA occlusion. (**i**) Illustration showing bilateral STA-RA-MCA bypasses and prolonged right ICA occlusion. (**j**–**l**) A postoperative right common carotid artery DSA demonstrated that the right ICA GIA was occluded (**j**) and that the right RA graft was patent (**k**, **l**). (**m**, **n**) Postoperative left common carotid artery angiogram demonstrated the patency of the left RA graft (Reproduced from: Zhu W, Tian YL, Zhou LF, Song DL, Xu B, Mao Y. Treatment strategies for complex internal carotid artery (ICA) aneurysms: direct ICA sacrifice or combined with extracranial-to-intracranial bypass. World Neurosurg. 2011;75:476–84)

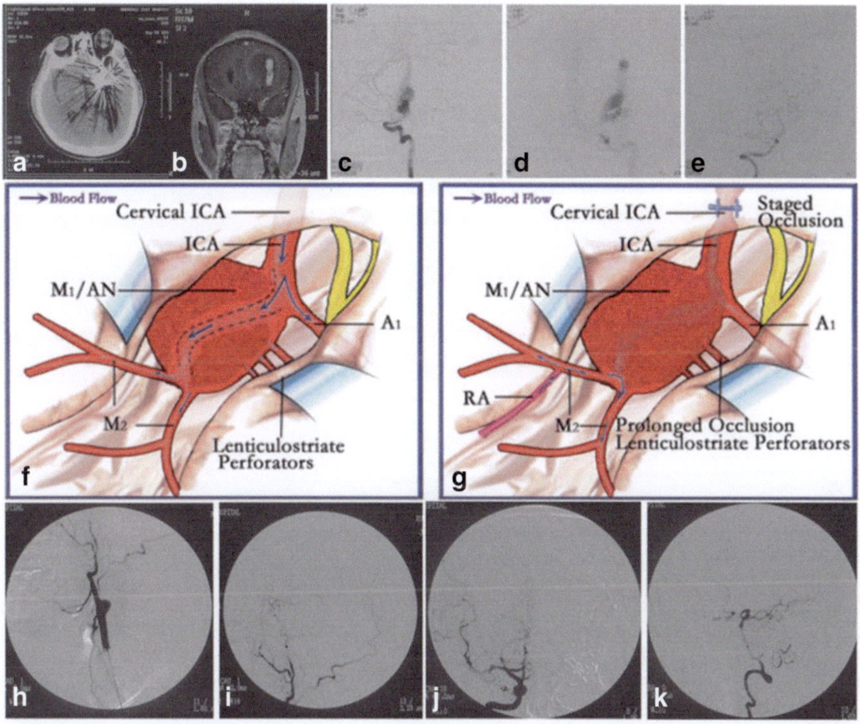

Fig. 7.4 (**a**) CT showed a partially coiled giant aneurysm in a 56-year-old man. (**b**) The MRI revealed a giant serpentine aneurysm. (**c–e**) DSA confirmed that the aneurysm originated from the left M1 segment. (**f, g**) The diagram shows the surgical procedure. Intraoperative findings showed that LSA perforators were involved. The cervical ICA was sacrificed via staged occlusion after a left STA-RA-M3 bypass. The aneurysm was obliterated after complete intraluminal thrombosis, and an STA-RA-M3 bypass supplied the blood flow in the MCA territory. The LSA perforators were occluded in a prolonged fashion. (**h–k**) Postoperative DSA demonstrated the obliteration of the aneurysm. (**h**) Right ICA angiogram. (**i**) The left angiogram showed occlusion of the left ICA. (**j**) A left CCA angiogram showed that the left MCA territory was supplied by STA-RA-M3 bypass. (**k**) Left VA angiogram (Modified from: Zhu W, Liu P, Tian Y, Gu Y, Xu B, Chen L, Zhou L, Mao Y. Complex middle cerebral artery aneurysms: a new classification based on the angioarchitecture and surgical strategies. Acta Neurochir. 2013; 155(8): 1481–91)

recurrent aneurysm without ischemic syndromes. The 13-year follow-up DSA (Fig. 7.5e, f) showed well-developed collateral vessels supplied by the bypasses. Recently, the 18-year follow-up DSA showed occlusion of the GIAs and complete replacement of the blood flow supply beyond the GIAs by double STA bypasses (Fig. 7.5g, h).

Case 4

A 53-year-old man was admitted to our hospital with an intermittent headache. The imaging studies demonstrated a giant M1 thrombotic Sup-C aneurysm (Fig. 7.6a–d). A left pterion craniotomy was performed, and the parietal branch of the STA was preserved. Because of the M1-M2 bifurcation involvement in this patient, we chose

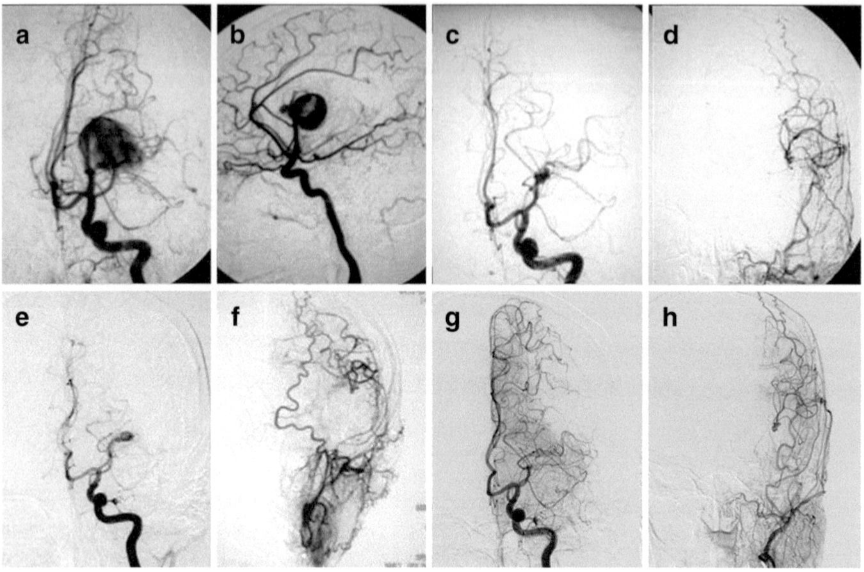

Fig. 7.5 (**a**, **b**) DSA 18 years ago revealed a giant left serpentine aneurysm. (**c, d**) The 2-year follow-up showed a small recurrence in the proximal end of the aneurysm. (**e**, **f**) The 13-year follow-up DSA showed reduced recurrent aneurysm and well-developed collateral vessels supplied by the bypasses. (**g**, **h**) The 18-year follow-up DSA showed occlusion of the GIAs and complete replacement of the blood flow supply beyond the GIAs by double STA bypasses

an aneurysm resection strategy followed by combination bypass, including STA parietal branch-M2 inferior branch anastomosis with M1-M2 superior branch reanastomosis, to reconstruct the bifurcation (Fig. 7.6e–g). The intraoperative MEP signal from the right limbs was attenuated >80% after the aneurysm had been resected but recovered 60% after the bifurcation had been reconstructed (Stage 1 warning). The final MEP results showed a 20% decrease compared with the baseline. The patient was neurologically intact after surgery. A follow-up angiogram at 10 months demonstrated the obliteration of the aneurysm and patency of both stomas (Fig. 7.6h, i).

7.4 Advances

7.4.1 Noninvasive Optimal Vessel Analysis (NOVA)

A common issue in bypass surgery is precisely evaluating the blood flow volume of the donor, recipient, graft, and planned occluded parent vessels. This information may be critical for choosing a bypass technique and ensuring effectiveness. Amin-Hanjani and Charbel et al. applied the MRI NOVA technique to quantitatively analyze the blood vessels' flow rate in bypass surgery [118]. Theoretically, the

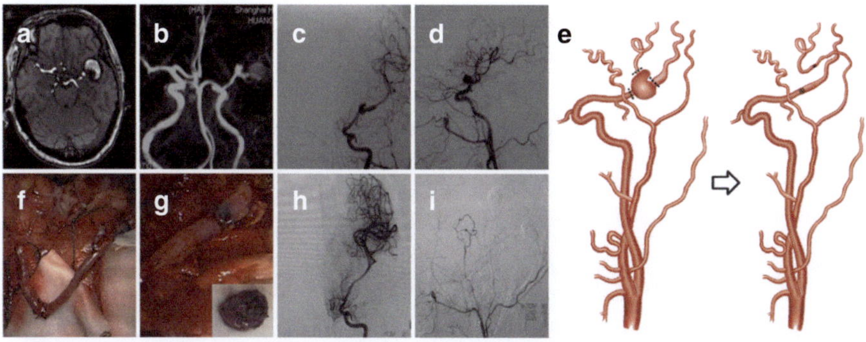

Fig. 7.6 (**a–d**) Imaging studies demonstrating a giant M1 thrombotic aneurysm originating from the superior wall distal to LSAs. (**e**) Diagram showing the intraoperative procedure. (**f, g**) Intraoperative photographs showing aneurysm resection, followed by combination bypass, including superficial temporal artery parietal branch-M2 inferior branch anastomosis with M1-M2 superior branch reanastomosis. (**h, i**) Follow-up angiograms showing total obliteration of the aneurysm and continued patency of the bypass (Reproduced from: Ni W, Yang H, Xu B, Xu F, Jiang H, Lei Y, et al. Proximal Middle Cerebral Artery Aneurysms: Microsurgical Management and Therapeutic Results. World Neurosurg. 2019;122:e907-e16)

appropriate type of bypass technique can be determined based on the measured flow rates. However, after bypass surgery, blood flow changes are based on remodeling in the vascular network's overall hemodynamics rather than the flow of a single artery. Thus, it is still necessary to perform brain metabolism and functional assessments. The evaluation scheme of NOVA needs to be further improved in future research. An example of NOVA is illustrated in Fig. 7.7 for Case 3 at the 13-year follow-up. The majority of the blood flow of the STA went through the bypass to supply the revascularized territory.

7.4.2 High-Resolution Vessel Wall MRI (HR-VW MRI)

Atherosclerosis of an intracranial aneurysm wall is a major surgical challenge. First, atherosclerosis may prevent the full closure of the aneurysm clip and result in incomplete obliteration because of plaque formation. Moreover, plaques often break off after clipping, leading to ischemic events and eventual infarction. A recent prospective study showed that ischemic events discovered on diffusion-weighted imaging (DWI) occurred among 71% of patients post-clipping [119]. Therefore, preoperative assessment of the aneurysmal wall structure is of great importance in surgical planning.

3.0 T high-resolution HR-VW MRI, acquired using a 3D CUBE T1WI sequence, is promising for the screening of regional intracranial vessel wall inflammation reactions or atherosclerosis, including intracranial aneurysms [120]. Aneurysm wall enhancement is determined by comparing Gd-enhanced images with nonenhanced images. The wall enhancement features on Gd-enhanced images are classified as

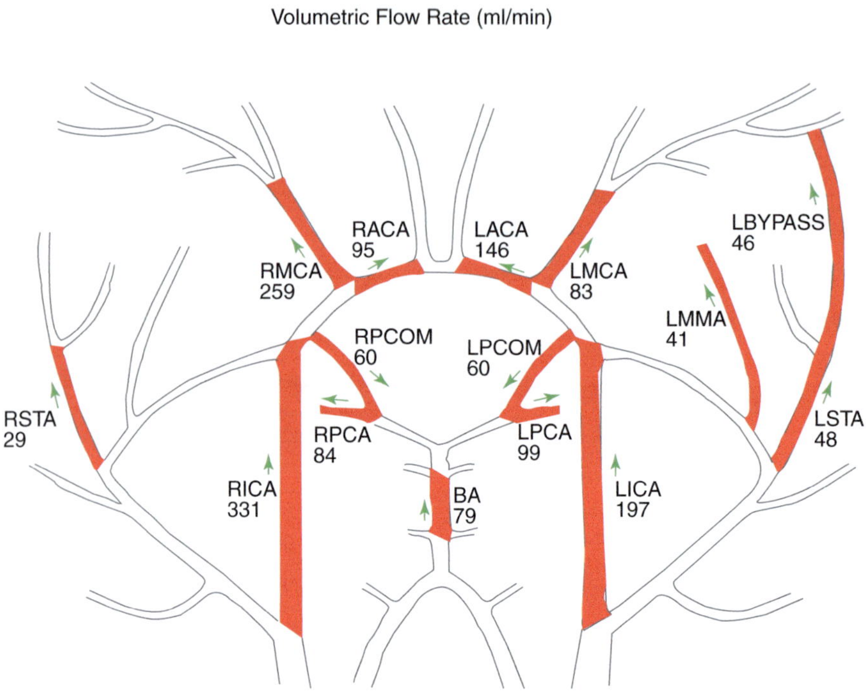

Fig. 7.7 The NOVA analysis for Case 3 at 13-year follow-up

follows: negative (no wall enhancement), uniform wall enhancement (UWE; the whole wall was homogeneously enhanced), or focal wall enhancement (FWE; part of the wall was strongly enhanced, and the rest was minimally or not enhanced).

First, we confirmed that wall enhancement (both UWE and FWE) strongly indicated inflammatory infiltration of the UIA wall because it was significantly correlated with high expression of inflammatory markers. Similarly, we found wall enhancement to be significantly related to irregular shape and large size, suggesting active UIA wall remodeling and unstable wall structure [121]. Second, we verified that FWE was a promising radiological biomarker for atherosclerotic plaques in UIAs. The potential reason for this may be that atherosclerosis after the initial inflammatory reaction leads to hypoxia, followed by denser and deeper extension into the UIA wall of pre-existing vasa vasorum caused by proliferating neovascularization, resulting in much stronger FWE [122]. Therefore, in the case of FWE, prominent atherosclerotic plaques may exist, and there may be a higher risk of postoperative ischemic events caused by plaque breakdown. Moreover, direct clipping may be inapplicable in cases of FWE; thus, bypass surgery or endovascular treatment should be applied. Unlike FWE, UWE may indicate rich vasa vasorum but fewer atherosclerotic plaques (Case 5).

7.4.3 The Hybrid Operating Room

The modern hybrid operation room was first used to treat congenital heart disease in the early twenty-first century. In 2011, Murayama et al. applied a hybrid operating room to diagnose and treat neurosurgical diseases [123]. The development of a modern hybrid operating room may provide an immediate cure for complex cerebrovascular disease by combining endovascular and microsurgical techniques in a single procedure and in a multidisciplinary environment. The hybrid treatment concept not only is simple for providing preoperative/intraoperative embolization and intraoperative angiography to assist surgery but also allows comprehensive integration of functional brain imaging, navigation techniques, and cerebral hemodynamic and neurophysiological monitoring techniques. The hybrid treatment concept relies on the best evidence-driven perioperative medical care offered by physicians' close teamwork in neurosurgery, neurointervention, neuroanesthesia, neuroelectrophysiology, and neuroradiology to render the hybrid operation room a genuinely safe and efficient surgical platform for treating cerebrovascular disease [124]. In Case 5, we illustrated a case of complicated ICA GIA treated by multiple procedures.

7.5 Case Illustration

Case 5
A 17-year-old female presented with impaired visual acuity in the left eye that had persisted for 1 year. The physical examination showed blindness of the left eye without other neurological deficits. The preoperative CT and MRI showed a right sellar region lesion with a flow void sign inside and UWE (Fig. 7.8a–f). A GIA at the ophthalmic segment of the left ICA was identified by DSA (Fig. 7.8g–i). Considering the patient's young age, we performed open surgery to secure the aneurysm by clipping in the hybrid operating room. Intraoperatively, we observed rich vasa vasorum on the aneurysmal wall without apparent atherosclerosis (Fig. 7.8j). The optic nerve was heavily compressed by the GIA (Fig. 7.8k). A left anterior clinoid process resection was performed using an ultrasound curet (Fig. 7.8l). We temporarily clipped the posterior communicating artery (PComA, Fig. 7.8m), and a balloon-assisted retrograde suction decompression technique was applied (Fig. 7.8n, o). The GIA was decompressed and dissected from the optic nerve and dura adhesion (Fig. 7.8p). Two long permanent clips were placed to secure the neck (Fig. 7.8q). Intraoperative DSA showed satisfactory clipping results (Fig. 7.8r).

However, the 6-month follow-up DSA revealed recurrence of the GIA (Fig. 7.9a, b). The patient was treated by coiling (Fig. 7.9c, d). One year later, DSA showed a relapse of the GIA (Fig. 7.10a, b). We then performed an ECA-RA-MCA bypass and proximal ICA occlusion for this patient in the hybrid operating room (Fig. 7.10c). However, intraoperative DSA showed backflow from the PComA (Fig. 7.10d). Therefore, several coils were placed in the left PComA to block the backflow

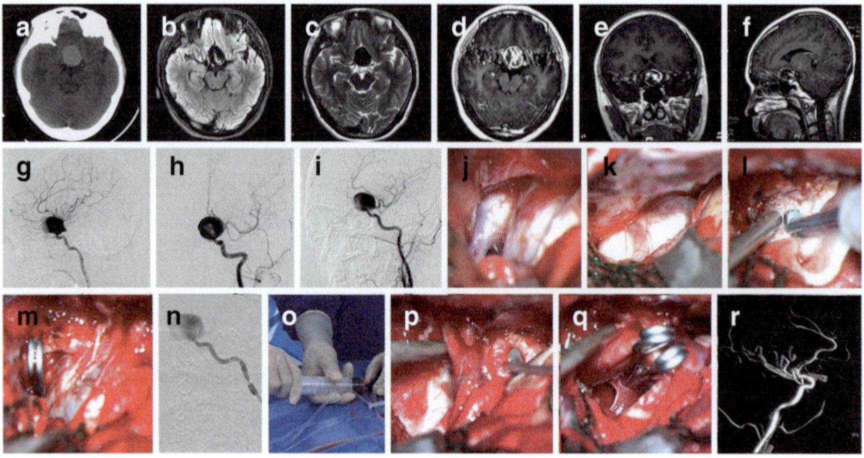

Fig. 7.8 (**a–c**) The preoperative CT and MRI showed a right seller region lesion with a flow void sign inside. (**d–f**) The wall enhancement of the GIA was relatively uniform. (**g–i**) DSA diagnosed a GIA at the ophthalmic segment of the left ICA. (**j**) Rich vasa vasorum without apparent atherosclerosis could be found on the aneurysmal wall. (**k**) The optic nerve was heavily compressed by the GIA. (**l**) A left anterior clinoid process resection was performed using an ultrasound curet. (**m**) We temporarily clipped the PComA. (**n, o**) The balloon-assisted retrograde suction decompression technique was applied. (**p**) The GIA was decompressed and dissected from the optic nerve and dura adhesion. (**q**) Two long permeant clips were placed to secure the neck. (**r**) Intraoperative DSA showed satisfactory clipping results

(Fig. 7.10e). The GIA was finally cured with bypass and did not recur at the 1-year follow-up (Fig. 7.10f).

7.6 Controversies

There is beauty in simplicity. We advocated using the fewest procedures to cure GIAs to minimize the treatment burden of the patient. Therefore, as we suggested in the bypass strategy, preoperative imaging and hemodynamic evaluation, and comprehensive application of intraoperative monitoring techniques, are essential in every case. Temporary occlusion is necessary during the clipping and bypass procedures. The collateral circulation and tolerance of ischemia while the parent is temporarily occluded is usually evaluated according to preoperative BOT. Under general anesthesia, however, these preoperative analyses may be unreliable because the anesthetized brain's metabolic demand is less than that of the awake brain. MEP monitoring may be useful for identifying a safe time window for prolonged temporary occlusion during GIA clipping surgery, thereby avoiding unnecessary bypass [81, 109]. This technique can be used to identify patients who may endure prolonged temporary occlusion so reconstructive clipping can be performed under general anesthesia without bypass (Fig. 7.11). MEP monitoring may also be used to

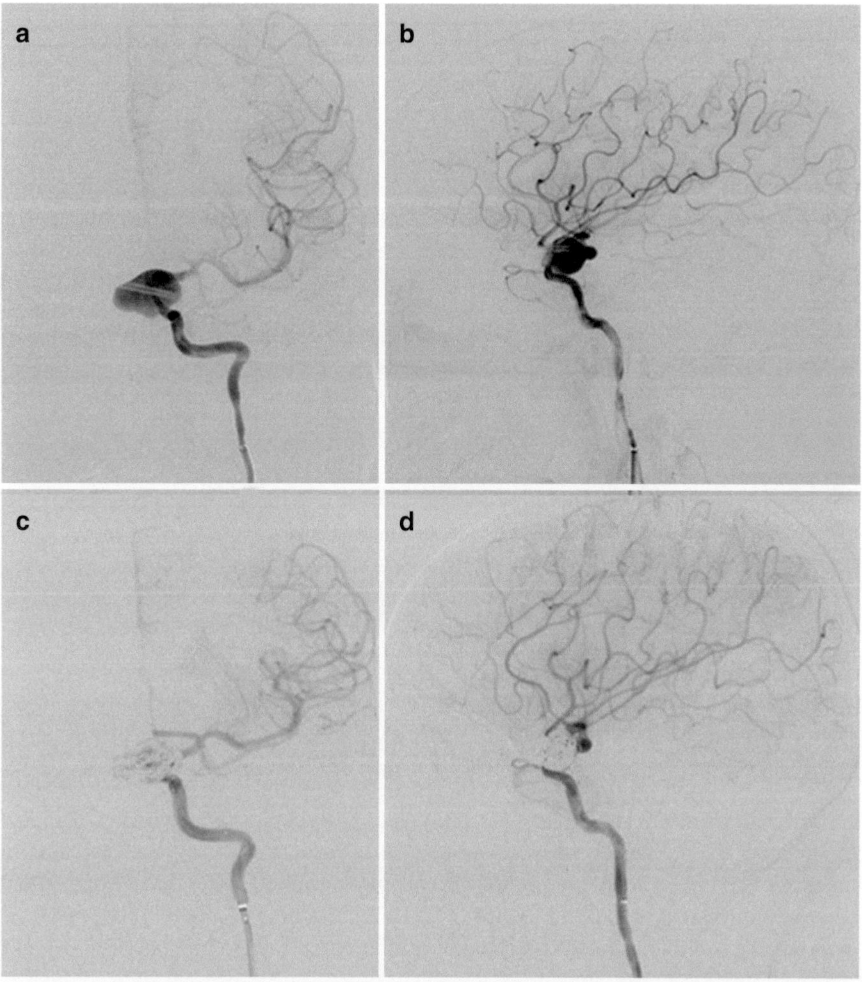

Fig. 7.9 (**a**, **b**) The 6-month follow-up DSA showed a recurrence of the GIA. (**c**, **d**) The patient was then treated by coiling

evaluate the therapeutic effect of bypass surgery. A significant decrease in or permanent disappearance of MEPs may indicate an immediate postoperative motor deficiency, whereas MEPs' recovery after opening the bypass may indicate a good outcome (Fig. 7.12) [50, 81, 109]. With the advancement of HR-VW MRI and hybrid operating rooms, we can apply this strategy to simplify the surgical procedure with more confidence (Case 6). Although still controversial, partial trapping with distal outflow occlusion after flow-replacement bypass for treating complex intracranial aneurysms represents a useful strategy as a last resort measure, especially in MCA and PICA aneurysms [125].

Additionally, the reshuffling of the conventional combinations of anastomoses and suturing techniques has led to the invention of more creative and efficient

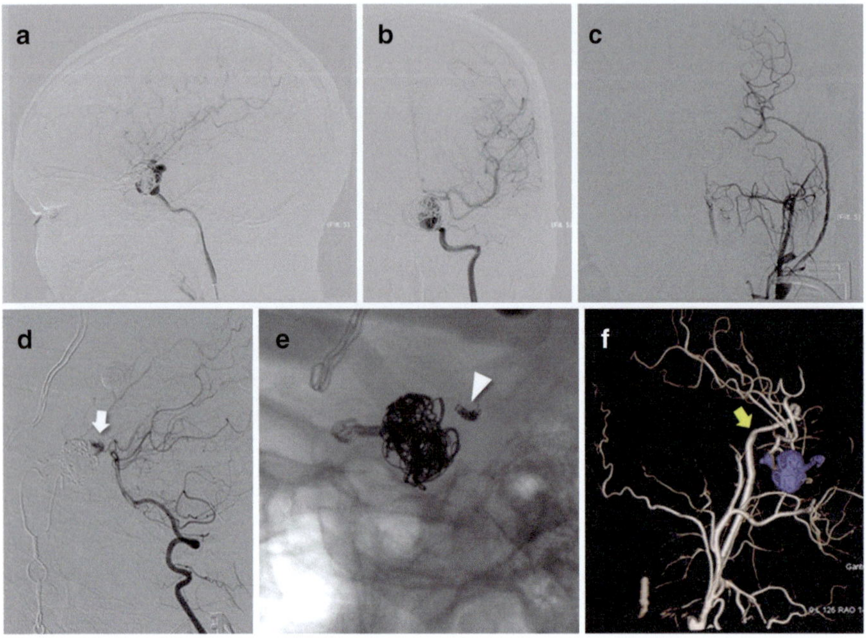

Fig. 7.10 (**a**, **b**) One year later, DSA showed a relapse of the GIA. (**c**) ECA-RA-MCA bypass and proximal ICA occlusion were performed for this patient. (**d**) Intraoperative DSA showed backflow (*white arrow*) from the PComA. (**e**) Several coils (*white arrowhead*) were placed in the left PComA to block the backflow. (**f**) The GIA was finally cured with bypass (*yellow arrow*)

bypass techniques, the so-called fourth generation bypasses, for repairing complex lesions that cannot be otherwise managed [24]. For example, by creating the so-called middle communicating artery, we can cure complex MCA aneurysms with a minimal ischemic period (Case 7) [24, 126, 127]. Although computer hemodynamic analysis is a promising technique for predicting complex cerebral vascular disease treatment modalities and outcomes, a viable product for performing such analysis is still lacking [48, 49]. We believe that, in the near future, with the development of cloud-based supercomputing technology, real-time computer hemodynamic analysis techniques for clinical application to improve GIA surgery safety might become available.

7.7 Case Illustration

Case 6

A 53-year-old female was found to have a right MCA GIA 4 years prior, which was enlarged at follow-up. Preoperative MRA and DSA showed a right MCA giant serpentine aneurysm (Fig. 7.13a–c). The preoperative HR-VW MRI showed narrow flow channels surrounded by thrombosis. The enhancement wall of the aneurysm

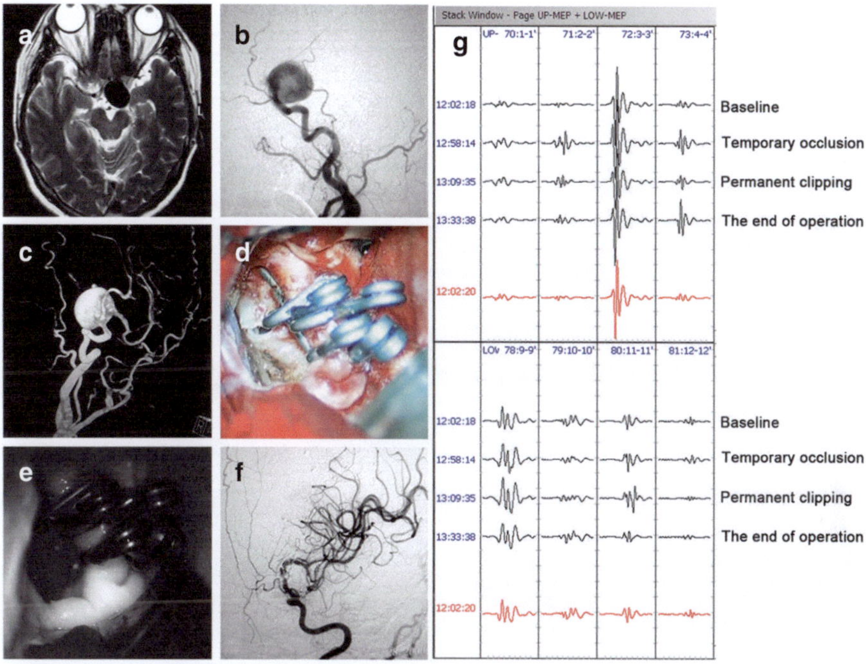

Fig. 7.11 (**a**) Preoperative MRI shows a mass lesion after the orbit on the left side. (**b**, **c**) DSA and three-dimensional (3D) reconstructed images reveal a giant right ICA aneurysm at the ophthalmic segment. (**d**) The "multiple clipping" technique was used to secure the aneurysm. (**e**, **f**) Intraoperative ICGVA and postoperative DSA showed the parent artery's patency and complete obliteration of the aneurysm. (**g**) MEPs remained stable during the operation (Reproduced from: Song J, Lang L, Zhu W, Gu Y, Xu B, Cai J, et al. Application of intraoperative motor evoked potential monitoring during giant internal carotid artery aneurysm surgery using prolonged temporary occlusion. Acta Neurochir (Wien). 2015;157:1833–40)

was relatively uniform, but focal enhancement could be observed on the temporal side of the aneurysm body (Fig. 7.13d–f). The giant size, distinctive neck anatomy, and brain parenchyma of the outflow tract posed technical challenges in treatment. A bypass plan using STA branches was considered preoperatively. During the operation, we placed a temporary clip on the inflow tract of the aneurysm and dissected the aneurysm body with caution (Fig. 7.13f). Since there was no change in the MEPs of SSEPs during prolonged temporary occlusion (>30 min) under normal blood pressure, we changed the surgical plan to simple aneurysm resection. We cut open the GIA (Fig. 7.13g), removed the heavy thrombosis inside for decompression, and observed a large area of atherosclerotic plaques on the temporal side, in line with the preoperative HR-VW MRI findings (Fig. 7.13h). The outflow tract was identified and clipped (Fig. 7.13i). The aneurysm was totally removed, and the inflow and outflow tracts were both secured using permanent clips (Fig. 7.13j, k). After hemostasis, we closed as usual. The MEPs and SSEPs were stable during the whole operation (Fig. 7.13l, m), and intraoperative DSA showed no delay in the right MCA blood flow (Fig. 7.13n). The 1-year follow-up CTA showed no

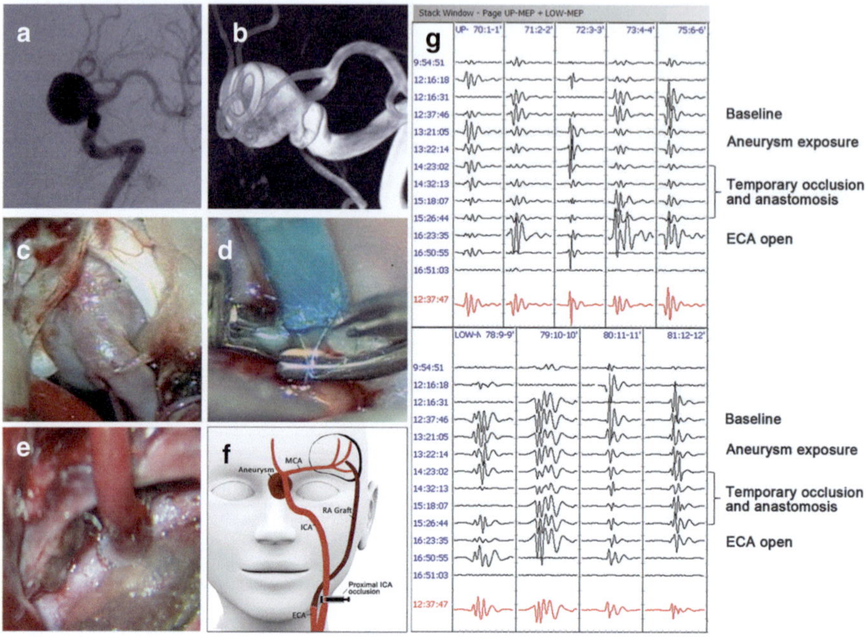

Fig. 7.12 (**a**, **b**) DSA and 3D reconstructed images reveal a giant right ICA aneurysm at the ophthalmic segment. (**c**) Aneurysm exposure after craniotomy. (**d**, **e**) RA-MCA end-to-side anastomosis. (**f**) Treatment strategy, including ECA-RA bypass and chronic proximal left ICA occlusion. (**g**) MEPs changed slightly when exposing the aneurysm without temporary clipping. MEP attenuation was observed when anastomosis was performed. MEPs recovered after opening the ECA at the end of the bypass procedure (Reproduced from: Song J, Lang L, Zhu W, Gu Y, Xu B, Cai J, et al. Application of intraoperative motor evoked potential monitoring during giant internal carotid artery aneurysm surgery using prolonged temporary occlusion. Acta Neurochir (Wien). 2015;157:1833–40.)

recurrence (Fig. 7.13o), and MRI showed no ischemia signal (Fig. 7.13p). The patient did not have any neurological deficits postoperatively or at follow-up.

Case 7

A 21-year-old man was incidentally found to have an intracranial lesion on physical examination. The imaging studies demonstrated a giant M1 thrombotic aneurysm (Fig. 7.14a–d). The patient underwent microsurgical exploration of the aneurysm via an enlarged, modified pterional approach. After the aneurysm was exposed, we found that three M2 branches were involved (Fig. 7.14e). Three clips were applied to occlude the neck of the aneurysm and preserve the patency of the inferior branch of the M2 segment. Next, a combined bypass was performed, including an STA parietal branch-M2 middle branch end-to-side anastomosis and an MCA superior branch-M2 middle branch end-to-end anastomosis (Fig. 7.14f–h). Intraoperative MEP monitoring indicated that the right limb signal had attenuated >80% after the aneurysm was clipped and recovered 60% after the recovery of blood flow following the reconstruction of the middle communicating artery. The patient had a slight neurologic deficit at discharge but had recovered at the 3-month follow-up. A

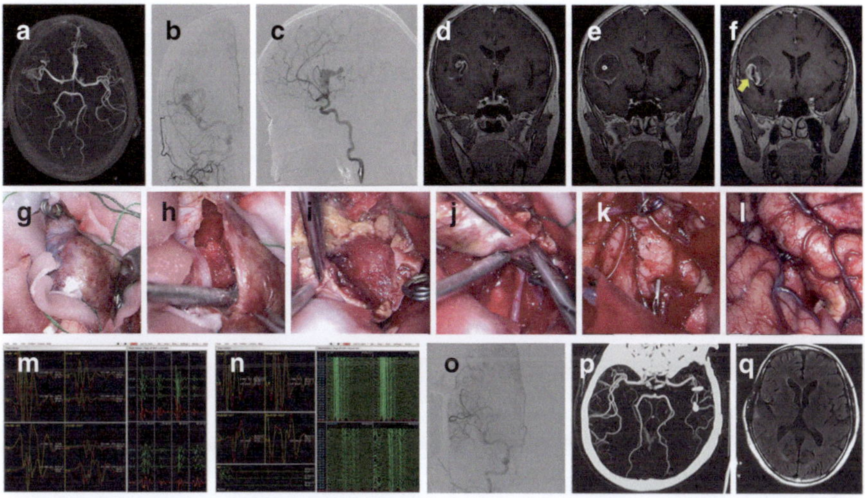

Fig. 7.13 (**a–c**) Preoperative MRA and DSA showed a right MCA giant serpentine aneurysm. (**d–f**) The preoperative HR-VW MRI showed narrow flow channels surrounded by thrombosis. The enhancement wall of the aneurysm was relatively uniform on the wall, but focal enhancement (*yellow arrow*) could be observed on the temporal side of the aneurysm body. (**g**) During the operation, a temporary clip was placed on the inflow tract of the aneurysm. (**h**) The aneurysm was incised to remove the heavy thrombosis inside for decompression. (**i**) A large portion of atherosclerotic plaques on the temporal side. (**j**) The outflow tract was identified and clipped. (**k**, **l**) The aneurysm was removed, and the inflow and outflow tracts were both secured using permanent clips. (**m**, **n**). The MEPs and SSEPs were stable during the whole operation. (**o**) Intraoperative DSA showed no delay in right MCA blood flow. (**p**) The 1-year follow-up CTA showed no recurrence. (**q**) MRI showed no ischemia signal

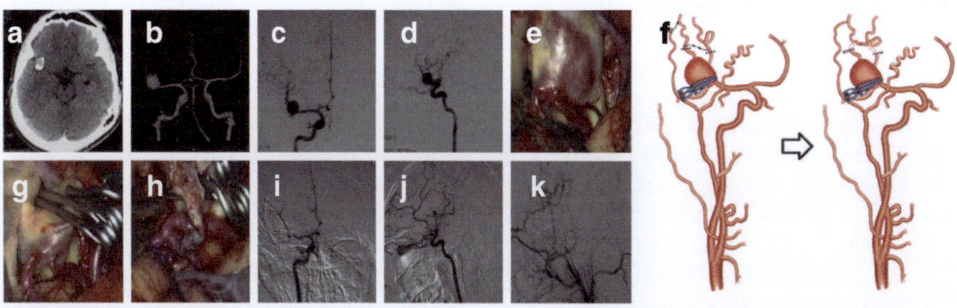

Fig. 7.14 (**a–d**) Imaging studies demonstrating a giant M1 aneurysm originating from the superior wall distal to LSAs. (**e**) Intraoperative photograph showing a GIA with three M2 branches. (**f**) Diagram showing the intraoperative procedure. (**g**) Intraoperative photograph showing three clips occluding the aneurysm's neck and preserving the patency of the inferior branch of M2. (**h**) Intraoperative photograph showing combined bypass, including the superficial temporal artery parietal branch-M2 middle branch end-to-side anastomosis and MCA M2 superior branch-M2 middle branch end-to-end anastomosis (creating the so-called middle communicating artery). (**i–k**) Follow-up DSA showed total obliteration of the aneurysm and continued patency of the bypass (Reproduced from: Ni W, Yang H, Xu B, Xu F, Jiang H, Lei Y, et al. Proximal Middle Cerebral Artery Aneurysms: Microsurgical Management and Therapeutic Results. World Neurosurg. 2019;122:e907-e16)

postoperative follow-up angiogram at 22 months demonstrated the obliteration of the aneurysm and patency of the stomas (Fig. 7.14i–k).

References

1. Hanel RA, Spetzler RF. Surgical treatment of complex intracranial aneurysms. Neurosurgery. 2008;62:1289–97; discussion 97-9
2. Locksley HB. Natural history of subarachnoid hemorrhage, intracranial aneurysms and arteriovenous malformations. Based on 6368 cases in the cooperative study. J Neurosurg. 1966;25:219–39.
3. Dengler J, Rufenacht D, Meyer B, Rohde V, Endres M, Lenga P, et al. Giant intracranial aneurysms: natural history and 1-year case fatality after endovascular or surgical treatment. J Neurosurg. 2019:1–9.
4. Wong GK, Teoh J, Chan EK, Ng SC, Poon WS. Intracranial aneurysm size responsible for spontaneous subarachnoid haemorrhage. Br J Neurosurg. 2013;27:34–9.
5. Thines L, Proust F, Marinho P, Durand A, van der Zwan A, Regli L, et al. Giant and complex aneurysms treatment with preservation of flow via bypass technique. Neurochirurgie. 2016;62:1–13.
6. Telles JPM, Solla DJF, Yamaki VN, Rabelo NN, da Silva SA, Caldas JGP, et al. Comparison of surgical and endovascular treatments for fusiform intracranial aneurysms: systematic review and individual patient data meta-analysis. Neurosurg Rev. 2020.
7. Spiessberger A, Strange F, Fandino J, Marbacher S. Microsurgical clipping of basilar apex aneurysms: a systematic historical review of approaches and their results. World Neurosurg. 2018;114:305–16.
8. da Silva HB, Messina-Lopez M, Sekhar LN. Bypasses and reconstruction for complex brain aneurysms. Methodist Debakey Cardiovasc J. 2014;10:224–33.
9. Balik V, Yamada Y, Talari S, Kei Y, Sano H, Suyama D, et al. State-of-art in surgical treatment of dissecting posterior circulation intracranial aneurysms. Neurosurg Rev. 2018;41:31–45.
10. Lawton MT, Quinones-Hinojosa A, Chang EF, Yu T. Thrombotic intracranial aneurysms: classification scheme and management strategies in 68 patients. Neurosurgery. 2005;56:441–54; discussion 54
11. Steinberg GK, Drake CG, Peerless SJ. Deliberate basilar or vertebral artery occlusion in the treatment of intracranial aneurysms. Immediate results and long-term outcome in 201 patients. J Neurosurg. 1993;79:161–73.
12. Wiebers DO, Whisnant JP, Huston J 3rd, Meissner I, Brown RD Jr, Piepgras DG, et al. Unruptured intracranial aneurysms: natural history, clinical outcome, and risks of surgical and endovascular treatment. Lancet. 2003;362:103–10.
13. Chancellor B, Raz E, Shapiro M, Tanweer O, Nossek E, Riina HA, et al. Flow diversion for intracranial aneurysm treatment: trials involving flow diverters and long-term outcomes. Neurosurgery. 2020;86:S36–s45.
14. Nasr DM, Flemming KD, Lanzino G, Cloft HJ, Kallmes DF, Murad MH, et al. Natural history of vertebrobasilar dolichoectatic and fusiform aneurysms: a systematic review and meta-analysis. Cerebrovasc Dis. 2018;45:68–77.
15. Can A, Mouminah A, Ho AL, Du R. Effect of vascular anatomy on the formation of basilar tip aneurysms. Neurosurgery. 2015;76:62–6.
16. Lonjon M, Pennes F, Sedat J, Bataille B. Epidemiology, genetic, natural history and clinical presentation of giant cerebral aneurysms. Neurochirurgie. 2015;61:361–5.
17. Xu K, Yu T, Guo Y, Yu J. Study and therapeutic progress on intracranial serpentine aneurysms. Int J Med Sci. 2016;13:432–9.
18. Enomoto Y, Egashira Y, Matsubara H, Yoshimura S, Iwama T. Long-term outcome of endovascular therapy for large or giant thrombosed intracranial aneurysms. World Neurosurg. 2020;144:e507–e12.

19. Lawton MT, Abla AA, Rutledge WC, Benet A, Zador Z, Rayz VL, et al. Bypass surgery for the treatment of dolichoectatic basilar trunk aneurysms: a work in progress. Neurosurgery. 2016;79:83–99.
20. Mascitelli JR, Lawton MT, Hendricks BK, Nakaji P, Zabramski JM, Spetzler RF. Analysis of wide-neck aneurysms in the Barrow ruptured aneurysm trial. Neurosurgery. 2019;85:622–31.
21. Campos JK, Ball BZ, Cheaney Ii B, Sweidan AJ, Hasjim BJ, Hsu FPK, et al. Multimodal management of giant cerebral aneurysms: review of literature and case presentation. Stroke Vasc Neurol. 2020;5:22–8.
22. Luzzi S, Gragnaniello C, Giotta Lucifero A, Del Maestro M, Galzio R. Microneurosurgical management of giant intracranial aneurysms: datasets of a twenty-year experience. Data Brief. 2020;33:106537.
23. Luzzi S, Gragnaniello C, Giotta Lucifero A, Del Maestro M, Galzio R. Surgical management of giant intracranial aneurysms: overall results of a large series. World Neurosurg. 2020;144:e119–e37.
24. Lawton MT, Lang MJ. The future of open vascular neurosurgery: perspectives on cavernous malformations, AVMs, and bypasses for complex aneurysms. J Neurosurg. 2019;130:1409–25.
25. Lozano CS, Lozano AM, Spears J. The changing landscape of treatment for intracranial aneurysm. Can J Neurol Sci. 2019;46:159–65.
26. Dandapat S, Mendez-Ruiz A, Martínez-Galdámez M, Macho J, Derakhshani S, Foa Torres G, et al. Review of current intracranial aneurysm flow diversion technology and clinical use. J Neurointerv Surg. 2021;13:54–62.
27. Liang F, Yang Y, Luo L, Liao B, Zhang G, Ou S, et al. Endovascular treatment of complex middle cerebral artery aneurysms using TuBridge flow diverters. Interv Neuroradiol. 2020;26:539–46.
28. Wakhloo AK, Gounis MJ. Revolution in aneurysm treatment: flow diversion to cure aneurysms: a paradigm shift. Neurosurgery. 2014;61(Suppl 1):111–20.
29. Walcott BP, Stapleton CJ, Choudhri O, Patel AB. Flow diversion for the treatment of intracranial aneurysms. JAMA Neurol. 2016;73:1002–8.
30. Wagner A, Cortsen M, Hauerberg J, Romner B, Wagner MP. Treatment of intracranial aneurysms. Reconstruction of the parent artery with flow-diverting (silk) stent. Neuroradiology. 2012;54:709–18.
31. Patel PD, Chalouhi N, Atallah E, Tjoumakaris S, Hasan D, Zarzour H, et al. Off-label uses of the pipeline embolization device: a review of the literature. Neurosurg Focus. 2017;42:E4.
32. Cruz JP, Chow M, O'Kelly C, Marotta B, Spears J, Montanera W, et al. Delayed ipsilateral parenchymal hemorrhage following flow diversion for the treatment of anterior circulation aneurysms. AJNR Am J Neuroradiol. 2012;33:603–8.
33. Yeomans J, Sandu L, Sastry A. Pipeline flex embolisation device with shield technology for the treatment of patients with intracranial aneurysms: periprocedural and 6 month outcomes. Neuroradiol J. 2020;33:471–8.
34. Lv X, Yang H, Liu P, Li Y. Flow-diverter devices in the treatment of intracranial aneurysms: a meta-analysis and systematic review. Neuroradiol J. 2016;29:66–71.
35. Arrese I, Sarabia R, Pintado R, Delgado-Rodriguez M. Flow-diverter devices for intracranial aneurysms: systematic review and meta-analysis. Neurosurgery. 2013;73:193–9; discussion 9-200
36. Hokari M, Kazumara K, Nakayama N, Ushikoshi S, Sugiyama T, Asaoka K, et al. Treatment of recurrent intracranial aneurysms after clipping: a report of 23 cases and a review of the literature. World Neurosurg. 2016;92:434–44.
37. Abla AA, McDougall CM, Breshears JD, Lawton MT. Intracranial-to-intracranial bypass for posterior inferior cerebellar artery aneurysms: options, technical challenges, and results in 35 patients. J Neurosurg. 2016;124:1275–86.
38. Cenzato M, Bortolotti C. The role of extra- and intracranial bypass in the treatment of complex aneurysms. J Neurosurg Sci. 2016;60:70–82.
39. Wessels L, Fekonja LS, Vajkoczy P. Bypass surgery of complex middle cerebral artery aneurysms-technical aspects and outcomes. Acta Neurochir. 2019;161:1981–91.

40. Yasargil MG, Yonekawa Y. Results of microsurgical extra-intracranial arterial bypass in the treatment of cerebral ischemia. Neurosurgery. 1977;1:22–4.
41. Wessels L, Hecht N, Vajkoczy P. Bypass in neurosurgery-indications and techniques. Neurosurg Rev. 2019;42:389–93.
42. Raper DMS, Rutledge WC, Winkler EA, Meisel K, Callen AL, Cooke DL, et al. Controversies and advances in adult intracranial bypass surgery in 2020. Oper Neurosurg (Hagerstown). 2020;20:1–7.
43. Amin-Hanjani S, Alaraj A, Charbel FT. Flow replacement bypass for aneurysms: decision-making using intraoperative blood flow measurements. Acta Neurochir. 2010;152:1021–32; discussion 32
44. Zarrinkoob L, Ambarki K, Wahlin A, Birgander R, Eklund A, Malm J. Blood flow distribution in cerebral arteries. J Cereb Blood Flow Metab. 2015;35:648–54.
45. Roh SW, Ahn JS, Sung HY, Jung YJ, Kwun BD, Kim CJ. Extracranial-intracranial bypass surgery using a radial artery interposition graft for cerebrovascular diseases. J Korean Neurosurg Soc. 2011;50:185–90.
46. Hanakita S, Lenck S, Labidi M, Watanabe K, Bresson D, Froelich S. The occipital artery as an alternative donor for low-flow bypass to anterior circulation after internal carotid artery occlusion failure prior to Exenteration for an atypical cavernous sinus meningioma. World Neurosurg. 2018;109:10–7.
47. Mao Y. Revascularization with the occipital artery to treat aneurysms in the posterior circulation. World Neurosurg. 2014;82:e415–6.
48. Zhu FP, Zhang Y, Higurashi M, Xu B, Gu YX, Mao Y, et al. Haemodynamic analysis of vessel remodelling in STA-MCA bypass for Moyamoya disease and its impact on bypass patency. J Biomech. 2014;47:1800–5.
49. Zhu F, Karunanithi K, Qian Y, Mao Y, Xu B, Gu Y, et al. Assessing surgical treatment outcome following superficial temporal artery to middle cerebral artery bypass based on computational haemodynamic analysis. J Biomech. 2015;48:4053–8.
50. Alaraj A, Ashley WW Jr, Charbel FT, Amin-Hanjani S. The superficial temporal artery trunk as a donor vessel in cerebral revascularization: benefits and pitfalls. Neurosurg Focus. 2008;24:E7.
51. Kaku Y, Takei H, Miyai M, Yamashita K, Kokuzawa J. Surgical treatment of complex cerebral aneurysms using interposition short vein graft. Acta Neurochir Suppl. 2016;123:65–71.
52. Zaki Ghali MG, Srinivasan VM, Britz GW. Maxillary artery to intracranial bypass. World Neurosurg. 2019;128:532–40.
53. Yu Z, Shi X, Brohi SR, Qian H, Liu F, Yang Y. Measurement of blood flow in an intracranial artery bypass from the internal maxillary artery by intraoperative duplex sonography. J Ultrasound Med. 2017;36:439–47.
54. Eguchi T. Long vein graft for EC/IC bypass surgery. Neurol Med Chir (Tokyo). 1983;23:931–8.
55. Sekhar LN, Tariq F, Mai JC, Kim LJ, Ghodke B, Hallam DK, et al. Unyielding progress: treatment paradigms for giant aneurysms. Clin Neurosurg. 2012;59:6–21.
56. Sekhar LN, Duff JM, Kalavakonda C, Olding M. Cerebral revascularization using radial artery grafts for the treatment of complex intracranial aneurysms: techniques and outcomes for 17 patients. Neurosurgery. 2001;49:646–58; discussion 58-9
57. Sanai N, Zador Z, Lawton MT. Bypass surgery for complex brain aneurysms: an assessment of intracranial-intracranial bypass. Neurosurgery. 2009;65:670–83; discussion 83
58. Lang MJ, Kan P, Baranoski JF, Lawton MT. Side-to-side superficial temporal artery to middle cerebral artery bypass technique: application of fourth generation bypass in a case of adult Moyamoya disease. Oper Neurosurg (Hagerstown). 2020;18:480–6.
59. Natarajan SK, Zeeshan Q, Ghodke BV, Sekhar LN. Brain bypass surgery for complex middle cerebral artery aneurysms: evolving techniques, results, and lessons learned. World Neurosurg. 2019;130:e272–e93.
60. Rennert RC, Steinberg JA, Strickland BA, Ravina K, Bakhsheshian J, Fredrickson V, et al. Extracranial-to-intracranial bypass for refractory Vertebrobasilar insufficiency. World Neurosurg. 2019;126:552–9.

61. Zhu W, Liu P, Tian Y, Gu Y, Xu B, Chen L, et al. Complex middle cerebral artery aneurysms: a new classification based on the angioarchitecture and surgical strategies. Acta Neurochir. 2013;155:1481–91.
62. Zhong J, Ding M, Mao Q, Wang B, Fu H. Evaluating brain tolerability to carotid artery occlusion. Neurol Res. 2003;25:99–103.
63. Zhang Z, Lv X, Wu Z, Li Y, Yang X, Jiang C, et al. Clinical and angiographic outcome of endovascular and conservative treatment for giant cavernous carotid artery aneurysms. Interv Neuroradiol. 2014;20:29–36.
64. Asai K, Imamura H, Mineharu Y, Tani S, Adachi H, Narumi O, et al. X-ray angiography perfusion analysis for the balloon occlusion test of the internal carotid artery. J Stroke Cerebrovasc Dis. 2015;24:1506–12.
65. Sivakumaran R, Mohamed AZ, Akhunbay-Fudge CY, Edwards RJ, Renowden SA, Nelson RJ. Internal carotid artery test balloon occlusion using single photon emission computed tomography scan in the management of complex cerebral aneurysms and skull base tumors: a 20-year review. World Neurosurg. 2020;139:e32–e7.
66. Sattur MG, Welz ME, Bendok BR, Miller JW. Balloon occlusion testing to assess retinal collateral and predict visual outcomes in the management of a fusiform intraorbital ophthalmic artery aneurysm: technical note and literature review. Oper Neurosurg (Hagerstown). 2019;16:60–6.
67. Lejeune JP, Thines L, Proust F, Riegel B, Koussa M, Decoene C. Selective microsurgical treatment of giant intracranial aneurysms. Neurochirurgie. 2016;62:30–7.
68. Zhu W, Tian YL, Zhou LF, Song DL, Xu B, Mao Y. Treatment strategies for complex internal carotid artery (ICA) aneurysms: direct ICA sacrifice or combined with extracranial-to-intracranial bypass. World Neurosurg. 2011;75:476–84.
69. Yu-Tse L, Ho-Fai W, Cheng-Chi L, Chu-Mei K, Yi-Chou W, Tao-Chieh Y. Rupture of symptomatic blood blister-like aneurysm of the internal carotid artery: clinical experience and management outcome. Br J Neurosurg. 2012;26:378–82.
70. Yang M, Wu J, Ma L, Pan L, Li J, Chen G, et al. The value of syngo DynaPBV neuro during neuro-interventional hypotensive balloon occlusion test. Clin Neuroradiol. 2015;25:387–95.
71. Xu J, Xu L, Wu Z, Chen X, Yu J, Zhang J. Fetal-type posterior cerebral artery: the pitfall of parent artery occlusion for ruptured P2 segment and distal aneurysms. J Neurosurg. 2015;123:906–14.
72. Torigai T, Mase M, Ohno T, Katano H, Nisikawa Y, Sakurai K, et al. Usefulness of dual and fully automated measurements of cerebral blood flow during balloon occlusion test of the internal carotid artery. J Stroke Cerebrovasc Dis. 2013;22:197–204.
73. Charbel FT, Zhao M, Amin-Hanjani S, Hoffman W, Du X, Clark ME. A patient-specific computer model to predict outcomes of the balloon occlusion test. J Neurosurg. 2004;101:977–88.
74. Allen JW, Alastra AJ, Nelson PK. Proximal intracranial internal carotid artery branches: prevalence and importance for balloon occlusion test. J Neurosurg. 2005;102:45–52.
75. Barker DW, Jungreis CA, Horton JA, Pentheny S, Lemley T. Balloon test occlusion of the internal carotid artery: change in stump pressure over 15 minutes and its correlation with xenon CT cerebral blood flow. AJNR Am J Neuroradiol. 1993;14:587–90.
76. Kuribara T, Mikami T, Iihoshi S, Miyata K, Kim S, Kawata Y, et al. Ischemic tolerance evaluated by computed tomography perfusion during balloon test occlusion. J Stroke Cerebrovasc Dis. 2020;29:104807.
77. Mathews D, Walker BS, Purdy PD, Batjer H, Allen BC, Eckard DA, et al. Brain blood flow SPECT in temporary balloon occlusion of carotid and intracerebral arteries. J Nucl Med. 1993;34:1239–43.
78. Sudhakar KV, Sawlani V, Phadke RV, Kumar S, Ahmed S, Gujral RB. Temporary balloon occlusion of internal carotid artery: a simple and reliable clinical test. Neurol India. 2000;48:140–3.
79. Bailes JE, Deeb ZL, Wilson JA, Jungreis CA, Horton JA. Intraoperative angiography and temporary balloon occlusion of the basilar artery as an adjunct to surgical clipping: technical note. Neurosurgery. 1992;30:949–53.

80. Barr JD, Lemley TJ, McCann RM. Carotid artery balloon test occlusion: combined clinical evaluation and xenon-enhanced computed tomographic cerebral blood flow evaluation without patient transfer or balloon reinflation: technical note. Neurosurgery. 1998;43:634–7; discussion 7-8
81. Chen L, Lang L, Zhou L, Song D, Mao Y. Bypass or not? Adjustment of surgical strategies according to motor evoked potential changes in large middle cerebral artery aneurysm surgery. World Neurosurg. 2012;77:398.E1–6.
82. Ricci G, Ricci A, Gallucci M, Zotta D, Scogna A, Costagliola C, et al. Combined endovascular and microsurgical approach in the treatment of giant paraclinoid and vertebrobasilar aneurysms. J Neurosurg Sci. 2005;49:1–6.
83. Skrap M, Petralia B, Toniato G. Temporary balloon occlusion during the surgical treatment of giant paraclinoid and vertebrobasilar aneurysms. Acta Neurochir. 2010;152:435–42.
84. Dashti R, Laakso A, Niemela M, Porras M, Hernesniemi J. Microscope-integrated near-infrared indocyanine green videoangiography during surgery of intracranial aneurysms: the Helsinki experience. Surg Neurol. 2009;71:543–50; discussion 50
85. Raabe A, Nakaji P, Beck J, Kim LJ, Hsu FP, Kamerman JD, et al. Prospective evaluation of surgical microscope-integrated intraoperative near-infrared indocyanine green videoangiography during aneurysm surgery. J Neurosurg. 2005;103:982–9.
86. Jing Z, Ou S, Ban Y, Tong Z, Wang Y. Intraoperative assessment of anterior circulation aneurysms using the indocyanine green video angiography technique. J Clin Neurosci. 2010;17:26–8.
87. Li J, Lan Z, He M, You C. Assessment of microscope-integrated indocyanine green angiography during intracranial aneurysm surgery: a retrospective study of 120 patients. Neurol India. 2009;57:453–9.
88. Ma CY, Shi JX, Wang HD, Hang CH, Cheng HL, Wu W. Intraoperative indocyanine green angiography in intracranial aneurysm surgery: microsurgical clipping and revascularization. Clin Neurol Neurosurg. 2009;111:840–6.
89. Gruber A, Dorfer C, Standhardt H, Bavinzski G, Knosp E. Prospective comparison of intraoperative vascular monitoring technologies during cerebral aneurysm surgery. Neurosurgery. 2011;68:657–73; discussion 73
90. Imizu S, Kato Y, Sangli A, Oguri D, Sano H. Assessment of incomplete clipping of aneurysms intraoperatively by a near-infrared indocyanine green-video angiography (Niicg-Va) integrated microscope. Minim Invasive Neurosurg. 2008;51:199–203.
91. Moon HS, Joo SP, Seo BR, Jang JW, Kim JH, Kim TS. Value of indocyanine green videoangiography in deciding the completeness of cerebrovascular surgery. J Korean Neurosurg Soc. 2013;53:349–55.
92. Ozgiray E, Akture E, Patel N, Baggott C, Bozkurt M, Niemann D, et al. How reliable and accurate is indocyanine green video angiography in the evaluation of aneurysm obliteration? Clin Neurol Neurosurg. 2013;115:870–8.
93. Roessler K, Krawagna M, Dörfler A, Buchfelder M, Ganslandt O. Essentials in intraoperative indocyanine green videoangiography assessment for intracranial aneurysm surgery: conclusions from 295 consecutively clipped aneurysms and review of the literature. Neurosurg Focus. 2014;36:E7.
94. Sharma M, Ambekar S, Ahmed O, Nixon M, Sharma A, Nanda A, et al. The utility and limitations of intraoperative near-infrared indocyanine green videoangiography in aneurysm surgery. World Neurosurg. 2014;82:e607–13.
95. Wang S, Liu L, Zhao Y, Zhang D, Yang M, Zhao J. Evaluation of surgical microscope-integrated intraoperative near-infrared indocyanine green videoangiography during aneurysm surgery. Neurosurg Rev. 2010;34:209–15.
96. Bailes JE, Tantuwaya LS, Fukushima T, Schurman GW, Davis D. Intraoperative microvascular Doppler sonography in aneurysm surgery. Neurosurgery. 1997;40:965–70; discussion 70-2

97. Woydt M, Greiner K, Perez J, Krone A, Roosen K. Intraoperative color duplex sonography of basal arteries during aneurysm surgery. J Neuroimaging. 1997;7:203–7.
98. Stendel R, Pietila T, Al Hassan AA, Schilling A, Brock M. Intraoperative microvascular Doppler ultrasonography in cerebral aneurysm surgery. J Neurol Neurosurg Psychiatry. 2000;68:29–35.
99. Siasios I, Kapsalaki EZ, Fountas KN. The role of intraoperative micro-Doppler ultrasound in verifying proper clip placement in intracranial aneurysm surgery. Neuroradiology. 2012;54:1109–18.
100. Kapsalaki EZ, Lee GP, Robinson JS 3rd, Grigorian AA, Fountas KN. The role of intraoperative micro-Doppler ultrasound in verifying proper clip placement in intracranial aneurysm surgery. J Clin Neurosci. 2008;15:153–7.
101. Marchese E, Albanese A, Denaro L, Vignati A, Fernandez E, Maira G. Intraoperative microvascular Doppler in intracranial aneurysm surgery. Surg Neurol. 2005;63:336–42; discussion 42
102. Cui H, Wang Y, Yin Y, Wan J, Fei Z, Gao W, et al. Role of intraoperative microvascular Doppler in the microsurgical management of intracranial aneurysms. J Clin Ultrasound. 2011;39:27–31.
103. Rodriguez-Hernandez A, Lawton MT. Flash fluorescence with indocyanine green videoangiography to identify the recipient artery for bypass with distal middle cerebral artery aneurysms: operative technique. Neurosurgery. 2012;70:209–20.
104. Esposito G, Durand A, Van Doormaal T, Regli L. Selective-targeted extra-intracranial bypass surgery in complex middle cerebral artery aneurysms: correctly identifying the recipient artery using indocyanine green videoangiography. Neurosurgery. 2012;71:ons274–84; discussion ons84–5
105. Guo L, Gelb AW. The use of motor evoked potential monitoring during cerebral aneurysm surgery to predict pure motor deficits due to subcortical ischemia. Clin Neurophysiol. 2011;122:648–55.
106. Horiuchi K, Suzuki K, Sasaki T, Matsumoto M, Sakuma J, Konno Y, et al. Intraoperative monitoring of blood flow insufficiency during surgery of middle cerebral artery aneurysms. J Neurosurg. 2005;103:275–83.
107. Neuloh G, Schramm J. Monitoring of motor evoked potentials compared with somatosensory evoked potentials and microvascular Doppler ultrasonography in cerebral aneurysm surgery. J Neurosurg. 2004;100:389–99.
108. Sakuma J, Suzuki K, Sasaki T, Matsumoto M, Oinuma M, Kawakami M, et al. Monitoring and preventing blood flow insufficiency due to clip rotation after the treatment of internal carotid artery aneurysms. J Neurosurg. 2004;100:960–2.
109. Song J, Lang L, Zhu W, Gu Y, Xu B, Cai J, et al. Application of intraoperative motor evoked potential monitoring during giant internal carotid artery aneurysm surgery using prolonged temporary occlusion. Acta Neurochir. 2015;157:1833–40.
110. Yue Q, Zhu W, Gu Y, Xu B, Lang L, Song J, et al. Motor evoked potential monitoring during surgery of middle cerebral artery aneurysms: a cohort study. World Neurosurg. 2014;82:1091–9.
111. Ni W, Yang H, Xu B, Xu F, Jiang H, Lei Y, et al. Proximal middle cerebral artery aneurysms: microsurgical management and therapeutic results. World Neurosurg. 2019;122:e907–e16.
112. Tian Y, Zhu W, Mao Y. Surgical strategies for treatment of complex anterior cerebral artery aneurysms. World Neurosurg. 2014;81:304–5.
113. Abla AA, Lawton MT. Anterior cerebral artery bypass for complex aneurysms: an experience with intracranial-intracranial reconstruction and review of bypass options. J Neurosurg. 2014;120:1364–77.
114. Balik V, Yamada Y, Talari S, Kei Y, Sano H, Sulla I, et al. State-of-art surgical treatment of dissecting anterior circulation intracranial aneurysms. J Neurol Surg A Cent Eur Neurosurg. 2017;78:67–77.

115. Baranoski JF, Przybylowski CJ, Mascitelli JR, Lang MJ, Lawton MT. Anterior inferior cerebellar artery bypasses: the 7-bypass framework applied to ischemia and aneurysms in the cerebellopontine angle. Oper Neurosurg (Hagerstown). 2020;19:165–74.
116. Tjahjadi M, Niemelä M, Kivelev J, Serrone J, Maekawa H, Jahromi BR, et al. Presigmoid approach to vertebrobasilar artery aneurysms: a series of 31 patients and review of the literature. World Neurosurg. 2016;92:313–22.
117. Chang SW, Abla AA, Kakarla UK, Sauvageau E, Dashti SR, Nakaji P, et al. Treatment of distal posterior cerebral artery aneurysms: a critical appraisal of the occipital artery-to-posterior cerebral artery bypass. Neurosurgery. 2010;67:16–25; discussion 25–6
118. Helthuis JHG, van Doormaal TPC, Amin-Hanjani S, Du X, Charbel FT, Hillen B, et al. A patient-specific cerebral blood flow model. J Biomech. 2020;98:109445.
119. Shinagawa K, Matsushige T, Okazaki T, Ishii D, Ichinose N, Sakamoto S, et al. Asymptomatic ischemic risks in microsurgical clipping for unruptured intracranial aneurysms in anterior circulation. World Neurosurg. 2017;108:418–26.
120. Quan K, Song J, Yang Z, Wang D, An Q, Huang L, et al. Validation of wall enhancement as a new imaging biomarker of unruptured cerebral aneurysm. Stroke. 2019;50:1570–3.
121. Edjlali M, Gentric JC, Regent-Rodriguez C, Trystram D, Hassen WB, Lion S, et al. Does aneurysmal wall enhancement on vessel wall MRI help to distinguish stable from unstable intracranial aneurysms? Stroke. 2014;45:3704–6.
122. Lindenholz A, van der Kolk AG, Zwanenburg JJM, Hendrikse J. The use and pitfalls of intracranial vessel wall imaging: how we do it. Radiology. 2018;286:12–28.
123. Murayama Y, Irie K, Saguchi T, Ishibashi T, Ebara M, Nagashima H, et al. Robotic digital subtraction angiography systems within the hybrid operating room. Neurosurgery. 2011;68:1427–32; discussion 33
124. Song J, Li P, Tian Y, An Q, Liu Y, Yang Z, et al. One-stage treatment in a hybrid operation room to cure brain arteriovenous malformation: a single-center experience. World Neurosurg. 2020.
125. Esposito G, Fierstra J, Regli L. Distal outflow occlusion with bypass revascularization: last resort measure in managing complex MCA and PICA aneurysms. Acta Neurochir. 2016;158:1523–31.
126. Frisoli FA, Catapano JS, Baranoski JF, Lawton MT. The middle communicating artery: a novel fourth-generation bypass for revascularizing trapped middle cerebral artery bifurcation aneurysms in 2 cases. J Neurosurg. 2020:1–8.
127. Catapano JS, Frisoli FA, Cadigan MS, Farhadi DS, Nguyen CL, Lawton MT. Double-barrel superficial temporal artery-M2 middle cerebral artery bypass and creation of a middle communicating artery via M2-M2 end-to-end reimplantation for trapping of a dolichoectatic middle cerebral artery aneurysm: 2-dimensional operative video. Oper Neurosurg (Hagerstown). 2020;19:E521–E2.

Chapter 8
Contralateral Clipping of Multiple Intracranial Aneurysms

Manas Panigrahi, Chirag Patel, Pratik Koradia, and Y. B. V. K. Chandrasekhar

8.1 Introduction

The reported incidence of multiple intracranial aneurysms (MIA) is approximately 7–35% of all intracranial aneurysms [1]. Bilateral intracranial aneurysm (BIA) constitute 20–40% of all MIA [2] and more often than not, present symmetrically along the ICA. Bilateral middle cerebral artery aneurysms have been reported to account for 1% of all intracranial aneurysms [3]. The primary goal in the management of MIAs is to secure the ruptured aneurysm and to treat as many of the remaining lesions as possible without affecting the outcome of the patient. Reported risks of aneurysm management include bleeding from one of the incidental aneurysms, vasospasm, and other complications related to the sub-arachnoid hemorrhage (SAH) [4]. Although the choice of treatment depends on the aneurysm characteristics, patient condition, and the infrastructure and post-operative monitoring available. Established treatment strategies for bilateral MIAs include (a) bilateral sequential craniotomy and clipping in two stages, (b) unilateral craniotomy and clipping of multiple aneurysm including contra lateral aneurysm, and (c) clipping of ipsilateral ruptured aneurysm and addressing contralateral side aneurysms with endovascular options. However, criteria for selecting the contralateral approach are still debatable. In this chapter we elaborate management of bilateral MIAs by unilateral craniotomy. The current chapter emphasizes on parameters to be considered during selecting cases for contralateral clipping and outcome comparisons.

M. Panigrahi (✉) · C. Patel · P. Koradia · Y. B. V. K. Chandrasekhar
Department of Neurosurgery, Krishna Institute of Medical Sciences, Secunderabad, Telangana, India

Y. Kato, A. Ansari (eds.), *Cerebrovascular Surgery*, Advances and Technical Standards in Neurosurgery 44, https://doi.org/10.1007/978-3-030-87649-4_8

8.2 Selection Criteria for Contralateral Clipping of Aneurysm

Clipping of MIAs, including contralateral aneurysm is now feasible, especially when the aneurysm originates between distal dural ring till the bifurcation of MCA. However, selection criteria for patient with contralateral ICA (Ophthalmic, communicating and ICA bifurcation) and MCA bifurcation vary. Although, computed tomography (CT) of brain and cerebral angiography are investigations of choice, magnetic resonance imaging (MRI) brain is also increasingly employed to plan and execute clipping of MIAs. Patient selection criteria for clipping for clipping of MIA (including contralateral ICA and MCA aneurysm) are summarized in the following:

8.2.1 Selection Criteria for Contralateral Ophthalmic Segment ICA Aneurysm Clipping

Ophthalmic segment of ICA extends from origin of ophthalmic artery to origin of posterior communicating artery (PCOM) and carries ophthalmic segment of ICA aneurysm and aneurysm that originate at superior hypophyseal artery. The reported incidence of aneurysms in the carotid-ophthalmic region is 0.5–11% of all intracranial aneurysms [5]. An approach to the aneurysm from the contralateral side may provide a better view. To plan the side of approach, many radiographic landmarks such as a visual system (length of optic nerve, position of optic chiasm, and displacement of the optic nerve), surrounding structures (anterior clinoid process, tuberculum sellae, dural ring and the cavernous sinus), and vessels (the ICA, ophthalmic artery, and superior hypophyseal arteries) have been used previously [6].

1. *The distance between the anterior aspect of the optic chiasm and the limbus sphenoidale* (Fig. 8.1)
   The surgical route for contralateral clipping of ICA-ophthalmic segment aneurysms is through the interoptic space and prechiasmatic cistern. However, in some cases, the presence of a prefixed chiasm or short interoptic distance limits the accessibility to these aneurysms. Andrade-Barazarte et al. [7] described contralateral clipping of ICA opthalmic aneurysm was feasible through the interoptic route in patients with a median prechiasmatic cistern of 5.7 mm and a median interoptic space of 10.5 mm.
2. *The distance between the bilateral optic nerves at the entrance to the optic canal* (Fig. 8.1)
   Contralateral clipping of ophthalmic aneurysm is also feasible if the median interoptic distance is 10.5 mm (range, 7.6–15.9 mm) [7].
3. The inter-relation of the optic nerve and the ICA is expressed as a/b, where a is the distance from the midline to the optic nerve and b is the distance from the midline to the ICA (Fig. 8.2).

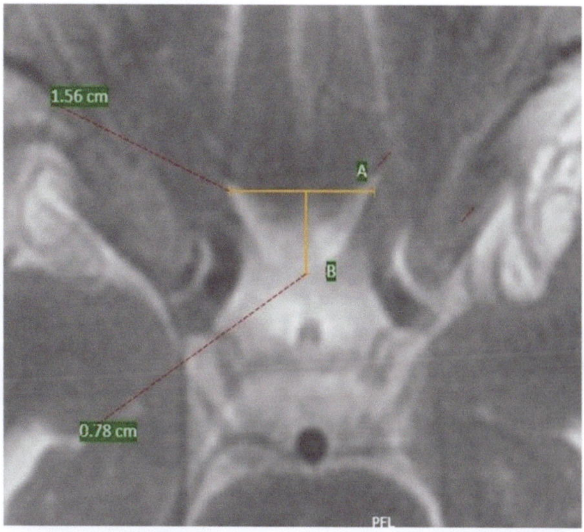

Fig. 8.1 The distance between the anterior aspect of the optic chiasm and the limbus sphenoidale

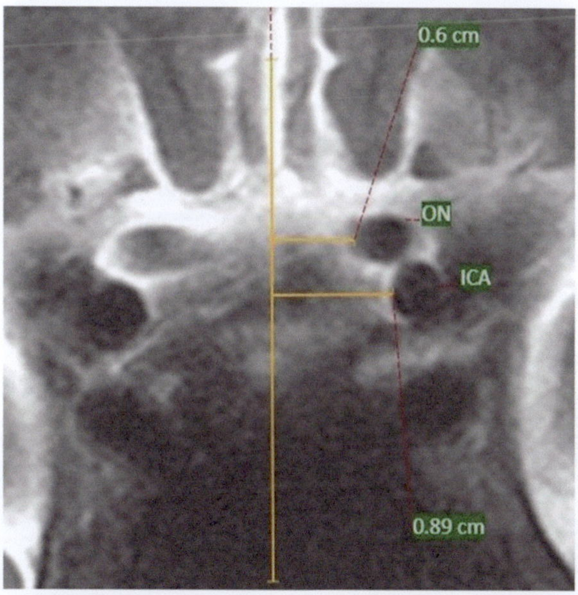

Fig. 8.2 The inter-relation of the optic nerve and the ICA is expressed as a/b, where a is the distance from the midline to the optic nerve and b is the distance from the midline to the ICA

If a/b is 1.0, the optic nerve approximately overlaps the ICA. If a/b is less than 1.0, the ICA is lateral and if greater than 1.0, ICA is medial to optic nerve. The median distance between both ICAs reported in various studies was 14.7 mm (10.4–21.4 mm).

4. *The distance between the tip of both ACPs and bilateral ICA* (Fig. 8.3) Although, the reported mean distance between bilateral ACP tips is 26.2 mm (22.5–31.5), but no correlation has been reported between the median distance

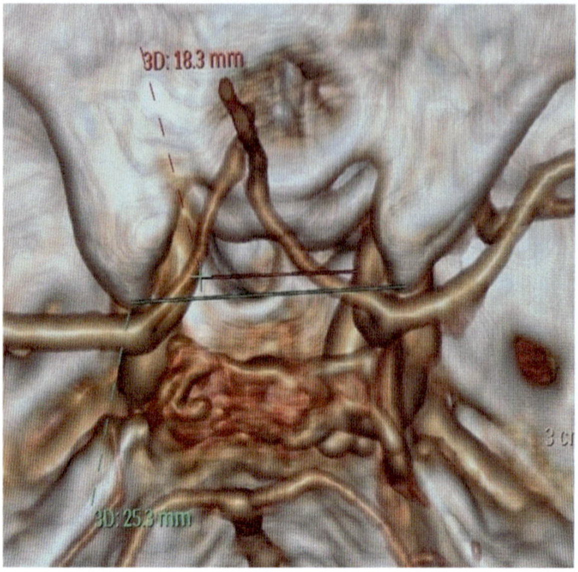

Fig. 8.3 The distance between the tip of both ACPs and Bilateral ICA

of both ICAs at the level of the tuberculum sellae and the median distance between the tip of both ACPs.

5. *The size of the aneurysm and neck*
   Contralateral approach is also indicated for small (>7 mm, up to 15 mm and mean diameter of neck 2.9 mm) and medially located aneurysms [8, 9]. Larger aneurysms may require complex surgical techniques that involve extreme mobilization of the contralateral optic nerve, with resultant visual defect, hence contralateral approach is avoided in large aneurysms.
6. *Morphology of aneurysm*
   Contralateral approach is preferred if the aneurysms were saccular with simple configurations. However, complex aneurysms (giant, fusiform, bilobulate, ruptured aneurysms, the presence of wall irregularities, and calcifications) are preferably clipped through ipsilateral craniotomy [10, 11].
7. *The direction of the aneurysm from the ICA wall on anteroposterior angiogram* (Fig. 8.4)
   Contralateral clipping of ICA-ophthalmic aneurysms is preferred for medial, superior, and superomedial aneurysms. Whereas aneurysms arising from the lateral wall of the ophthalmic segment and projecting superolaterally or laterally should be approached via an ipsilateral craniotomy to avoid injury to optic nerve, obtain proximal vascular control, better visualization of the aneurysm [12]. Moreover, drilling of the bone is not required when direction of aneurysm was between 30 and 160° and the aneurysm neck was more than 1 mm away from distal dural ring [13].
8. *Distance of the proximal neck of the aneurysm from the medial side of the estimated distal dural ring on the lateral angiogram*

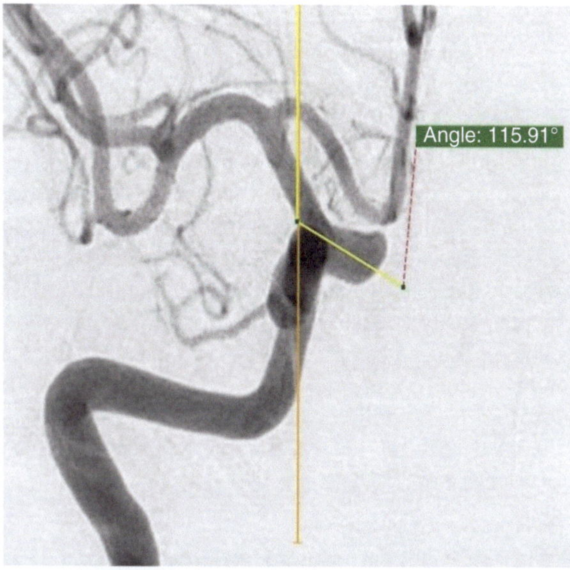

Fig. 8.4 The direction of the aneurysm from the ICA wall on anteroposterior angiogram

Oikawa et al. [14] described in detail about the identification of dural ring in angiogram lateral view at the level of tuberculum sellae meningioma. Bone drilling was not required when distance of neck of aneurysm from distal dural ring was more than 1 mm. Drilling would be needed if distance is shorter than 1 mm. Because bone drilling of the optic canal (aneurysm side) has a potential risk of causing injury to the optic nerve and ICA, it is useful in estimating the difficulty of the procedure. If distance exceeds 1.5 mm (the width of a Sugita clip blade), temporary clipping of the ICA locally in the meantime is preferable while permanent clipping of the aneurysm neck is performed. The aneurysms very close to the dural ring are best approached ipsilaterally because of the minimal space available proximal to the aneurysm neck. The ipsilateral approach is also recommended when distance has a negative value, which means that the aneurysm is located in the carotid cave or in the cavernous sinus [1].

9. *Rupture side craniotomy*
   Managing a ruptured aneurysm through a contralateral approach may be challenging due to poor visualization of the vessel and aneurysm secondary to hematoma, and higher risk of intra-operative rupture, therefore ruptured aneurysms should be approached from the ipsilateral side [3, 15].
10. *Brain edema*
    A contralateral approach should not be performed in patients with severe SAH, tight brain, and edema to avoid the risk of inflicting additional injuries to the surrounding neurovascular structures as a result of excessive brain retraction and difficult dissection [16].

8.2.2 Selection Criteria for Contralateral Communicating Segment ICA Aneurysm Clipping

Criteria for communicating segment ICA aneurysm are similar to that described for ophthalmic segment aneurysm with reference to the size of the aneurysm and neck, morphology of aneurysm, brain edema, and side of craniotomy. Additionally, condition of the parent vessels and the collateral circulation should also be taken into account. Fetal posterior communicating artery (PCoA) and/or an abnormal P1 increases the risk of post-surgical cerebral infarction. Operative side should be ipsilateral to the abnormality, thus ensuring PCoA is not obstructed. Whereas contralateral approach can be opted for a PCoA aneurysm that is medial, posteromedial, and inferior, lateral, and inferior lateral projections. Mobilization and rotation of the ICA prior to clipping, avoids occlusion of the PCoA for inferolaterally projecting PComA aneurysms.

8.2.3 Selection Criteria for Contralateral ICA Bifurcation Aneurysm Clipping

Clinical criteria for clipping of communicating segment ICA aneurysm are also similar to ophthalmic segment aneurysm. In the era of minimally invasive approaches and retractor-less brain surgery, an apparent disadvantage of the contralateral approach is the need for significant frontal lobe retraction. The ICA bifurcation represents the highest point of the circle of Willis, and this height may be indicative of the potential need of frontal lobe retraction for access to aneurysms located beyond the contralateral ICA bifurcation. Andrade-Barazarte et al. described a median height of the ICA bifurcation of 11 mm (4–16 mm) allows performing the contralateral approach without excessive frontal lobe retraction.

8.2.4 Selection Criteria for Contralateral MCA Bifurcation Aneurysm Clipping

Parameters to be considered for contralateral clipping of MCA bifurcation aneurysm are the length of the M1 segment, the size of the aneurysm, and the orientation of the aneurysm.

1. *Length of M1 segment of MCA*
   Oshiro et al. described exposure of the MCA bifurcation was possible only if the M1 segment was 14 mm or shorter, while the ICA terminus was the most consistently exposed location. Both Vajda et al. and Lynch and Andrade-Barazarte ascribed their inability to clip aneurysms at the contralateral MCA bifurcation due to a long M1 segment [6].

2. *Direction of aneurysm*

   The aneurysm can be easily found when it is pointing forward or downward. In contrast, with the body of the aneurysm pointing backward, and is parallel to the M1 segment's main stem, it is difficult to dissect, expose, and clip the aneurysm, particularly for an aneurysm with a wide neck [17]. Aneurysms pointing inferior are more difficult to control from the contralateral approach because the MCA regularly covers the neck region of the aneurysm and visualization of the perforating branches is poor. Aneurysms pointing in lateral, anterior or posterior directions are also difficult to clip from the contralateral side, because further inferior extension of the neck may be difficult to recognize. Importantly, when the body of the aneurysm points toward the insula, the clipping of the aneurysm from the contralateral approach will be blocked by the M1 segment; the aneurysm thus cannot be completely exposed in the operation field, and may damage the perforator vessels. In these cases, the operation has some limitations, and the appropriate technique should be selected carefully [18].

8.3 Surgical Nuances While Clipping of Multiple Intracranial Aneurysm Including Contralateral ICA and MCA Bifurcation Aneurysm

Selection for clipping of multiple bilateral intracranial aneurysm needs to be careful. The following selection criteria may help the surgeon plan the clipping:

8.3.1 Proximal ICA Control

Contralateral approach has the disadvantage of difficulty in securing the proximal ICA; therefore, techniques for proximal arterial control in the operative field include the following:

Techniques for Proximal Arterial Control

1. Proximal control at the neck and exposure of the proximal cervical ICA
2. Contralateral drilling of ACP and temporary clipping of ICA.
3. Adenosine induced-transient cardiac arrest

Systemic flow arrest by pharmacological mechanisms (adenosine, sodium nitroprusside) or invasive procedures (open chest-circulatory arrest) have been previously described to obtain proximal control of complex aneurysm, during intra-operative rupture or deep located aneurysms [19]. The main principle of these procedures is to induce profound hypotension leading to a decrease in the intramural pressure of the aneurysm, softening the aneurysm sac and making it amenable for safe clip placement. Adenosine is an endogenous purine nucleoside widely used for cardiac arrhythmias due to its negative chronotropic and dromotropic effects, as well as its relative short half-life. Transient cardiac arrest induced by adenosine has been used during cardiac surgery, embolization of arteriovenous malformations, complex aneurysms, and intra-operative aneurysm rupture [20].

8.3.2 Placement of Proximal ICA Balloon by Angiographic Guidance

- Side of craniotomy usually ipsilateral to ruptured aneurysm and if any mass effect due to aneurysm rupture.
- Most of aneurysm amenable with pterional craniotomy. Pterion and medial part of the sphenoid wing are drilled down to the lateral edge of the superior orbital fissure, thus flattening the bone connecting the anterior and middle cranial fossae.
- Wide opening of sylvian fissure, basal cisterns, and lamina terminalis for drain CSF and making the brain lax.
- Carotid—ophthalmic aneurysms, a generous clinoidectomy was carried out and the underlying aneurysm was well visualized.
- Clipping to be attempted first for ruptured aneurysm.
- Intra-operative flow in the parent artery can be confirmed with fluorescence microscope, ICG or Doppler probe.

8.3.3 MCA Bifurcation Aneurysm Clipping

- Contralateral clipping of MCA aneurysms has been described but is not practiced widely because of long dissection distances, limited view, and impaired maneuverability in the operative corridor and complications such as intra-operative aneurysm rupture. Contralateral clipping of MCA aneurysms is widely debated but are practiced due to prevalence of MCA aneurysms, the limitations of endovascular therapy, and patient preference for less invasive management.
- The side of the craniotomy is selected ipsilateral to the larger or more complex of the two MCA aneurysms, placing the smaller or simpler aneurysm on the contralateral side.
- Pterion and medial part of the sphenoid wing are drilled down to the lateral edge of the superior orbital fissure, thus flattening the bone connecting the anterior and middle cranial fossae.
- The contralateral approach starts at the ipsilateral ICA bifurcation, identification of A1 ACA, followed all the way to the anterior communicating artery complex.
- Cerebrospinal fluid is release by the fenestration of the lamina terminalis resulting in the slackening of the brain, which is followed by frontal retraction. Once

the chiasmatic and lamina terminalis cisterns are opened extensively, incision of the arachnoidal trabeculations (between the inferior frontal lobe and optic nerve) is performed. This arachnoidal dissection aims to open the sub-frontal corridor by extending anteriorly to the optic canal to free the frontal lobe.

- Exposure of contraletral A1 ACA is achieved by Mobilization of the frontal lobe either with a fixed or with dynamic retraction leading to the ICA bifurcation, rising above the plane of the optic apparatus. The carotid cistern when opened widely helps to visualize the origin of M1 MCA and arachnoid of the sylvian cistern.
- The dissection then proceeds distally along the M1 MCA where the anterior temporal artery originates from the inferior wall of M1 MCA and courses inferiorly, a useful landmark to visualize than the M1 MCA.
- Inferiorly and anteriorly projecting aneurysms are often visible in the surgical window, hence visualization and permanent clipping is achieved with a simple straight clip.
- On the contrary, laterally projecting aneurysms are challenge to visualize with the parent arteries obstructing the surgeons' view of the aneurysm neck. The aneurysm and/or the parent arteries may are mobilized by temporarily clipping of the M1 segment and t thereby softening of the aneurysm.
- A curved clip with its tips curving downward across the neck is preferable for laterally projecting aneurysms. A second curved clip, with the tips curving upward across the neck and intersecting the blades of the first clip, may be needed when the first clip does not completely occlude the neck.
- Exposure of superiorly projecting aneurysms that hide behind the medial orbital gyrus is done by mobilizing the aneurysm inferiorly and/or retracting the frontal lobe superiorly, or perhaps by resecting a small portion of overlying gyrus.

8.4 Outcome and Failure to Clip Contralateral Aneurysm in MIA

- Contralateral clipping of ICA-opht segment aneurysms has a reported good patient outcome rate of 74–85% of at three-month follow-up [21].
- Contralateral clipping of MCA aneurysms has a reported rate of good outcomes of 83% to 91% in previous series. Similar to that other studies demonstrated good outcome in 86% at three months follow up [16].
- Jinlu Yu et al. reported ten patients with bilateral middle cerebral artery aneurysms. All ten cases of bilateral middle cerebral artery aneurysms were successfully clipped and recovered well at discharge. The GOS scores at the half-year follow-ups included nine cases of five points and one case of four points. Follow-up on CT Angiography at one-year follow-ups showed that the clippings of the aneurysms complete without remnants at the necks of the aneurysms.
- Hugo Andrade-Barazarte reported that of the 30 patients who underwent a contralateral approach; 15 patients (50%) had multiple intracranial aneurysms and

15 patients had a single aneurysm on the contralateral side of the craniotomy. All patients underwent direct microsurgical treatment via a lateral supraorbital approach. A total of 28 patients (93%) had a good outcome and 2 (7%) patients had a poor outcome at discharge and at three-month follow-up. Of the two poor outcomes, one was related to posthemorrhagic vasospasm and the other to poor preoperative clinical grade [7].
- Vajda et al. [22] reported a failure rate of 5% of contralateral clipping mainly caused by arachnoid adhesions surrounding the aneurysm neck, complex shape, deep location or in the presence of a prefixed chiasm.

8.5 Advantages of Single Stage Clipping of Bilateral MIA

- The contralateral approach for bilateral MCA aneurysms in selected patients spares performing an additional craniotomy and all its related phases (bilateral opening and closure).
- It decreases the costs and surgical time.
- Decrease the chance of rupture in the post-operative period in which hypertension therapy may be required for vasospasm.

8.6 Disadvantages

The risk of olfactory dysfunction after performing a contralateral approach for MCA aneurysms has been reported in nearly 58% of patients. However, the risk of experiencing olfactory dysfunctions is not unique to the contralateral approach, since it may occur even in a unilateral approach for ipsilateral anterior circulation aneurysms in up to 4% of cases. In order to reduce the rate of olfactory disturbances, prolonged retraction of the frontal lobe should be avoided, and sharp dissection of the arachnoid adhesions surrounding the olfactory nerve should be used to allow better mobilization of the frontal lobe [22, 23].

8.7 Authors Experience and Case Example of Clipping of Multiple Bilateral Intracranial Aneurysms

Over the last four years, the authors have successfully performed clipping of contralateral side aneurysm in eight patients. Five out of eight cases have multiple bilateral intracranial aneurysms. (Illustrated Cases, Figs. 8.5 and 8.6). The above mentioned selection criteria were important tools for patient selection and pre-surgical counselling, especially for contralateral clippings. The five patients had total 16 aneurysms that included contralateral ophthalmic segment ICA, M1, supraclinoid ICA

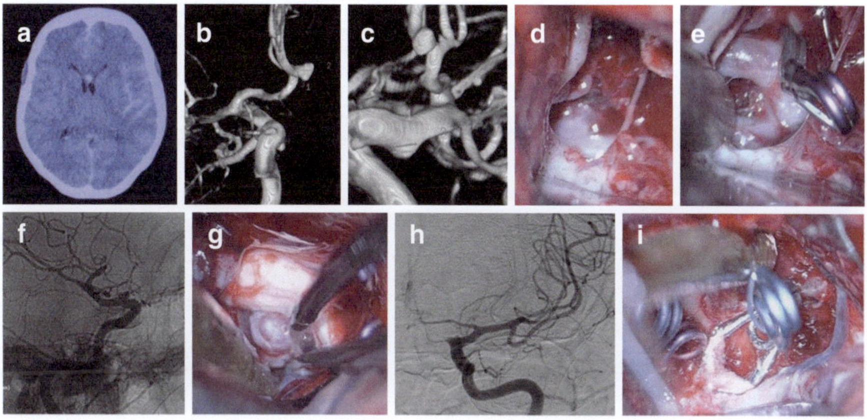

Fig. 8.5 65-year-old female patient with acute severe headache. On further evaluation patient have multiple bilateral intracranial aneurysms with rupture. (**a**) Ct brain suggestive of diffuse SAH at interhemispheric and left sylvian fissure. (**b**, **c**) 3D DSA showing ACOM aneurysm and small aneurysm at A1–A2 junction. (**d**, **e**) Intra-operative picture of ACOM and A1–A2 junction aneurysm. (**f**) DSA lateral projection showing right supra clinoid ICA aneurysm. (**g**) Intra-operative picture of right supraclinoid ICA aneurysm. (**h**) DSA showing left supraclinoid ICA aneurysm. (**i**) Intra-operative picture showing clipped left supra clinoid aneurysm

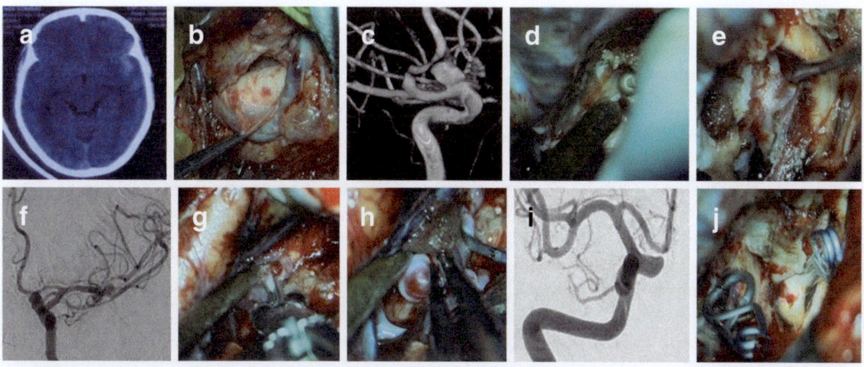

Fig. 8.6 43-year-old female presented with severe acute headache. (**a**) CT brain suggestive of left sylvian fissure SAH. (**b**) Left cervical ICA exposure for proximal control. (**c**) 3D DSA s/o lest ophthalmic ICA aneurysm. (**d**) Drilling of the left clinoid process. (**e**) Intra-operative showing clipping of left clinoid aneurysm. (**f–h**) DSA showing left MCA bifurcation and M1 segment aneurysm and intra-operative picture showing aneurysm. (**i, j**) DSA showing medially directed right ICA-ophthalmic segment aneurysm. Intra-operative picture showing clipping of aneurysms

and ICA bifurcation aneurysms. Side of craniotomy was according to brain hematoma, ruptured aneurysm and projection and morphology of aneurysms. All patients recovered well during the latest follow-up. Three cases have associated pathology was ipsilateral tubercullum sella and suprasellar meningioma along with contralateral paraclinoid aneurysms. All three cases were operated in single stage with side of craniotomy of the side of tumor and clipping of contralateral paraclinoid aneurysms. All three cases were successfully addressed tumor and aneurysms without any complication. Encouragingly, none of the eight patients we operated reported post-operative anosmia, probably because we opted for sharp dissection to avoid traction of olfactory tracts. Importantly, we were able to clip all selected contralateral aneurysms.

8.8 Conclusion

Although rare, multiple bilateral intracranial aneurysms are a stiff challenge for a Neurosurgeon. Patient selection when done meticulously, clipping of multiple intracranial aneurysms including contralateral side aneurysms is feasible and safe. Thus becoming a single stage, cost effective management strategy. Additionally, clipping is cost effective and reduces the morbidity in patients with multiple intracranial aneurysms.

References

1. Kaminogo M, Yonekura M, Shibata S. Incidence and outcome of multiple intracranial aneurysms in a defined population. Stroke. 2003;34(1):16–21.
2. Inagawa T. Incidence and risk factors for multiple intracranial saccular aneurysms in patients with subarachnoid hemorrhage in Izumo City, Japan. Acta Neurochir. 2009;151(12):1623–30.
3. McMahon JH, Morgan MK, Dexter MA. The surgical management of contralateral anterior circulation intracranial aneurysms. J Clin Neurosci. 2001;8(4):319–24.
4. Yao Z, Hu X, Ma L, You C, He M. Timing of surgery for aneurysmal subarachnoid hemorrhage: a systematic review and meta-analysis. Int J Surg. 2017;48:266–74.
5. Nakao S, Kikuchi H, Takahashi N. Successful clipping of carotid-ophthalmic aneurysms through a contralateral pterional approach. Report of two cases. J Neurosurg. 1981;54(4):532–6.
6. Oshiro EM, Rini DA, Tamargo RJ. Contralateral approaches to bilateral cerebral aneurysms: a microsurgical anatomical study. J Neurosurg. 1997;87(2):163–9.
7. Andrade-Barazarte H, Kivelev J, Goehre F, et al. Contralateral approach to internal carotid artery ophthalmic segment aneurysms: angiographic analysis and surgical results for 30 patients. Neurosurgery. 2000;77(1):104–12; discussion 112
8. Chandela S, Chakraborty S, Ghobrial GM, Jeddis A, Sen C, Langer DJ. Contralateral mini-craniotomy for clipping of bilateral ophthalmic artery aneurysms using unilateral proximal carotid control and Sugita head frame. World Neurosurg. 2011;75(1):78–82; discussion 41-72
9. Nishio S, Matsushima T, Fukui M, Sawada K, Kitamura K. Microsurgical anatomy around the origin of the ophthalmic artery with reference to contralateral pterional surgical approach to the carotid-ophthalmic aneurysm. Acta Neurochir. 1985;76(3–4):82–9.
10. de Sousa AA, Filho MA, Faglioni W Jr, Carvalho GT. Unilateral pterional approach to bilateral aneurysms of the middle cerebral artery. Surg Neurol. 2005;63(Suppl 1):S1–7.
11. Hongo K, Watanabe N, Matsushima N, Kobayashi S. Contralateral pterional approach to a giant internal carotid-ophthalmic artery aneruysm: technical case report. Neurosurgery. 2001;48(4):955–7; discussion 957-959

12. Perneczky A, Knosp E, Vorkapic P, Czech T. Direct surgical approach to infraclinoidal aneurysms. Acta Neurochir. 1985;76(1–2):36–44.
13. Kakizawa Y, Tanaka Y, Orz Y, Iwashita T, Hongo K, Kobayashi S. Parameters for contralateral approach to ophthalmic segment aneurysms of the internal carotid artery. Neurosurgery. 2000;47(5):1130–6; discussion 1136-1137
14. Oikawa S, Kyoshima K, Kobayashi S. Surgical anatomy of the juxta-dural ring area. J Neurosurg. 1998;89(2):250–4.
15. Inci S, Akbay A, Ozgen T. Bilateral middle cerebral artery aneurysms: a comparative study of unilateral and bilateral approaches. Neurosurg Rev. 2012;35(4):505–17; discussion 517-508
16. Rodriguez-Hernandez A, Gabarros A, Lawton MT. Contralateral clipping of middle cerebral artery aneurysms: rationale, indications, and surgical technique. Neurosurgery. 2012;71(1 Suppl Operative):116–23; discussion 123-114
17. Hopf NJ, Stadie A, Reisch R. Surgical management of bilateral middle cerebral artery aneurysms via a unilateral supraorbital key-hole craniotomy. Minim Invasive Neurosurg. 2009;52(3):126–31.
18. Horiuchi T, Nitta J, Nakagawa F, Hongo K. Horizontal contralateral approach for the distal anterior cerebral artery aneurysm: technical note. Surg Neurol. 2009;72(1):65–8.
19. Groff MW, Adams DC, Kahn RA, Kumbar UM, Yang BY, Bederson JB. Adenosine-induced transient asystole for management of a basilar artery aneurysm. Case report. J Neurosurg. 1999;91(4):687–90.
20. Perneczky A, Fries G. Endoscope-assisted brain surgery: Part 1—evolution, basic concept, and current technique. Neurosurgery. 1998;42(2):219–24; discussion 224-215
21. Fries G, Perneczky A, van Lindert E, Bahadori-Mortasawi F. Contralateral and ipsilateral microsurgical approaches to carotid-ophthalmic aneurysms. Neurosurgery. 1997;41(2):333–42; discussion 342-333
22. Vajda J, Juhasz J, Pasztor E, Nyary I. Contralateral approach to bilateral and ophthalmic aneurysms. Neurosurgery. 1988;22(4):662–8.
23. Park J, Lee SH, Kang DH, Kim JS. Olfactory dysfunction after ipsilateral and contralateral pterional approaches for cerebral aneurysms. Neurosurgery. 2009;65(4):727–32; discussion 732

Chapter 9
Moyamoya Disease-Standards and Advances in Revascularization Procedure and Peri-operative Management

Miki Fujimura

9.1 Introduction

Moyamoya disease (MMD) is a chronic, occlusive cerebrovascular disease with unknown etiology characterized by progressive stenosis at the terminal portion of the internal carotid artery (ICA) and the abnormal vascular network formation at the base of the brain [1]. MMD is known to have a characteristic nature to convert the vascular supply for the cerebral tissue from intracranial/internal carotid (*IC*) system to extracranial/external carotid (*EC*) system, the so called *IC-EC conversion system* [2, 3], which is well documented by Suzuki's angiographic staging in the initial report of MMD [1]. The Suzuki's angiographic staging may not reflect the severity of MMD but it well describes the exact self-compensatory pathophysiology of this entity, including its long-term temporal profile [3]. Insufficiency of this "*IC-EC conversion system*" could clinically lead to cerebral ischemia and/or intracranial hemorrhage from the fragile vascular networks, the so called moyamoya vessels.

While considering the basic pathology of MMD as a gradual conversion of the vascular supply from *IC* to *EC* system, extracranial-intracranial bypass such as superficial temporal artery-middle cerebral artery (STA-MCA) bypass may have a perfect concept to complement the "*IC-EC conversion system*" of MMD [3]. In fact, STA-MCA bypass has been established as a preferred surgical procedure for ischemic-onset MMD patients by improving cerebral hemodynamics [2–4]. Furthermore, recent evidence indicates that STA-MCA bypass has a potential role for preventing re-bleeding in hemorrhagic-onset MMD patients [5, 6]. In this chapter, the author sought to demonstrate the standard surgical procedure of STA-MCA

M. Fujimura (✉)
Department of Neurosurgery, Hokkaido University Graduate School of Medicine, Sapporo, Hokkaido, Japan
e-mail: fujimur@med.hokudai.ac.jp

Y. Kato, A. Ansari (eds.), *Cerebrovascular Surgery*, Advances and Technical Standards in Neurosurgery 44, https://doi.org/10.1007/978-3-030-87649-4_9

bypass with indirect pial synangiosis for adult MMD and its pitfall during the early postoperative period, introducing the characteristic peri-operative hemodynamic condition of adult MMD patients after surgery, such as local cerebral hyperperfusion and intrinsic hemodynamic ischemia by watershed shift phenomenon, defined as a paradoxical cerebral blood flow (CBF) decrease at the adjacent cerebral cortex near the site of the anastomosis.

9.2 Surgical Indication of STA-MCA Bypass for MMD

9.2.1 Concept of Surgical Revascularization for MMD

Concept of the revascularization surgery for MMD includes not only the vascular reconstruction by STA-MCA anastomosis, but also the consolidation for the future neovascularization by indirect pial synangiosis [2, 3]. Surgical procedures of indirect pial synangiosis include lots of variations such as encephalo-duro-arterio-synangiosis (EDAS), encephalo-myo-synangiosis, encephalo-duro-myo-synangiosis (EDMS), and multiple burr hole surgery [4, 7, 8]. The concept of the revascularization surgery, either direct or indirect bypass procedure, is to facilitate the physiological conversion of the vascular supply for the brain from *IC* system to the *EC* system [2, 4]. Now it is well-known that the STA-MCA bypass not only prevents recurrent stroke by improving CBF in ischemic MMD patients, but also could ameliorate the hemodynamic stress to the vulnerable collateral anastomosis including choroidal anastomosis, and thus reduce the risk of re-bleeding from the affected vessels in hemorrhagic-onset patients with adult MMD [5, 6, 9, 10].

9.2.2 Best Surgical Indication of STA-MCA Bypass for MMD

Current surgical indication for MMD in our institute is highlighted in Table 9.1. STA-MCA bypass has been reported a preferred surgical procedure for the ischemic-onset MMD patients, which provides long-term effect of stroke prevention and the improvement of the outcome of cognitive impairment [2, 4, 7, 8]. Although there is no multicenter randomized control trial to evaluate the efficacy of STA-MCA bypass for ischemic-onset MMD patients, multiple meta-analyses indicated the effectiveness of STA-MCA bypass for MMD patients with ischemic symptoms [11, 12]. Indirect revascularization procedure such as EDAS is also recommended for pediatric MMD, but simultaneous use of direct bypass procedure has been considered as an essential item for adult patients [4, 7]. As for the hemorrhagic-onset MMD patients, there had been a controversy whether STA-MCA bypass could have a potential role for preventing re-bleeding, but the Japan Adult Moyamoya (JAM) Trial, a randomized controlled trial which investigated the impact of STA-MCA

Table 9.1 Current indication of STA-MCA bypass for moyamoya disease

Type of the onset	Required items for surgical indication
Ischemia	Ischemic symptoms (TIA, minor completed stroke)
	Hemodynamic compromise (decreased CBF/CVR)
	Independent ADL (mRS 0-2)
	Absence of major brain damage
Hemorrhage	Adult (16–65 years old)
	Within 1 year after hemorrhage (1–12 months) Independent ADL (mRS 0-2)
	Absence of major brain damage
	Posterior location of the hemorrhagic site

TIA transient ischemic attack, *CBF* cerebral blood flow, *CVR* cerebrovascular reactivity, *ADL* activity of daily living, *mRS* modified Rankin Scale

bypass for preventing re-bleeding in hemorrhagic MMD patients, strongly suggested the efficacy of STA-MCA bypass for preventing re-bleeding in hemorrhagic-onset MMD patients [5, 6]. The inclusion criteria of JAM trial represented as follows. (1) Adult patient (aged from 16 to 65 years old), (2) STA-MCA bypass within 1–12 months after the onset of hemorrhage, (3) independent activity of daily living (modified Rankin Scale of 0–2), and (4) absence of major cortical damage [5]. The initial report of JAM trial indicated that the annual re-bleeding tares of the surgically treated group (2.7%) was significantly lower than that in non-surgical group (7.6%/year, $p = 0.042$) [5]. Moreover, the second report of JAM trial with the pre-specified subgroup analysis further suggested that annual re-bleeding rate of the MMD patients with posterior hemorrhage was as high as 17.1% per year, and STA-MCA bypass significantly reduced the risk of re-bleeding in patients with posterior hemorrhage ($p = 0.001$) [6]. Taken together, ischemic-onset MMD and/or adult MMD patients with posterior hemorrhage may have a best surgical indication for STA-MCA bypass on the affected hemisphere.

9.2.3 Controversy Issues of the Surgical Indication for MMD

STA-MCA bypass for asymptomatic MMD patients is currently not recommended because the natural history of this patient population is undetermined [4, 7]. To address this critical question, Asymptomatic Moyamoya Registry (AMORE); a multicenter observational study is currently undertaken in Japan to clarify the natural history of asymptomatic patients with MMD [13]. Alternatively, more recent supplemental analysis of JAM trial indicated that the development of choroidal anastomosis, which is defined as dilatation and extension of choroidal collateral toward the medullary arteries, was significantly associated with posterior hemorrhage in MMD patients [9], and choroidal anastomosis is a strong indicator for hemorrhagic presentation [10]. Choroidal anastomosis was also found to be more prominent in hemorrhagic-onset MMD patients as compared to ischemic-onset patients [14]. More surprisingly, another supplemental analysis of JAM trial examined the effect of choroidal anastomosis on de novo hemorrhage in adult MMD, and the authors found that annual de novo bleeding risk of the non-hemorrhagic/choroidal anastomosis-positive hemisphere was as high as 5.8% per year [15]. These results raise the question whether asymptomatic hemispheres with choroidal anastomosis should be treated by STA-MCA bypass for reducing the substantial risk of de novo hemorrhage. This issue should be solved by future prospective multicenter study.

9.3 Surgical Procedure of STA-MCA Bypass for Adult MMD

9.3.1 Standard Procedure of Direct/Indirect Combined Revascularization

Intra-operative finding of the representative case of an adult patient with hemorrhagic-onset MMD is shown (Fig. 9.1). Under general anesthesia, the head is positioned at 80° by three-point fixture. Skin incision is usually made along with the donor STA approximately 8–10 cm in length, a skin flap is inverted by L-shape when I use of parietal STA as donor or by question-marked incision (frontal STA as donor). Craniotomy is performed around the Sylvian fissure end, and the stump of the STA is prepared as semi-fish mouth shape with 1.6 mm (Fig. 9.1). Then the stump of STA is anastomosed by 10-0 or 11-0 nylon monofilament suture to the M4 segment of the MCA, approximately 0.6 mm in diameter (Fig. 9.1). After reperfusion, the patency of STA-MCA anastomosis is confirmed by intra-operative indocyanine green (ICG) video-angiography and Doppler ultrasonography (arrows in Fig. 9.1). The STA-MCA bypass is followed by indirect pial synangiosis with EDMS. The inner layer of the free bone flap is routinely drilled out for avoiding postoperative compression of the brain surface by the temporal muscle pedicle, and a wide bone window is made on the side of EDMS flap insertion [16]. The temporal muscle is usually split out into two layers. The bone flap is fixed both by two pieces of titanium plates (ThinFlap®, SHINOBI®) and a bio-absorbable plate; LactoSorb® (82% Poly-L-Lactic Acid and 18% Poly-Glycolic Acid). The author has been employing this combined revascularization procedure since 2004, with long-term favorable outcomes. The bypass could be visualized by standard MR angiography of 1.5 or 3 T (arrow in Fig. 9.2) without affecting brain parenchyma. Serial CBF measurement by ^{123}I-IMP SPECT indicated typical temporal profile of postoperative hemodynamic change, as characterized by the relatively localized CBF increase near the site of the anastomosis on postoperative day (POD) 1 (arrow in Fig. 9.2) and subsequent favorable distribution of CBF in a wider territory of the ipsilateral ACA/MCA territories on POD 7 (Fig. 9.2).

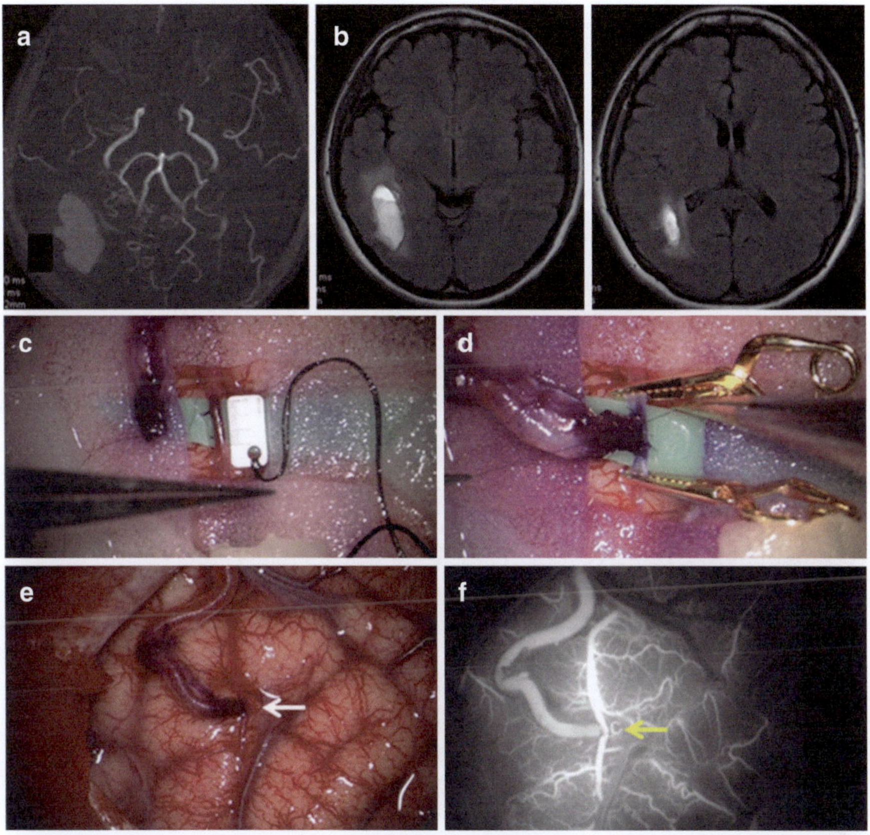

Fig. 9.1 (**a**) Representative pre-operative finding of magnetic resonance (MR) angiography (**a**) and MR imaging with fluid attenuated inversion recovery (**b**) of a 38-year-old woman with hemorrhagic-onset MMD. Intra-operative view of direct/indirect combined revascularization. Surgical view before (**c**), during (**d**), and after left STA-MCA bypass (**e**, **f**). Indocyanine green video-angiography demonstrated apparently patent bypass with favorable distribution of bypass flow (*arrow* in **f**)

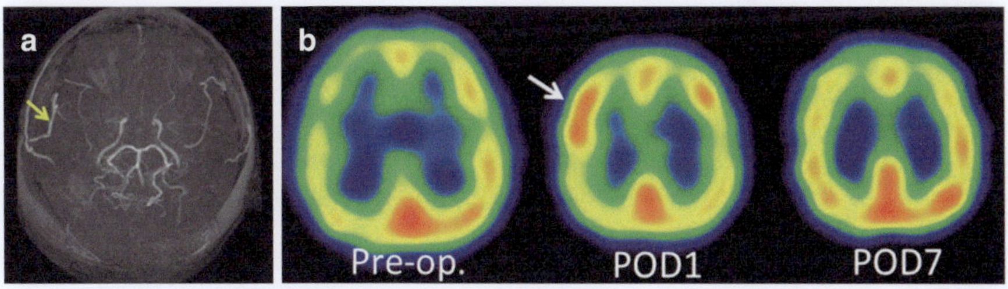

Fig. 9.2 Postoperative MR angiography demonstrated that the right STA-MCA bypass was patent (*arrow* in **a**). Serial CBF measurement by N-isopropyl-p-[^{123}I] iodoamphetamine single-photon emission computed tomography (^{123}I-IMP SPECT) (**b**) indicating typical temporal profile of post-operative hemodynamic change, as characterized by the relatively localized CBF increase near the site of the anastomosis on POD 1 (*arrow*) and subsequent distribution of CBF in a wider territory of the ipsilateral MCA territory

9.4 Intrinsic Peri-Operative Hemodynamics and Optimal Peri-Operative Management

9.4.1 Ischemic Complication of Combined Revascularization Procedure for MMD

Surgical complications of the STA-MCA bypass for MMD generally include peri-operative cerebral infarction and cerebral hyperperfusion (CHP) syndrome (Table 9.2). Peri-operative ischemic stroke could be caused by various factors such as intra-operative hypotension and/or hypocapnia by inadequate general anesthesia, anemia, and surgical procedure [4, 7]. Peri-operative ischemic complications are categorized into three distinct mechanisms; thrombo-embolism at the site of the microvascular anastomosis [17], intrinsic hemodynamic ischemia by "watershed shift phenomenon" [18–20], and mechanical compression of the brain surface by swollen temporal muscle pedicle used for additional indirect pial synangiosis [21]. Among them, "watershed shift phenomenon" is a characteristic pathophysiological condition after STA-MCA bypass for MMD, which is initially proposed by Professor Heros [22]. Watershed shift ischemia is defined as a paradoxical CBF decrease at the adjacent cortex near the site of local CHP [18, 19]. Possible mechanism underling watershed shift phenomenon is that retrograde blood supply from STA-MCA bypass could conflict with the anterograde CBF from more proximal MCA, resulting in the transient CBF decrease at the cortex supplied by the adjacent branch of MCA [20]. Clinical outcome of watershed shift ischemia is generally favorable but its simultaneous occurrence with CHP could make the peri-operative pathology more complex and difficult, since the management of each condition is contradictory [18, 19]. To avoid ischemic complications, it is essential to maintain proper

Table 9.2 Surgical complications of STA-MCA bypass for moyamoya disease

1. *Peri-operative cerebral ischemia*
(a) Thrombo-embolism from anastomosis site
(b) Watershed shift ischemia (paradoxical CBF decrease near local CHP)
(c) Cortical compression by swollen temporal muscle pedicle (combined surgery)
2. *Cerebral hyperperfusion syndrome*
(a) Focal neurological deterioration (BP-dependent worsening)
(b) Epileptic seizure
(c) Hemorrhagic conversion (intracerebral hemorrhage)
3. *Others*
(a) Chronic subdural hematoma
(b) Wound problem
(c) Cardio-pulmonary complication during BP lowering

BP blood pressure, *CBF* cerebral blood flow

peri-operative hydration and blood pressure control with prompt hemoglobin concentration maintenance [4, 7]. Efficacy of the anti-platelet agent during the peri-operative period is controversial among MMD patients, but recent multiple studies strongly suggested the advantage of aspirin administration to reduce the risk of peri-operative complication after STA-MCA bypass for MMD [23, 24].

9.4.2 Significance of Transient Local Cerebral Hyperperfusion (CHP) in Adult MMD Patients

CHP syndrome is one of the most serious complications after STA-MCA bypass for MMD [16, 25–30]. Excessive local increase in CBF at the site of the STA-MCA bypass is known to result in local hyperemia associated with vasogenic edema and/or delayed intracerebral hemorrhage in MMD, especially in adult patients. Most common clinical presentation of local CHP is transient neurological deteriorations without causing permanent neurological deficit in most cases [26, 28], but it could also lead to epileptic seizure and/or delayed intracerebral hemorrhage in a rare occasion [29]. Blood pressure dependent worsening of the focal neurological sign has a diagnostic value for CHP syndrome in adult MMD. Although the CHP syndrome after low flow bypass including STA-MCA anastomosis was considered relatively rare until the early 2000, we have reported for the first time that the incidence of CHP syndrome after STA-MCA bypass was significantly higher in MMD patients than that in atherosclerotic occlusive cerebrovascular disease patients undergoing same STA-MCA bypass procedure [25]. Representative finding of local CHP is shown in Fig. 9.3. ^{123}I-IMP SPECT 1 day after the left STA-MCA bypass with indirect pial synangiosis revealed intense focal increase of CBF at the site of the anastomosis (arrows in Fig. 9.3). Under strict blood pressure control with the administration of minocycline hydrochloride and edaravone, a free radial scavenger, the patient remained asymptomatic for 7 days, when local CHP was ameliorated by ^{123}I-IMP SPECT.

Prognosis of local CHP is generally favorable, but it could again lead to delayed intracerebral hemorrhage and/or intractable seizure in a rare occasion. Kameyama and colleagues reported the significance of quantitative CBF analysis in the early postoperative period of STA-MCA bypass for adult MMD patients. They indicated that pathological threshold of postoperative local CBF increase ratio was 184.5% for CHP syndrome and 241.3% for hemorrhagic CHP syndrome [31]. Based on these findings, quantitative CBF analysis at the site of the anastomosis could provide critical information to perform prompt peri-operative management for adult MMD patients. Regarding the prediction of CHP after STA-MCA bypass for MMD, multiple risk factors were recently reported. The indicators for postoperative CHP phenomenon or CHP syndrome are as follows; adult-onset or elderly patient's age [28, 30], onset of hemorrhagic [16, 28], operation on the dominant hemisphere [32, 33], decreased CBF before surgery [31] or increased cerebral blood volume before surgery [30], diameter mismatch between donor and recipient arteries [33], poorer

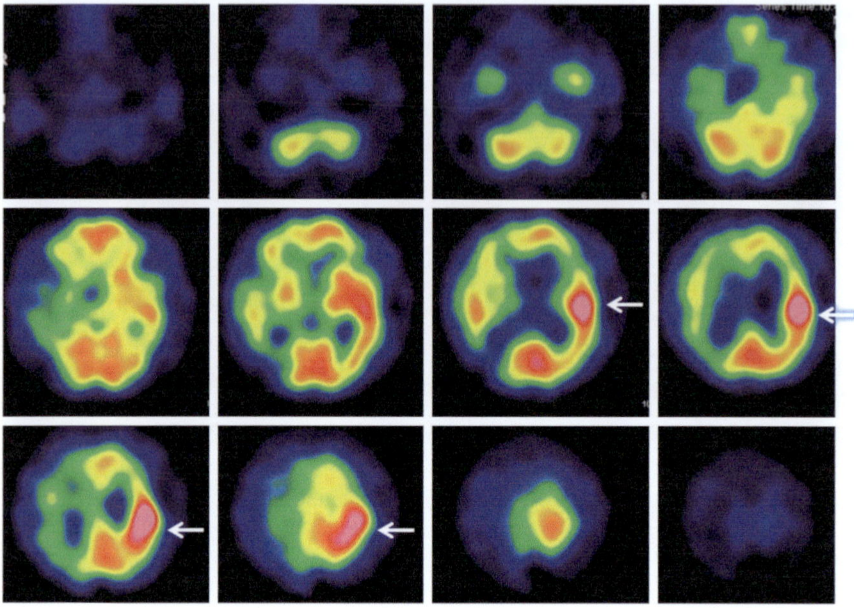

Fig. 9.3 ^{123}I-IMP SPECT after left STA-MCA bypass in 60-year old man, indicating remarkable local cerebral hyperperfusion at the site of the anastomosis (*arrows*)

intra-operative distribution pattern by ICG video-angiography or by brain surface thermography [34, 35], and lower total protein levels or higher hematocrit concentration in the pre-operative blood examination [36]. Regarding the involvement of genetic background, Tashiro et al. found that MMD patients with the *RNF213* gene polymorphism c.14576G>A [37, 38], have significantly higher risk for prolonged/delayed CHP [39]. More recently, Nishizawa and colleagues attempted to predict CHP after STA-MCA bypass by three-dimensional time-of-flight (3D-TOF) MR angiography in adult MMD patients, indicating that the signal intensity of the intracranial major arteries, including the decreased signal intensity of the peripheral cortical arteries on pre-operative 3D-TOF MR angiography could identify adult MMD patients at higher risk for CHP after direct revascularization surgery [40]. Based on these observations, it is essential to manage adult MMD patients with higher risk of CHP under more strict blood pressure to avoid deleterious effect of local CHP during the early postoperative period.

9.4.3 Limitation of the Current Peri-Operative Management Strategy

Beneficial effect of the blood pressure lowering is established to counteract with the deleterious impact of CHP phenomenon [41], but the excessive blood pressure decrease has a substantial risk for peri-operative ischemic stroke at the remote area, either ipsilateral or contralateral hemisphere, from STA-MCA bypass [33]. To manage the complex hemodynamic condition in the early postoperative period in MMD patients, the author and colleagues previously reported that moderate but prophylactic blood pressure lowering between 110 and 130 mmHg of the systolic blood pressure could significantly reduce the risk of CHP syndrome, without increasing the incidence of ischemic complication, after STA-MCA for MMD patients [18, 33, 41]. Alternatively, the prophylactic use of pharmacological agents was reported to be beneficial to prevent CHP syndrome in the previous literatures. Minocycline hydrochloride and/or edaravone (a free radical scavenger) significantly reduced the incident of CHP syndrome in MMD patients [33, 42]. The author and colleagues introduced minocycline hydrochloride, a neuro-protective antibiotic, to prevent both CHP syndrome and cerebral ischemia at the remote area [33]. Nevertheless, concomitant manifestation of local CHP with cerebral ischemia at the remote area, such as contralateral hemisphere and/or adjacent cortex affected by "watershed shift phenomenon," is still a major issue that can result in peri-operative neurological deterioration [18]. Therefore, mechanism underlying peri-operative pathologies including CHP after revascularization surgery should be further investigated in the future study.

9.5 Conclusion

STA-MCA bypass has a potential role for preventing stroke recurrence and/or rebleeding in patients with MMD. Long-term outcome of STA-MCA bypass for MMD is generally favorable, but thorough understanding of the unique pathophysiological condition of MMD and prompt peri-operative management is essential to avoid surgical complications including CHP syndrome and concomitant cerebral ischemia.

Declarations

Funding This study was supported by JSPS KAKENHI grant number 20K09362 (Miki Fujimura).

Conflicts of interest The authors have nothing to declare.

References

1. Suzuki J, Takaku A. Cerebrovascular 'moyamoya' disease. Disease showing abnormal net-like vessels in base of brain. Arch Neurol. 1969;20:288–99.
2. Fujimura M, Tominaga T. Lessons learned from moyamoya disease: outcome of direct/indirect revascularization surgery for 150 affected hemispheres. Neurol Med Chir (Tokyo). 2012;52:327–32.

3. Fujimura M, Tominaga T. Current status of revascularization surgery for moyamoya disease: special consideration for its 'internal carotid-external carotid (IC-EC) conversion' as the physiological reorganization system. Tohoku J Exp Med. 2015;236:45–53.
4. Research Committee on the Pathology and Treatment of Spontaneous Occlusion of the Circle of Willis, Health Labour Sciences Research Grant for Research on Measures for Intractable Diseases. Guidelines for diagnosis and treatment of moyamoya disease (Spontaneous Occlusion of the Circle of Willis). Neurol Med Chir (Tokyo). 2012;52:245–66.
5. Miyamoto S, Yoshimoto T, Hashimoto N, Okada Y, Tsuji I, Tominaga T, et al. Effects of extracranial-intracranial bypass for patients with hemorrhagic moyamoya disease: results of the Japan Adult Moyamoya Trial. Stroke. 2014;45:1415–21.
6. Takahashi JC, Funaki T, Houkin K, Inoue T, Ogasawara K, Nakagawara J, et al. Significance of the hemorrhagic site for recurrent bleeding: prespecified analysis in the Japan Adult Moyamoya Trial. Stroke. 2016;47:37–43.
7. Tominaga T, Suzuki N, Miyamoto S, Koizumi A, Kuroda S, Takahashi JC, et al. Recommendations for the management of moyamoya disease: A statement from Research Committee on Spontaneous Occlusion of the Circle of Willis (Moyamoya Disease) [2nd edition]. Surg Cereb Stroke. 2018;46:136–40. (In Japanese)
8. Cho WS, Kim JE, Kim CH, Ban SP, Kang HS, Son YJ, et al. Long-term outcomes after combined revascularization surgery in adult moyamoya disease. Stroke. 2014;45:3025–31.
9. Funaki T, Takahashi JC, Houkin K, Kuroda S, Takeuchi S, Fujimura M, et al. Angiographic features of hemorrhagic moyamoya disease with high recurrence risk: a supplementary analysis of the Japan Adult Moyamoya Trial. J Neurosurg. 2018;128:777–84.
10. Funaki T, Takahashi JC, Houkin K, Kuroda S, Takeuchi S, Fujimura M, et al. High rebleeding risk associated with choroidal collateral vessels in hemorrhagic moyamoya disease: analysis of a nonsurgical cohort in the Japan Adult Moyamoya Trial. J Neurosurg. 2019;130(2):337–673. https://doi.org/10.3171/2017.9.JNS17576.
11. Jeon JP, Kim JE, Cho WS, Bang JS, Son YJ, Oh CW. Meta-analysis of the surgical outcomes of symptomatic moyamoya disease in adults. J Neurosurg. 2018;128:793–9.
12. Qian C, Yu X, Li J, Chen J, Wang L, Chen G. The efficacy of surgical treatment for the secondary prevention of stroke in symptomatic moyamoya disease: a meta-analysis. Medicine (Baltimore). 2015;94:e2218.
13. Kuroda S, AMORE Study Group. Asymptomatic moyamoya disease: literature review and ongoing AMORE study. Neurol Med Chir (Tokyo). 2015;55:194–8.
14. Funaki T, Takahashi JC, Houkin K, Kuroda S, Fujimura M, Tomata Y, et al. Effect of choroidal collateral vessels on de novo hemorrhage in moyamoya disease: analysis of nonhemorrhagic hemispheres in the Japan Adult Moyamoya Trial. J Neurosurg. 2019;132:408–14. https://doi.org/10.3171/2018.10.JNS181139.
15. Fujimura M, Funaki T, Houkin K, Takahashi JC, Kuroda S, Tomata Y, et al. Intrinsic development of choroidal and thalamic collaterals in hemorrhagic-onset moyamoya disease: case-control study of the Japan Adult Moyamoya Trial. J Neurosurg. 2019;130:1453–9. https://doi.org/10.3171/2017.11.JNS171990.
16. Tokairin K, Kazumata K, Uchino H, Ito M, Ono K, Tatezawa R, et al. Post-operative intracerebral hemorrhage after combined revascularization surgery in moyamoya disease: profiles and clinical associations. World Neurosurg. 2018;120:e593–600. https://doi.org/10.1016/j.wneu.2018.08.132.
17. Fujimura M, Kaneta T, Tominaga T. Efficacy of superficial temporal artery-middle cerebral artery anastomosis with routine postoperative cerebral blood flow measurement during the acute stage in childhood moyamoya disease. Childs Nerv Syst. 2008;24:827–32.
18. Tu XC, Fujimura M, Rashad S, Mugikura S, Sakata H, Niizuma K, et al. Uneven cerebral hemodynamic change as a cause of neurological deterioration in the acute stage after direct revascularization for moyamoya disease: cerebral hyperperfusion and remote ischemia caused by the 'watershed shift'. Neurosurg Rev. 2017;40:507–12.

19. Tashiro R, Fujimura M, Kameyama M, Mugikura S, Endo H, Takeuchi Y, et al. Incidence and risk factors of the watershed shift phenomenon after superficial temporal artery-middle cerebral artery anastomosis for adult moyamoya disease. Cerebrovasc Dis. 2019;47:178–87.
20. Hayashi T, Shirane R, Fujimura M, Tominaga T. Postoperative neurological deterioration in pediatric moyamoya disease. Watershed shift and hyperperfusion. J Neurosurg Pediatr. 2010;6:73–81.
21. Fujimura M, Kaneta T, Shimizu H, Tominaga T. Cerebral ischemia owing to compression of the brain by swollen temporal muscle used for encephalo-myo-synangiosis in moyamoya disease. Neurosurg Rev. 2009;32:245–9.
22. Heros RC, Scott RM, Kistler JP, Ackerman RH, Conner ES. Temporary neurological deterioration after extracranial-intracranial bypass. Neurosurgery. 1984;15:178–85.
23. Schubert GA, Biermann P, Weiss C, Seiz M, Vajkoczy P, Schmiedek P, et al. Risk profile in extracranial/intracranial bypass surgery—the role of antiplatelet agents, disease pathology, and surgical technique in 168 direct revascularization procedures. World Neurosurg. 2014;82:672–7.
24. Zhao Y, Zhang Q, Zhang D, Zhao Y. The effect of aspirin in the postoperative management of adult ischemic moyamoya disease. World Neurosurg. 2017;105:728–31.
25. Fujimura M, Shimizu H, Inoue T, Mugikura S, Saito A, Tominaga T. Significance of focal cerebral hyperperfusion as a cause of transient neurologic deterioration after EC-IC bypass for moyamoya disease: comparative study with non-moyamoya patients using n-isopropyl-p-[(123)i]iodoamphetamine single-photon emission computed tomography. Neurosurgery. 2011;68:957–65.
26. Fujimura M, Kaneta T, Mugikura S, Shimizu H, Tominaga T. Temporary neurologic deterioration due to cerebral hyperperfusion after superficial temporal artery-middle cerebral artery anastomosis in patients with adult-onset moyamoya disease. Surg Neurol. 2007;67:273–82.
27. Kim JE, Oh CW, Kwon OK, Park SQ, Kim SE, Kim YK. Transient hyperperfusion after superficial temporal artery/middle cerebral artery bypass surgery as a possible cause of postoperative transient neurological deterioration. Cerebrovasc Dis. 2008;25:580–6.
28. Fujimura M, Mugikura S, Kaneta T, Shimizu H, Tominaga T. Incidence and risk factors for symptomatic cerebral hyperperfusion after superficial temporal artery-middle cerebral artery anastomosis in patients with moyamoya disease. Surg Neurol. 2009;71:442–7.
29. Fujimura M, Shimizu H, Mugikura S, Tominaga T. Delayed intracerebral hemorrhage after superficial temporal artery-middle cerebral artery anastomosis in a patient with moyamoya disease: possible involvement of cerebral hyperperfusion and increased vascular permeability. Surg Neurol. 2009;71:223–7.
30. Uchino H, Kuroda S, Hirata K, Shiga T, Houkin K, Tamaki N. Predictors and clinical features of postoperative hyperperfusion after surgical revascularization for moyamoya disease: a serial single photon emission CT/positron emission tomography study. Stroke. 2012;43:2610–6.
31. Kameyama M, Fujimura M, Tashiro R, Sato K, Endo H, Niizuma K, et al. Significance of quantitative cerebral blood flow measurement in the acute stage after revascularization surgery for adult moyamoya disease: implication for the pathological threshold of local cerebral hyperperfusion. Cerebrovasc Dis. 2019;48:217–25.
32. Hwang JW, Yang HM, Lee H, Lee HK, Jeon YT, Kim JE, et al. Predictive factors of symptomatic cerebral hyperperfusion after superficial temporal artery-middle cerebral artery anastomosis in adult patients with moyamoya disease. Br J Anesth. 2013;110:773–9.
33. Fujimura M, Niizuma K, Inoue T, Sato K, Endo H, Shimizu H, et al. Minocycline prevents focal neurologic deterioration due to cerebral hyperperfusion after extracranial-intracranial bypass for moyamoya disease. Neurosurgery. 2014;74:163–70.
34. Horie N, Fukuda Y, Izumo T, Hayashi K, Suyama K, Nagata I. Indocyanine green videoangiography for assessment of postoperaive hyperperfusion in moyamoya disease. Acta Neurochir. 2014;156:919–26.

35. Nakagawa A, Fujimura M, Arafune T, Sakuma I, Tominaga T. Clinical implications of intraoperative infrared brain surface monitoring during superficial temporal artery-middle cerebral artery anastomosis in patients with moyamoya disease. J Neurosurg. 2009;111:1158–64.
36. Katsuki M, Fujimura M, Tashiro R, Tomata Y, Nishizawa T, Tominaga T. Pre-operative higher hematocrit and lower total protein levels are independent risk factors for cerebral hyperperfusion syndrome after superficial temporal artery-middle cerebral artery anastomosis with pial synangiosis in adult moyamoya disease patients—case-control study. Neurosurg Rev. 2021;44(4):2191–200. https://doi.org/10.1007/s10143-020-01395-z.
37. Kamada F, Aoki Y, Narisawa A, Abe Y, Komatsuzaki S, Kikuchi A, et al. A genome-wide association study identifies RNF213 as the first moyamoya disease gene. J Hum Genet. 2011;56:34–40.
38. Liu W, Morito D, Takashima S, Minoehary Y, Kobayashi H, Hitomi T, et al. Identification of RNF213 as a susceptibility gene for moyamoya disease and its possible role in vascular development. PLoS One. 2011;6:e22452.
39. Tashiro R, Fujimura M, Katsuki M, Nishizawa T, Tomata Y, Niizuma K, et al. Prolonged/delayed cerebral hyperperfusion in adult moyamoya disease patients with RNF213 gene polymorphism c.14576G>A (rs112735431) after superficial temporal artery-middle cerebral artery anastomosis. J Neurosurg. 2020;23:1–8. https://doi.org/10.3171/2020.6.JNS201037. Online ahead of print
40. Nishizawa T, Fujimura M, Katsuki M, Mugikura S, Tashiro R, Sato K, et al. Prediction of cerebral hyperperfusion after superficial temporal artery-middle cerebral artery anastomosis by three-dimensional-time-of-flight magnetic resonance angiography in adult patients with moyamoya disease. Cerebrovasc Dis. 2020;49:396–403.
41. Fujimura M, Inoue T, Shimizu H, Saito A, Mugikura S, Tominaga T. Efficacy of prophylactic blood pressure lowering according to a standardized postoperative management protocol to prevent symptomatic cerebral hyperperfusion after direct revascularization surgery for moyamoya disease. Cerebrovasc Dis. 2012;33:436–45.
42. Uchino H, Nakayama N, Kazumata K, Kuroda S, Houkin K. Edaravone reduces hyperperfusion-related neurological deficits in adult moyamoya disease: historical control study. Stroke. 2016;47:1930–2.

Chapter 10
Carotid Endarterectomy

Takayuki Hara and Yurie Rai

10.1 Introduction

Stroke is the second leading cause of death worldwide. One of the main causes of stroke is carotid artery stenosis. Stenosis with atherosclerosis in the carotid artery can cause stroke by hemodynamic ischemia or artery to artery embolism. Carotid artery stenosis has been often treated with surgical interventions. Carotid intervention was first successfully performed in 1951 by excision of the diseased carotid artery segment and an end-to-end anastomosis of internal carotid artery and common carotid artery [1, 2]. Since then, carotid endarterectomy (CEA) has been evolved with introduction of temporary shunt system in 1956 [3], eversion endarterectomy in 1970 [4], and electroencephalogram monitoring in 1980 [5]. In 1980s and 1990s several randomized control trials (RCTs) have proven efficacy of CEA compared to medical treatment in symptomatic and asymptomatic patients [6–11]. Since carotid artery stenting (CAS) was appeared in 1990s, several RCTs has been conducted [12–18]. As the devices have been developed, treatment outcomes of CAS have been improved, and CAS has been shown to be equally beneficial to CEA with some conditions [17, 18]. By its curability and long-stand stroke preventive effect, however, CEA is still first choice of treatment for symptomatic severe carotid stenosis [19]. Here, we review the recent RCTs for CEA, explain the perioperative management, and show surgical techniques with illustrations.

T. Hara (✉) · Y. Rai
Department of Neurosurgery, Toranomon Hospital, Minato-ku, Tokyo, Japan
e-mail: thara@toranomon.gr.jp

Y. Kato, A. Ansari (eds.), *Cerebrovascular Surgery*, Advances and Technical Standards in Neurosurgery 44, https://doi.org/10.1007/978-3-030-87649-4_10

10.2 Evidence of CEA

10.2.1 CEA for Symptomatic Carotid Stenosis

For symptomatic carotid stenosis, two large RCTs, European Carotid Surgery Trial (ECST), and North American Symptomatic Carotid Endarterectomy Trial (NASCET) compared CEA with medical treatment.

In ECST, 3024 carotid stenosis patients with transient or mild symptomatic ischemic vascular event on the distribution of one or both carotid arteries were allocated to medical treatment only or CEA. As a result, ipsilateral stroke or perioperative death with more than 80% stenosis was 20.6% in medical group and 6.8% in CEA group (<0.0001) [8].

NASCET was started in 1987 in North America. Patients who experienced transient ischemic attack (TIA) or nondisabling stroke within 120 days were assigned to optimal medical care alone or optimal medical care plus CEA. The results showed that cumulative risk of any ipsilateral stroke at 2 years with 70–99% stenosis were 26% in medical group and 9% in surgical group ($P < 0.001$) on the condition that the treatments were conducted in the centers with the rate of less than 6% for stroke and death occurring within 30 days of operation [6]. Also, the ipsilateral stroke risk at 5 years with 50–69% stenosis were 22.2% in medical group and 15.7% in surgical group, whose difference became statistically significant ($P = 0.045$) if the surgeons have lower rates of complications than 2% [7]. Efficacy of CEA in symptomatic patients with less than 50% stenosis has not been proved.

Mata-analysis of ECST and NASCET focused on clinical subgroups and timing of surgery was reported in 2004 [20]. CEA was especially beneficial in men, patients aged 75 years or older, and patients who underwent surgery within 2 weeks of their last symptoms, and fell rapidly with increasing delay (see Timing of Surgery).

10.2.2 CEA for Asymptomatic Carotid Stenosis

For asymptomatic carotid stenosis, Asymptomatic Carotid Atherosclerosis Study (ACAS) began in 1987. Medical treatment and CEA were compared in 1662 patients with asymptomatic carotid stenosis of 60% or greater. The aggregate risk over 5 years for ipsilateral stroke and any perioperative stroke or death was 11.0% in medical group and 5.1% in CEA group ($P = 0.004$), which proved the efficacy of CEA if it was performed with less than 3% perioperative morbidity and mortality [9].

Another trial for asymptomatic stenosis, Asymptomatic Carotid Surgery Trial (ACST), was started in 1993. It compared deferral of any carotid procedure and immediate CEA in asymptomatic patients with at least 60%. The risk of perioperative events and strokes was 10.9% in deferral CEA group and 6.9% in immediate CEA group at 5 years ($P = 0.0001$) and 17.9% and 13.4% at 10 years ($P = 0.009$)

[10, 11]. Contrary to the trials in symptomatic patients, these ACST showed no significant association between the risk of stroke and the percentage of stenosis, and CEA was effective for both males and females.

With a recent progress of intensive medical therapy, however, the superiority of CEA to medical therapy becomes equivocal in asymptomatic patients [21]. In practice, CEA is recommended only when the stenosis is more severe (70–99%) or the patients have a particular high risk of stroke (progression of stenosis, the detection of asymptomatic carotid embolism, carotid plaque vulnerability, reduced cerebrovascular reserve, and the presence of silent embolic infarcts) [22]. Other than these risk factors, we should consider the comorbidities and life expectancy of the patients and also the surgeons' experience so as to get maximum benefit from CEA. In our opinion, the indication of CEA for asymptomatic patients should depend not only upon guidelines, but also upon the tailor-made medicine.

Updated guidelines for the treatment of carotid stenosis from American Heart Association (AHA), Society of Vascular Surgery (SVS), and European society of vascular surgeons (ESVS) are listed in Table 10.1 [23–26].

10.2.3 CEA vs. CAS

Since CAS was first performed in 1994, several RCTs comparing CEA and CAS have been reported. The first RCT comparing CAS to CEA was Stent and Angioplasty with Patients at High Risk for Endarterectomy (SAPPHIRE) trial [13]. The trial focused on the patients at high risk for CEA who have at least one of the following risk factors: positive stress test; age older than 80 years; contralateral carotid occlusion; pulmonary dysfunction; high cervical lesion; repeat carotid operation; congestive heart failure and/or known severe left ventricular dysfunction; open heart surgery needed within 6 weeks; recent myocardial infarction; unstable angina; contralateral laryngeal nerve palsy; radiation therapy to the neck. In this trial, CAS is proved not to be inferior to CEA at 1 year and also at 3 years' follow-up [13]. For patients without high risk for CEA, Endarterectomy Versus Angioplasty in Patients with Symptomatic Severe Carotid Stenosis Trial (EVA-3S) [14], Stent-Protected Angioplasty versus Carotid Endarterectomy (SPACE) [15], and International Carotid Stenting Study (ICSS) [16] compared CAS and CEA for symptomatic stenosis. All of these three trials failed to show the non-inferiority of CAS to CEA. We need to note that these three trials did not require the use of protection devices in CAS, and the surgeons were not selected strictly. Contrary to these three trials, recent RCTs reported the equal benefit of CEA and CAS. One of these RCTs is Carotid Revascularization Endarterectomy versus Stenting Trial (CREST). The trial compared CAS with embolic protection devices and CEA in symptomatic patients (>50% stenosis), and asymptomatic patients (>70% stenosis). There was no significant difference in the primary end point: 4-year rates of stroke, myocardial infarction, or death of any cause during the periprocedural period or any ipsilateral stroke within 4 years after randomization (7.2% in CAS and 6.8% in

Table 10.1 Guidelines of CEA

	AHA guidelines (2014 for symptomatic, 2011 for asymptomatic)	SVS guidelines (2011)	ESVS/ESC guidelines (2017)
Symptomatic	For patients with a TIA or ischemic stroke within the past 6 months and ipsilateral severe (70–99%) carotid artery stenosis as documented by noninvasive imaging, CEA is recommended if the perioperative morbidity and mortality risk is estimated to be <6%. (class I, level of evidence A)	In most patients with carotid stenosis who are candidates for intervention, CEA is preferred to CAS for reduction of all-cause stroke and periprocedural death (grade I, level of evidence B).	CEA is recommended in symptomatic patients with 70–99% carotid stenosis, provided the procedural death/stroke rate is <6% (class I, level of evidence A).
	For patients with a TIA or ischemic stroke within the past 6 months and ipsilateral moderate (50–69%) carotid artery stenosis as documented by catheter-based imaging or noninvasive imaging with corroboration (e.g., magnetic resonance angiogram or computed tomography angiogram), CEA is recommended depending on patient-specific factors like age, sex, comorbidities, if the perioperative morbidity and mortality risk is estimated to be <6% (class I, level of evidence B).	Data from CREST suggest that patients aged <70 years may be better treated by CAS, but these data need further confirmation.	CEA should be considered in symptomatic patients with 50–69% carotid stenosis, provided the procedural death/stroke rate is <6% (class IIa, level of evidence A).

Table 10.1 (continued)

	AHA guidelines (2014 for symptomatic, 2011 for asymptomatic)	SVS guidelines (2011)	ESVS/ESC guidelines (2017)
Asymptomatic	Selection of asymptomatic patients for carotid revascularization should be guided by an assessment of comorbid conditions, life expectancy, and other individual factors and should include a thorough discussion of the risks and benefits of the procedure with an understanding of patient preferences (class I, level of evidence C).	Neurologically asymptomatic patients with equal or more than 60% diameter stenosis should be considered or CEA for reduction of long-term risk of stroke, provided the patient has a 3- to 5-year life expectancy and perioperative stroke/ death rates can be equal or less than 3% (grade I, level of evidence A).	In "average surgical risk" patients with an asymptomatic 60–99% stenosis, CEA should be considered in the presence of clinical and/or more imaging characteristics that may be associated with an increased risk of late ipsilateral stroke, provided the perioperative stroke/death rates are <3% and the patient's life expectancy is >5 years (class IIa, level of evidence B).
	It is reasonable to perform CEA in asymptomatic patients with more than 70% stenosis if the risk of perioperative stroke, MI, and death is low. (class IIa, level of evidence A)		

CEA, $P = 0.51$), and the rates did not differ depending on symptomatic status ($P = 0.84$) or sex ($P = 0.34$). However, an interaction between age and treatment efficacy was detected ($P = 0.02$); CAS tended to show greater efficacy at younger than 70 years, and CEA at older. Moreover, periprocedural complication rate differed between CAS and CEA: the stroke rate was higher in CAS (4.1% and 2.3%, $P = 0.01$), and the myocardial infarction rate was higher in CEA (1.1% and 2.3%, $P = 0.03$). The rate of ipsilateral stroke was low in both groups (2.0% and 2.4%, $P = 0.85$) [17].

Another RCT showing efficacy of CAS is Asymptomatic Carotid Trial (ACT) one reported in 2016. The study targeted asymptomatic patients with at least 70% stenosis aged 79 years or younger without high risk for CEA, and compared CAS with embolic protection and CEA. In this study, CAS was noninferior to CEA for the prevention of ipsilateral stroke and death until 5-year follow-up period [18]. Today some new RCTs (CREST-2, ECST-2, and ACST-2) are now ongoing. In these trials, not only CEA vs CAS but also best medical treatment (BMT) vs interventions (CEA/CAS) are being compared. Indication of intervention should be reconsidered based on the upcoming trials' results.

10.3 Theoretical Background of CEA

Most of the carotid plaques are known to be limited to carotid bifurcation. The reason of this localization is not clear, but shear stress seems to play an important role in the formation of atheromatous plaque. In the carotid bifurcation, blood stream changes its direction, which can induce shear stress to the vessel wall [27–29]. In addition, Hori et al. reported that the characteristics of artery change from elastic to muscular artery at the bifurcation, and this histological change can also affect atheromatous formation [30]. They mentioned this change ended up to 20 mm distal from the bifurcation and plaque formation was also terminated up to 25 mm distal from bifurcation in most of the cadaver cases even with severe atherosclerosis.

Theoretically, in other words, we can remove almost all plaques with CEA when we expose distal ICA more than 25 mm from the bifurcation, although there are some exceptions.

10.4 Timing of Surgery

It is not well-known which timing is best for CEA after stroke or TIA. Concerning about TIA, risk for stroke onset after TIA increases by time, especially within 14 days. It has been reported that stroke occurs in 5–8% of patients with 50–99% carotid stenosis within 48 h after the index TIA, 4–17% within 72 h, 8–22% within 7 days, and 11–25% within 14 days [31–38], which indicate early (<14 days) intervention is beneficial to prevent stroke in TIA (or minor stroke) patients [20]. But the effectiveness of urgent (<24, or 48 h) CEA is still controversial. The 2017 Clinical Guidelines of European Society for Vascular Surgery states that patients with 50–99% stenosis who present with crescendo TIA should be considered for an urgent CEA, preferably within 24 h [39], but a systemic analysis demonstrated that CEA within 48 has a beneficial effect for crescendo TIA patients, but its effectiveness was not different between CEA within 24 h and after 24 h [40]. In addition, for the patients who have large infarct volume (≥1/3 of MCA territory) and severe disability (modified Rankin score ≥3), CEA should be deferred to minimize the risks of postoperative parenchymal hemorrhage [41]. Recent report shows urgent (<48 h) CEA leads to worse functional outcome if it is applied to the patients with moderate to severe strokes (NIHSS >10) [42].

In summary, the patients who have symptomatic 50–99% carotid stenosis should undergo CEA.

1. Within 14 days if the symptom is TIA or minor stroke and within 48 h is better if possible.
2. After 30 days if the symptom is severe (mRS ≥ 3 or NIHSS>10) or infarct volume is large (≥1/3 of MCA territory).

10.5 Imaging

10.5.1 Carotid Ultrasonography (CUS)

CUS is less invasive and suitable for screening. It can also evaluate plaque fragility by its echo-lucency. Hypoechoic (echo-lucent) plaque seems lipid-rich fragile plaque, whereas hyperechoic plaque seems elastic, and/or calcified stable plaque. Doppler-CUS gives us the peak systolic velocity (PSV) of the blood stream, which helps us to estimate the severity of stenosis. PSV > 125 cm/s means >50% stenosis, and PSV > 200–230 cm/s means >70% stenosis [43, 44].

10.5.2 Magnetic Resonance Imaging (MRI) and Angiography (MRA) (Fig. 10.1)

MRI/MRA is also less invasive imaging modality and gives us much more information about plaque characteristics with higher reproducibility than CUS. We can grasp the plaque extension, which is helpful to decide the range of distal ICA

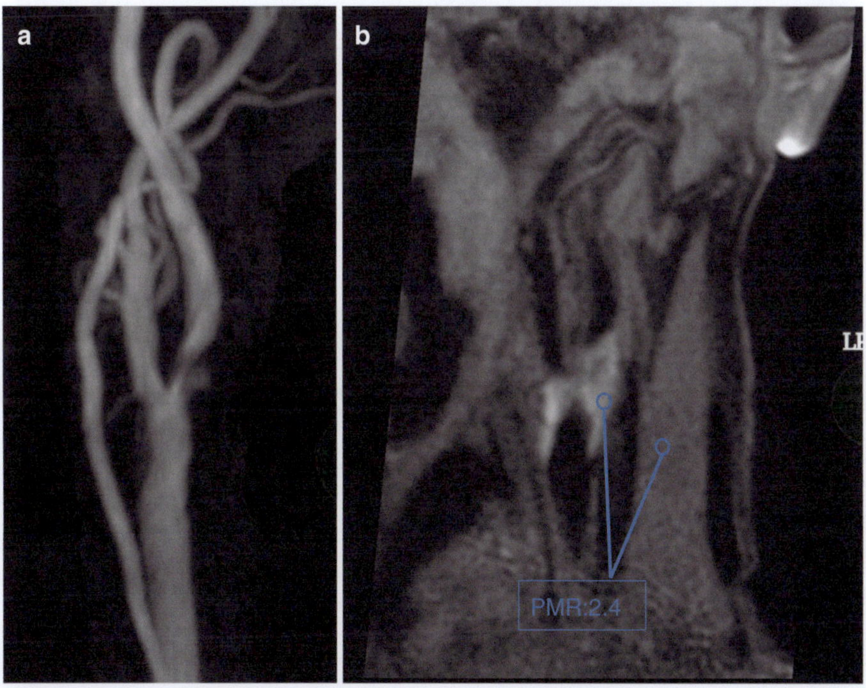

Fig. 10.1 Magnetic resonance angiography (MRA) of carotid artery. (**a**) time-of-flight (TOF) image. (**b**) black-blood (BB) image. In this patient, plaque/muscle ratio (PMR) was 2.4, which indicated fragile plaque

exposure during CEA [45]. With black-blood MRI (BB-MRI), moreover, plaque vulnerability can be evaluated. The plaque-to-muscle (sternocleidomastoid muscle) signal intensity ratio (plaque/muscle ratio [PMR]) is widely used and PMR > 3 is thought to be very fragile, PMR 1–3 be fragile, whereas PMR <1 is stable [46, 47].

10.5.3 Computed Tomography Angiography (CTA) (Fig. 10.2)

CTA needs contrast medium and X-ray exposure, which means more invasive than CUS and MRI, but much less invasive than digital subtraction angiography (DSA) because of no necessity of catheter procedure. Using three-dimensional (3D) CTA with bone images, surgical simulation becomes possible. We routinely measure mandibular angle to bifurcation length (M-B length) and according to this length, skin incision is designed in CEA.

10.5.4 Other Imaging Modalities

Conventional DSA is not always necessary for CEA patients, considering its risk. Brain MRI is to be done just prior to surgery to check the presence of fresh infarction in the ipsilateral brain and MRA is also to be done to check tandem lesion distal to the CEA site, and also to estimate the collateral blood flow from contralateral ICA or posterior circulation through circle of Willis during cross clamping. In our institute, cerebral blood flow (CBF) evaluation with single photon emission CT (SPECT) becomes mandatory to estimate the risk of postoperative cerebral hyperperfusion syndrome (CHS) if the patient seems to have hemodynamic compromise [48, 49]. The patients who have severe hypoperfusion preoperatively tend to suffer from CHS.

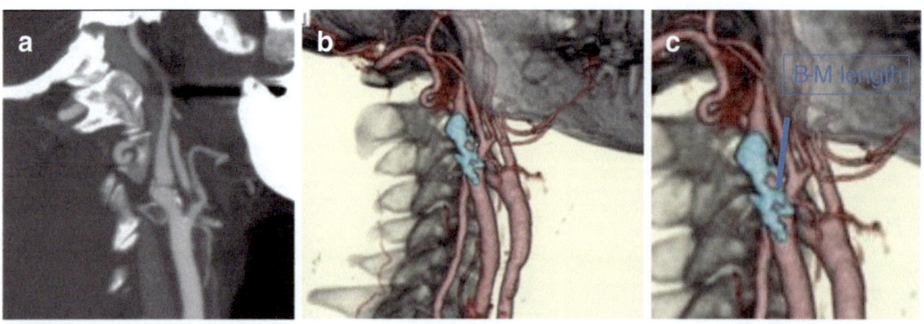

Fig. 10.2 Computed Tomography Angiography (CTA) of carotid artery. (**a**) Maximum intensity projection (MIP) image. (**b**) 3D-CTA shows anatomical landmarks around the lesion. (**c**) Mandibular-Bifurcation length (M-B length) is useful to estimate the bifurcation point before CEA

10.6 Anatomy of CEA (Fig. 10.3)

It is essential to know the surgical anatomy quite well before we start real surgery. In CEA, anatomy itself is not complicated. We do surgery inside the "carotid triangle," which is surrounded by three muscles (sternocleidomastoid, omohyoid, and posterior belly of digastric muscle), and other than arteries and veins, we should know the running course of two important nerves: hypoglossal nerve and superior laryngeal nerve. Descending branch of hypoglossal nerve (ansa cervicalis) could be cut without any symptoms, but a damage to superior laryngeal nerve can cause hoarseness and/or dysphagia. Different from hypoglossal nerve, branches of this nerve are very fine and cannot usually be identified during surgery, so comprehending the anatomy of this nerve and avoiding the rough dissection around this nerve (especially near the external carotid artery) lead to functional preservation.

10.7 Preoperative Management

10.7.1 Risk Management of General Anesthesia

Many patients who need CEA have some comorbidities such as other atheromatous vessel disease, pulmonary disease, and renal failure. In particular, those who have coronary artery disease (CAD) likely to develop myocardial infarction (MI) after

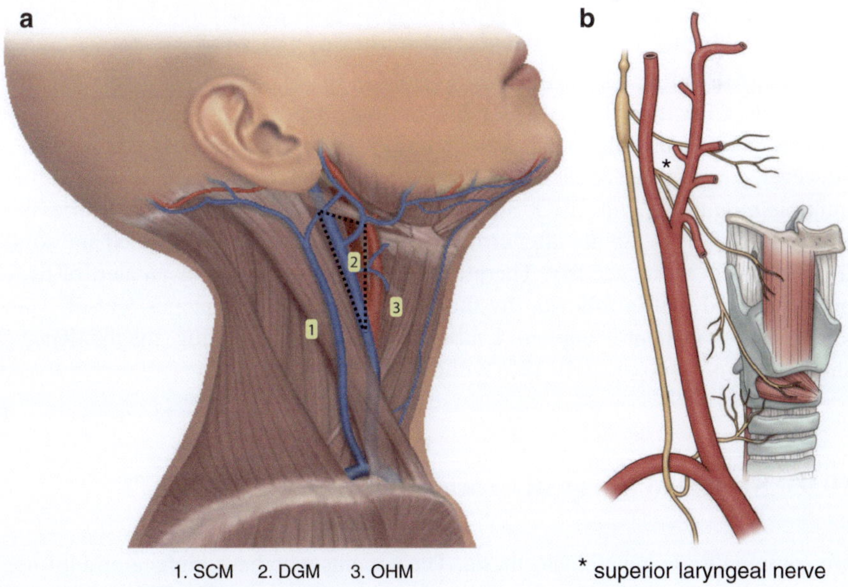

Fig. 10.3 Anatomy of CEA. (**a**) Carotid triangle is a triangle which was surrounded by three muscles. *SCM* sternocleidomastoid muscle, *DGM* digastric muscle, *OHM* omohyoid muscle. (**b**) Nerves around carotid arteries. Note the branches of superior laryngeal nerves run very close to external carotid and superior laryngeal nerve

CEA, so that careful checkup of CAD with ECG with physical load test, myocardial perfusion scintigraphy, or coronary 3D-CTA is necessary. If CAD coexists, intervention to it should take a priority if there is a time before CEA.

10.7.2 Antiplatelet Therapy

Cessation of antiplatelet therapy increases the risk of perioperative stroke and MI, so single or also dual antiplatelet therapy should continue just before CEA. On the other hand, anticoagulation therapy for atrial fibrillation can be stopped before surgery because the combination of antiplatelet and anticoagulation therapy may increase the risk of postoperative bleeding [50].

10.8 Neurophysiological Monitoring and Shunt Usage

Routine shunt or selective shunt usage during cross clamping is still controversial. Routine use of shunting system may increase the risk of intimal injury, dissection, and thrombosis formation by its insertion and removal [51], and shunt system disturbs the surgical view, which makes exposure of distal plaque end sometimes difficult. To select the patients who definitely require the shunt, neurophysiological monitoring becomes mandatory. Electroencephalography (EEG) [52, 53], Transcranial Doppler flowmetry (TCD) [54, 55], Near-infrared spectroscopy (NIRS) [56–58], Somatosensory evoked potential (SSEP) [59–61], and Motor evoked potential (MEP) [62, 63] have been applied as a single or multiple monitoring [64, 65] during CEA, and their efficacy has been reported for the selection of shunt-required patients and also for the prediction of the postoperative functional status. However, cut-off value of each monitoring has not been established. In our institute, multiple monitoring with EEG, SSEP, and MEP has been used. To our impression, EEG change occurs rapidly after cross clamp, but it cannot be quantified and sometimes recovers spontaneously. Therefore, we use EEG change as an alert of hypoperfusion, and if it is followed by the SSPE and/or MEP changes (cut-off value <50%), internal shunt is applied. Under this multiple monitoring, the incidence of shunt usage is approximately 10% without false negative.

10.9 Standard Surgical Procedure (Figs. 10.4–10.7)

We commonly use general anesthesia. The patients who have high carotid bifurcation needs nasal intubation. To lift up the mandibular angle, neck tends to be extended with vertex down position, but it has a risk to worsen the cervical spondylosis (CS). Those who have a history of CS or have myelopathic symptoms in the

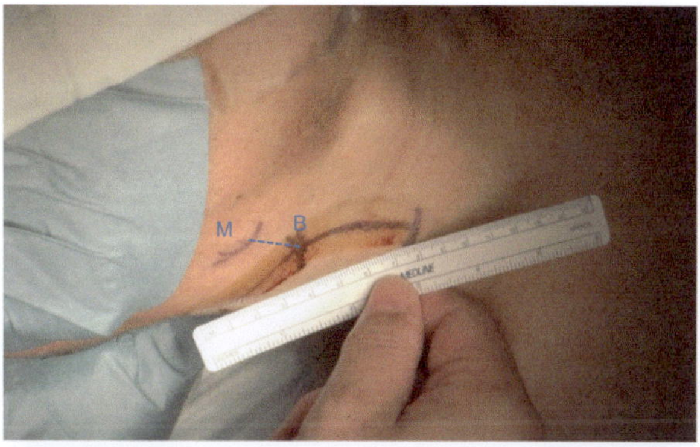

Fig. 10.4 Skin incision. According to the B-M length in 3D-CTA, carotid bifurcation is marked first. Skin incision is made 4 cm above and 4 cm below this point (total 8 cm)

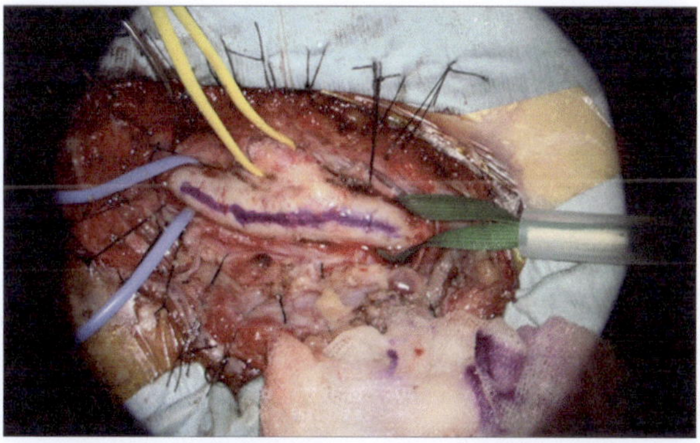

Fig. 10.5 Exposure of carotid arteries with hitch-up method. Note carotid sheath was hitched up to the surface, which makes retractors unnecessary. Carotid artery is exposed more than 2.5 cm distal and 2 cm proximal from the bifurcation in all cases

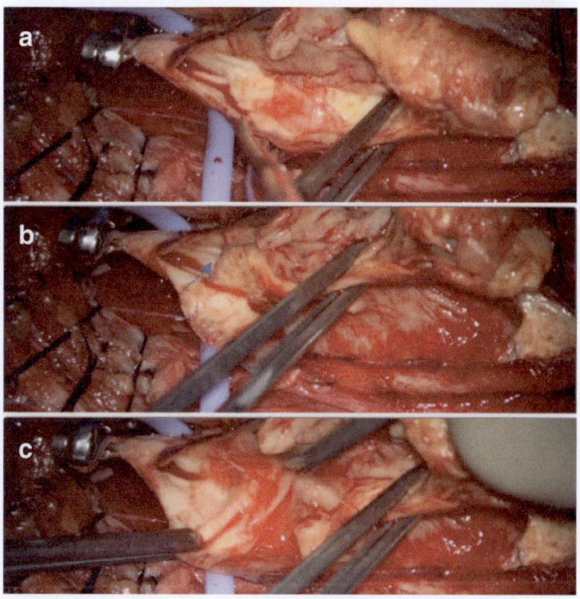

Fig. 10.6 Removal of the plaque at the distal end. (**a**): Sharp cut is sometimes necessary at the border of plaque and normal intima. (**b**) Plaque should be dissected toward vertical direction (*dotted arrow*). (**c**) After plaque removal. Note no intimal flap was made, which makes taking suture unnecessary

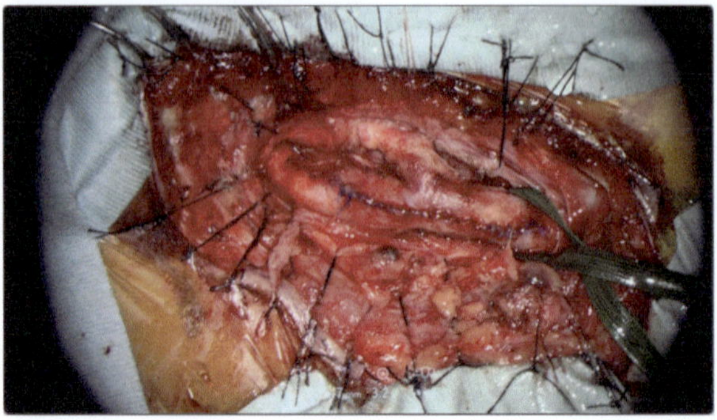

Fig. 10.7 Primary closure with 6-0 Nylon. Small suture bite-to-stich interval in the ICA is important to prevent postoperative restenosis

preoperative neck extension test, we should not keep the patients in the vertex down position. Instead, we can get similar surgical working space by lifting up the mandibular bone with blunt hooks even in the normal head positioning.

According to B-M length measured by the preoperative CT angiography, first we mark the carotid bifurcation on the skin. Skin incision is made 4 cm above and 4 cm below the marking of bifurcation (total 8 cm) along with the anterior margin of sternocleidomastoid muscle (SCM). After cutting the skin and platysma muscle, SCM is exposed. First, dissection is to be done between SCM and omohyoid muscle to expose common carotid artery (CCA). Anterior margin of SCM is hitched up laterally to expose the carotid sheath, and internal jugular vein is not always to be exposed. Carotid sheath is cut and hitched upward together with carotid arteries to get shallow surgical field. Common facial vein is cut during this exposure, but care should be taken no to cut the hypoglossal nerve which sometimes runs very close to this vein. How to identify the hypoglossal nerve is to follow the ansa cervicalis or to dissect just below the posterior belly of digastric muscle, which could easily be found just below the parotid gland. The patient who has high carotid bifurcation requires us some effort to expose the distal end of plaque. We have used tailor-made mouth piece to achieve mandibular subluxations [66] but recently it is thought to be enough to dissect SCM and parotid gland as much as possible and lift up the mandible with blunt hooks with nasal intubation. We commonly expose the carotid artery at least 2.5 cm distal to the bifurcation, 2 cm proximal to it according to the literature mentioned above [30], but it can be modified by refereeing the plaque imaging in MRA [45]. To visualize the distal end of the plaque clearly even in case of shunt usage, we think 5 mm more to be exposed from the distal edge of the plaque, and more exposure leads to less possibility of acute postoperative occlusion of distal ICA. After systemic heparinization with activated clotting time (ACT) >250 s, cross clamp is made. According to the intraoperative monitoring, we selectively use internal shunt. The plaque is removed from CCA to ICA. ECA plaque is easily pulled out without additional arteriotomy, but ICA plaque end should not be pulled out blindly. With adequate exposure, ICA plaque end must be visually confirmed and removed totally with gentle dissection. Most of the plaques can be dissected from normal intima at their ends by splitting the margin with micro-scissors and move the plaques laterally. Tacking suture is done with 6-0 nylon only when the intimal flap formation is recognized at the distal end of dissection (rare). Vessel wall is closed with 5-0 Nylon running suture from both sides and overlapped 5 mm at the midpoint of suture line. Prior to total declamping, ECA and CCA clips are released temporally to prevent air embolism to ICA and secure the hemostasis. Additional stitches are requested when the arterial bleeding occurs from suture line, but small oozing can be stopped with gentle compression and heparinization reversal (after total declamping), or hemostatic agent (Floseal®). After checking the patency of ICA with Doppler sonography or flowmetry, wound is closed with layer-by-layer.

10.10 Controversial Issue

10.10.1 Eversion or Standard CEA?

Eversion CEA is first described by DeBakey et al. in 1959 [67]. This technique is known to be superior to standard CEA in terms of short surgical time and less frequent restenosis [68]. Instead, shunt insertion is more challenging and access to high lesion is difficult. Moreover, eversion CEA requires full dissection around carotid bulb and distal ICA that may lead to cranial nerve palsies. We prefer standard CEA because Asian people usually have high carotid bifurcation and shunt insertion is requested for approximately 10% of patients in our series with multiple neurophysiological monitoring.

10.10.2 Primary Closure or Patch Angioplasty?

Primary closure is a simple method and can reduce the clamp time but may increase the incidence of acute occlusion or restenosis. Patch angioplasty is thought to reduce these complications even though longer operation time and rare complication of vein graft rupture and patch infection were reported [69–71]. Patch material is made from an autologous vein, bovine pericardium, or synthetic material including polytetrafluoroethylene (PTFE), dacron, polyurethane, and polyester. The difference of patch material does not affect the outcome so much [72]. In our institute, patch angioplasty is not mandatory because we have rarely encountered restenosis after CEA (1%) with primary closure. We have used as small suture bite-to-stich interval as possible and tried not to involve the adventitia in the suture, which may lead to prevent acute occlusion or restenosis (Fig. 10.7). On the other hand, those who have originally small diameter in ICA (especially women) or CEAs after restenosis are treated with patch angioplasty (Hemashield patch graft), so this technique should be ready to use whenever necessary.

10.10.3 Restenosis After CEA

It has been reported that restenosis occurs in 5–22% after CEA [73–75]. Restenosis is defined as more than 50% of stenosis after more than 30 days postoperatively [76]. Pathophysiology of early restenosis (within 2 years after CEA) is thought not to be atherosclerosis, but to be inflammation and neo-intimal hyperplasia, so it is not likely to cause artery to artery embolism even though the stenosis becomes severe. But late restenosis (>2 years after CEA) is deemed similar to primary atherosclerotic lesion that can become an embolic source [77]. There is no clear guideline to treat post-CEA restenosis, but controlling the risk factors is most essential. Vascular risk factors (hyperlipidemia, hypertension, smoking, and metabolic syndrome), and female gender have been described as risk factors [75], so best medical treatment (BMT) should continue and careful follow-up is necessary to the patients who have those factors. If the restenosis becomes severe (>70%) and symptomatic, reintervention should be taken into consideration [39]. Re-do CEA and CAS seems to be the same effect for the prevention of ipsilateral stroke [78, 79], but its choice must depend upon pathophysiology of stenosis mentioned above. If the restenosis occurs in early phase (<2 years) and intimal hyperplasia is suspected with plaque imaging, CAS has a priority because plaque rupture is hard to occur during stenting procedure. On the other hand, CEA with patch angioplasty may be better to the lesion which has been caused more than 3 years after initial CEA and has a sign of atheromatous plaque in the echo or MRI imaging.

10.11 Postoperative Management

The patients are recovered from anesthesia soon after surgery, but those who have been treated with dual antiplatelet therapy (DAPT) are kept anesthetized overnight to prevent postoperative bleeding. Patients are strictly monitored in the intensive care unit (ICU) or rooms comparable to ICU. Postoperative airway obstruction due to a carotid rupture or wound hematoma can occur mainly within 24 h postoperatively, which sometimes becomes fatal. If it occurs, emergency wound reopening and decompression should be performed. Blood pressure is kept under 80–100% of preoperative value until the SPECT denies postoperative hyperperfusion. If the hyperperfusion is recognized in SPECT, strict control of blood pressure should be continued for at least 4–7 days even if it is asymptomatic, because it can cause massive and sometimes fatal intracranial hemorrhage. Single antiplatelet therapy (SAPT) is restarted soon after surgery and continues thereafter [80–82].

10.12 Complication and its Management

10.12.1 Myocardial Infarction

This is most common systemic complication in CEA. As mentioned before, preoperative screening is essential to avoid this complication, but if preoperative coronary evaluation was insufficient, electrocardiogram (ECG) monitoring should be continued for a few days postoperatively. It is important to recognize that carotid artery stenosis is a part of systemic vascular disease, and vascular surgeons must keep in touch with cardiologists.

10.12.2 Nerve Palsies

Hypoglossal nerve and superior laryngeal nerve palsy can be occurred in CEA. The latter one, especially, can cause hoarseness and dysphagia and affect the quality of life. Most of the symptoms will recover within 3 months, but not completely in some patients. To avoid superior laryngeal nerve palsy, care should be taken not to dissect the tissue around ECA and superior thyroid artery too much, because this nerve usually runs just behind these arteries.

10.12.3 Cerebral Hyperperfusion Syndrome (CHS)

CHS has been reported in 0.2–18.9% of cases following CEA, but recent report showed less incidence (1.9%) [83]. It is well-known that the patients whose cerebral blood flow was severely decreased before surgery have dysregulation of cerebral vascular system and have a tendency of CHS [49]. The major symptoms of CHS include headache, restless, and seizure that appear in parallel with blood pressure elevation [48]. It is also reported that intracerebral hemorrhage (ICH) can be caused by CHS, and this ICH sometimes becomes fatal even though the incidence is quite low (0.37%) [83]. This complication is preventable, so screening the patient who is prone to CHS and postoperative BP control (<100% of preoperative value) with CBF evaluation (SPECT) are essential.

10.13 CEA for High Risk Patients (Advanced)

High risk for CEA is defined in Table 10.2. Comorbidities listed in this table are the risks for general anesthesia and if they are poorly controlled, CEA with general anesthesia becomes contraindication. As for risks for anatomical factors, most of

Table 10.2 High risk for CEA

Anatomical factors	Comorbidities
Previous neck surgery or tracheostomy	Severe CHF
Restenosis after CEA	Severe CAD
Previous radiation therapy	Severe pulmonary disease
Contralateral carotid occlusion	CKD
Contralateral laryngeal nerve palsy[a]	
High carotid bifurcation (above C2 vertebra)	

CHF chronic heart failure, *CAD* coronary artery disease, *CKD* chronic renal failure
[a]True contraindication for CEA among anatomical factors (personal opinion)

them can be overcome and not contraindication. For example, it has been reported that CEA for carotid stenosis with previous radiation therapy has longer stroke prevention with less restenosis than CAS, whereas cranial nerve palsy was more common [84–86]. CEA for contralateral carotid occlusion (CCO) seems not to be contraindication, because some reports demonstrated that perioperative stroke risk was not different between CCO and non-CCO patients, under routine or selective shunt [87, 88]. In our institute, among anatomical factors listed in Table 10.2, only contralateral laryngeal nerve palsy is thought to be contraindication of CEA. In case of previous neck surgery or tracheostomy, we usually use microscope to do meticulous dissection around carotid artery when adventitia and surrounding tissues are tightly adhered, although all of these patients have not been treated only with CEA.

10.14 Summary

CEA is a surgery for stroke prevention, whose efficacy is supported by many RCTs and whose recommendation level is quite high. Even though the devices and techniques of CAS progress, CEA seems to be golden standard for the intervention for carotid stenosis by its curability. To warrant its superiority, low complication rate is required, so CEA surgeons should continue to brush up their knowledge and skills. On the other hand, CEA, CAS and medical therapy are no longer competitive, but complementary treatment, so vascular surgeons should also catch up the current status of other two options and become able to change their surgical indication flexibly to give an optimal treatment to the patients.

Conflict of Interest Authors do not have any conflict of interest in this manuscript.

References

1. Carrea R, Molins M, Murphy G. Surgery of spontaneous thrombosis of the internal carotid in the neck; carotido-carotid anastomosis; case report and analysis of the literature on surgical cases. Medicina (B Aires). 1955;15:20–9.
2. Morris DR, Ayabe K, Inoue T, Sakai N, Bulbulia R, Halliday A, Goto S. Evidence-based carotid interventions for stroke prevention: state-of-the-art review. J Atheroscler Thromb. 2017;24:373–87.
3. Cooley DA, Al-Naaman YD, CAC. Surgical treatment of atherosclerotic occlusion of the internal carotid artery. J Neurosurg. 1956;13:500–6.
4. Samuel N. A simple technic for carotid endarterectomy. Am J Surg. 1970;120:275–8.
5. Callow AD. An overview of the stroke problem in the carotid territory. Am J Neurosurg. 1980;140:181–91.
6. North American Symptomatic Carotid Endarterectomy Trial Collaborators, HJM B, Taylor DW, Haynes RB, Sackett DL, Peerless SJ, Ferguson GG, Fox AJ, Rankin RN, Hachinski VC, EM WDO. Beneficial effect of carotid endarterectomy in symptomatic patients with high-grade carotid stenosis. N Engl J Med. 1991;325:445–53.
7. Barnett HJ, Taylor DW, Eliasziw M, Fox AJ, Ferguson GG, Haynes RB, Rankin RN, Clagett GP, Hachinski VC, Sackett DL, Thorpe KE, Meldrum HESJD. Benefit of carotid endarterectomy in patients with symptomatic moderate or severe stenosis. New Engl J Med. 1998;339:1415–25.
8. Warlow C, Farrell B, Fraser A, Sandercock P, Slattery J. Randomised trial of endarterectomy for recently symptomatic carotid stenosis: final results of the MRC European Carotid Surgery Trial (ECST). Lancet. 1998;351:1379–87.
9. Mayberg MR. Endarterectomy for asymptomatic carotid artery stenosis. JAMA. 1995;273:1459.
10. Halliday A, Mansfield A, Marro J, Peto C, Peto R, Potter J, Thomas D, MRC Asymptomatic Carotid Surgery Trial (ACST) Collaborative Group. Prevention of disabling and fatal strokes by successful carotid endarterectomy in patients without recent neurologic symptoms: randomized controlled trial. Lancet. 2004;363:1491–502.
11. Halliday A, Harrison M, Hayter E, Kong X, Mansfi A, Marro J, Pan H, Peto R, Potter J. 10-Year stroke prevention after successful carotid endarterectomy for asymptomatic stenosis (ACST-1): a multicentre randomised trial. Lancet. 2010;376:1074–84.
12. Yadav JS. Carotid stenting in high-risk patients: design and rationale of the SAPPHIRE trial. Cleve Clin J Med. 2004;71:45–6.
13. Gurm HS, Yadav JS, Fayad P, et al. Long-term results of carotid stenting versus endarterectomy in high-risk patients. N Engl J Med. 2008;358:1572–9.
14. Mas J-L, Chatellier G, Beyssen B, et al. Endarterectomy versus stenting in patients with symptomatic severe carotid stenosis. N Engl J Med. 2006;355:1660–71.
15. SPACE Collaborative Group, Ringleb PA, Allenberg J, Brückmann H, Eckstein HH, Fraedrich G, Hartmann M, Hennerici M, Jansen O, Klein G, Kunze A, Marx P, Niederkorn K, Schmiedt W, Solymosi L, Stingele R, HW ZH. 30 day results from the SPACE trial of stent-protected angioplasty versus carotid endarterectomy in symptomatic patients: a randomised non-inferiority trial. Lancet. 2006;368:1239–47.
16. International Carotid Stenting Study Investigators, Ederle J, Dobson J, et al. Carotid artery stenting compared with endarterectomy in patients with symptomatic carotid stenosis (International Carotid Stenting Study): an interim analysis of a randomised controlled trial. Lancet. 2010;375:985–97.
17. Brott TG, Hobson RW, Howard G, et al. Stenting versus endarterectomy for treatment of carotid-artery stenosis. N Engl J Med. 2010;363:11–23.
18. Rosenfield K, Matsumura JS, Chaturvedi S, Riles T, Ansel GM, Metzger DC, Wechsler L, Jaff MR, Gray W, Investigators ACTI. Randomized trial of stent versus surgery for asymptomatic carotid stenosis. N Engl J Med. 2016;374:1011–20.

19. Orrapin S, Rerkasem K. Carotid endarterectomy for symptomatic carotid stenosis. Cochrane Database Syst Rev. 2017;6(6):CD001081. https://doi.org/10.1002/14651858.CD001081.pub3.
20. Rothwell PM, Eliasziw M, Gutnikov SA, Warlow CP, Barnett HJM. Endarterectomy for symptomatic carotid stenosis in relation to clinical subgroups and timing of surgery. Lancet. 2004;363:915–24.
21. Keyhani S, Cheng EM, Hoggatt KJ, et al. Comparative effectiveness of carotid endarterectomy vs initial medical therapy in patients with asymptomatic carotid stenosis. JAMA Neurol. 2020;77(9):1–12. https://doi.org/10.1001/jamaneurol.2020.1427.
22. Bogiatzi C, Azarpazhooh MR, Spence JD. Choosing the right therapy for a patient with asymptomatic carotid stenosis. Expert Rev Cardiovasc Ther. 2020;18:53–63.
23. Brott TG, Halperin JL, Abbara S, et al. 2011 ASA/ACCF/AHA/AANN/AANS/ACR/ASNR/CNS/SAIP/SCAI/SIR/SNIS/SVM/SVS Guideline on the management of patients with extracranial carotid and vertebral artery disease. Circulation. 2011;124:54–130.
24. Kernan WN, Ovbiagele B, Black HR, et al. Guidelines for the prevention of stroke in patients with stroke and transient ischemic attack: a guideline for healthcare professionals from the American Heart Association/American Stroke Association. Stroke. 2014;45:2160–236.
25. Aboyans V, Ricco JB, Bartelink MLEL, et al. 2017 ESC Guidelines on the diagnosis and treatment of peripheral arterial diseases, in collaboration with the European Society for Vascular Surgery (ESVS). Eur Heart J. 2018;39:763–816.
26. Ricotta JJ, Aburahma A, Ascher E, Eskandari M, Faries P, Lal BK. Updated Society for Vascular Surgery guidelines for management of extracranial carotid disease. J Vasc Surg. 2011;54:e1–e31.
27. Kjaernes M, Svindland A, Walløe L, Wille SO. Localization of early atherosclerotic lesions in an arterial bifurcation in humans. Acta Pathol Microbiol Scand A. 1981;89:35–40.
28. LoGerfo FW, Nowak MD, Quist WC, Crawshaw HM, Bharadvaj BK. Flow studies in a model carotid bifurcation. Arteriosclerosis. 1981;1:235–41.
29. Motomiya M. Flow patterns in the human carotid artery bifurcation. Stroke. 1984;15:50–6.
30. Hori E, Hayashi N, Hamada H, Masuoka T, Kuwayama N, Hirashima Y, Origasa H, Ohtani O, Endo S. A development of atheromatous plaque is restricted by characteristic arterial wall structure at the carotid bifurcation. Surg Neurol. 2008;69:586–90.
31. Marnane M, Prendeville S, McDonnell C, Noone I, Barry M, Crowe M, Mulligan N, Kelly PJ. Plaque inflammation and unstable morphology are associated with early stroke recurrence in symptomatic carotid stenosis. Stroke. 2014;45:801–6.
32. Merwick Á, Albers GW, Arsava EM, et al. Reduction in early stroke risk in carotid stenosis with transient ischemic attack associated with statin treatment. Stroke. 2013;44:2814–20.
33. Mono ML, Steiger I, Findling O, et al. Risk of very early recurrent cerebrovascular events in symptomatic carotid artery stenosis: clinical article. J Neurosurg. 2013;119:1620–6.
34. Johansson EP, Arnerlöv C, Wester P. Risk of recurrent stroke before carotid endarterectomy: The ANSYSCAP Study. Int J Stroke. 2012;8:220–7.
35. Bonifati DM, Lorenzi A, Ermani M, Refatti F, Gremes E, Boninsegna C, Filipponi S, Orrico D. Carotid stenosis as predictor of stroke after transient ischemic attacks. J Neurol Sci. 2011;303:85–9.
36. Ois A, Cuadrado-Godia E, Rodríguez-Campello A, Jimenez-Conde J, Roquer J. High risk of early neurological recurrence in symptomatic carotid stenosis. Stroke. 2009;40:2727–31.
37. Purroy F, Montaner J, Molina CA, Delgado P, Ribo M, Álvarez-Sabín J. Patterns and predictors of early risk of recurrence after transient ischemic attack with respect to etiologic subtypes. Stroke. 2007;38:3225–9.
38. Fairhead JF, Mehta Z, Rothwell PM. Population-based study of delays in carotid imaging and surgery and the risk of recurrent stroke. Neurology. 2005;65:371–5.
39. Naylor AR, Ricco JB, de Borst GJ, et al. Editor's choice—management of atherosclerotic carotid and vertebral artery disease: 2017 Clinical practice guidelines of the European Society for Vascular Surgery (ESVS). Eur J Vasc Endovasc Surg. 2018;55:3–81.

40. Fereydooni A, Gorecka J, Xu J, Schindler J, Dardik A. Carotid endarterectomy and carotid artery stenting for patients with crescendo transient ischemic attacks: a systematic review. JAMA Surg. 2019;154:1055–63.
41. Pini R, Faggioli G, Vacirca A, Dieng M, Goretti M, Gallitto E, Mascoli C, Ricco J-B, Gargiulo M. The benefit of deferred carotid revascularization in patients with moderate-severe disabling cerebral ischemic stroke. J Vasc Surg. 2021;73:117–24.
42. Mihindu E, Mohammed A, Smith T, Brinster C, Sternbergh WC 3rd, Bazan HA. Patients with moderate to severe strokes (NIHSS score >10) undergoing urgent carotid interventions within 48 hours have worse functional outcomes. J Vasc Surg. 2019;69:1471–81.
43. Koga M, Kimura K, Minematsu K, Yamaguchi T. Diagnosis of internal carotid artery stenosis greater than 70% with power doppler duplex sonography. Am J Neuroradiol. 2001;22: 413–7.
44. Grant EG, Benson CB, Moneta GL, et al. Carotid artery stenosis: gray-scale and doppler US diagnosis—Society of Radiologists in Ultrasound Consensus Conference. Radiology. 2003;229:340–6.
45. Yoshida K, Endo H, Sadamasa N, Narumi O, Chin M, Inoue K, Mitsudo K, Yamagata S. Evaluation of carotid artery atherosclerotic plaque distribution by using long-axis high-resolution black-blood magnetic resonance imaging: clinical article. J Neurosurg. 2008;109:1042–8.
46. Takemoto K, Ueba T, Takano K, Abe H, Hirata Y, Higashi T, Inoue T, Sakata N, Yoshimitsu K. Quantitative evaluation using the plaque/muscle ratio index panels predicts plaque type and risk of embolism in patients undergoing carotid artery stenting. Clin Neurol Neurosurg. 2013;115:1298–303.
47. Eto A, Kinoshita Y, Matsumoto Y, Kiyomi F, Iko M, Nii K, Tsutsumi M, Sakamoto K, Aikawa H, Kazekawa K. Relationship between the carotid plaque T1 relaxation time and the plaque-to-muscle signal intensity ratio on black-blood magnetic resonance imaging scans. J Stroke Cerebrovasc Dis. 2016;25:2580–4.
48. Farooq MU, Goshgarian C, Min J, Gorelick PB. Pathophysiology and management of reperfusion injury and hyperperfusion syndrome after carotid endarterectomy and carotid artery stenting. Exp Transl Stroke Med. 2016;8:1–8.
49. Manojlovic V, Budakov N, Budinski S, Milosevic D, Nikolic D. Cerebrovacular reserve predicts the cerebral hyperperfusion syndrome after carotid endarterectomy. J Stroke Cerebrovasc Dis. 2020;29(12):105318. https://doi.org/10.1016/j.jstrokecerebrovasdis.2020.105318.
50. Becker RC, Caprini JA, Dunn AS, et al. Perioperative bridging anticoagulation in patients with atrial fibrillation. N Engl J Med. 2015;373:823–33.
51. Chongruksut W, Vaniyapong T, Rerkasem K. Routine or selective carotid artery shunting for carotid endarterectomy (and different methods of monitoring in selective shunting). Cochrane Database Syst Rev. 2014;2014(6):CD000190. https://doi.org/10.1002/14651858.CD000190.pub3.
52. Mcgrail KM. Intraoperative use of electroencephalography as an assessment of cerebral blood flow. Neurosurg Clin N Am. 1996;7:685–92.
53. Schneider JR, Droste JS, Schindler N. Carotid endarterectomy with routine electroencephalography and selective shunting : influence of contralateral internal carotid artery occlusion and utility in prevention of perioperative strokes. J Vasc Surg. 2002;35:1114–22.
54. Yun W. Cerebral monitoring during carotid endarterectomy by transcranial Doppler ultrasonography. Ann Surg Treat Res. 2017;92:105–9.
55. Ackerstaff RGA, Moons KGM, Van De Vlasakker CJW, Moll FL, Vermeulen FEE, Algra A, Spencer MP. Association of intraoperative transcranial doppler monitoring variables with stroke from carotid endarterectomy. Stroke. 2000;31:1817–23.
56. Kondov S, Beyersdorf F, Sch J, Benk C. Outcome of near-infrared spectroscopy e guided selective shunting during carotid endarterectomy in general anesthesia. Ann Vasc Surg. 2019;61:170–7.

57. Pennekamp CWA, Immink RV, Den Ruijter HM, Kappelle LJ, Bots ML, Buhre WF, Moll FL, De Borst GJ. Near-infrared spectroscopy to indicate selective shunt use during carotid endarterectomy. Eur J Vasc Endovasc Surg. 2013;46:397–403.
58. Mille T, Tachimiri ME, Klersy C, Ticozzelli G, Bellinzona G, Blangetti I, Pirrelli S, Lovotti M, Odero A. Near infrared spectroscopy monitoring during carotid endarterectomy : which threshold value is critical ? Eur J Vasc Endovasc Surg. 2004;27:646–50.
59. Amantini A, Bartelli M, De Scisciolo G, Lombardi M, Macucci M, Rossi R, Pratesi C, Pinto F. Monitoring of somatosensory evoked potentials during carotid endarterectomy. J Neurosurg. 1992;239:241–7.
60. Crammond DJ, Thirumala PD. Diagnostic value of somatosensory evoked potential changes during carotid endarterectomy: a systematic review and meta-analysis. JAMA Neurol. 2015;72:73–80.
61. Seidel K, Jeschko ÃJ, Schucht ÃP, et al. Somatosensory evoked potential and transcranial Doppler monitoring to guide shunting in carotid endarterectomy. J Neurol Surg A Cent Eur Neurosurg. 2021;82(4):299–307.
62. Uchino H, Nakamura T, Kuroda S, Houkin K, Murata JI, Saito H. Intraoperative dual monitoring during carotid endarterectomy using motor evoked potentials and near-infrared spectroscopy. World Neurosurg. 2012;78:651–7.
63. Malcharek MJ, Ulkatan S, Marinò V, et al. Intraoperative monitoring of carotid endarterectomy by transcranial motor evoked potential: a multicenter study of 600 patients. Clin Neurophysiol. 2013;124:1025–30.
64. Koyama S, Chonan M, Niizuma K, Kon H, Abe M, Matsuo S, Sasaki T, Nishijima M. Intraoperative monitoring for carotid endarterectomy using regional saturation of oxygen, motor evoked potential and somatosensory evoked potential : reference to necessity of internal shunt. Surg Cereb Stroke. 2014;42:340–6.
65. Alcantara SD, Wuamett JC, Ii JCL, Ulkatan S, Bamberger P, Mendes D, Benvenisty A, Todd G, York N, York N. Outcomes of combined somatosensory evoked potential, motor evoked potential, and electroencephalography monitoring during carotid endarterectomy. Ann Vasc Surg. 2014;28:665–72.
66. Yoshino M, Fukumoto H, Mizutani T, Yuyama R, Hara T. Mandibular subluxation stabilized by mouthpiece for distal internal carotid artery exposure in carotid endarterectomy. J Vasc Surg. 2010;52:1401–4.
67. DE BAKEY ME, CRAWFORD ES, COOLEY DA, MORRIS GCJ. Surgical considerations of occlusive disease of innominate, carotid, subclavian, and vertebral arteries. Ann Surg. 1959;149:690–710.
68. Antonopoulos CN, Kakisis JD, Sergentanis TN, Liapis CD. Eversion versus conventional carotid endarterectomy: a meta-analysis of randomised and non-randomised studies. Eur J Vasc Endovasc Surg. 2011;42:751–65.
69. Archie JP, Barnes RW, Robicsek F, Bock R, AbuRahma AF, Sobel M, Clagett GP. Carotid endarterectomy saphenous vein patch rupture revisited: selective use on the basis of vein diameter. J Vasc Surg. 1996;24:346–52.
70. Archie JP. A fifteen-year experience with carotid endarterectomy after a formal operative protocol requiring highly frequent patch angioplasty. J Vasc Surg. 2000;31:724–35.
71. Naylor R. Management of prosthetic patch infection after CEA. J Cardiovasc Surg (Torino). 2016;57:137–44.
72. Orrapin S, Benyakorn T, Howard DP, Siribumrungwong B, Rerkasem K. Patches of different types for carotid patch angioplasty. Cochrane Database Syst Rev. 2021;2:CD000071.
73. Sadideen H, Taylor PR, Padayachee TS. Restenosis after carotid endarterectomy. Int J Clin Pract. 2006;60:1625–30.
74. Bekelis K, Moses Z, Missios S, Desai A, Labropoulos N. Indications for treatment of recurrent carotid stenosis. Br J Surg. 2013;100:440–7.
75. Stilo F, Montelione N, Calandrelli R, Distefano M, Spinelli F, Di Lazzaro V, Pilato F. The management of carotid restenosis: a comprehensive review. Ann Transl Med. 2020;8:1272–2.

76. Lal BK, Beach KW, Roubin GS, et al. Restenosis after carotid artery stenting and endarterectomy: a secondary analysis of CREST, a randomised controlled trial. Lancet Neurol. 2012;11:755–63.
77. Domanin M, Gallo D, Vergara C, Biondetti P, Forzenigo LV, Morbiducci U. Prediction of long term restenosis risk after surgery in the carotid bifurcation by hemodynamic and geometric analysis. Ann Biomed Eng. 2019;47:1129–40.
78. Archie JPJ. Reoperations for carotid artery stenosis: role of primary and secondary reconstructions. J Vasc Surg. 2001;33:495–503.
79. Tu J, Wang S, Huo Z, Wu R, Yao C, Wang S. Repeated carotid endarterectomy versus carotid artery stenting for patients with carotid restenosis after carotid endarterectomy: systematic review and meta-analysis. Surgery. 2015;157:1166–73.
80. Glotzer OS, Rojas E, Bouchard DR, Hill SS, Harad FT, Zhang Z, Bowser KE. Carotid restenosis following endarterectomy in patients managed with single antiplatelet therapy versus dual antiplatelet therapy. Vasc Endovascular Surg. 2020;55:209–15.
81. Kretschmer G, Pratschner T, Prager M, Wenzl E, Polterauer P, Schemper M, Ehringer H, Minar E. Antiplatelet treatment prolongs survival after carotid bifurcation endarterectomy. Analysis of the clinical series followed by a controlled trial. Ann Surg. 1990;211:317–22.
82. Bischof G, Pratschner T, Kail M, Mittlböck M, Turkof E, Puig S, Polterauer P, Kretschmer G. Anticoagulants, antiaggregants or nothing following carotid endarterectomy? Eur J Vasc Surg. 1993;7:364–9.
83. Moulakakis KG, Mylonas SN, Sfyroeras GS, Andrikopoulos V. Hyperperfusion syndrome after carotid revascularization. J Vasc Surg. 2009;49:1060–8.
84. Renard R, Davaine J-M, Couture T, Jayet J, Tresson P, Gaudric J, Chiche L, Koskas F. Surgical repair of radiation-induced carotid stenosis. J Vasc Surg. 2020;72:959–67.
85. Giannopoulos S, Texakalidis P, Jonnalagadda AK, Karasavvidis T, Giannopoulos S, Kokkinidis DG. Revascularization of radiation-induced carotid artery stenosis with carotid endarterectomy vs. carotid artery stenting: a systematic review and meta-analysis. Cardiovasc Revasc Med. 2018;19:638–44.
86. Fokkema M, Den Hartog AG, Bots ML, Van Der Tweel I, Moll FL, De Borst GJ. Stenting versus surgery in patients with carotid stenosis after previous cervical radiation therapy: systematic review and meta-analysis. Stroke. 2012;43:793–801.
87. Kong J, Li J, Ye Z, Fan X, Wen J, Zhang J, Liu P. Carotid endarterectomy with routine shunt for patients with contralateral carotid occlusion. Ann Thorac Cardiovasc Surg. 2017;23:227–32.
88. Samson RH, Cline JL, Showalter DP, Lepore MR, Nair DG. Contralateral carotid artery occlusion is not a contraindication to carotid endarterectomy even if shunts are not routinely used. J Vasc Surg. 2013;58:935–40.

Chapter 11
Carotid Angioplasty and Stenting for Occlusive Diseases

Shigeru Miyachi

11.1 Introduction

Carotid artery stenting (CAS) is a valuable treatment option instead of carotid endarterectomy (CEA) for high-risk patients with carotid stenosis [1, 2]. However, the use of CAS has diminished due to the inferiority of CAS compared with CEA in recent randomized controlled trials (EVA-3S [3], SPACE [4], ICSS [5]). The results of these trials have actually restricted the application of CAS in Western countries [6]. However, CAS has been recently reevaluated and thought better due to the higher safety and efficacy thanks to the development of devices, strategies, and various protection methods. Properly protected CAS based on risk management and the careful evaluation of plaque images has dramatically improved the clinical results. In this chapter, the indication, strategy, technique, complication, and pitfall of CAS are described.

11.2 Medical Treatments

The first-line treatment of carotid artery stenosis is medication. Antiplatelet agents are indispensable to prevent stroke with the effect avoiding thrombogenesis at the stenotic lesion. Statins are also effective in the prevention of the increase of plaque due to atherosclerosis. These are prescribed together with advice about life-style risks such as smoking and medical management of co-existing diabetes and hypertension [1, 7]. The patients with carotid artery stenosis tend to have coronary and

S. Miyachi (✉)
Department of Neurological Surgery, Aichi Medical University, Nagakute, Japan
e-mail: miyachi.shigeru.752@mail.aichi-med-u.ac.jp

Y. Kato, A. Ansari (eds.), *Cerebrovascular Surgery*, Advances and Technical Standards in Neurosurgery 44, https://doi.org/10.1007/978-3-030-87649-4_11

peripheral artery stenotic diseases together as general atherosclerotic disorders. Managements of anti-thrombogenesis and anti-atherosclerosis are also important to reduce the risk of ischemic events of these lesions.

11.3 Indication of CAS

Revascularization of extracranial carotid artery stenosis is mainly applied for the patients with ischemic events in spite of maximum medical treatments. The methods for reconstruction of carotid artery are carotid endarterectomy (CEA) and CAS. Acceptable indication of CAS is defined according to the AHA Guide line [1] as follows.

1. Symptomatic stenosis (>50%) that is surgically difficult to access.
2. Symptomatic severe stenosis in patients with a significant medical disease* that would make the patient at high risk for surgery.
3. Severe stenosis associated with contralateral carotid artery occlusion requiring treatment before undergoing cardiac surgery.
4. Severe underlying carotid artery stenosis revealed after recanalization of carotid occlusion after recanalization for acute stroke.
5. Extracranial pseudoaneurysm, dissecting aneurysm.
6. Asymptomatic severe stenosis (>80%) or preocclusive stenosis (>90%).

   *: significant comorbid conditions

   (a) Congestive heart failure (CHF), class III/IV
   (b) Left ventricular ejection fraction (CVEF) <30%
   (c) Unstable angina
   (d) Contralateral carotid occlusion
   (e) Recent myocardial infarction (MI)
   (f) Previous CEA with recurrent stenosis
   (g) Prior radiation treatment to the neck
   (h) Other high-risk conditions for CEA

Contraindication of CAS is as follows.

1. Carotid stenosis with angiographically visible intraluminal thrombus.
2. Carotid stenosis that cannot be safely reached or crossed by an endovascular approach.
3. Contraindication (allergy) of Iodine contrast.
4. Severe chronic renal failure.
5. Carotid stenosis with totally surrounding calcification.
6. Severe aortic valve stenosis.

However, recent technical development of CAS has resolved these difficulties in some particular cases. Particularly the complete protection method with proximal and distal balloon protection enables to perform CAS without thrombus migration. As for the approaches, trans-brachial, trans-radial, and direct carotid approach will be useful for the cases difficult to access transfemorally.

For the patients with inconvenience of contrast materials, no or less contrast CAS should be adopted. Iodixanol (Visipaque®) (isosmotic contrast) is useful to avoid the worsening of renal function, and no contrast CAS under transcutaneous ultrasound navigation is possible for those with contraindication of iodine [8]. However, the shell-type full calcification is hardly dilated and occasionally causes stent trap and fracture. The patients with severe aortic valve stenosis usually develop high grade cardiac dysfunction and they have a high risk of acute fatal cardiac failure after CAS due to extremely poor output induced by hypotension and bradycardia based on the carotid-body (vagal) reflex. Therefore, the cases with shell-type calcification or severe aortic valve stenosis are of absolute contraindication of CAS.

11.4 Preoperative Evaluation

The success of CAS depends on the best strategy, adequate device selection, and proper maneuver based on the preoperative risk management. We should evaluate the general condition and plaque properties to avoid the perioperative complications. As mentioned above, the patients with carotid stenosis have coexisting atherosclerotic lesions in whole body. Cardiac evaluation like electrocardiogram and cardiac ultrasound is required to rule out coronary and valve diseases. Examination to detect the atherosclerotic circulation disorder of lower limbs such as Ancle-Brachial Index (ABI) or Pulse Wave Velocity (PWV) is also useful to check the peripheral arteriosclerosis obliterans (ASO). Plaque imaging is essential to detect the fragile, high-risk plaque (Fig. 11.1). The most reliable plaque image is T1-weighted image and time-of-flight (TOF) image on black blood MR imaging. Conventional ultrasound and IVUS (Intravascular ultrasound) are also helpful. Particularly virtual histology (VH) of IVUS brings valuable information of the contents of plaque. The characters of plaque are demonstrated in four patterns in VH. Fibrous plaque is shown in green color, lipid plaque in yellow, calcification in white, necrotic core in red, respectively. Massive lipid plaque has high risk of plaque protrusion and liquid oil embolization, and large rate of necrotic tissue may cause plaque rupture and debris migration [8].

For particular cases with hemodynamic compromise, all the investigators evaluated the intracranial hemodynamic status of the patients using SPECT to predict post-procedural hyperperfusion syndrome.

11.5 Treatment Method and Maneuver

1. Preoperative management

   Patients for CAS are usually medicated with dual antiplatelet therapy (Clopidogrel and Aspirin) for 14 days prior to stenting. Anti-hypertensive medications should be held on the morning of procedure to prevent the excessive hypotensive reaction due to the carotid body reflex.

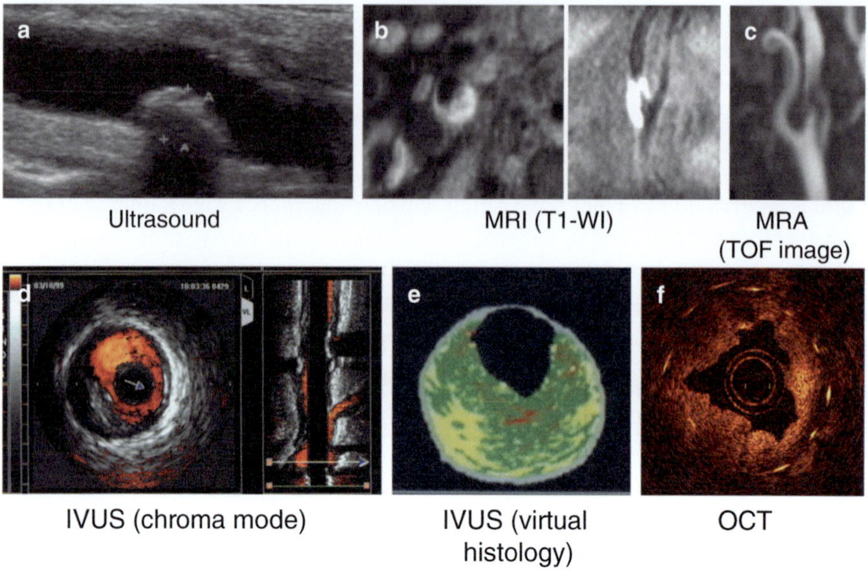

Fig. 11.1 Various methods for plaque imaging. Ultrasound (**a**), MRI (**b**), MRA (**c**), intravascular ultrasound (IVUS) (**d**, **e**), OCT (**f**)

2. Standard procedure of CAS (Figs. 11.2 and 11.3)

   Patients are sedated and groin puncture is performed under the local anesthesia. Usually, 8 or 9 Fr sheath is placed in the femoral artery, and an iliac artery angiogram from the sheath is performed to confirm no branch injury and no dissection in the access route. After the sheath insertion, general heparinization is started with bolus intravenous injection of approximately 100 units/kg of heparin (more than 200 s. on ACT monitoring). Then a guide catheter is advanced in the common carotid artery in the affected side. When proximal protection method is applied, 9 Fr Balloon guide catheter is necessary. After taking the angiogram to check the lesion and intracranial vessels, the size of the diameter of concerned vessels is measured. A distal embolic protection device (EPD) is prepared and the tip of the lead wire is appropriately reshaped to facilitate the lesion cross. It is inserted to the guide catheter and is passed through the lesion. After the EPD is deployed sufficiently distal to the lesion, an angiography is taken to check its position. If necessary, IVUS is inserted and the color Doppler and virtual histology images are obtained. The exact vessel and lesion diameter is also measured in the IVUS image. In case of distal balloon protection, whether the carotid flow is completely ceased with balloon inflation should be confirmed. Under effective protection, predilatation balloon catheter, usually sized in 3 mm balloon diameter and 40-mm length, is advanced along the wire of EPD system, and was slowly inflated at the lesion for 10–20 s. Just before the inflation of balloon 0.5 mg of atropine sulfate is injected to avoid the bradycardia. After the

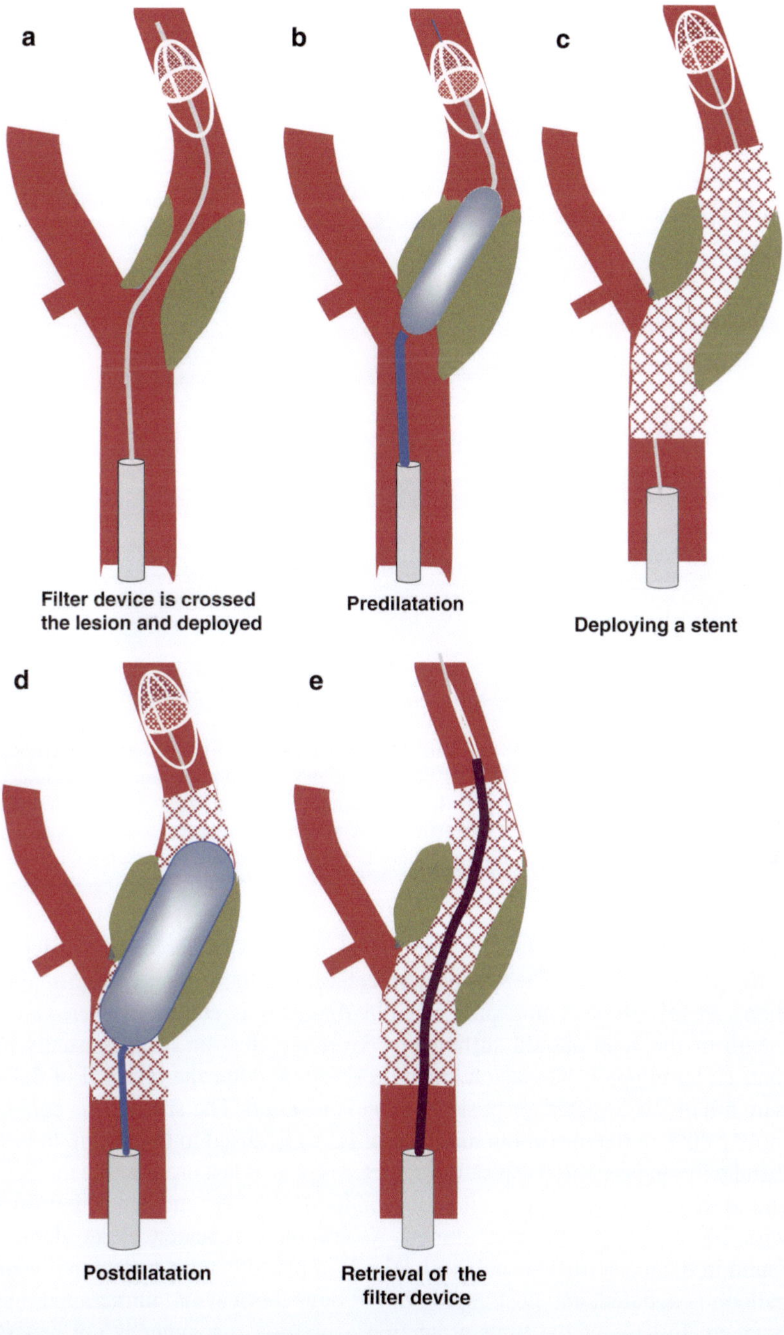

Fig. 11.2 Standard CAS under the filter protection. Filter embolic protection device is crossed the lesion and is released at the distal internal carotid artery (ICA) (**a**). After the predilatation with balloon catheter (**b**) stent is deployed (**c**). After postdilatation (**d**) and checking the carotid angiogram, the filter device is retrieved by pulling it within the outer sheath (**e**) (Quoted from Ref. [8])

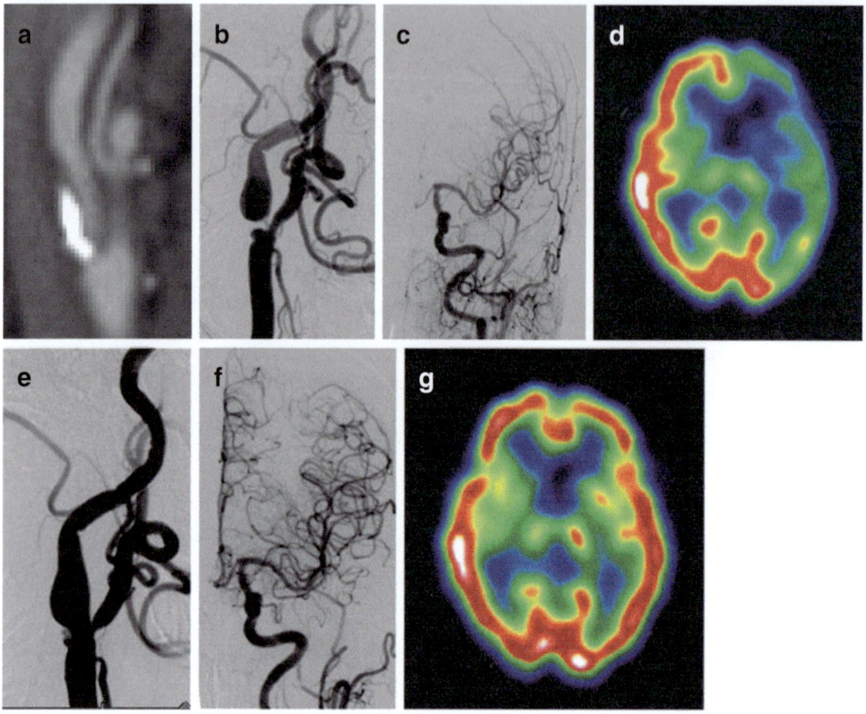

Fig. 11.3 A case of CAS for calcified hard plaque under distal filter protection method. The enhanced CT showed a partially calcified plaque (**a**), and carotid angiogram demonstrated the severe stenosis at the origin of left ICA (**b**). Intracranial circulation was very impaired (**c**) and SPECT showed the hypoperfusion of the ipsilateral hemisphere (**d**). After stenting the stenosis was well improved (**e**), and hemodynamic condition was found to improve remarkably on postoperative angiogram (**f**) and SPECT (**g**)

balloon catheter was deflated and retrieved, a self-expandable stent is deployed at the proper position. The size of stent is based on the diameter of normal common carotid artery; 1 mm plus of CCA diameter is commonly selected. The length of the stent should sufficiently cover the stenotic lesion; usually more than 10 mm longer than lesion length is selected. After the removal of delivery wire a balloon catheter for postdilatation is inserted. The size of this balloon is mostly 80% of the maximum diameter of ICA just distal to the lesion. In case of distal balloon protection aspiration catheter is placed just proximal to the balloon end after removing the postdilatation balloon catheter, and blood is aspirated with 20–30 ml syringe, and filtered. Aspiration is repeated till no debris are found in the mesh filter (usually 60–80 mL of blood is aspirated). Finally, distal balloon is deflated, and post-angiogram of both cervical and intracranial images is taken. In case of the filter protection aspiration maneuver is not necessary except for the cases with no flow phenomenon with clogged mesh due to the

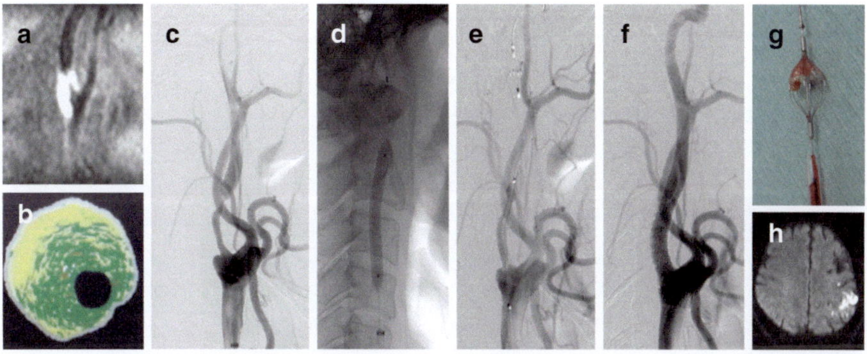

Fig. 11.4 A case of no flow phenomenon in CAS for lipid-rich fragile plaque. Preoperative plaque evaluation showed a high-risk plaque expressed as the high intensity lesion on MRI-T1 image (**a**) and lipid-rich plaque on IVUS (**b**). Left carotid angiogram showed nearly total occlusion at the origin of ICA (**c**). Balloon dilatation and stenting was performed under the filter protection with Angioguard (Cordis) (**d**). The angiogram taken after postdilatation showed no flow of ICA due to the filter clogging (**e**). After aspiration of large amounts of debris in the filter as much as possible, filter was retrieved. Final angiogram showed the lesion was found to be well dilated (**f**). Massive debris with the fragments of plaque was observed in the retrieved filter (**g**), but post-MRI showed multiple ipsilateral symptomatic ischemic lesions due to the showering of overflowed debris (**h**)

massive debris (Fig. 11.4). After confirming the well dilatation of the lesion, no plaque protrusion, no thrombus formation, and no intracranial branch occlusion, all the devices are retrieved. When dilating the lesion, if major hypotension and bradycardia is encountered, catecholamine is administered.

3. Protection methods

   There is general consensus that protection should prevent ischemic complications in CAS, and insufficient or inadequate protection may result in major adverse events. There are two types of protection devices (filter and balloon) and two protection strategies (distal and proximal). Usual protection methods are listed as follows [9].

   (a) Distal balloon [PercuSerge(Guardwire plus)]
   (b) Distal filter [Filterwire, Spider]
   (c) Double balloon (ICA + ECA balloons)
   (d) Proximal (balloon) + ECA balloon [Parodi, Mo.Ma Ultra]*
   (e) Proximal + distal balloon (Seatbelt & Airbag: S & A)
   (f) Proximal + distal filter
   (g) Triple balloon (proximal + double (ICA + ECA) balloon)

Each device has own merits and demerits (Table 11.1). Distal balloon protection requires temporary occlusion of carotid flow, but it is effective for debris collection without leakage through the occlusion site [11]. Filter protection systems are widely available and easily maneuverable, and can preserve carotid flow during the procedure. However, filter systems have limitations based on

Table 11.1 Comparison among protection methods

	Distal filter	Distal balloon (Guardwire)	Seatbelt and airbag	Parodi, Mo.Ma.
Guide catheter	8 Fr Guide	8 Fr Guide	9 Fr Balloon guide	9 Fr Balloon guide, Mo.Ma.
Leion cross	Easy (MGW)	Difficult[a]	Difficult[a]	Easy (MGW)
Maneuverability	Easy	Easy	Easy	Difficult[b]
Complexity	Low	Low	High	Very high
Carotid flow during protection	Intact	Arrest	Arrest	Reversed#, arrest
Intolerance	None	Possible	Possible	Possible
Position check#	Possible	Impossible	Impossible	Possible
Protection ability (reliability)	Middle	High	Very high	Very high

Abbreviation: *MGW* crossing with microguide wire
[a]In case of severe tortuous stenosis
[b]Positioning
#: On using Parodi method
#: Angiography during protection worked

their structure. In cases that develop the no flow and/or overflow phenomenon during the procedure according to a previous study [12]. The no flow phenomenon is caused by filter clogging due to excessive amounts of debris shed from the plaque [13]. No flow may result in the passage of debris through the filter mesh because the increased forward pressure may extrude the accumulated debris and cause leak or overflow from gaps in the filter sleeve, resulting in cerebral showering embolism [2, 14].

**Proximal Balloon Technique*

The proximal protection method was invented by Parodi et al., but a modification of Parodi's method has been generally used [10]. A 9 Fr balloon catheter is initially placed in the common carotid artery to block forward flow and a Guardwire® (PercuSerge) balloon (Medtronic AVE, Santa Rosa, CA) is placed in the most proximal side of the external carotid artery (ECA) for the protection of retrograde flow from the ECA to ICA. This system can be substituted by Mo.Ma Ultra system (Fig. 11.5). Then, a 4 Fr short sheath is inserted into the femoral vein and is connected to the hemostatic valve of the balloon catheter via a connection tube inserted into the filter tube for transfusion. Thus, a continuous arteriovenous shunt system is created to aspirate debris ejected during lesion crossing and angioplasty. Using this proximal and ECA protection method with retrograde aspiration, the lesion is crossed with a distal protection device and placed in the proper position of the distal ICA. After the distal protection device is deployed, stenting of the carotid lesion is performed. Proximal protection and aspiration are continued until the end of the procedure. This double protection method using proximal protection (seatbelt) and a distal protection device (airbag) was

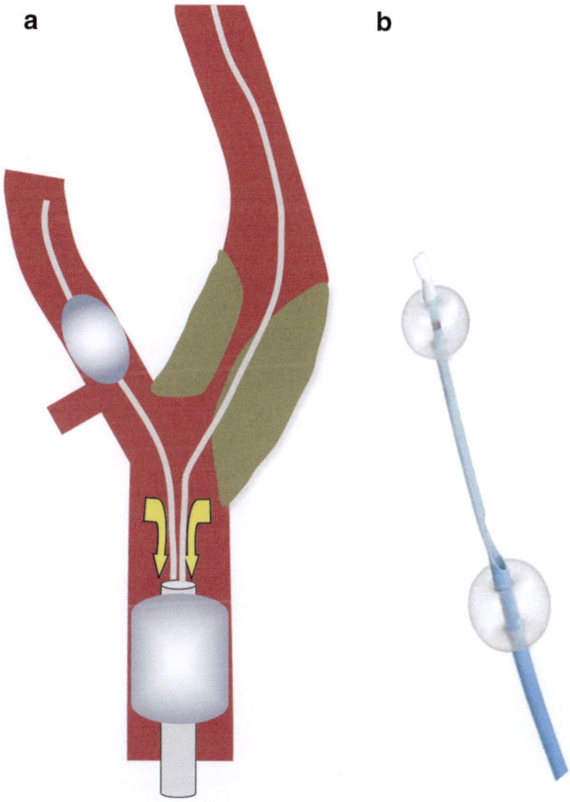

Fig. 11.5 A schema of Parodi method. Balloon catheter is placed in the external carotid artery (ECA) through the balloon guide catheter and continuous arteriovenous shunt system is created to aspirate debris ejected during lesion crossing and angioplasty (**a**). This system is substituted for Mo.Ma Ultra system (Metronic) (**b**) (Quoted from Ref. [8])

called the modified "Seatbelt and Airbag method" (Figs. 11.6, 11.7, and 11.10). This type of proximal protection is used to cross the lesion in high-risk cases, where there is nearly total occlusion or there is a floating thrombus. Multiple protection methods that combine two balloons or a filter and balloon are used to improve the degree of protection.

The most reliable method to achieve complete protection is considered to be a multiple protection system. The most popular and stable multiple protection system involves proximal protection with a balloon in the common and external carotid arteries, and intentional reversed flow to the venous system [15]. However, for cases requiring the highest risk management triple protection method with three balloons should be considered (Figs. 11.8 and 11.9).

4. Measures to complement the protection

   CAS for lesions with plaque that have a thin fibrous cap and rich necrotic core (vulnerable plaque) are associated with an elevated risk of ischemic complications even under filter protection; however, the complication rate was significantly reduced by the use of balloon protection. There are measures that can be taken to reduce the amount of debris shed from high-risk plaques. Excessive dilatation of the balloon is considered to release a large amount of debris due to

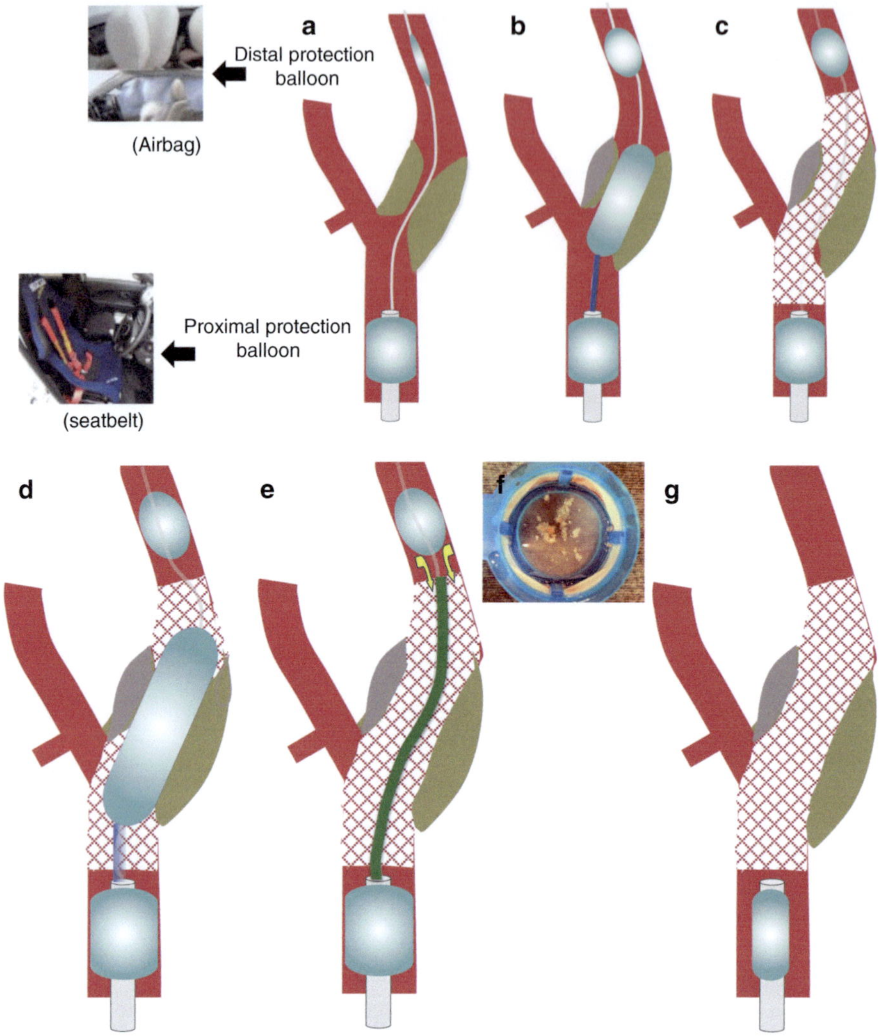

Fig. 11.6 CAS under the proximal and distal protection (Seatbelt & Airbag method). A distal balloon protection device (Guradwire (Percu Serge®) system) is placed and distal to the lesion under the proximal flow control with balloon guide catheter (**a**). Both balloons are inflated and predilatation (**b**), stenting (**c**), and postdilatation (**d**) is performed. Aspiration catheter is inserted, and floating debris in the lumen is aspirated together with blood (**e**). The blood containing the debris is filtered (**f**), and when no debris is detected, balloons are deflated and all the systems are withdrawn (**g**) (Quoted from Ref. [8])

the destruction of the intima and fibrous cap. Therefore, dilatation of the balloon to less than 80% of the expected diameter is recommended in the expert consensus statement [1]. However, it is possible that such modest dilatation with remnant stenosis may increase the rate of restenosis or the recurrence of symptoms.

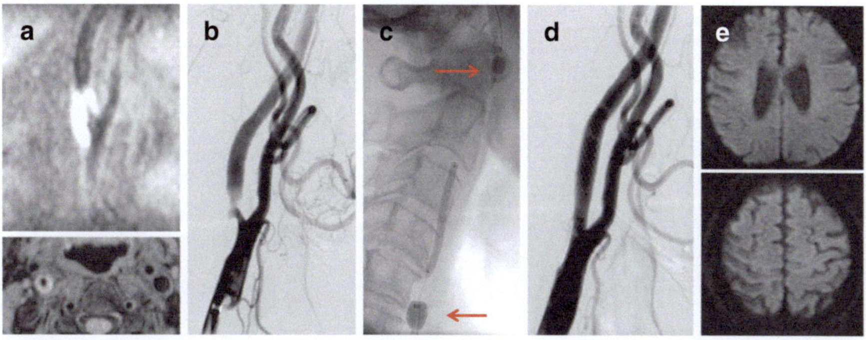

Fig. 11.7 A case of CAS for high-risk plaque under Seatbelt and Airbag protection method. Preoperative MRI showed a stenosis at the origin of right ICA, and plaque imaging showed marked high intensity lesion (**a**). Carotid angiogram showed severe stenosis (**b**). Under the Seatbelt and Airbag protection with distal and proximal balloons (*arrows*), stenting was performed (**c**). Post-angiogram showed successful dilatation of the lesion (**d**). Postoperative MRI showed no ischemic lesions (**e**)

5. Selection of stent

   Stents used for carotid angioplasty are roughly divided to two types by strut structure, closed cell and open cell types. Carotid wall stent (Boston Scientifics) is a representative closed stent, and Precise (Cordis) and Protégé (Medtronic) are open cell stents. The selection criteria are mainly based on the plaque characteristics and the angioarchitecture of the lesion. Table 11.2 shows the difference between both type stents. The newly developed stent, double-layer micromesh stent (Fig. 11.10), is useful for the lesion with the high risk of plaque protrusion.

6. Perioperative management

   The postoperative management of circulation is important. In some particular cases, severe bradycardia and hypotension due to carotid body reflex are encountered after the stenting or postdilatation. If such reaction is critical and persistent, rapid administration of catecholamine and temporary pacing are required. Newly developed neurological symptoms, particularly hemiparesis, aphasia and verbal dysfunction should be frequently checked at least postoperative 24 h. Convulsion and hyperactive, abnormally exciting state should be paid much attention because such symptoms often suggest hyperperfusion syndrome. If there is a high risk of hemorrhage due to hyperperfusion, rapid sedation and hypotensive management is mandatory.

   Heparinization will be naturally neutralized or small amount of general heparinization is continued for 24 h (15,000–20,000 units per day). The dual antiplatelet agents should be taken at least 6 months postoperatively if the patient does not suffer from the hemorrhagic tendency.

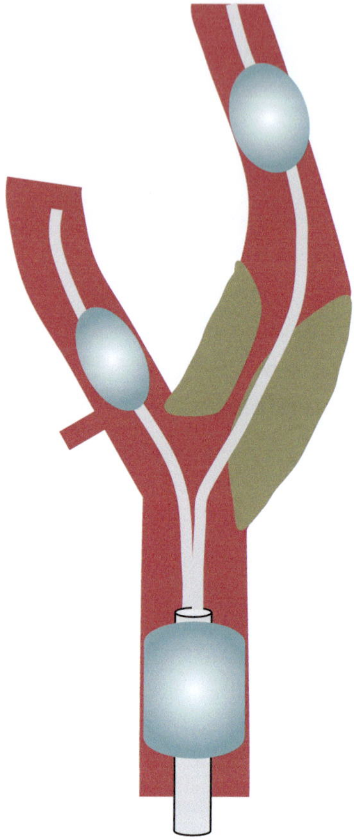

Fig. 11.8 A schema of triple protection. Two balloon catheters are placed both ECA and ICA under the flow control of balloon guide catheter. The complete stuck of carotid flow is obtained with this system. Quoted from Ref. 8

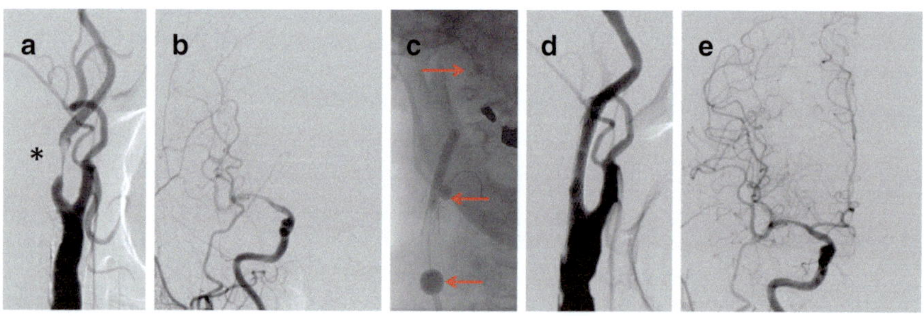

Fig. 11.9 A case of CAS for the lesion with thrombus under triple protection method. Right carotid angiogram showed sever stenosis with floating thrombus (**a**: *asterisk*) and impaired intracranial circulation (**b**). Under the tripe protection (**c**: *arrows*) stenting was successfully performed (**d**) with the marked improvement of intracranial flow (**e**). New ischemic lesions were not found in post-operative MRI

Table 11.2 Comparison between closed and open cell stents

		Closed cell stent	Open cell stent
Stent profile	Strut design	Closed mesh	Open (partial connection)
	Size variation	Less	More
	Radial force	Middle	Large
	Lumen holding	Very well	Well[a]
	Foreshortening	Yes	No
	Positioning	Arrangement required	Easy
	Prediction of total length	Difficult	Easy
	Resheath	Possible	Impossible
	Pass of devices	Easy	Occsionally difficult[b]
Recommended lesion	Fragile plaque	○	△
	Thin fibrous cap	○	△
	Jerry-fish thrombus	○	△
	Ulceration	○	△
	Calcification (local)	△	○
	Tortuous vessel	△	○
	Dissection	○	△
Angiographic result	Shape of cross section	Round	Ovale, irregular[c]
	Conformability to vessel wall	Occsionally poor[d]	Well
	Prevention of plaque protrusion	Well[e]	Poor
	Tapering	Possible	None
	Coning	Possible[f]	None
	Fructure of strut	None	Possible[g]
	Position stability	Occasionally unstable[h]	Stable
	Intimal hyperplasia (restenosis)	More	Less

[a]Occasionally collapse
[b]Due to the stent fructure
[c]With deformity (internal folding)
[d]In curved lesion, calcified plaque, big caliver difference
[e]Particularly with stent with micromesh
[f]In tandem lesion, malpositioning
[g]Stuck into soft plaque
[h]Shortening, migration to CCA

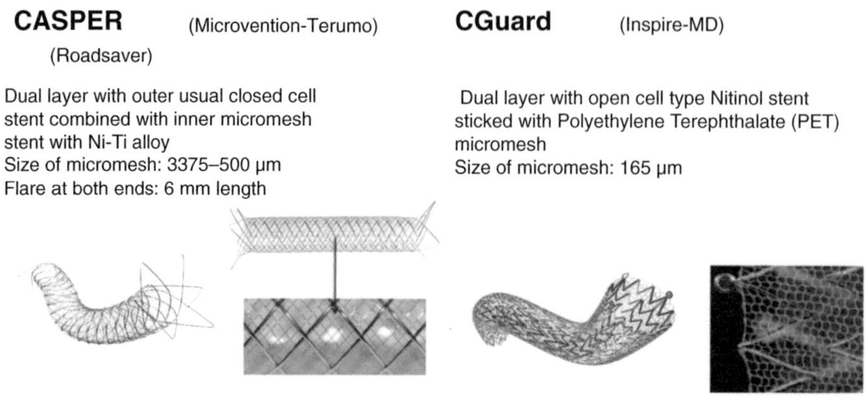

Fig. 11.10 Double-layer micromesh stents. CASPER® (Roadsaver®) (Microvention-Terumo): Dual layer with outer usual closed cell stent combined with inner micromesh stent with Ni-Ti alloy. CGuard (Inspire MD): Dual layer with open cell type Nitinol stent sticked with Polyethylene Terephthalate (PET) micromesh

11.6 The Importance of Tailored CAS

It is very important to evaluate the true characteristics of plaque and to discriminate high-risk plaques. Symptomatic patients tend to have high-risk plaque such as floating thrombus, nearly total occlusion, very soft and vulnerable plaque or a thin fibrous cap based on plaque imaging. Such patients should be intentionally treated using strict debris control, and perioperative management should be based on risk assessment. In this situation, a combined protection method using proximal protection and aspiration is useful [8, 9]. Protection methods should be selected from many options and that combined methods should be based on the plaque contents and lesion morphology in each case [16]. In addition, the access route should be changed from transfemoral to transbrachial depending on the condition of the aortic arch and the severity of atherosclerosis. From a hemodynamic point of view, a strategy of staged CAS [17] and postoperative management to avoid post-procedural hyperperfusion should be tailored by the preoperative cerebral perfusion data including symptoms and hemodynamic imaging. Thus, tailored CAS based on individual preoperative risk management is important to perform CAS safely and effectively.

References

1. ACCF/SCAI/SVMB/SIR/ASITN Clinical Expert Consensus Document Committee on Carotid Stenting. ACCF/SCAI/SVMB/SIR/ASITN 2007 clinical expert consensus document on carotid stenting. J Am Coll Cardiol. 2007;49:151–5.
2. Bates ER, Babb JD, Casey DE Jr, Cates CU, Duckwiler GR, Feldman TE, Gray WA, Ouriel K, Peterson ED, Rosenfield K, Rundback JH, Safian RD, Sloan MA, White CJ. Clinical Expert

Consensus. ACCF/SCAI/SVMB/SIR/ASITN 2007 Clinical Expert Consensus Document on carotid stenting. Vasc Med. 2007;12:35–83.
3. EVA-3S Investigators. Endarterectomy vs. angioplasty in patients with symptomatic severe carotid stenosis (EVA-3S) trial. Cerebrovasc Dis. 2004;18:62–5.
4. SPACE Collaborative Group, Ringleb PA, Allenberg J, Brückmann H, Eckstein HH, Fraedrich G, Hartmann M, Hennerici M, Jansen O, Klein G, Kunze A, Marx P, Niederkorn K, Schmiedt W, Solymosi L, Stingele R, Zeumer H, Hacke W. 30 Day results from the SPACE trial of stent-protected angioplasty versus carotid end- arterectomy in symptomatic patients: a randomised non-inferiority trial. Lancet. 2006;368:1239–47.
5. International Carotid Stenting Study investigators, Ederle J, Dobson J, Featherstone RL, Bonati LH, van der Worp HB, de Borst GJ, Lo TH, Gaines P, Dorman PJ, Macdonald S, Lyrer PA, Hendriks JM, McCollum C, Nederkoorn PJ, Brown MM. Carotid artery stenting compared with endarterectomy in patients with symptomatic carotid stenosis (International Carotid Stenting Study): an interim analysis of a randomised controlled trial. Lancet. 2010;375:985–97.
6. Gurm HS, Yadav JS, Fayad P, Katzen BT, Mishkel GJ, Bajwa TK, Ansel G, Strickman NE, Wang H, Cohen SA, Massaro JM, Cutlip DE, SAPPHIRE Investigators. Long-term results of carotid stenting versus endarterectomy in high-risk patients. N Engl J Med. 2008;358:1572–9.
7. Harrigan MR, Deveikis JP. Extracranial angioplasty and stenting. In: Harrigan MR, Deveikis JP, editors. Handbook of cerebrovascular disease and neurointerventional technique. 3rd ed. Cham: Humana; 2018. p. 501–30.
8. Miyachi S. Carotid artery stenosis. In: Miyachi S, editor. Tactics, techniques and spirits of neuroendovascular therapy. Osaka: Medicus Shuppan; 2015. p. 280–321.
9. Miyachi S, Taki W, Sakai N, Nakahara I, The Japanese CAS Survey Investigators. Historical perspective of carotid stenting in Japan—analysis of 8,092 cases in the Japanese survey. Acta Neurochir. 2012;154:2127–37.
10. Parodi JC, Schönholz C, Ferreira LM, Mendaro E, Ohki T. "Seat belt and air bag" technique for cerebral protection during carotid stenting. J Endovasc Ther. 2002;9:20–4.
11. Higashida RT, Popma JJ, Apruzzese P, Zimetbaum P, MAVErIC I and II Investigators. Evaluation of the medtronic exponent self-expanding carotid stent system with the medtronic guardwire temporary occlusion and aspiration system in the treatment of carotid stenosis: combined from the MAVErIC (Medtronic AVE Self-expanding CaRotid Stent System with distal protection In the treatment of Carotid stenosis) I and MAVErIC II trials. Stroke. 2010;41:e102–9.
12. Jansen O, Fiehler J, Hartmann M, Brückmann H. Protection or nonprotection in carotid stent angioplasty: the influence of interventional techniques on outcome data from the SPACE trial. Stroke. 2009;40:841–6.
13. Tsurumi A, Miyachi S, Hososhima O, Izumi T, Ohshima T, Matsubara N, Kinkori T, Naito T, Yoshida J. Can periprocedural hypotension in carotid artery stenting be predicted? A carotid morphologic autonomic pathologic scoring model using virtual histology. Interv Neuroradiol. 2009;15:17–28.
14. Yoshimura S, Yamada K, Kawasaki M, Asano T, Kanematsu M, Takamatsu M, Hara A, Iwama T. High-intensity signal on time-of-flight magnetic resonance angiography indicates carotid plaques at high risk for cerebral embolism during stenting. Stroke. 2011;42:3132–7.
15. Stabile E, Salemme L, Sorropago G, Tesorio T, Nammas W, Miranda M, Popusoi G, Cioppa A, Ambrosini V, Cota L, Petroni G, Della Pietra G, Ausania A, Fontanelli A, Biamino G, Rubino P. Proximal endovascular occlusion for carotid artery stenting: results from a prospective registry of 1,300 patients. J Am Coll Cardiol. 2010;55:1661–7.
16. Gray WA, Chaturvedi S, Verta P, Investigators and the Executive Committees. Thirty-day outcomes for carotid artery stenting in 6320 patients from 2 prospective, multicenter, high-surgical-risk registries. Circ Cardiovasc Interv. 2009;2:159–66.
17. Yoshimura S, Kitajima H, Enomoto Y, Yamada K, Iwama T. Staged angioplasty for carotid artery stenosis to prevent postoperative hyperperfusion. Neurosurgery. 2009;64:122–8.

Chapter 12
Complex Intracranial Aneurysms

Shuntaro Togashi and Hiroaki Shimizu

12.1 Introduction

Several characteristics of complex intracranial aneurysms have been reported: (1) large or giant; (2) broad neck; (3) intra–aneurysmal thrombus; (4) calcified or atherosclerotic neck; (5) branches or perforators originating from the aneurysmal dome or neck; (6) recurrence after previous clipping or coil embolization; (7) absence of collateral circulation; and (8) non-saccular morphology, such as in the case of, for example, fusiform/serpentine, mycotic, or dissecting/blood-blister-like aneurysms [1]. In most cases, these aneurysms are unsuitable for standard microsurgical clipping or endovascular coil embolization.

Although recent advances in endovascular procedures, including stent-assisted coil embolization and flow diverter stenting, may yield favorable outcomes in some cases [2, 3], there remain many challenging cases in which microsurgical management may represent the optimal form of treatment. Most of these complex aneurysms require parent artery occlusion (PAO) [4], flow alteration [5], and blind-alley formation [6] with cerebral revascularization to prevent ischemic complications and maintain the cerebral blood flow in the distal territory. Herein, we describe microsurgical aneurysmal clipping and PAO/flow alteration/blind-alley formation procedures using various bypass techniques to treat complex intracranial aneurysms.

S. Togashi (✉) · H. Shimizu
Department of Neurosurgery, Akita University Graduate School of Medicine, Akita, Akita, Japan
e-mail: togashi@med.akita-u.ac.jp; nshrk@med.akita-u.ac.jp

Y. Kato, A. Ansari (eds.), *Cerebrovascular Surgery*, Advances and Technical Standards in Neurosurgery 44, https://doi.org/10.1007/978-3-030-87649-4_12

12.2 Standards

12.2.1 Giant/Large Middle Cerebral Artery Bifurcation Aneurysms

Giant/large middle cerebral artery (MCA) bifurcation aneurysms are often difficult to treat with simple clipping due to the cortical branches or lenticulostriate arteries (LSA) arising from the aneurysm neck or dome. Such aneurysms may also have a sclerotic aneurysmal wall that precludes clipping.

When clipping is not indicated, a superficial temporal artery (STA)-MCA bypass to the distal MCA branches followed by PAO is usually the next best choice. Complex MCA bifurcation aneurysms may be treated by clipping the neck together with one of the M2 branches arising from the aneurysm dome following protection with a bypass. This strategy of preserving the outflow of M1 to one of the M2 branches can effectively prevent infarction in the LSA territory. On the other hand, PAO at the most distal part of M1, occluding its anterograde flow, may cause infarction in the LSA territory due to abrupt blood flow reduction of M1 [7]. It is important to plan a bypass and PAO strategy such as to maintain adequate blood flow in the LSAs.

Case presentation (Fig. 12.1): A 59-year-old man suffered a World Federation of Neurosurgical Societies (WFNS) Grade IV subarachnoid hemorrhage (SAH). Initial computed tomography (CT) revealed right-dominant SAH. Preoperative digital subtraction angiography (DSA) demonstrated a giant MCA aneurysm (45 mm in diameter). The distal branches and perforators were unclear on angiography. Because the brain damage was minimal on diffusion-weighted imaging (DWI), surgery to exclude the aneurysm was performed on the same day. Intraoperatively, the M2 inferior trunk originated from the aneurysm dome, and neck clipping was considered difficult. Following the STA-MCA double bypass to both the M2 areas, the aneurysm was investigated under temporary occlusion of the most distal part of M1 (26 min) to finally perform clipping on the neck of the aneurysm with occlusion of the M2 inferior trunk while maintaining anterograde blood flow to the M2 superior trunk. Postoperative DWI revealed an acute infarction in the right LSA territory, probably due to a prolonged temporary occlusion of the distal M1 which caused blood flow reduction of M1 to make the LSA territories ischemia. The patient's condition improved postoperatively, and he was transferred to a rehabilitation hospital with a modified Rankin scale (mRS) score of 3.

12.2.2 Unruptured Symptomatic Intracavernous Giant/Large Internal Carotid Artery Aneurysms

Giant/large internal carotid artery (ICA) aneurysms of the intracavernous portion may cause visual dysfunction and cranial nerve (III, IV, and VI) palsy [8]. Whether cranial nerve palsy improves after treatment depends on the duration of symptoms [9], and the best early surgical indication is recommended.

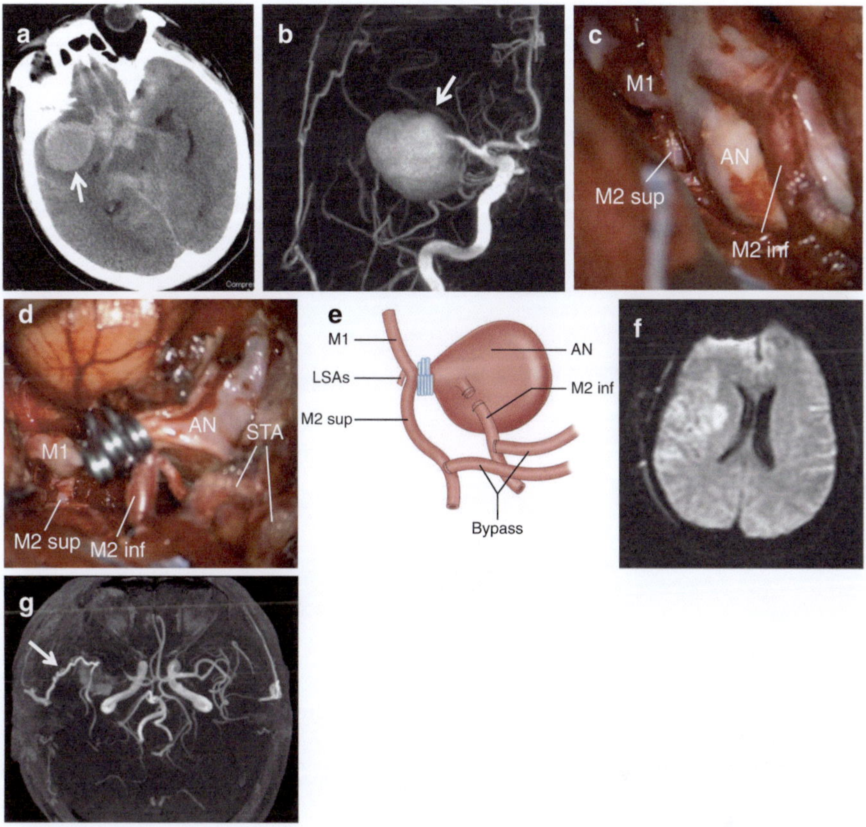

Fig. 12.1 (**a**) Preoperative computed tomography image representing a right-dominant subarachnoid hemorrhage. A giant right middle cerebral artery (MCA) aneurysm was suspected in the right temporal lobe (*arrow*). (**b**) Digital subtraction angiography (DSA) showing a giant MCA aneurysm (45 mm in diameter). The M2 superior trunk originated from the aneurysm neck (*arrow*), but the M2 inferior trunk was unclear. (**c–e**) Intraoperative photographs and the schema showing that the M2 inferior trunk originated from the aneurysm dome (**c**); neck clipping was performed with occlusion of the M2 inferior trunk while maintaining anterograde blood flow to the M2 superior trunk following superior temporal artery-MCA double bypasses (**d**, **e**). (**f**) Postoperative diffusion-weighted image showing the right lenticulostriate artery territory infarction, probably due to prolonged temporary occlusion of the M1. (**g**) Postoperative magnetic resonance angiography showing a patent bypass and disappearance of the aneurysm

Following microsurgical clipping, the symptoms caused by the aneurysms may be alleviated by a decrease in the mass effect and loss of pulsation due to aneurysmal size reduction. Such effects are difficult to achieve with coil embolization [10]. Although flow diversion is a superior treatment that can improve cranial nerve palsy, it has been reported to be associated with 5.3% morbidity and 10.7% mortality [11]. Therefore, PAO, which can immediately and reliably obliterate the blood flow on the proximal side of the aneurysm, remains an effective surgical option.

Case presentation (Fig. 12.2 [12]): A 56-year-old man presented with left abducens nerve palsy. Magnetic resonance angiography (MRA) revealed bilateral ICA

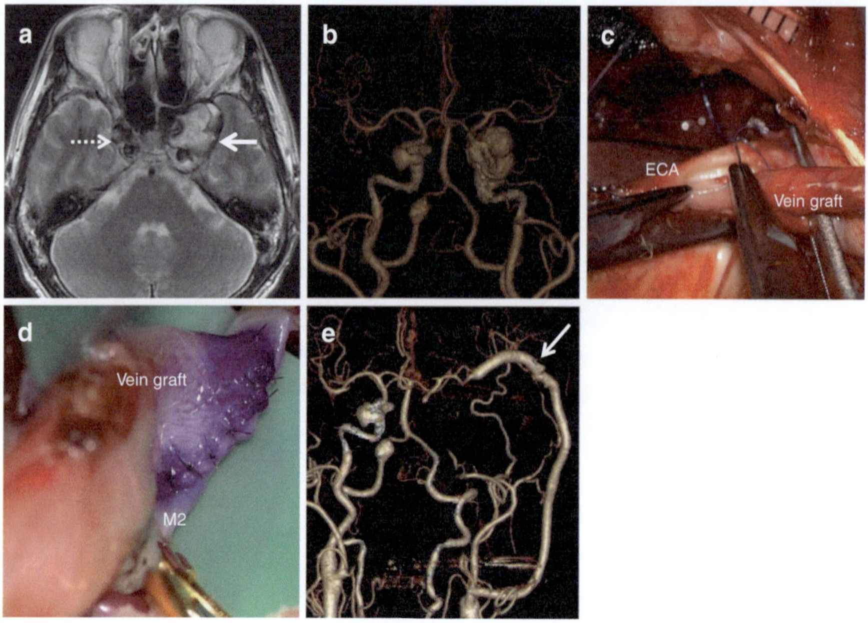

Fig. 12.2 (**a**) A T2-weighted image showing the bilateral internal carotid artery (ICA) aneurysms of the intracavernous portion (*arrow* and *dot arrow*). (**b**) Magnetic resonance angiography (MRA) showing the bilateral ICA aneurysms and the right vertebral artery aneurysm. (**c**, **d**) Intraoperative photographs showing cervical external carotid artery (ECA)-vein graft anastomosis (**c**) and M2-vein graft anastomosis (**d**). (**e**) Postoperative MRA demonstrating a patent vein graft between the left ECA and M2, and disappearance of the left ICA aneurysm (Reprinted from reference [12] under permission)

aneurysms and a right vertebral artery (VA) fusiform aneurysm. The left symptomatic giant ICA aneurysm (50 mm in diameter) of the intracavernous portion was treated with PAO (ligation of the ICA at the cervical portion) following a saphenous vein graft bypass from the cervical external carotid artery to M2. An STA–MCA bypass to the distal branch of the M2 was performed prior to the vein graft bypass to minimize ischemia during temporary occlusion of the recipient M2 [13]. The patient was discharged without any complications.

12.2.3 Ruptured Intradural Vertebral Artery Dissecting Aneurysms

This type of aneurysm has been reported to have a high incidence of rebleeding and a high mortality rate in a previous study [14]. Therefore, the treatment of such aneurysms should be carried out as early as possible, as previously emphasized. In recent years, endovascular internal trapping has been increasingly selected as a first-line treatment because it is less invasive and can be performed immediately following a diagnosis [15]. However, this procedure includes a risk of medullary infarction (MI) due to perforator occlusion, which may affect patient outcomes [16]. Although microsurgical trapping may often prevent ischemic complications by avoiding occlusion of the perforators from the VA or posterior inferior cerebellar artery (PICA) to the medulla, it is not always possible depending on the anatomical structures.

Revascularization surgery, such as an occipital artery (OA)-PICA bypass or PICA-PICA bypass, is often required if the PICA is involved in the dissection of the VA [17]. When patient conditions do not allow for a surgical intervention, PAO proximal to the dissection may be the treatment of choice; however, it carries the risk of rebleeding due to retrograde flow from the contralateral VA.

Case presentation (Fig. 12.3): A 55-year-old man suffered a WFNS Grade I SAH. Initial MRA and DSA demonstrated a right VA dissecting aneurysm located on the midline. An OA-PICA bypass was performed because the large PICA originated from the aneurysm wall. Subsequently, the dissecting part was completely occluded by internal trapping using a coil. Postoperative DWI showed right dorso-lateral MI, and the patient presented with dysphagia and right ataxia. The patient was transferred to a rehabilitation hospital with an mRS score of 2.

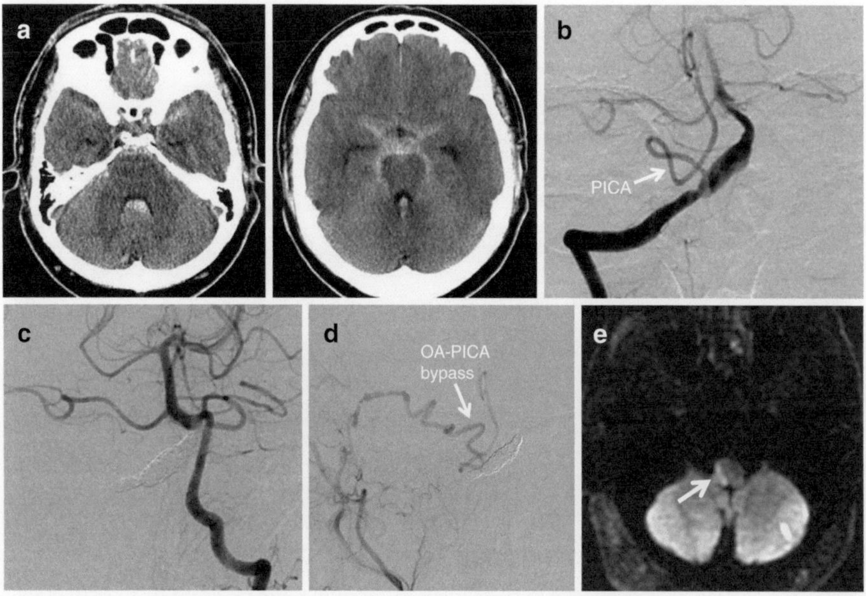

Fig. 12.3 (**a**) Preoperative computed tomography showing subarachnoid hemorrhage and intra-fourth ventricle hemorrhage. (**b**) Digital subtraction angiography (DSA) showing a right vertebral artery (VA) dissecting aneurysm located on the midline. The surgical strategy included an internal trapping following an occipital artery (OA)-posterior inferior cerebellar artery (PICA) bypass given that the large PICA originated from the aneurysm wall. (**c**, **d**) Postoperative DSA showing complete occlusion of the right VA dissecting part (**c**) and a patent bypass (**d**). The region distal from the VA union was well supplied by the left VA. (**e**) Postoperative diffusion-weighted image showing the right dorso-lateral medullary infarction

12.3 Advances

12.3.1 Recurrent Intradural ICA Aneurysms Following Previous Coil Embolization

As long-term follow-ups after coil embolization increase, recurrent aneurysms due to incomplete obliteration and coil compaction are being increasingly reported [18]. Surgical procedures may be challenging in most cases because it is difficult to identify the entire structure of the aneurysm due to the previously placed coil mass [19]. A bypass surgery to prevent ischemic complications is often carried out either to prolong temporary occlusion time or to permanently provide alternative blood flow following sacrifice of the related arterial branch.

Case presentation (Fig. 12.4): A 61-year-old woman had suffered from SAH 4 years prior. The ruptured left ICA-posterior communicating (IC-PC) aneurysm was

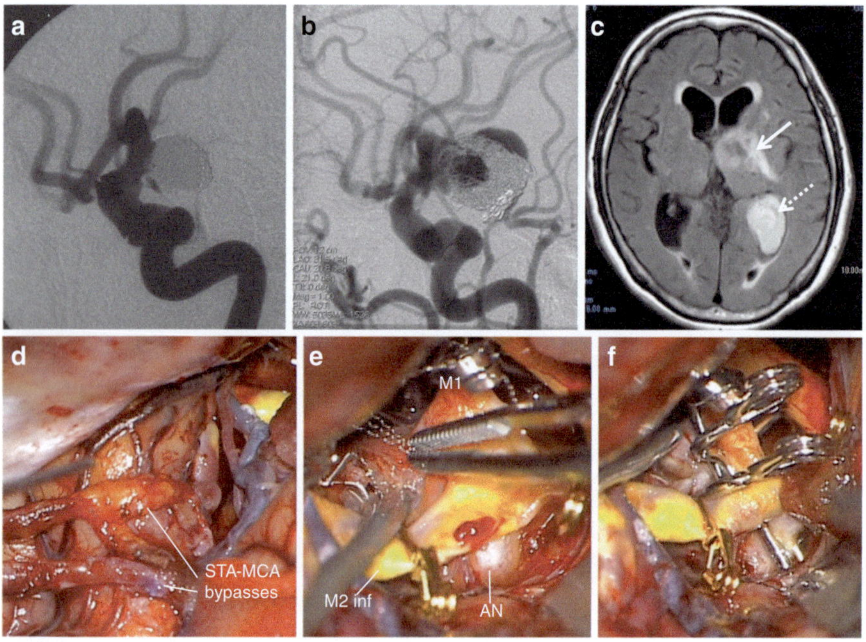

Fig. 12.4 (**a**) Digital subtraction angiography (DSA) showing a ruptured left internal carotid artery-posterior communicating artery (IC-PC) aneurysm which was successfully treated by simple coil embolization. (**b**) DSA 4 years after the surgery showing the left IC-PC aneurysm that had regrown and rebleeding. (**c**) A fluid-attenuated inversion-recovery image showing the left anterior choroidal artery territory infarction (*arrow*) and the left intraventricular hemorrhage (*dot arrow*). (**d–f**) Intraoperative photographs showing the superficial temporal artery-middle cerebral artery double bypasses as an insurance bypass (**d**) and aneurysm neck clipping following partial removal of the previous coil (**e**, **f**)

successfully treated using simple coil embolization. However, the IC-PC aneurysm gradually enlarged and rebled to cause SAH as well as right hemiparesis due to infarction in the left anterior choroidal artery (AchA) 4 years later. Removal of a part of the coil followed by neck clipping was planned. Bypass and PAO were the second choice of treatment when clipping was not possible. STA-MCA double bypass to the M3 portions was first performed. Because the AchA was already obstructed, the aneurysm neck was clipped after coil removal, including the origin of the AchA, and the anterograde flow of the ICA was preserved. No adverse events were observed during the postoperative period, and the patient was discharged to a rehabilitation hospital with an mRS score of 3.

12.3.2 Giant/Large Distal ACA Aneurysms

Giant/large distal ACA aneurysms that require distal revascularization surgery are difficult to treat using standard bypass techniques. In such cases, A3-A3 bypass is useful when the recipient artery and contralateral A3 are sufficiently close. A short interposition STA graft may be useful for anastomosing bilateral A3s, which are apart [20].

Case presentation (Fig. 12.5 [12]): A 68-year-old man presented with multiple infarctions in the right ACA territory. DSA revealed a right giant ACA aneurysm. Notably, both ACAs were supplied by the unpaired ACA, and there was stenosis of the right ACA just proximal to the aneurysm. Intra-aneurysmal thrombus was suspected as the embolic source, and microsurgical obliteration of the aneurysm was performed. The aneurysm was trapped following an A3-A3 bypass using a short-interpositioned STA graft. The postoperative course was favorable, and the patient was discharged with no clinical symptoms.

12.3.3 Unruptured Symptomatic Giant/Large Basilar Trunk Saccular Aneurysms

Giant/large basilar trunk saccular aneurysms may cause neurological symptoms due to compression of the brainstem or surrounding cranial nerves and are sometimes life-threatening. Such aneurysms are mostly challenging for microsurgical clipping while preserving perforators or other branches. Although flow diverter stents have recently become a new treatment option, they lack long-term follow-up data. According to previously published literature [21], a flow alteration method using various bypasses to the superior cerebellar artery and/or posterior cerebral artery (PCA) combined with PAO can be effective in reducing the aneurysm and improving the symptoms.

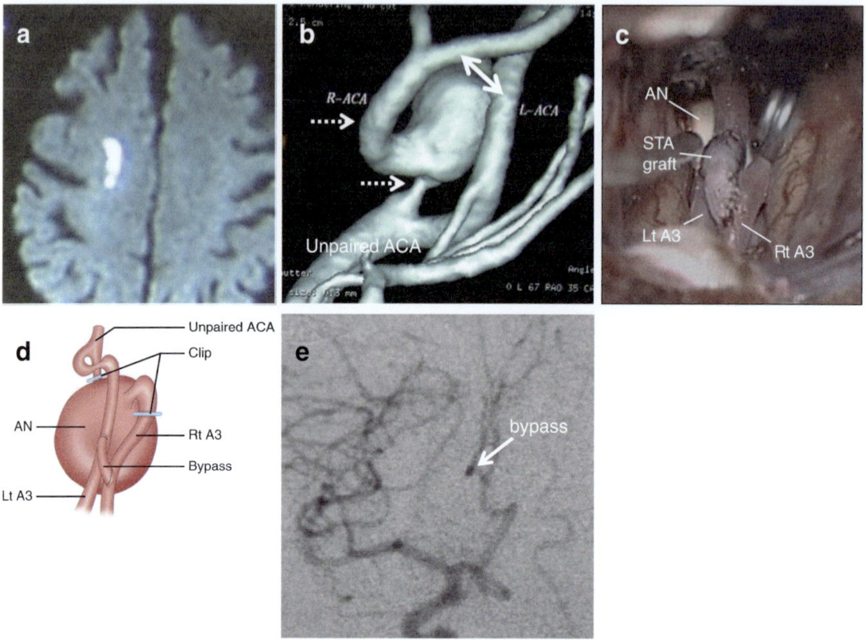

Fig. 12.5 (**a**) A diffusion-weighted image showing the right frontal lobe infarction. (**b**) Digital subtraction angiography (DSA) showing the right anterior cerebral artery (ACA) aneurysm. Bilateral ACAs are supplied by the unpaired ACA and a stenotic lesion is observed in the right ACA just proximal to the aneurysm. The surgical strategy included trapping of the aneurysm (*dot arrows*) followed by an A3-A3 bypass (*double arrow*). (**c**, **d**) Intraoperative photograph (**c**) and schema (**d**) showing the A3-A3 bypass using an interposed superficial temporal artery graft due to the differences in depth of both A3s. (**e**) Postoperative DSA showing a patent bypass and disappearance of the aneurysm (Reprinted from reference [12] under permission)

Case presentation (Fig. 12.6 [12]): A 46-year-old man presented with progressive dysphagia, dysarthria, and right upper motor paresis over the course of 3 months. Magnetic resonance T2-weighted imaging showed an aneurysm that severely compressed the brainstem. DSA revealed a giant basilar trunk aneurysm protruding from basilar fenestration. The right anterior inferior cerebellar artery (AICA) originated just proximal to the aneurysm. Because both curative clipping and coiling were considered difficult, a flow alteration strategy was selected for aneurysmal flow reduction. Maintenance of adequate flow to the basilar perforators was thought to be a key of this surgery.

Using a transpetrosal presigmoid approach, a left STA short saphenous vein graft--PCA bypass was performed to introduce sufficient blood flow to replace basilar artery blood flow. The basilar trunk was occluded just proximal to the origin of the right AICA to make an outflow of the bypass flow toward the AICA and preserve basilar perforators. Postoperative images revealed a decrease in the size of the aneurysm, and the patient's clinical symptoms gradually improved.

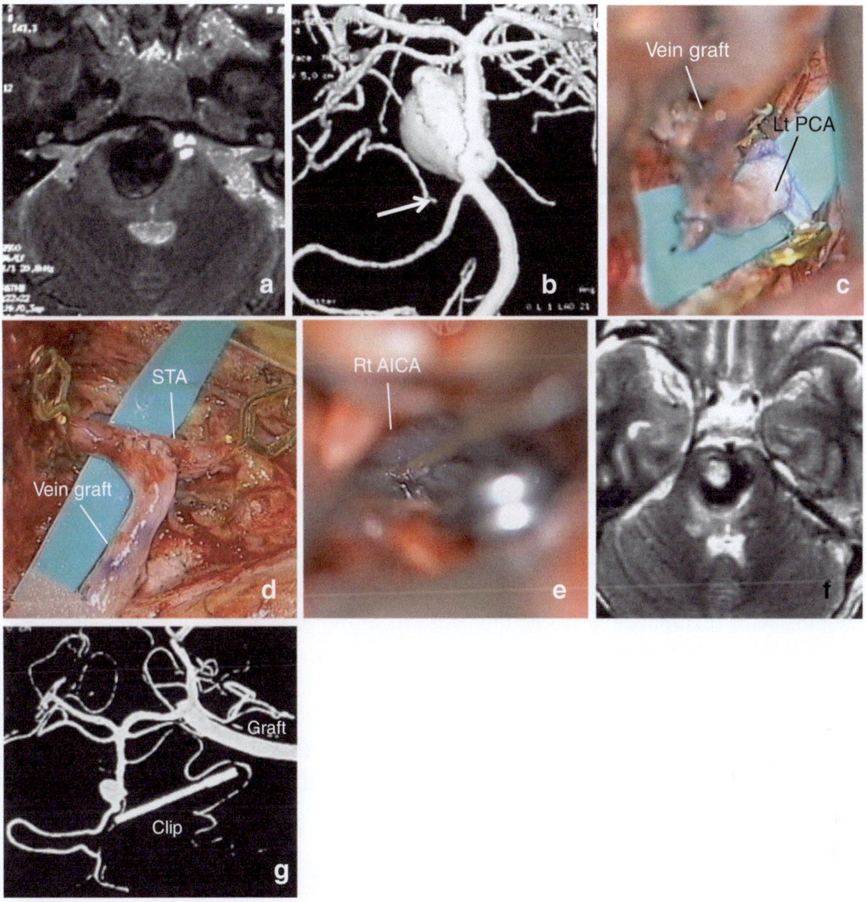

Fig. 12.6 (**a**) A T2-weighted image showing an aneurysm which severely compressed the brainstem. (**b**) Digital subtraction angiography (DSA) showing the giant basilar trunk aneurysm protruding from a basilar fenestration. The right anterior inferior cerebellar artery (AICA) originates just distal to the aneurysm (*arrow*). (**c–e**) Intraoperative photographs showing left posterior cerebral artery-vein graft anastomosis (**c**) and superficial temporal artery-vein graft anastomosis (**d**). The basilar trunk was occluded just proximal to the origin of the right AICA (**e**) to create an outflow of the bypass flow toward to the AICA and preserve basilar perforators. (**f**) A T2-weighted image 1 month after the surgery showing the decreased aneurysm size. (**g**) Left carotid angiogram showing a patent bypass graft and an occluded basilar trunk just proximal to the origin of the right AICA. The right AICA made an outflow of the bypass flow and the aneurysm decreased in size (Reprinted from reference [12] under permission)

12.4 Controversies

12.4.1 Bypass Selection upon Therapeutic ICA Occlusion

Simple ICA ligation without distal revascularization resulted in cerebral infarction in 26% of patients, 46% of which were fatal according to an analysis of several reports [22]; therefore, the PAO procedure is usually combined with reconstructive bypass surgery, such as a STA-MCA bypass or high-flow bypass using a saphenous vein graft or a radial artery graft [23, 24].

There are two approaches to planning which type of bypass surgery should be performed prior to PAO of the ICA. The selective approach uses preoperative balloon test occlusion (BTO) of the parent ICA to simulate an ischemic condition and selects either a low-or high-flow bypass according to the residual blood flow during BTO [25].

The universal approach uses a high-flow bypass for all patients who undergo PAO [26]. This is based on the consideration of possible errors in the selection and complications due to BTO.

We have applied a selective approach using preoperative BTO. Figure 12.7 demonstrates our criteria for bypass selection based on a previous study [4]. High-flow bypass is indicated for all patients with ischemic symptoms during BTO. In the absence of any ischemic symptoms, the bypass procedure was selected based on the percentage of residual flow, which was quantitatively assessed by single photon emission computed tomography (SPECT) during BTO. Residual flow of less than 70–75% indicated a high-flow bypass, while residual flow between 75 and 90% indicated a STA-MCA bypass. Simple PAO without bypass may be possible for patients with residual flow exceeding 90% in terms of immediate good outcomes; however, considering the long-term risk of aneurysm induction on collateral arteries, a STA-MCA bypass was applied in most patients, except in elderly patients or patients with systemic surgical risks.

Postoperative quantitative SPECT demonstrated that cerebral blood flow and cerebrovascular reactivity to acetazolamide on the surgical and non–surgical sides did not differ significantly [4].

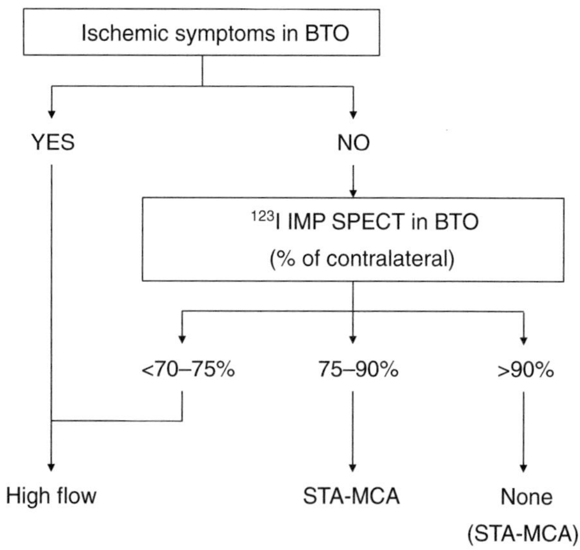

Fig. 12.7 Balloon test occlusion criteria in our institution for bypass selection in parent artery occlusion

However, BTO is associated with a 3.2% complication rate [6], and the process is cumbersome because of the use of SPECT during BTO. Further improvements in bypass selection are warranted.

12.4.2 *PAO Strategy: Coiling or Clipping?*

12.4.2.1 Intracavernous Giant/Large ICA Aneurysms

In most cases of intracavernous giant/large ICA aneurysms, a cervical ICA ligation is appropriate as a PAO after EC-IC bypass. Usually, there are no major branches arising from the cervical ICA to the origin of the ophthalmic artery, and spontaneous thrombotic formation is expected. However, in approximately 10–20% of cases, several collateral circulations, such as the meningohypophyseal trunk or vidian artery, may be observed between the external carotid artery and the ICA during BTO, providing intense aneurysmal opacification [27]. In these cases, coil embolization of the ICA just proximal to the aneurysm was used to avoid residual blood flow to the aneurysm in our institution. However, it has not been clarified if this strategy is correct and further evaluation is necessary.

12.4.2.2 Paraclinoid Giant/Large ICA Aneurysms

In cases of paraclinoid giant/large ICA (C2) aneurysms, cervical ICA ligation is unsuitable for PAO due to the remaining collateral circulation via the ophthalmic artery to the aneurysm. In these cases, PAO of the ICA between the ophthalmic artery and aneurysm is theoretically necessary. This can be achieved either by clip occlusion after anterior clinoidectomy or coil embolization, usually together with the aneurysm.

On the other hand, PAO for C1 portion aneurysms should be performed with clip occlusion because the critical branches, including the posterior communicating artery, anterior choroidal artery, and direct ICA perforators originate from the C1 portion of the ICA. If a coil is used for PAO of the C1 portion of the ICA, thromboembolic infarction of these branches may occur [28]. Clip trapping or proximal clipping is preferred for PAOs in C1 portion aneurysms.

12.4.2.3 Intradural VA Dissecting Aneurysms

Although endovascular internal trapping is frequently chosen as the first-line treatment for this type of aneurysm, postoperative MI may occur in 30–47% of cases [16, 29, 30]. Several risk factors for MI have been previously reported. Endo et al. reported that the long segment of the VA coiling (15.7 ± 6.0 mm) was significantly associated with MI [29]. Ikeda et al. reported that the length of the coil mass proximal to the dilated portion of more than 5.8 mm was associated with a higher incidence of MI

[30]. In contrast, Aihara et al. reported that the length of trapping was not the primary risk factor for MI, and proximal VA stumps were associated with MI. Preservation of the origin of the anterior spinal artery may also reduce the risk of MI [16].

In some cases, clip ligation of the dissected VA may outperform internal trapping with a coil to preserve perforators to the medulla; however, this is not necessarily possible in all patients, and it remains controversial which method is the best to occlude dissected VA.

12.4.3 *Surgical Strategy for Fusiform Giant Partially Thrombosed Basilar Trunk Aneurysms*

Unclippable fusiform giant partially thrombosed basilar trunk aneurysms are among the most challenging types in the treatment of neurovascular disorders. Although the optimal therapeutic strategy for these aneurysms remains unclear, flow alteration or blind-alley methods have been reported to be effective treatments by several authors [5, 6]. The purpose of both methods is to reduce the intra-aneurysmal flow or aneurysmal wall shear stress by altering the pathological hemodynamics. If collateral circulation is insufficient to maintain an adequate distal blood supply, a bypass surgery for one or more distal main vessels is required. However, it remains difficult to predict how much bypass flow is appropriate to preserve distal blood flow and how rapidly intraluminal thrombus formation progresses.

Recently, computational fluid dynamics (CFD) models have become available to predict the territories that are likely to be ischemic upon PAO and simulate postoperative flows following a planned flow alteration procedure [31]. Further advances in this field are expected to create a universal prediction model for the treatment of challenging complex aneurysms in the future.

12.5 Conclusion

We have described various treatments such as PAO, flow alteration, and blind-alley formation combined with bypass surgery. To prevent aneurysmal rupture and ischemic complications, case-by-case multi-modal evaluations and careful surgical strategy planning are indispensable.

References

1. Nussbaum ES, Kallmes KM, Lassig JP, et al. Cerebral revascularization for the management of complex intracranial aneurysms: a single-center experience. J Neurosurg. 2018;131:1–11.
2. Roh H, Kim J, Bae H, et al. Comparison of stent-assisted and no-stent coil embolization for safety and effectiveness in the treatment of ruptured intracranial aneurysms. J Neurosurg. 2019;30:1–7.

3. Becske T, Brinjikji W, Potts MB, et al. Long-term clinical and angiographic outcomes following pipeline embolization device treatment of complex internal carotid artery aneurysms: five-year results of the Pipeline for Uncoilable or Failed Aneurysms Trial. Neurosurgery. 2017;80:40–8.
4. Shimizu H, Matsumoto Y, Tominaga T. Parent artery occlusion with bypass surgery for the treatment of internal carotid artery aneurysms: clinical and hemodynamic results. Clin Neurol Neurosurg. 2010;112:32–9.
5. Lee SH, Ahn JS, Kwun BD, et al. Surgical flow alteration for the treatment of intracranial aneurysms that are unclippable, untrappable, and uncoilable. J Korean Neurosurg Soc. 2015;58:518–27.
6. Wongsuriyanan S, Sriamornrattanakul K. Blind-alley formation and occipital artery-posterior inferior cerebellar artery bypass for the treatment of unclippable vertebral artery aneurysms with posterior inferior cerebellar artery involvement. W Neurosurg. 2020;138:e539–50.
7. Kivipelto L, Niemelä M, Meling T, et al. Bypass surgery for complex middle cerebral artery aneurysms: impact of the exact location in the MCA tree. J Neurosurg. 2014;120:398–408.
8. Date I. Symptomatic unruptured cerebral aneurysms: features and surgical outcome. Neurol Med Chir (Tokyo). 2010;50:788–99.
9. Yanaka K, Matsumaru Y, Mashiko R, et al. Small Unruptured cerebral aneurysms presenting with oculomotor nerve palsy. Neurosurgery. 2003;52:553–7; discussion 556.
10. Tan H, Huang G, Zhang T, et al. A retrospective comparison of the influence of surgical clipping and endovascular embolization on recovery of oculomotor nerve palsy in patients with posterior communicating artery aneurysms. Neurosurgery. 2015;76:687–94; discussion 694.
11. Raymond J, Gentric JC, Darsaut TE, et al. Flow diversion in the treatment of aneurysms: a randomized care trial and registry. J Neurosurg. 2017;127:454–62.
12. Shimizu H. Deep bypass surgery: basic techniques and tips. Jpn J Neurosurg (Tokyo). 2015;24:846–54.
13. Hongo K, Horiuchi T, Nitta J, et al. Double-insurance bypass for internal carotid aneurysm surgery. Neurosurgery. 2013;52:597–602; discussion 600.
14. Mizutani T, Aruga T, Kirino T, et al. Recurrent subarachnoid hemorrhage from untreated ruptured vertebrobasilar dissecting aneurysms. Neurosurgery. 1995;36:905–11; discussion 912.
15. Iihara K, Sakai N, Murao K, et al. Dissecting aneurysms of the vertebral artery: a management strategy. J Neurosurg. 2002;97:259–67.
16. Aihara M, Naito I, Shimizu T, et al. Predictive factors of medullary infarction after endovascular internal trapping using coils for vertebral artery dissecting aneurysms. J Neurosurg. 2018;129:107–13.
17. Shi L, Xu K, Sun X, et al. Therapeutic progress in treating vertebral dissecting aneurysms involving the posterior inferior cerebellar artery. Int J Med Sci. 2016;13:540–55.
18. Kole MK, Pelz DM, Kalapos P, et al. Endovascular coil embolization of intracranial aneurysms: important factors related to rates and outcomes of incomplete occlusion. J Neurosurg. 2005;102:607–15.
19. Daou B, Chalouhi N, Starke RM, et al. Clipping of previously coiled cerebral aneurysms: efficacy, safety, and predictors in a cohort of 111 patients. J Neurosurg. 2016;125:1337–43.
20. Labib MA, Gandhi S, Cavallo C, et al. Anterior cerebral artery bypass for complex aneurysms: advances in intracranial-intracranial bypass techniques. World Neurosurg. 2020;141:e42–54.
21. Yanagisawa T, Kinouchi H, Sasajima T, et al. Long-term follow-up for a giant basilar trunk aneurysm surgically treated by proximal occlusion and external carotid artery to posterior carotid artery bypass using a saphenous vein graft. J Stroke Cerebrovasc Dis. 2016;25:e212–3.
22. Linskey ME, Jungreis CA, Yonas H, et al. Stroke risk after abrupt internal carotid artery sacrifice: accuracy of preoperative assessment with balloon test occlusion and stable xenon-enhanced CT. AJNR Am J Neuroradiol. 1994;15:829–43.
23. Jafar JJ, Russell SM, Woo HH. Treatment of giant intracranial aneurysms with saphenous vein extracranial-to-intracranial bypass grafting: indications, operative technique, and results in 29 patients. Neurosurgery. 2002;51:138–44; discussion 144.

24. Sekhar LN, Duff JM, Kalavakonda C, et al. Cerebral revascularization using radial artery grafts for the treatment of complex intracranial aneurysms: techniques and outcomes for 17 patients. Neurosurgery. 2001;49:646–58; discussion 658.
25. Surdell DL, Hage ZA, Eddleman CS, et al. Revascularization for complex intracranial aneurysms. Neurosurg Focus. 2008;24:E21.
26. Mohit AA, Sekhar LN, Natarajan SK, et al. High-flow bypass grafts in the management of complex intracranial aneurysms. Neurosurgery. 2007;60(Suppl 1):ONS105–22; discussion ONS122: ONS105–122.
27. Allen JW, Alastra AJ, Nelson PK. Proximal intracranial internal carotid artery branches: prevalence and importance for balloon occlusion test. J Neurosurg. 2005;102:45–52.
28. Murakami K, Shimizu H, Matsumoto Y, et al. Acute ischemic complications after therapeutic parent artery occlusion with revascularization for complex internal carotid artery aneurysms. Surg Neurol. 2009;71:434–41; discussion 441.
29. Endo H, Matsumoto Y, Kondo R, et al. Medullary infarction as a poor prognostic factor after internal coil trapping of a ruptured vertebral artery dissection. J Neurosurg. 2013;118:131–9.
30. Ikeda H, Imamura H, Mineharu Y, et al. Effect of coil packing proximal to the dilated segment on postoperative medullary infarction and prognosis following internal trapping for ruptured vertebral artery dissection. Interv Neuroradiol. 2016;22:67–75.
31. Tsuji M, Ishikawa T, Ishida F, et al. Stagnation and complex flow in ruptured cerebral aneurysms: a possible association with hemostatic pattern. J Neurosurg. 2017;126:1566–72.

Chapter 13
Endovascular Treatment for Anterior Communicating Artery Aneurysms

Masataka Takeuchi, Atsushi Uyama, Takashi Matsumoto, and Kazuma Tsuto

13.1 Characteristics of the Anterior Communicating Artery Aneurysm

Anterior communicating artery aneurysms often have an anatomically complex shape. The majority of the aneurysms are small, often with a wide-neck and thin parent vessels. From these anatomical features, it has been pointed out that there are several cases of intraoperative aneurysm rupture, thromboembolism, incomplete occlusion, and recanalization. Intraoperative rupture in endovascular treatment of anterior communicating artery aneurysm is often reported to be around 4% [1, 2]. The analysis of intraoperative rupture of anterior communicating artery aneurysm lists ruptured aneurysms, 3 mm or less, small necks, and shallow domes as the risk factors.

There have been several reports that thromboembolic complications occur at approximately 6–7%. The risk factors include wide-neck carotid aneurysms, having the parent vessel and an aneurysm that are off-axis, and the use of concurrent stents. However, although the frequency of thromboembolic complications was high, several studies reported that the effect on the prognosis was small [3].

There are some reports that anterior communicating artery aneurysms are often recanalized after endovascular treatment. Finitsis et al. reported that 21.7% of ruptured anterior communicating artery aneurysms were recanalized and 10.2% were retreated. Furthermore, 23.5% of unruptured anterior communicating artery aneurysms were recanalized, and treatment had been performed in 8.8%. The average time to recurrence was 0.9 years (6 months to 3 years), and the risk factors are ruptured cerebral aneurysm and aneurysm less than 4 mm. It has been suggested that there is a risk of recanalization even after complete occlusion is noted

---

M. Takeuchi (✉) · A. Uyama · T. Matsumoto · K. Tsuto
Department of Neurosurgery, Seisho Hospital, Odawara, Kanagawa, Japan

Y. Kato, A. Ansari (eds.), *Cerebrovascular Surgery*, Advances and Technical Standards in Neurosurgery 44, https://doi.org/10.1007/978-3-030-87649-4_13

immediately after treatment [4]. In the examination of recurrence after endovascular treatment for cerebral aneurysm, the overall recurrence rate was 12.6%, while the recurrence rate of anterior communicating artery aneurysm was 22.3%. It has been reported that an anterior communicating artery aneurysm denotes a significant risk of recurrence along with middle cerebral artery aneurysm [5]. Therefore, it is necessary to provide a comparison with craniotomy for the assessment of the treatment indications and to obtain preoperative informed consent.

13.2 Treatment Strategy for Anterior Communicating Artery Aneurysm

It is notable that angiography is essential before surgery. It is of prime importance to confirm not only the shape of the aneurysm, but also the positional relationship with the surrounding blood vessels, the access route of the aneurysm, and the working angle, among others. For anterior communicating artery aneurysms that are projected anteriorly or posteriorly, the head position is often changed by raising the mandible to secure a working angle. It should also be remembered that the aneurysm and denture often overlap due to head position change. Endovascular treatment without an appropriate working angle has a high risk of complications; therefore, treatment indications need to be reconsidered in such cases. In addition, the angle between the internal carotid artery and the anterior communicating artery A1 and the angle between the anterior cerebral artery A1 and the axis of the aneurysm are important for safe endovascular treatment of the anterior communicating artery aneurysm. If the angle between the internal carotid artery and the anterior communicating artery A1 is sharp, the microcatheter will easily kick back when the microcatheter is deviated or embolized into the middle cerebral artery during microcatheter guidance. If the anterior cerebral artery A1 and the aneurysm are significantly off-axis, the risk of perforation during microcatheter induction is high. Since the anterior cerebral artery A1 often points anteriorly and inferiorly, caution is required for small aneurysms projecting upward or posteriorly.

The degree of the development of the bilateral anterior cerebral artery A1 and the anterior communicating artery is also important. If the bilateral A1 and the anterior communicating artery aneurysms are well developed, a bilateral approach and, in some cases, the blocking of the anterior communicating artery are considered. Choi et al. reported that the anterior communicating artery was occluded for anterior communicating artery aneurysm with bilateral A1 symmetry; however, it did not affect the complication of thromboembolism [6].

A stable backup of the guiding system is desirable; additionally, it is imperative that the guiding catheter and guiding sheath be placed as high as possible. The use of an intermediate catheter is considered when it is difficult to advance the guiding catheter or guiding sheath to a higher position due to the bending of the internal carotid artery. A 6 Fr intermediate catheter is used if possible in case of issues, such as intraoperative rupture.

Pre-shaping of the microcatheter is important. If the curve of the anterior cerebral artery A1 and the axis of the aneurysm are almost the same, it is possible to use simple shaping or a pre-shaped catheter. However, if the curve of the anterior cerebral artery A1 and the axis of the aneurysm are significantly deviated, it is necessary to have two or more shapes so that the tip of the microcatheter naturally projects into the aneurysm.

It is necessary to fill the coil as densely as possible in consideration of the recurrence rate. However, if the bifurcation from the internal carotid artery to the anterior cerebral artery A1 is at an acute angle, the microcatheter easily kicks back. In such a case, it may be necessary to fix the microcatheter with an assist balloon.

13.3 Indications for Treatment of Anterior Communicating Artery Aneurysm

Anterior communicating artery aneurysms often have an anatomically complex shape. There are numerous complications, such as intraoperative rupture and thromboembolism due to the characteristics of small aneurysms with thin parent blood vessels. In addition, problems, such as a high recanalization rate, have been pointed out. Therefore, it is important to select an appropriate case for safe treatment. Here are some points to check to determine the indication for endovascular treatment for anterior communicating artery aneurysms (Table. 13.1).

13.3.1 Case 1 Simple Technique

An 80-year-old woman with a family history of SAH exhibited a ruptured anterior communicating artery aneurysm that was projecting upward in a posterior manner. The angle between the internal carotid artery and the A1 origin of the anterior communicating artery was relatively linear. It was a relatively small aneurysm with a major axis of 4.3 mm × 2.9 mm. Additionally, the axis of the anterior cerebral artery A1 and the cerebral aneurysm was displaced (Fig. 13.1a). Therefore, two locations were steam shaped, from the internal carotid artery to the anterior

Table 13.1 Points to consider regarding the indication for the endovascular treatment of an anterior communicating artery aneurysm

• Shape of the aneurysm
• Bilateral anterior cerebral arteries, anterior communicating artery anatomy, and vessel diameter
• Angle from the internal carotid artery to the anterior cerebral artery A1
• Angle from the anterior cerebral artery A1 to the aneurysm
• Whether or not a working angle is secured with an angiography device

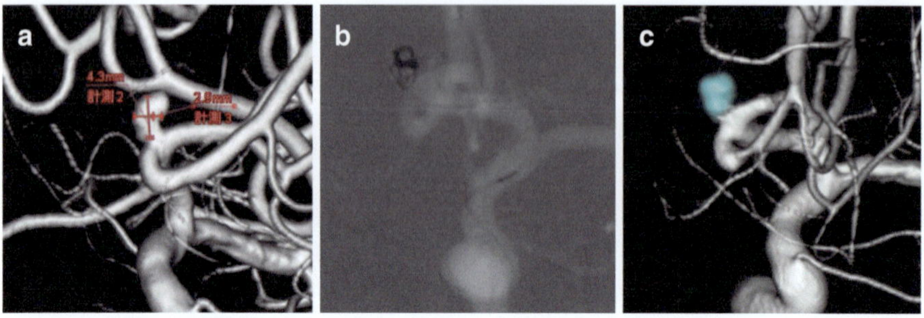

Fig. 13.1 Simple technique. Ruptured anterior communicating artery aneurysm. The axes of the small aneurysm, anterior cerebral artery A1, and the cerebral aneurysm are misaligned. Steam shapes of the microcatheter at the two sites were effective

cerebral artery A1 and from the anterior cerebral artery A1 to the aneurysm. The first coil was filled; however, the microcatheter was stable, and there was no kickback (Fig. 13.1b). Sufficient embolism was obtained without rupture during the operation (Fig. 13.1c).

Even during treatment with a simple technique, it is recommended to secure multiple access routes in order to prepare for potential issues such as intraoperative rupture and coil deviation. Assist balloon catheters are useful for controlling the blood flow during intraoperative rupture, and it is necessary to prepare an assist balloon even when treatment with a simple technique is performed. Regarding the handling of the assist balloon, there are methods, such as preparing and placing it on the table or guiding it to the internal carotid artery or the anterior cerebral artery A1 and putting it on standby.

13.3.2 Double Catheter Technique

A 66-year-old woman visited our institution with a ruptured anterior communicating artery aneurysm, which was significantly irregular (Fig. 13.2a). The bilateral anterior cerebral arteries A1 were symmetric, and two microcatheters were inserted from both A1s for embolization. One microcatheter was removed because it was necessary to fill the piecemeal with a coil and move the microcatheter into the aneurysm bleb. This facilitated microcatheter operation, and the aneurysm bleb was embolized (Fig. 13.2b). Although it was irregular, sufficient embolism was obtained (Fig. 13.2c).

This technique is useful for wide-neck carotid aneurysms, large aneurysms, and irregular anterior cerebral aneurysms. The insertion of two microcatheters from one side should be confirmed by frequent angiography, paying close attention to thromboembolism. In addition, it is desirable to remove one of the microcatheters judged to be unnecessary in the latter half of the treatment, from the standpoint of thromboembolism.

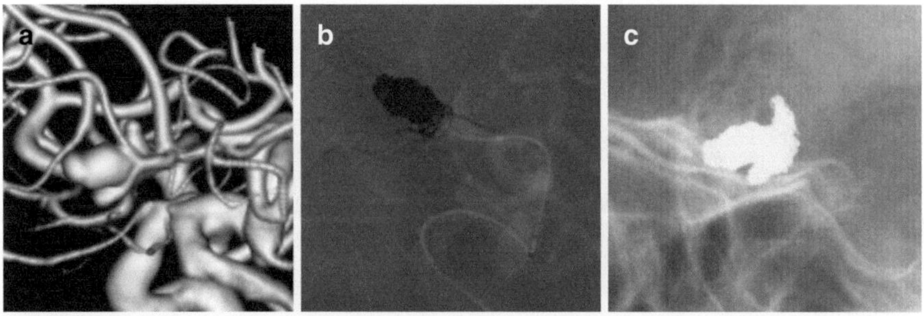

Fig. 13.2 Double catheter technique. Ruptured anterior communicating artery aneurysm. It was observed to be very irregular. After embolizing the tip with a double catheter, one microcatheter was removed. A microcatheter was operated to embolize the aneurysm bleb

13.3.3 Balloon Assist Technique

A 69-year-old woman presented with a ruptured anterior communicating artery that was observed to bulge superiorly and inferiorly from the anterior communicating artery. Additionally, a bleb was observed in the upper part (Fig. 13.3a). An assist balloon was placed in the anterior communicating artery. The right side of the A1-A2 junction was confirmed from the frontal tube and the left side of the A1-A2 junction was visually confirmed from the lateral tube (Fig. 13.3b). Additionally, sufficient embolism was obtained in the upper bleb, and the anterior communicating artery and bilateral A2 could be preserved (Fig. 13.3c).

Since the diameter of the parent vessel is small, the balloon assist technique has not been recommended because there is concern about vascular damage due to balloon dilation. In recent years, small-diameter balloon catheters have been developed and are frequently used. The important criterion in the balloon assist technique is the angle from the anterior cerebral artery A1 to the A2 or the anterior communicating artery. The balloon should be placed such that it can cover the aneurysm neck ideally; however, the guidance method should be determined in consideration of the bifurcation angle. It is frequently guided from the ipsilateral anterior cerebral artery A1 to A2. However, depending on the anatomical structure, guidance may be provided from the contralateral anterior cerebral artery A1 to the anterior cerebral artery A2 via the anterior communicating artery. Since vascular extension often occurs when the balloon is guided, a roadmap is often required again when the microcatheter is guided into the aneurysm. At the end of the embolization, it is necessary to confirm that the blood flow obstruction does not occur due to the return of the extended vessels.

13.3.4 Stent Assist Technique

A 76-year-old woman visited our institution with an unruptured anterior cerebral aneurysm. The aneurysm and the anterior communicating artery overlap in large aneurysms over 10 mm, making it difficult to secure a sufficient working angle. An

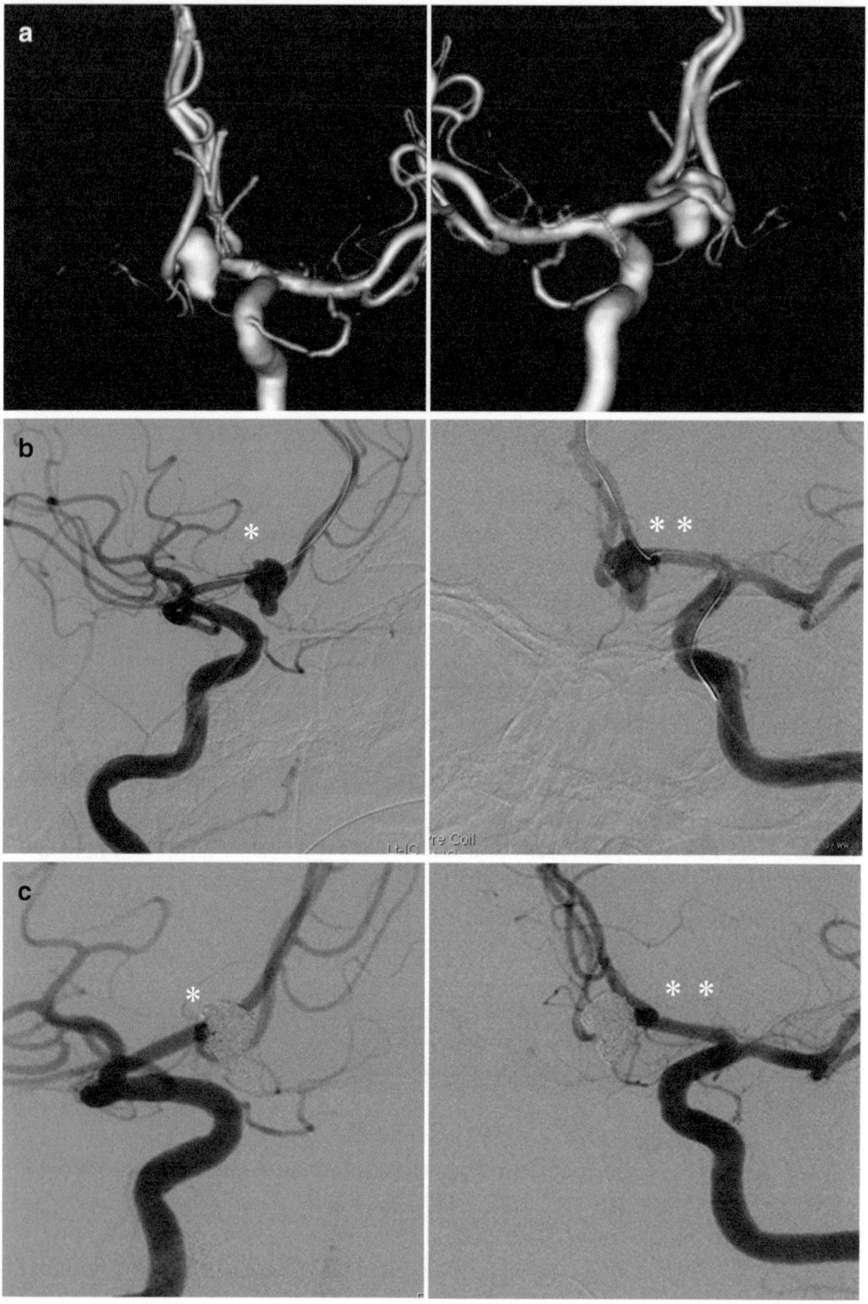

Fig. 13.3 Balloon assist technique. Ruptured anterior communicating artery aneurysm. Superior and inferior bulges were observed. An assist balloon was dilated into the anterior communicating artery and embolized. *Asterisk* Rt A1-A2 junction, *Double asterisk* Lt A1-A2 junction

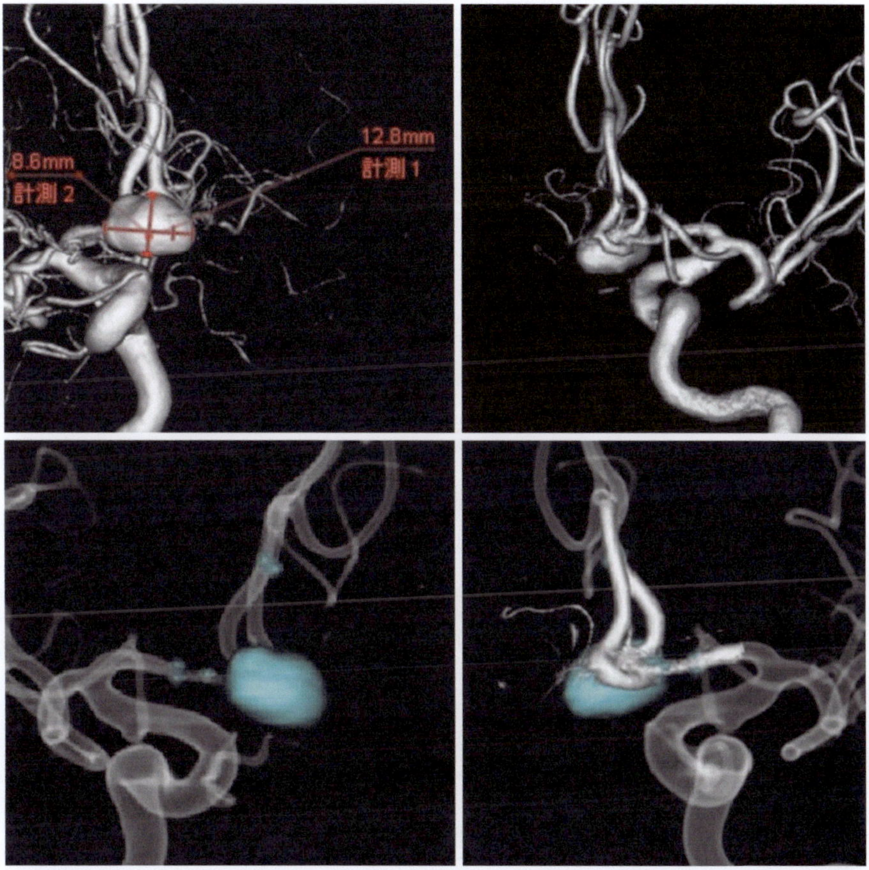

Fig. 13.4 Stent assist technique. Unruptured anterior cerebral aneurysm. When the size is 10 mm or more, securing a working angle becomes a challenge. The combined use of VRD made it possible to preserve the anterior communicating artery and the bilateral anterior cerebral artery A2

embolic microcatheter was inserted into the cerebral aneurysm, and a VRD was placed from the right anterior cerebral artery A2. The bilateral anterior cerebral artery A2 and the anterior communicating artery were preserved, and sufficient embolism was obtained (Fig. 13.4).

The stent assist technique was limited to cases, such as the assist balloon technique because the parent vessel diameter was small. However, small-diameter stents have been developed, and the indication has expanded. However, since the thromboembolic complications associated with stent placement have increased, the indications should be determined carefully and sufficient antithrombotic therapy is required. In combination with a stent, these methods involve a stent-jailing method and a trans-cell method. In the stent-jail method, the stent and the microcatheter jailed outside the stent are present in the narrow anterior cerebral artery A1, resulting in an impaired blood flow and poor stent dilation. As such, caution is required.

13.3.5 Postoperative Care

Anterior communicating artery aneurysms are observed to frequently recanalize after embolization. The risk is particularly high for ruptured aneurysms and small aneurysms. Recanalization is known to occur frequently within a year; therefore, sufficient follow-up is required. If possible, reassessments by cerebral angiography are ideal.

13.4 Characteristics of Anterior Communicating Artery Distal Aneurysms

The anterior cerebral artery distal aneurysm (ACA distal An) is most common at the branch of the anterior cerebral artery A2, the pericallosal artery, and the callosal marginal artery. Since it is located relatively close to the brain surface of the interhemispheric fissure, surgery is often selected [7]. However, endovascular treatment may be selected if the patient's general condition is poor and for the elderly. Liang et al. stated that the results of endovascular treatment of ACA distal An showed 1.1% for mortality and 0% for morbidity, and that endovascular treatment was safe and effective [8]. In addition, although ruptured aneurysms are often complicated by intracerebral hemorrhage, there is a report that the presence or absence of intracerebral hemorrhage does not affect the treatment prognosis [9]. It often occurs in the direction of anatomical and hemodynamic stress. Therefore, the catheter can be easily guided. However, the aneurysm is distally located, and the indwelling microcatheter becomes unstable.

13.4.1 Treatment Strategy for ACA Distal An

As with the anterior communicating artery aneurysm, the guiding catheter should be guided as high as possible in the internal carotid artery. The microcatheter guidance requires passing through the siphon, internal carotid and anterior cerebral arteries A1, A1-A2 junctions, and several flexions before reaching the ACA distal An. There are several branched vessels (ophthalmic artery, posterior communicating artery, anterior choroid plexus artery, and the Heubner artery) in between, and great care should be taken to avoid perforation with a microguide wire. The microguide wire requires shaping to pass through each flexion. However, it is often difficult to guide it into the final stage of the aneurysm; additionally, the guidance from the anterior cerebral artery A2 into the aneurysm is better performed by removing the microguide wire once and changing the shaping. At that time, the microcatheter that has passed through a steep angle may lose its deflection and advance at once. Therefore, it is recommended to carefully check it under fluoroscopy and slowly remove it. In addition, when guiding a microcatheter, pushability is often poor and torque is often difficult to transmit. To overcome this, setting an intermediate catheter (triple coaxial system) improves the operability of the microcatheter. When using an intermediate catheter, it is necessary to check the length of how far the microcatheter has come out of the intermediate catheter.

13.4.2 Treatment Indications for ACA Distal An

In the endovascular treatment of ACA distal An, adjunctive techniques, such as balloon assist and double catheter technique, are difficult because the parent vessels are thin. Whether it is possible with a simple technique is the most important factor in considering indication. Since several aneurysms are mounted on the origins of the callosal marginal arteries and pericallosal arteries, the selection of the first coil that creates framing is key. When the framing coil deviates from the parent vessel or the branch vessel, it is not indicated. As the filling coil, it is recommended to select a soft and short coil because the microcatheter is easy to kick back due to the thinness of the parent vessel.

13.4.3 Case 1

A 73-year-old woman presented with a ruptured ACA distal An, which was overriding the origin of the callosal marginal artery and the pericallosal artery.

The framing could subsequently be created with an inward coil. A feeling coil was added so as to not break the framing. The callosal marginal artery and pericallosal artery were preserved (Fig. 13.5).

13.5 The Future of ACA Distal An

Due to the development of the triple coaxial system, the development of small-diameter and flexible coils, and the application of flow diverter system, there have been a series of reports that the results of endovascular treatment are comparable to those of surgery. Going forward, the merit of endovascular treatment without craniotomy will be significant from the viewpoint of preserving higher functions. If the curability, safety, and durability of the treatment are ensured, it has the potential to

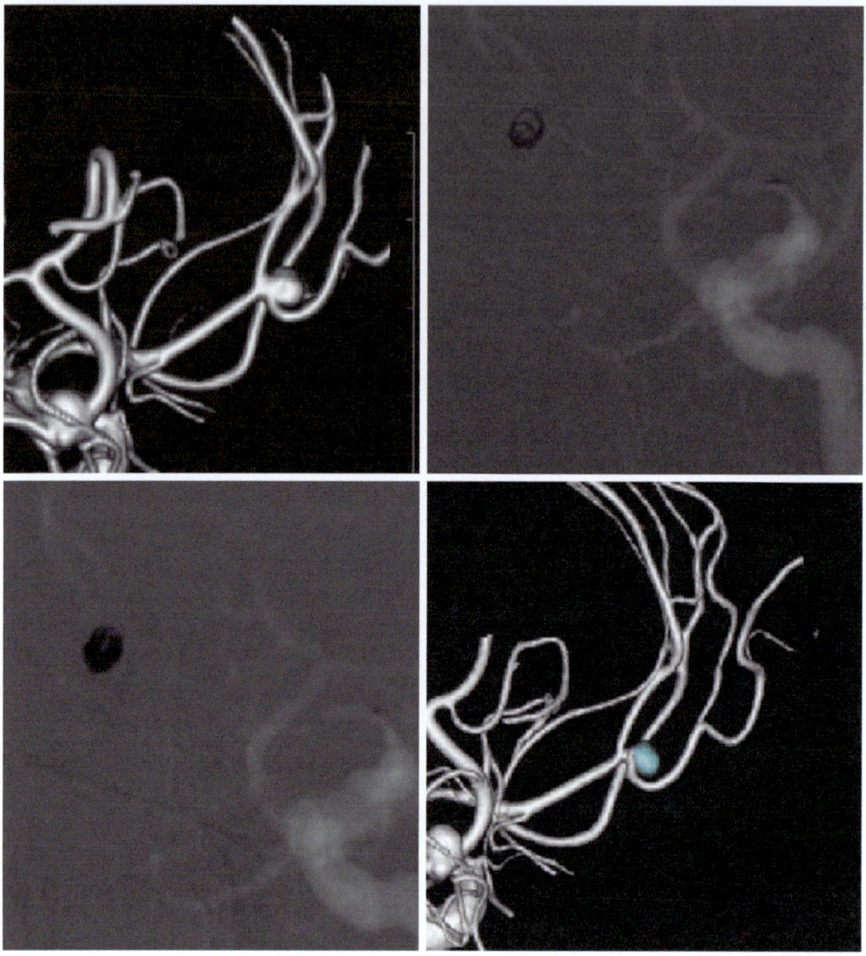

Fig. 13.5 ACA distal An. It is important to create a Fleming shape that preserves the branched vessels. Therefore, the double catheter technique is effective for irregular cerebral aneurysms. However, because it is a thin A2, embolic complications are also high

become the first-line treatment in the future, not only for the elderly and those with poor general condition.

References

1. Frang S, Brinjikji W, et al. Endovascular treatment of anterior communicating artery aneurysms: a systematic review and meta-analysis. AJNR Am J Neuroradiol. 2014;35(5):943–7.
2. Asif KS, Sattar A, et al. Consecutive endovascular treatment of 20 ruptured very small (<3 mm) anterior communicating artery aneurysms. Interv Neurol. 2016;5(1–2):57–64.

3. Fan L, Lin B, et al. Predicting intraprocedural rupture and thrombus formation during coiling of ruptured anterior communicating artery aneurysms. J Neurointerv Surg. 2017;9(4):370–5.
4. Finitsis S, Anxionnat R, et al. Endovascular treatment of ACom intracranial aneurysms. Report on series of 280 patients. Interv Neuroradial. 2010;16(1):7–16.
5. Huang DZ, Jiang B, et al. Risk factors for the recurrence of an intracranial saccular aneurysm following endovascular treatment. Oncotarget. 2017;8(20):33676–82.
6. Choi HH, Cho DY, Yoo HD, et al. Safety and efficacy of anterior communicating artery compromise during endovascular coil embolization of adjoining aneurysms. J Neurosurg. 2019;1(4):1068–76.
7. Lehecka M, Dashti R, et al. Distal anterior cerebral artery aneurysms. Acta Neurochir Suppl. 2010;107:15–26.
8. Liang L, Derelle AL, Merlot I, et al. Endovascular treatment of distal anterior cerebral artery aneurysms: long-term results. J Neuroradiol. 2018;47(1):33–7.
9. Oishi H, Nonaka S, et al. Feasibility and efficacy of endovascular therapy for ruptured distal anterior cerebral artery aneurysms. Neuro Med Chir (Tokyo). 2013;53:304–9.

Chapter 14
Management of Dural Arteriovenous Fistulas

Naoya Kuwayama

14.1 Standard Management

Dural arteriovenous fistulas (DAVF) are the acquired abnormal connection between the dural artery and the dural vein. The pathogenesis includes venous/sinus thrombosis, trauma, craniotomy (surgery), but still remains unknown in the majority of cases. The incidence has been reported as 0.16–1.0 per 100,000 person-year [1–3].

Among several classifications of DAVF, Borden Classification [4] and Cognard Classification [5] are important. These classifications are based on the pattern of the venous drainage, which is an essential factor to affect the severity of the diseases and treatment indication and strategy.

The involved sites include the cavernous sinus (CS), superior sagittal sinus (SSS), transverse-sigmoid sinus (TSS), confluence of sinuses (torcular herophili), tentorial sinus, anterior condylar confluence, anterior cranial fossa, craniocervical junction, convexity, and spinal dura mater.

Treatment indication is recommended by the clinical presentations of the hemorrhagic or venous ischemic events, progressive neurologic deficits or symptoms (ocular hypertension, gait disturbance and incontinence), aggressive hemodynamic features (such as vigorous cortical venous reflux), and the symptoms such as intractable tinnitus disturbing the patient's ADL.

Treatment options include observation, endovascular and surgical treatment, and stereotactic radiosurgery. Since the venous hypertension plays an important role in the clinical course of this disease, the main purpose of the treatment is to cure the venous congestion or reflux by means of decreasing the venous pressure.

N. Kuwayama (✉)
Department of Neurosurgery, University of Toyama, Toyama, Japan
e-mail: kuwa4090@alto.ocn.ne.jp

Y. Kato, A. Ansari (eds.), *Cerebrovascular Surgery*, Advances and Technical Standards in Neurosurgery 44, https://doi.org/10.1007/978-3-030-87649-4_14

14.1.1 Treatment Strategy

The lesions are divided into two types; the sinus type and the non-sinus type. The location of the sinus type includes the cavernous sinus (CS), superior sagittal sinus (SSS), transverse-sigmoid sinus (TSS), confluence (torcular herophili), tentorial sinus, and anterior condylar confluence. The location of the non-sinus type includes anterior cranial fossa, craniocervical junction, convexity, some of tentorial area, and spinal dura mater.

The principle of treatment of the sinus type is transvenous embolization (TVE), while that of the non-sinus type is transarterial embolization (TAE). In cases with difficulty of endovascular treatment, craniotomy and venous discontinuation will be an effective alternative treatment. The stereotactic radiosurgery will be the last choice of treatment in difficult cases, but it takes several months to obliterate the lesion. Because the difficult cases usually tend to need urgent treatment, we should not take an easy choice of the radiosurgery.

14.1.2 Transvenous Embolization (TVE)

Transvenous embolization includes two methods; selective TVE and whole sinus packing. The selective TVE is to occlude the localized inflow area of the blood flow (venous collector) in the involved sinus, keeping the physiological cerebral venous return to and from the sinus. This method is efficacious in the cases with localized AV shunt or localized venous collector, which can be seen frequently in the cavernous sinus. The whole sinus packing is to occlude the entire sinus. In case with diffuse AV shunt, the whole sinus packing is often required to cure the lesion.

When the brain still uses the involved sinus, the sinus blood flow should be maintained to keep the cerebral venous return, otherwise the treatment will cause the cerebral venous infarction. When the brain no longer uses the involved sinus, or the cortical venous reflux is apparent, the involved sinus can be occluded as a whole. In this case, the sinus occlusion will not affect at least the cerebral venous return.

The route of TVE is usually the trans-femoral trans-jugular vein. In case with the cavernous sinus DAVF, the first choice of the approach routes is the inferior petrosal sinus (IPS). The occluded IPS is sometimes seen but catheterization to the cavernous sinus via the occluded IPS is not difficult in majority of the cases. A microguidewire and a microcathter can proceed in the occluded IPS by rotating these devices with the sufficient backup of a guiding or distal access catheter. Other routes to the cavernous sinus include the inter-cavernous sinus (from the contralateral cavernous sinus), the superior petrosal sinus (from the ipsilateral/contralateral transverse sinus), and the superior ophthalmic vein (from the facial or superficial temporal vein). The distal access catheter will also be useful when the approach routes are very long.

The standard material of TVE is detachable coils. Onyx could be used in the involved sinus by cases, but it may cause the cranial nerve palsy in the cavernous sinus.

14.1.3 Transarterial Embolization (TAE)

Penetration of the liquid embolic materials from the arterial to the venous side can only cure the AV shunts. Proximal feeder occlusion using any materials will result in the recurrence of the shunts because the revascularization and recanalization of the fistula will occur soon after the feeder occlusion. Proximal occlusion can be effective when used as an adjunctive method of curative treatments. For example, the occipital artery can be occluded by coils before curative Onyx TAE from the middle meningeal artery or the middle meningeal artery can be occluded by coils before curative TVE of the cavernous sinus lesion.

Onyx and NBCA (*n*-butyl cyanoacrylate) are the liquid materials to achieve the curative TAE. NBCA is an adhesive polymerizing material (glue) to be used as a mixture with lipiodol. The lower the concentration of NBCA, the higher the viscosity of the material and the higher the temperature of the material, the lower the viscosity. Usually 20–30% mixture of NBCA is used with heating to achieve the easy penetration without adhering to the catheter. Onyx is a new precipitating material containing ethylene vinyl alcohol polymer, DMSO (dimethyl sulfoxide), and tantalum powder (for visualization). Initially it has been developed for AVM embolization, but has been found to be very effective also to DAVFs. Because Onyx is not an adhesive material, prolonged injection (even for hours) can be done and clinical results have been improved dramatically [6]. Plug and push method is very effective to penetrate the lesion to the draining veins or sinuses. A tip of a catheter is sometimes trapped in the Onyx mass in case with excessive embolization. A balloon catheter acts like a plug and is useful to prevent Onyx from coming back to the catheter. Since Onyx can easily proceed not only to the venous side but also to the other feeding arteries, the lesion sometimes will be obliterated completely by a single pedicle injection. However, one must be careful not to cause cranial nerve palsy (embolization of vasa nervorum) and cerebral infarction through the dangerous anastomosis between external and internal carotid and vertebral arteries. A profound knowledge about the functional microvascular anatomy is very important to prevent these complications.

The site of a good indication of Onyx is transverse-sigmoid sinus, superior sagittal sinus, confluence, and tentorial area. Onyx TAE in the anterior cranial base is feasible but not easy because the feeding pedicles arising from the ophthalmic artery are distal, small, and tortuous. Use of Onyx for DAVF of the cavernous sinus and anterior condylar confluence is very dangerous, causing cranial nerve palsy and cerebral infarction. NBCA is a reliable and effective material for the spinal lesion. Effectiveness of Onyx for the spinal lesion remains unknown.

14.1.4 Complications of Treatment

In general, hemodynamic status will dramatically change after obliteration of the AVF, regardless of the treatment method. Venous stasis and/or embolic materials as the foreign bodies in the veins are the potential cause of venous thrombosis both after TAE and TVE. Heparin infusion will be an essential treatment in the postoperative course to prevent the venous thrombosis. Cerebral hyperperfusion syndrome may occur after abrupt occlusion of the AV shunt in cases with high flow AVF. Important is the prediction and recognition of the hyperperfusion syndrome as an unexpected complication before treatment. Single photon emission CT or transcranial Doppler ultrasound will be very useful to detect the hyperperfusion phenomenon.

14.1.4.1 Complications of TAE

Migration of the Embolic Materials via the Arterial Anastomosis

One of the most important and critical complications is cerebral ischemia resulted from the migration of embolic materials via the so-called dangerous anastomosis between dural and pial arteries. Usually the dural branches of the external carotid artery have rich anastomosis with the dural and pial branches of the internal and vertebral arteries. Liquid embolic materials like NBCA and Onyx as well as particulate materials smaller than 200 μm easily migrate to the pial arteries via the network. One must care about the dangerous behavior of the liquid materials; it tends to come back the parent feeding pedicle vie the arterial network arising from the feeding artery itself (Fig. 14.1).

Migration of the Embolic Materials to the Venous Side

Onyx, particularly, tends to penetrate the arteriovenous fistula very easily and go to the venous side. This penetration is the essential phenomenon needed to the radical treatment and is the most advantageous point of Onyx. However, excessive penetration (migration) could occasionally result in the occlusion of the functioning cerebral veins (Fig. 14.2) causing potential venous infarction.

NBCA tends to make fragmentation in the venous side when the arterial blood flow comes from the other feeding arteries. If a block of fragment occludes the distal side of the draining vein, venous bleeding may occur due to the remaining arterial inflow.

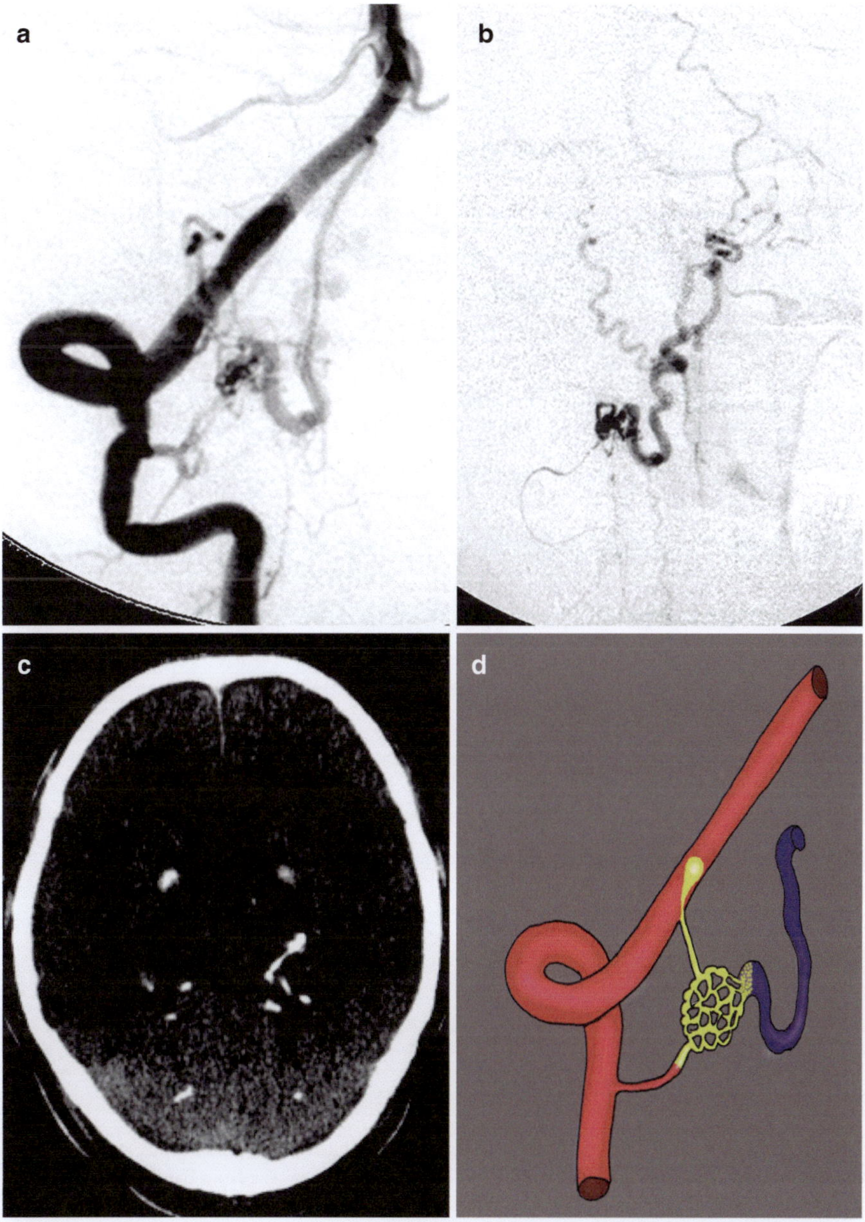

Fig. 14.1 A case with DAVF in the craniocervical junction showing NBCA migration. (**a**) Preoperative vertebral angiogram indicating DAVF fed by C2 segmental artery of the vertebral artery and drained into the cerebral vein in the brain stem. (**b**) Microangiogram from the feeding artery. (**c**) Postoperative CT scan indicating migration of the fragmented pieces of NBCA. (**d**) Schematic drawing of the mechanism of NBCA migration; injected NBCA came back to the distal parent vertebral artery via the network between the other feeding pedicle

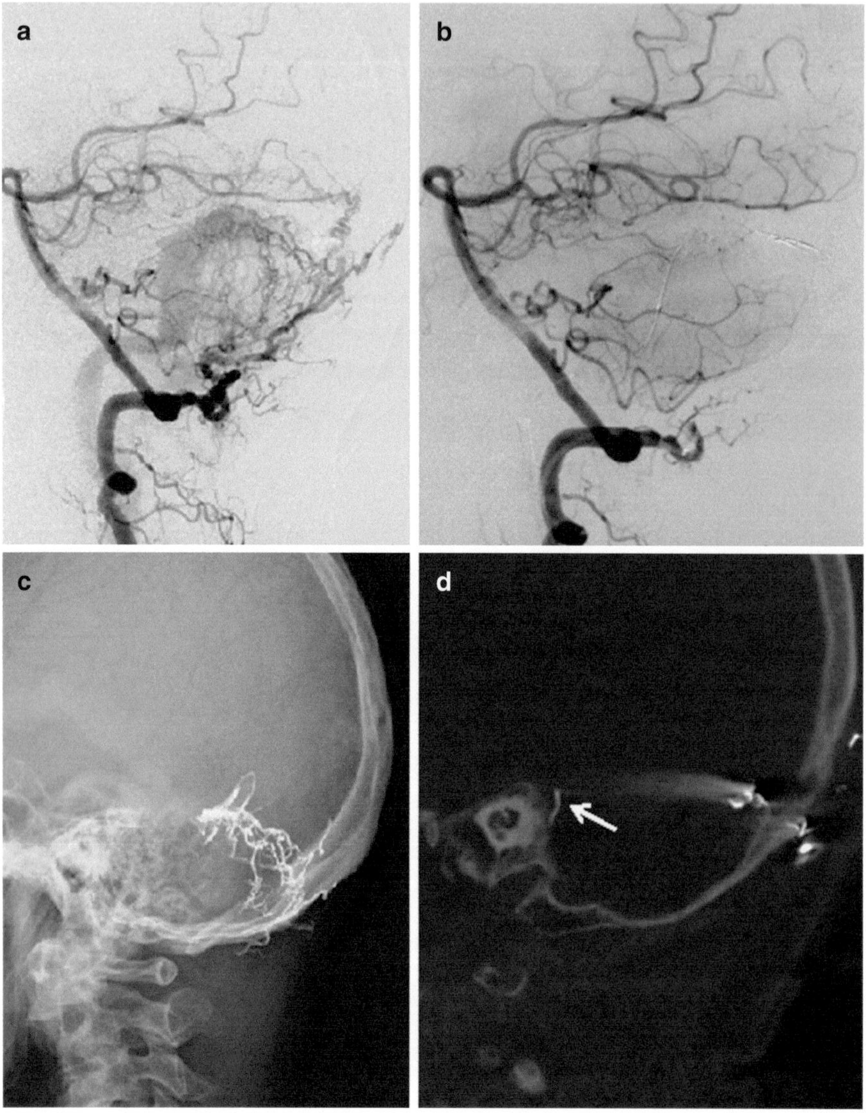

Fig. 14.2 A case with Borden type I DAVF involving the transverse-sigmoid sinus. The shunt was obliterated with Onyx injection from the distal occipital artery arising from the vertebral artery. A balloon catheter was inflated in the involved sinus to prevent Onyx migration to the sinus lumen. (**a**) Preoperative vertebral angiogram. (**b**) Postoperative vertebral angiogram indicating complete obliteration of the shunt. (**c**) Postoperative craniogram showing the Onyx cast. (**d**) Postoperative cone beam CT indicating Onyx migration to the tinny petrosal vein (*arrow*) from the superior petrosal sinus

Ischemia of the Vasa Nervorum

NBCA, Onyx, and small particulates (<200 μm) will cause cranial nerve palsy by migrating into the vasa nervorum. Many external carotid branches such as the middle meningeal, accessory meningeal, deep temporal arteries, and the artery of foramen rotundum give rise to branches which feed the cranial nerves around the middle fossa. The middle meningeal, ascending pharyngeal, occipital arteries, and posterior meningeal branch of the vertebral artery also feed the cranial nerves inside and outside of the posterior fossa. The inferolateral and meningohypophyseal trunks of the internal carotid artery feed many cranial nerves and have a rich collateral anastomosis between external carotid artery in the middle fossa.

14.1.4.2 Complications of TVE

Mass Effect to the Cranial Nerves

Excessive transvenous coil packing of the cavernous sinus causes III, IV, and V cranial nerve palsy and that of anterior condylar confluence causes XII nerve palsy. Sometimes, the delayed ocular palsy will occur and never recover [7]. This mechanism still remains unknown and one should remind.

Venous Infarction and Bleeding

Normal cerebral veins sometimes drain into the involved sinus in an antegrade fashion. Venous infarction will occur after the whole sinus packing by blocking the normal cerebral venous drainage (Fig. 14.3). Cortical venous drainage or retrograde

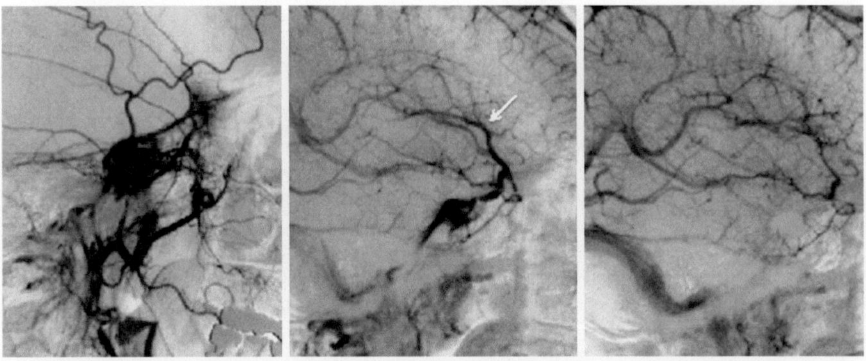

Fig. 14.3 A case with cavernous sinus DAVF treated with transvenous packing of the affected sinus. *Left*: Preoperative external carotid angiogram (*lateral view*) showing the shunt in the cavernous sinus. *Center*: Preoperative internal carotid angiogram (*lateral view*) showing the superficial middle cerebral veins are draining into the affected cavernous sinus in an antegrade fashion. *Right*: Venous phase of the postoperative common carotid angiogram (*lateral view*). Note one of the superficial middle cerebral veins (*arrow* in the *center figure*) was missing

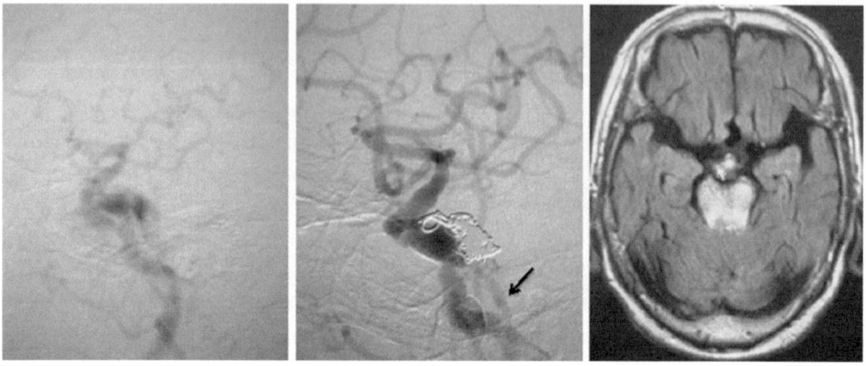

Fig. 14.4 A case with cavernous sinus DAVF treated by transvenous coil embolization. *Left*: Preoperative common carotid angiogram. *Center*: Postoperative common carotid angiogram showing incomplete obliteration of the affected cavernous sinus. Note the cavernous sinus was packed with coils but the inferior petrosal sinus was still opacified (*arrow*). *Right*: MRI (FLAIR) in the next day showing (venous) infarction of the entire brain stem, suggesting the postoperative change of the draining routes into the brain stem due to the incomplete transvenous occlusion of the cavernous sinus

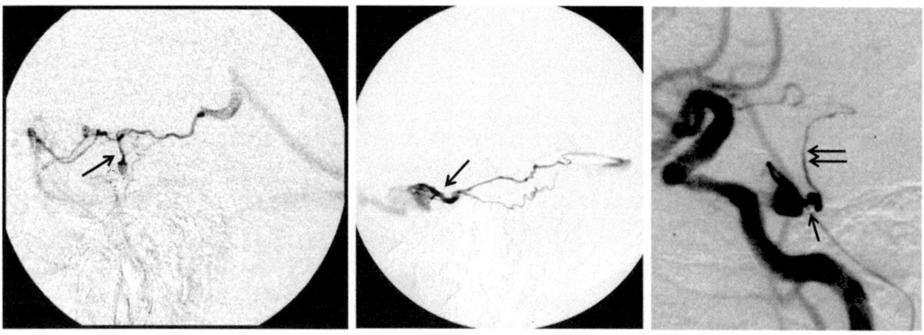

Fig. 14.5 Examples of the dangerous draining veins. *Left*: Cavernous sinus injection opaficied the uncal vein (*arrow*) connecting with deep cerebral veins (vein of Rosenthal and vein of Galen). *Center*: Cavernous sinus injection opaficied the petrosal vein (*arrow*). *Right*: Carotid angiogram showing the cavernous sinus DAVF draining only into the tinny vein of the brain stem (*double arrows*) via the bridging vein (*arrow*)

letpomeningeal venous drainage in sinus type is sometimes seen in Borden type II or III and Cognard type IIb. Transvenous sinus packing of these lesions have potent complication of venous bleeding from the residual cortical veins if the packing is incomplete (Fig. 14.4). One must obliterate, at first, the dangerous small draining veins like the uncal vein, petrosal vein, and bridging veins to the brain stem (Fig. 14.5).

14.2 Advances

Several topics at present will be shown with case presentation.

14.2.1 *Selective TVE*

Selective TVE is a recent trend. Advantage of this method is to spare the physiological cerebral venous return with a low cost, compared with the whole sinus packing. 3D-DSA can easily find the localized AV shunt (the shunting pouch or venous collector) in many cases with cavernous sinus DAVF (Fig. 14.6). Parallel sinus or small pouch is sometimes found in the case with transverse-sigmoid sinus DAVF (Fig. 14.7)

14.2.2 *Onyx Embolization*

Onyx has brought the paradigm shift in the treatment of DAVF of the transverse-sigmoid sinus, superior sagittal sinus, and confluence, especially in cases with Borden type I and II lesions. Curative treatment for these lesions was difficult before Onyx era because NBCA tended to result in a partial occlusion. Finally, sinus

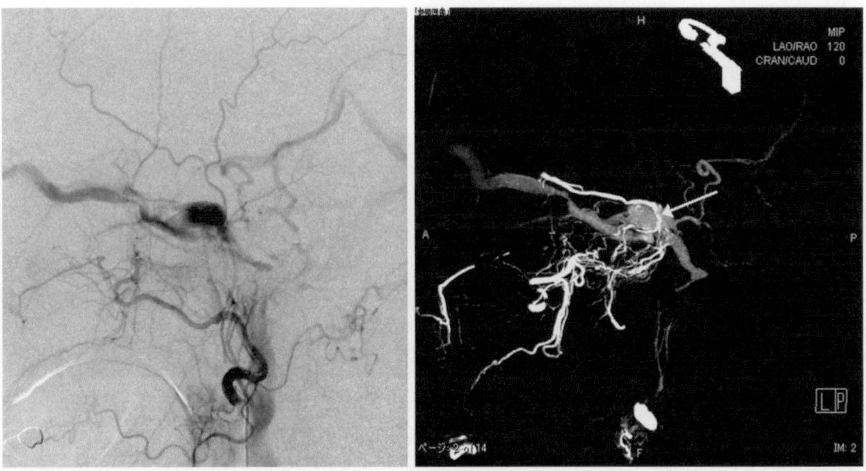

Fig. 14.6 A case with cavernous sinus DAVF. *Left*: external carotid angiogram showing the lesion fed by the dural branches of the external carotid artery, draining to the superior ophthalmic vein, inferior petrosal sinus, and the bridging vein connecting with the lateral mesencephalic vein. *Right*: a MIP image of 3D-DSA. Note the localized AV shunt point (venous collector) is clearly indicated (*arrow*)

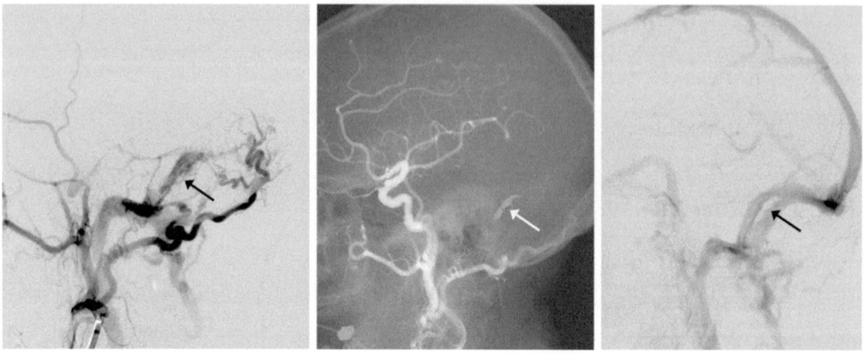

Fig. 14.7 A case of the sigmoid sinus DAVF with a shunting pouch in the parallel sinus. *Left*: lateral view of the external carotid angiogram showing the DAVF (*black arrow*) draining into the sigmoid sinus in an antegrade fashion. *Center*: arterial phase of the common carotid angiogram after selective transvenous embolization with coils (*white arrow*). *Right*: its venous phase. Note the patent sigmoid sinus after packing of the involved parallel sinus (*black arrow*)

packing was performed if necessary. Onyx has dramatically improved the obliteration rate of the shunts even in Borden type I lesion (Fig. 14.8). It also enables transarterial sinus packing instead of TVE (Fig. 14.9).

14.2.3 Spinal Dural and Epidural AV Shunts

Clinical entity of spinal "epidural" AVF has been newly proposed [8]. Recently, the concept of the angioarchitecture of the spinal dural and epidural AVF has changed and well been elucidated by the nation-wide survey in Japan [9]. The feeding arteries are usually the bilateral dorsal somatic arteries and the AV shunt is located in the dural lake on the ventral surface of the dura and drained into the radiculomedullary to the perimedullary veins and/or the paravertebral veins (Fig. 14.10). While, in the case with spinal "dural" AVF, the radiculomeningeal and/or prelaminar arteries connect with the bridging vein of the spinal dura and drained into the perimedullary vein. Previously it was said that the AV shunt located in the dural sleeve in the textbook. However, in the majority of cases with dural AVF, the AV shunt was located away from the dural sleeve in this report.

This nation-wide survey in Japan proved that dominant location of the spinal dural AVF was the thoracic level, while that of the spinal epidural AVF was lumbosacral level. Because the angioarchitecture of the feeding vessels of the epidural AVF is simpler, in general, than that of dural AVF, catheterization is usually easier in the epidural AVF. Successful rate of the surgery, tansarterial NBCA injection, or combination of these treatments was high. Effectiveness of Onyx for the spinal lesion remains unknown. When the endovascular treatment is failed or incomplete, surgical treatment should be followed.

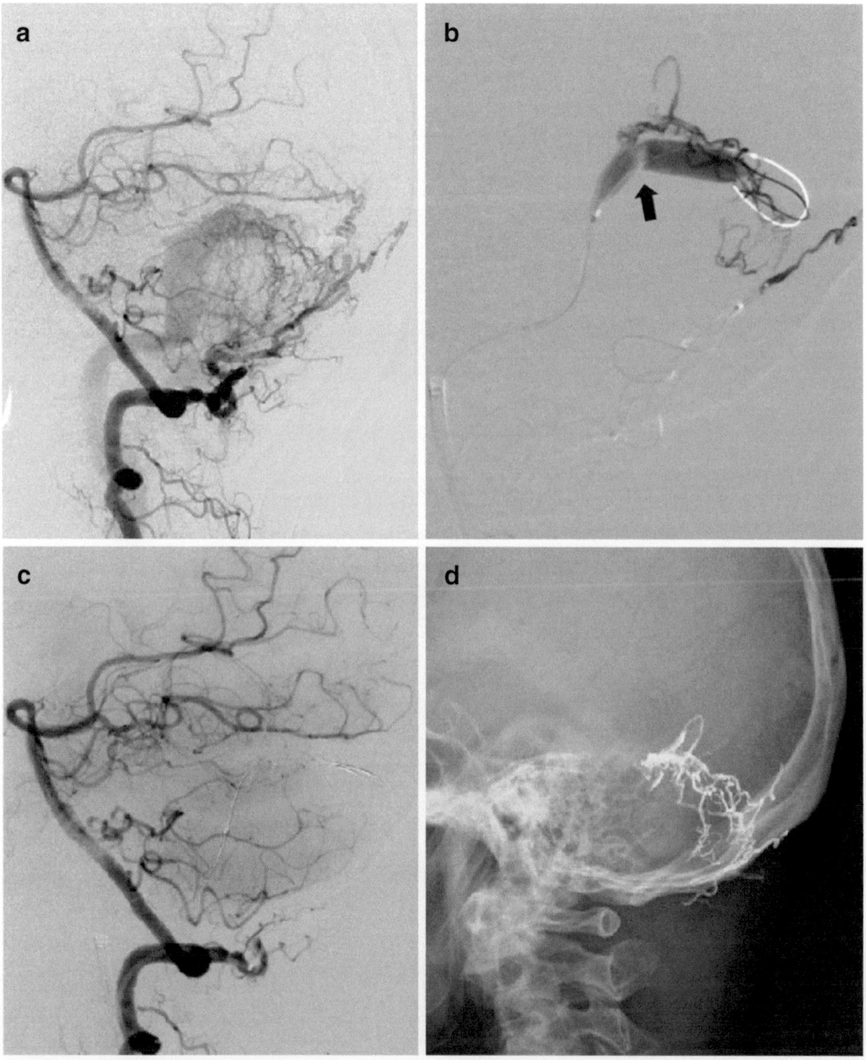

Fig. 14.8 The same case with Fig. 14.2 (Borden type I DAVF involving the transverse-sigmoid sinus). The shunt was obliterated with Onyx injection from the distal occipital artery. (**a**) Preoperative vertebral angiogram showing the transverse-sigmoid sinus DAVF fed by the occipital artery arising from the vertebral artery. (**b**) A sinus balloon (*arrow*) is inflated in the involved sinus during the Onyx injection from the occipital artery to avoid Onyx migration to the sinus lumen. (**c**) Postoperative vertebral angiogram. Note the DAVF was completely obliterated. (**d**) Postoperative craniogram showing the Onyx cast

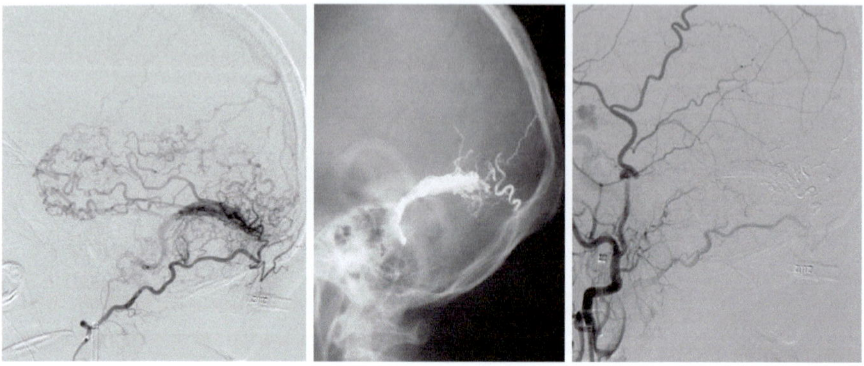

Fig. 14.9 A case of the transverse-sigmoid sinus DAVF with the so-called isolated sinus. *Left*: The occipital angiogram showing the DAVF (Borden type III, Cognard type IIa + b) with the vigorous cortical venous reflux. *Center*: Postoperative craniogram showing the Onyx cast which packed the entire sinus. *Right*: The left external carotid angiogram after the Onyx TAE showing the complete obliteration of the DAVF

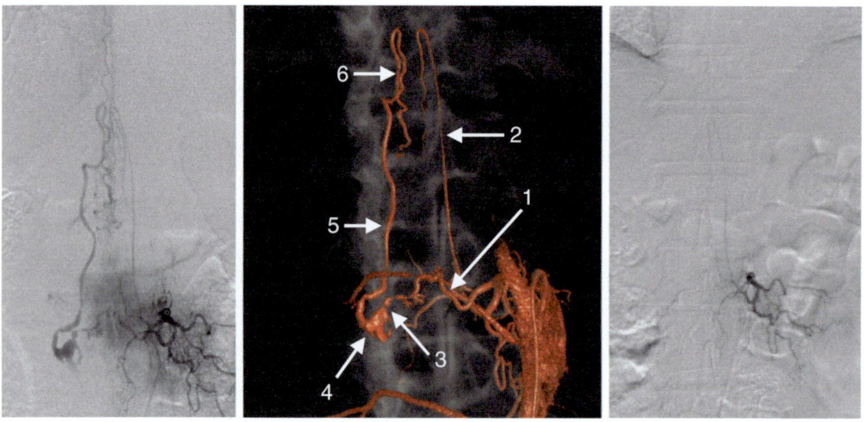

Fig. 14.10 A case with spinal epidural AVF. *Left*: No. 2 lumbar angiogram showing the epidural AVF fed by the dorsal somatic artery and draining into the venous lake on the dural surface. *Center*: 3D-DSA. (*1*) Dorsal somatic artery, (*2*) posterior spinal artery, (*3*) shunting point, (*4*) epidural venous lake (pouch), (*5*) radiculomedullary vein, (*6*) perimedullary vein. *Right*: postoperative angiogram. Note the shunt was completely obliterated with NBCA injection

14.3 Controversies

14.3.1 Timing of Treatment

Urgent treatment is mandatory in cases with the hemorrhagic onset, because re-bleeding rate is high [10]. Cortical venous reflux in cases with hemorrhagic onset is a potential risk of re-bleeding and is a strong reason of treatment. However, the bleeding risk of asymptomatic cases with cortical venous reflux is not high [11] and the necessity of the urgent treatment is controversial.

Treatment should not be delayed in cases with progressive (neurologic) symptoms such as diplopia and ocular hypertension in the cavernous sinus DAVF and congestive myelopathy in the spinal dural and epidural AVF.

Other symptoms such as headache, pulsatile tinnitus should be followed up conservatively because those symptoms do not harm the patients. In rare cases, intractable tinnitus in Borden type I fistulas may need to treat in order to improve the patients' mental status and activities of daily life.

14.3.2 Shunt Location and Treatment Modality

In the cavernous sinus DAVF, the priority of treatment is TVE. Recent trend is a selective TVE (targeted embolization). Multiplanar reconstruction (MPR) images of 3D-DSA help to find out the localization of the AV shunts (venous collector) and enable the selective TVE.

In the DAVF of transverse-sigmoid, superior sagittal sinuses and confluence, variety of treatment will be indicated according to its hemodynamic status. Recent topic is Onyx embolization for the Borden type I and II lesions. The sinus packing for the Borden type III lesions can be done both by TVE and transarterial Onyx injection.

Surgical treatment will be the first choice in the lesions of anterior cranial base and craniocervical junction. Also surgery with or without the endovascular treatment plays an important role in the treatment of tentorial DAVF and spinal dural and epidural AVF.

14.3.3 Surgical Treatment

Surgical treatment will be safer and the first choice in the region of anterior cranial fossa. Endovascular treatment (Onyx TAE) could be feasible but less safe. Craniotomy and clipping of the draining vein is a simple treatment. However, one must pay attention to the olfactory veins as draining routes running on the frontal base, not in the interhemispheric space.

Atypical angioarchitecture is a characteristic feature in the lesion of craniocervical junction. Feeding arteries include dural and pial branches and it is very difficult to differentiate these arteries. Even the anterior spinal artery often joins the fistula. Detection of the precise location of AV shunt (epidural, dural, or perimedullary) would be difficult by means of any diagnostic modality. Surgical exploration of the complex angioarchitecture is very effective and safe.

References

1. Al-Shahi R, Bhattacharya JJ, Currie DG, et al. Prospective populations-based detection of intracranial vascular malformations in adults: the Scottish Intracranial Vascular Malformation Study (SIVMS). Stroke. 2003;34:1163–9.
2. Kuwayama N. Epidemiologic survey of dural arteriovenous fistulas in Japan: clinical frequency and present status of treatment. Acta Neurochir Suppl. 2016;123:185–8. https://doi.org/10.1007/978-3-319-29887-0_26.
3. Murai S, Hiramatsu M, Suzuki E, et al. Trends in incidence of intracranial and spinal arteriovenous shunts: hospital-based surveillance in Okayama, Japan. Stroke. 2021;52(4):1455–9.
4. Borden JA, Wu JK, Shucart WA. A proposed classification for spinal and cranial dural arteriovenous fistulous malformations and implications for treatment. J Neurosurg. 1995;82:166–79.
5. Cognard C, Gobin YP, Pierot L, Bailly AL, Houdart E, Casasco A, Chiras J, Merland JJ. Cerebral dural arteriovenous fistulas: clinical and angiographic correlation with a revised classification of venous drainage. Radiology. 1995;194:671–80.
6. Gross BA, Albuquerque FC, Moon K, et al. Evolution of treatment and a detailed analysis of occlusion, recurrence, and clinical outcomes in an endovascular library of 260 dural arteriovenous fistulas. J Neurosurg. 2017;126:1884–93.
7. Kashiwazaki D, Kuwayama N, Akioka N, et al. Delayed abducens nerve palsy after transvenous coil embolization for cavernous sinus dural arteriovenous fistulae. Acta Neurochir. 2014;156:97–101.
8. Clarke MJ, Patrick TA, White JB, et al. Spinal arteriovenous malformations with parenchymal drainage: venous drainage variability and implications in clinical manifestations. Neurosurg Focus. 2009;26:E5. https://doi.org/10.3171/FOC.2009.26.1.E5.
9. Kiyosue H, Matsumaru Y, Niimi Y, et al. Angiographic and clinical characteristics of thoracolumbar spinal epidural and dural arteriovenous fistulas. Stroke. 2017;48:3215–22.
10. Söderman M, Pavic L, Ender G, et al. Natural history of dural arteriovenous shunts. Stroke. 2008;39:1735–9.
11. Storm RG, Botros JA, Refai D, et al. Cranial dural arteriovenous fistulae: asymptomatic cortical venous drainage portends less aggressive clinical course. Neurosurgery. 2009;64:241–8.

Chapter 15
Keyhole Approach in Cerebral Aneurysm Surgeries

Kentaro Mori and Sadayoshi Watanabe

15.1 Introduction

Routine treatment of intracranial cerebral aneurysms has increasingly adopted endovascular coiling rather than surgical clipping, but surgical clipping is still indicated to treat subsets of aneurysms with location and morphology unsuitable for endovascular treatment. Conventional fronto-temporal craniotomy and bifrontal craniotomy are considered the gold standards to approach cerebral aneurysms in the anterior circulation. Modern technological advances based on computer graphics techniques for preoperative simulation, endoscopy, exoscopy, and navigation with head-up display enable safe performance of less invasive open surgery, such as keyhole clipping [1]. This chapter describes surgical techniques, tips, and surgical indications for supraorbital keyhole clipping, and further discusses the pros and cons of keyhole surgery. Personally speaking, selection between the standard craniotomy and keyhole craniotomy should not be controversial but definite surgical indications for the keyhole approach for safe clipping should be established.

15.2 Pros and Cons of Keyhole Clipping Compared with Standard Craniotomy

We must appreciate the pros and cons of keyhole clipping surgery. The pros are minimum soft tissue damage and minimum hospital stay. Figure 15.1 shows the difference between standard craniotomy (right) and supraorbital keyhole craniotomy (left) in the

K. Mori (✉) · S. Watanabe
Department of Neurosurgery, Tokyo General Hospital, Nakano, Tokyo, Japan
e-mail: kentaro.mori@mt.strins.or.jp; s0530w@ybb.ne.jp

Y. Kato, A. Ansari (eds.), *Cerebrovascular Surgery*, Advances and Technical Standards in Neurosurgery 44, https://doi.org/10.1007/978-3-030-87649-4_15

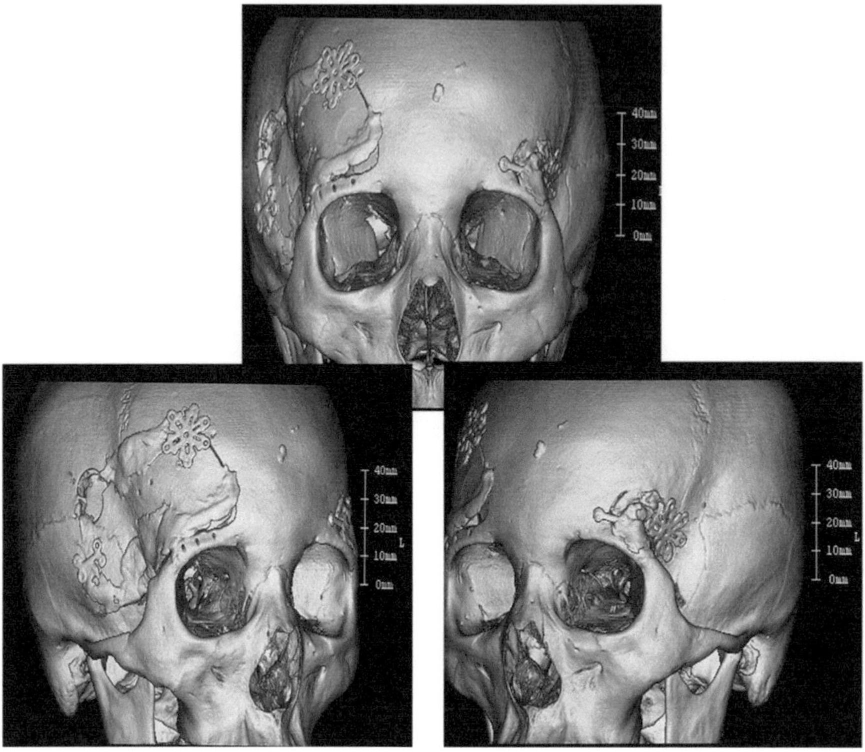

Fig. 15.1 Comparison of the sizes of standard fronto-temporal craniotomy (*right*) and supraorbital keyhole craniotomy (*left*) in the same patient

same patient. This illustrates the small size of supraorbital keyhole craniotomy with minimum soft tissue damage of keyhole approach compared with standard craniotomy. The cons are the narrow working angle that restricts multi-angled observation and manipulation of deeply located pathology. The pitfall of the keyhole approach is that the superficial middle cerebral artery cannot be harvested for precautionary bypass to the intracranial artery. Standard craniotomy is still the gold standard for clipping surgery because of the surgical flexibility such as potential for bypass, anterior clinoidectomy, and sinus reconstruction for complex cerebral aneurysms.

15.3 Surgical Indications of Clipping via the Supraorbital Keyhole Approach

Supraorbital keyhole clipping has been applied to middle cerebral artery and basilar artery aneurysms, but we recommend this technique for the subgroup of internal carotid artery (ICA) and anterior communicating artery (AcomA) aneurysms [2, 3].

Many neurosurgeons apply this keyhole approach to treat ruptured aneurysms, but I do not recommend this technique because brain swelling and dark bloody operative field caused by subarachnoid hemorrhage hinder safe clipping surgery. Consequently, we must know the pros and cons of keyhole clipping. I consider that only small ICAs of less than 10 mm in diameter and simple aneurysms are candidates for keyhole clipping for safety reasons. Anteriorly or inferiorly projecting AcomA aneurysm with height from the skull base of up to 13 mm is a good indication. Laterally projecting ICA aneurysm without badly attached anterior choroidal artery is also a good indication. The supraorbital keyhole approach cannot provide periosteal flap for closing the opened frontal sinus. If the frontal sinus is very large, the supraorbital keyhole approach is not recommended.

15.4 Preoperative Imaging and Surgical Simulation

The main targets of keyhole clipping are relatively small and simple cerebral aneurysms, so three-dimensional (3D) computed tomography angiography (CTA) is necessary but sufficient and catheter angiography is not required. However, keyhole mini-craniotomy is the minimum bone window to access a deeply situated aneurysm, so we should perform preoperative simulation with 3D CTA data to determine the optimal location and size of the keyhole. The 3D images of the aneurysm, cerebral arteries, and skull are merged into a single 3D image using computer workstation (Ziostation 2.4, Ziosoft, Inc.) (Fig. 15.5, *left*). The supraorbital keyhole should be located laterally to the supraorbital notch. Basically, keyhole clipping is a straight axis operation, so we should also determine the best head rotation angle from this simulation. In most cases, the width of the keyhole is 25–30 mm and the height is 22 mm (more than 20 mm). If the height is less than 20 mm, adequate light from the operating microscope cannot be introduced into the deep intracranial site.

15.5 Keyhole or Standard Craniotomy?

Several representative cases illustrate whether keyhole or standard craniotomy should be chosen.

15.5.1 ICA Aneurysm

The upper panels of Fig. 15.2 show the aneurysm is small and laterally projecting and the anterior choroidal artery is separated from the dome. The preoperative simulation image indicates the supraorbital keyhole approach is possible. The lower

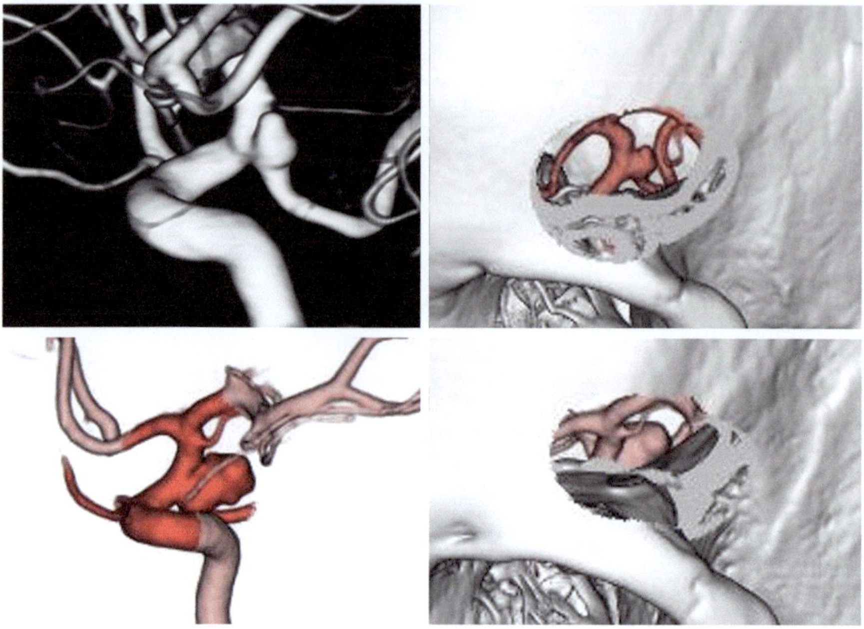

Fig. 15.2 Two cases of internal carotid-posterior communicating artery aneurysm. *Upper panels*: Small laterally projecting aneurysm and anterior choroidal artery separated from the dome. Preoperative simulation image indicates the supraorbital keyhole approach is possible. *Lower panels*: Low-laying aneurysm, which indicates the necessity of tentorial incision. The proximal neck is hidden by the anterior clinoid process, which indicates the necessity of anterior clinoidectomy. Standard fronto-temporal craniotomy was chosen

panels of Fig. 15.2 show the proximal neck of the aneurysm is hidden by the anterior clinoid process and the aneurysm is low-lying. Anterior clinoidectomy and resection of the tentorium were anticipated, so the standard fronto-temporal craniotomy was chosen.

15.5.2 Internal Carotid-Paraclinoid Aneurysm

The upper panels of Fig. 15.3 show the dome projecting upward with the space between the anterior clinoid process and the proximal neck. Anterior clinoidectomy seemed unnecessary for this aneurysm. Therefore, keyhole clipping was chosen. The lower panels of Fig. 15.3 show the aneurysm dome was embedded into the anterior clinoid process. Anterior clinoidectomy was considered to be definitely required, so standard fronto-temporal craniotomy (extradural approach) was chosen.

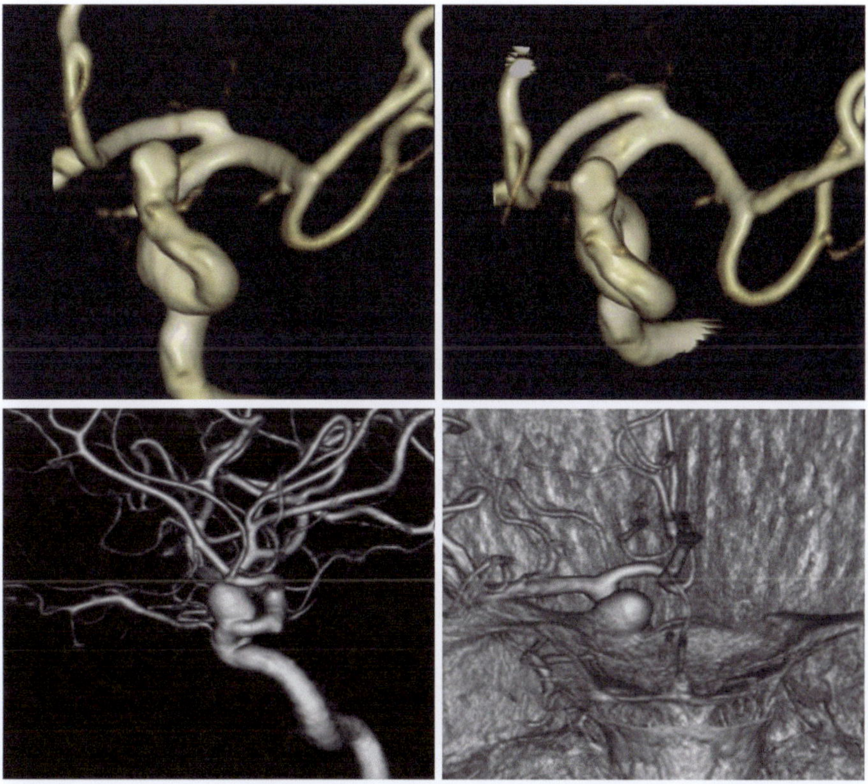

Fig. 15.3 Two cases of internal carotid-paraclinoid aneurysms. Upper panels: Dome seems separate from the anterior clinoid process. Supraorbital keyhole was chosen. Lower panels: Aneurysm dome is embedded into the anterior clinoid process. Anterior clinoidectomy was required, so standard fronto-temporal craniotomy was chosen

15.5.3 AcomA Aneurysm

The upper panel of Fig. 15.4 shows the dome projecting anteriorly without involving the A2. Supraorbital keyhole clipping was chosen. The lower panel of Fig. 15.4 shows the dome pointed upward and the bilateral A2 attached to the dome, so standard craniotomy (bifrontal) was chosen.

15.6 Surgical Technique of Supraorbital Keyhole Clipping

After induction of general anesthesia, the patient is positioned supine with the head away from the operative side at the angle determined by the preoperative simulation. The head is fixed with a Mayfield tri-pin holder. The motor evoked potential

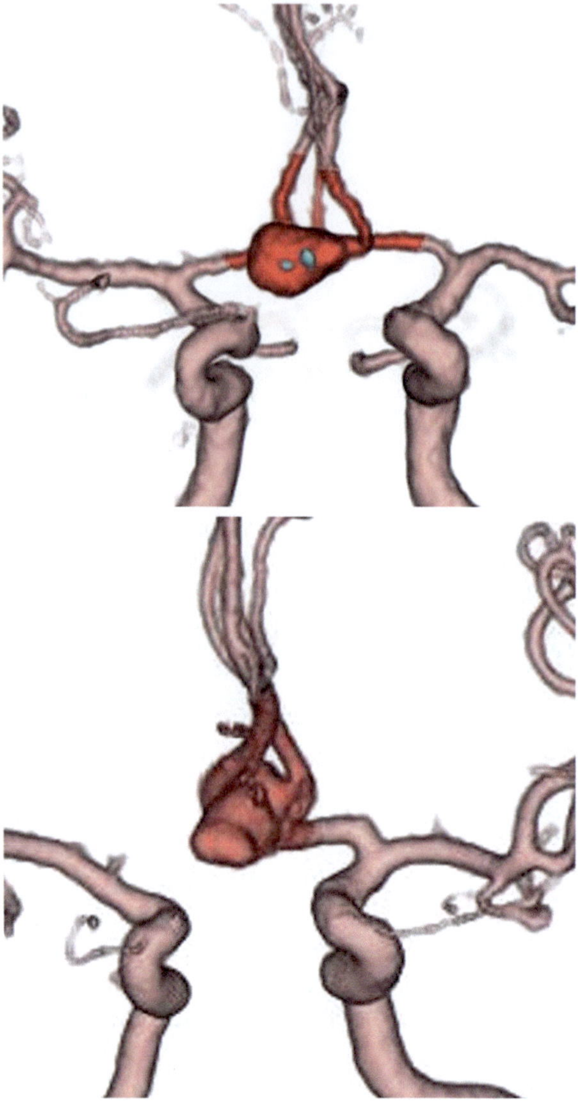

Fig. 15.4 Two cases of anterior communicating artery aneurysms. *Upper*: Aneurysm dome projects anteriorly without involving the A2, so supraorbital keyhole clipping was chosen. *Lower*: Aneurysm dome partially projecting upward and involving the bilateral A2, so standard craniotomy (bifrontal) was chosen

electrodes are set in the scalp. A slight chin-up position facilitates gravity retraction of the frontal lobe. The landmark structures such as the orbital limb, supraorbital notch, frontal sinus, and orbitozygomatic suture are marked on the face. The scheduled supraorbital keyhole is also marked on the face and then the skin incision just above the eyebrow is determined (Fig. 15.5, *right*). Surgical drapes should be tightly fixed with the Mayfield holder to retract the skin inferiorly using hooks. The operating microscope should be introduced from the step of skin incision. The eyebrow skin incision generally starts from just lateral to the supraorbital foramen and then about 40 mm laterally toward the end of the eyebrow. If the wrinkle just above

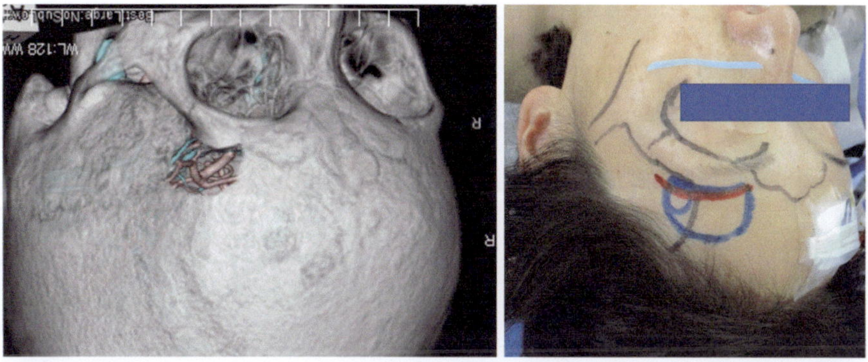

Fig. 15.5 Preoperative 3D CT multi-fusion image of left internal carotid artery aneurysm for preoperative simulation of supraorbital keyhole clipping (*left*) and the landmark structures, scheduled keyhole mini-craniotomy, and eyebrow skin incision (*right*)

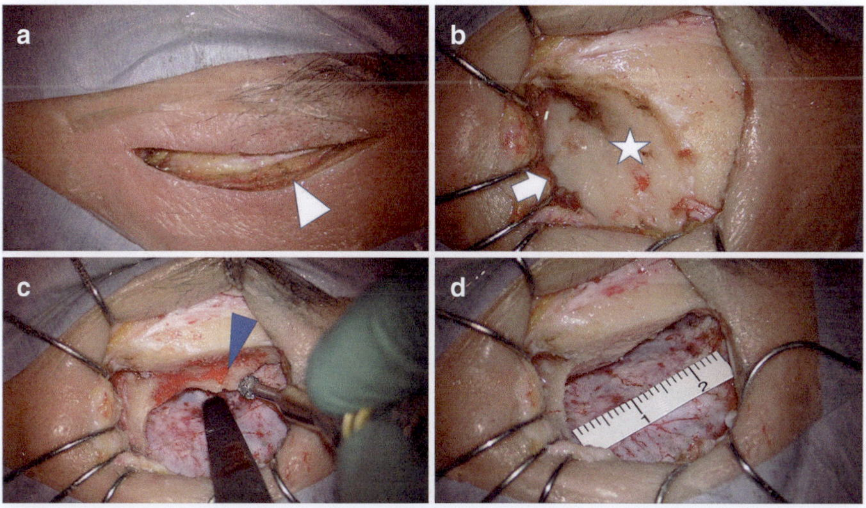

Fig. 15.6 Intraoperative photographs of clipping of left internal carotid-paraclinoid aneurysm via the supraorbital keyhole approach. (**a**) Eyebrow skin incision.(**b**) Subperiosteal exposure of the frontal bone, arrow showing the retracted temporal muscle, star showing the McCarty point. (**c**): Drilling the bony ridge over the orbital roof (*arrowhead*). (**d**) Supraorbital mini-craniotomy

the eyebrow is prominent, the skin incision follows the wrinkle (Figs. 15.6a and 15.8a). Skin incision along the wrinkle over the eyebrow is acceptable but should not pass too high from the eyebrow, otherwise the patient will suffer from postoperative frontal muscle weakness. After the skin incision, the frontalis muscle is incised using the monopolar coagulator (Fig. 15.6a). The skin and frontalis muscle are retracted together both superiorly and inferiorly. The subperiosteal dissection is made to expose the frontal bone and the anterior end of the temporal muscle fascia over the McCarthy point. The temporal muscle and its fascia are partially dissected

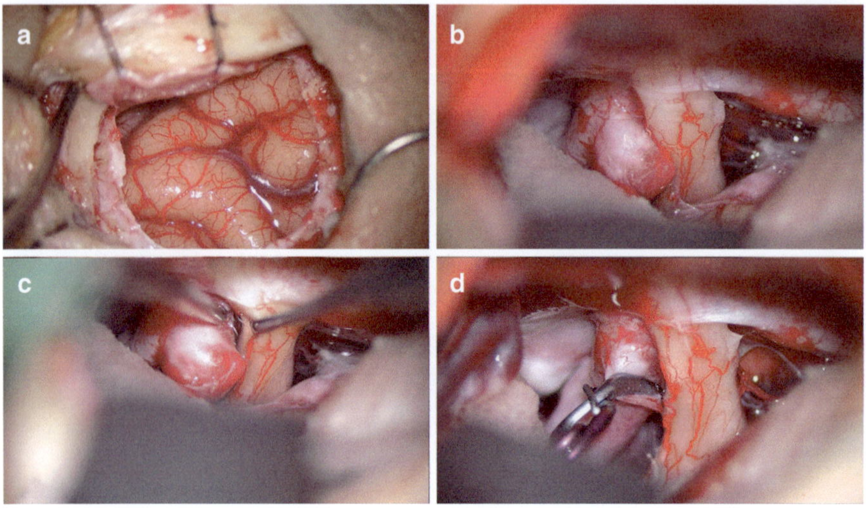

Fig. 15.7 Intraoperative photographs of clipping of left internal carotid-paraclinoid aneurysm via the supraorbital keyhole approach (continued). (**a**) After dural opening. (**b**) Left internal carotid-paraclinoid aneurysm attached to the left optic nerve. (**c**) Dissecting the paraclinoid aneurysm from the optic nerve (**d**) After aneurysm clipping

from the superior temporal line, and dissected and retracted inferiorly to expose the McCarty point (Figs. 15.6b and 15.8b). Burr hole is made at the McCarty point and then the supraorbital mini-craniotomy is performed. The dura mater is dissected from the frontal base and any bony ridge over the orbital roof (Juga) should be drilled away to flatten the frontal base (Figs. 15.6c, d and 15.8c, d). The dura mater is incised in curvilinear fashion (Fig. 15.7a). The frontal lobe is slightly retracted and the arachnoid membrane near the medial sylvian fissure is opened, then cerebrospinal fluid is aspirated until the brain become slightly slack. Then, the tip of the brain spatula is advanced little by little toward the carotid cistern. The carotid cistern is widely opened and cerebrospinal fluid is aspirated until the brain becomes slack enough to retract the brain more (Fig. 15.9a). Then, the medial sylvian fissure should be widely opened and the optic nerve dissected from the rectal gyrus (Fig. 15.9b). After this step, clipping procedures can be performed similarly to the pterional approach via standard craniotomy. I use Sugita titanium clip applier (Mizuho Corp.) because this device is thin enough for keyhole clipping. After the clipping, motor evoked potential, indocyanine green video-angiography, and Doppler sonography can be performed for safety as in the standard operation. After dural closure, I prefer to use a titanium pterion plate to cover the bone defect (Fig. 15.10a). The wound should be meticulously sutured in multi-layer fashion (Fig. 15.10b). After removal of the skin stitches, the wound is taped for 1 month for better cosmetic result.

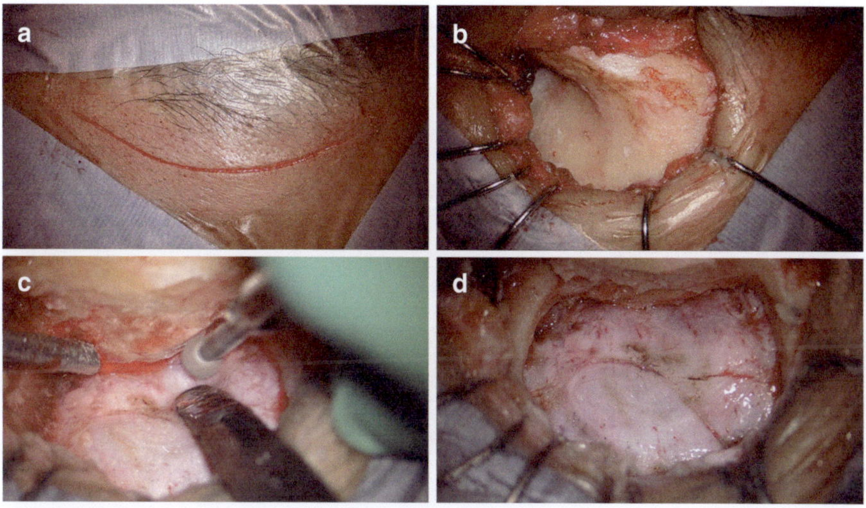

Fig. 15.8 Intraoperative photographs of clipping of anterior communicating artery aneurysm via the supraorbital keyhole approach. (**a**) Eyebrow skin incision. (**b**) Exposed left frontal bone. (**c**) Drilling the bony ridge over the orbital roof. (**d**) Supraorbital mini-craniotomy

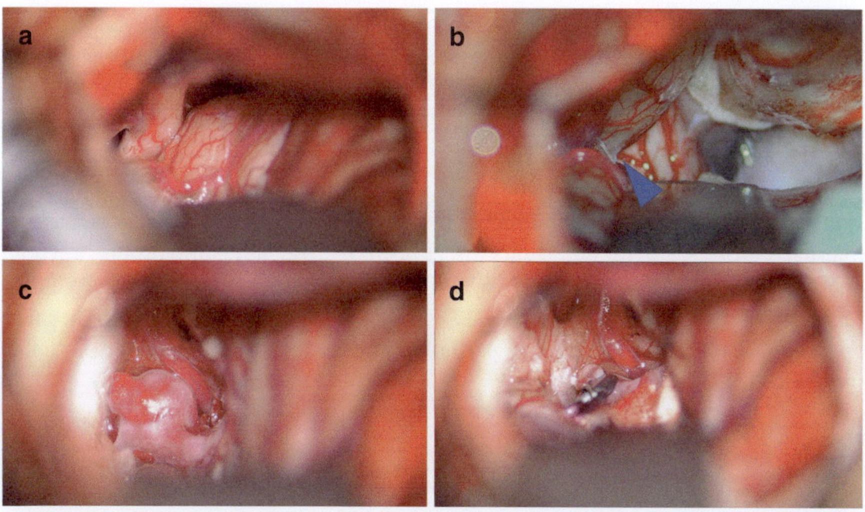

Fig. 15.9 Intraoperative photographs of clipping of anterior communicating artery aneurysm via the supraorbital keyhole approach (continued). (**a**) Opening of the left carotid cistern until the brain became slack. (**b**) Opening of the left medial sylvian fissure (arrowhead). (**c**) Dissection of the anterior communicating artery aneurysm after partial resection of the rectal gyrus. (**d**) Clipping the aneurysm

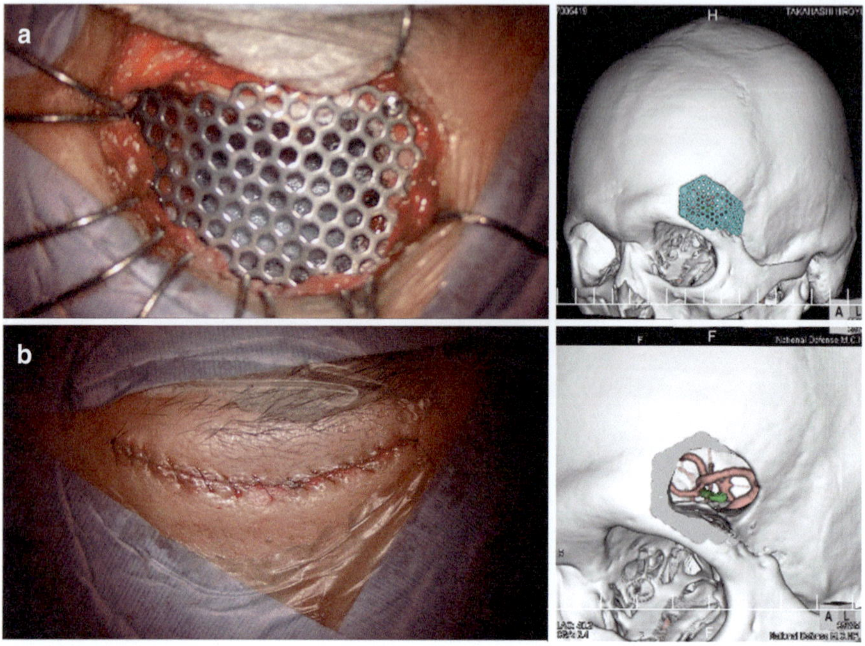

Fig. 15.10 Intraoperative photographs of clipping of anterior communicating artery aneurysm via the supraorbital keyhole approach and postoperative 3D images (continued). (**a**) Bony defect sealed by a titanium pterion plate. (**b**) After closure of the wound using 6–0 nylon

15.7 Representative Cases

Figures 15.6 and 15.7 show intraoperative photographs of a representative case of internal carotid-paraclinoid aneurysm clipped by the left supraorbital keyhole approach. Figures 15.8, 15.9, and 15.10 show intraoperative photographs of a representative case of AcomA aneurysm clipped by the left supraorbital keyhole approach. The rectal gyrus can be partially resected to expose the aneurysm complex (Fig. 15.9c).

15.8 Future Prospects

Pure endoscopic keyhole surgery and exoscopic surgery have been adopted more and more extensively in the field of neurosurgery. I mainly use the operating microscope and only use the endoscope to observe any small perforating artery and check the position of the clip blades and confirm complete clipping. One of the drawbacks of using the operating microscope during keyhole clipping is the relatively low illumination in the deep operative field. Choice of the modality for keyhole clipping may depend on the surgeon's experience and expertise.

15.9 Reminds

More details of the surgical indications, techniques, and surgical results of keyhole clipping have been published elsewhere [2, 3]. The supraorbital keyhole approach and keyhole concept were established by Alex Perneczky (1945–2009). He noted that the keyhole concept is not to reduce the size of craniotomy to a real keyhole but rather make the minimal craniotomy large enough to access deeply situated intracranial pathologies [4]. Keyhole clipping is not established as a safe surgical method. Consequently, less invasive keyhole clipping may suddenly be changed to maximum invasive surgery. Therefore, strict surgical indications and preoperative simulation are mandatory for safe keyhole surgery. If any disadvantages or complicated procedures are identified, standard craniotomy should be chosen for safe clipping. Keyhole surgery is performed for the benefit of the patient not for the neurosurgeon.

References

1. Toyooka T, Otani N, Wada K, Tomiyama A, Takeuchi S, Fujii K, et al. Head-up display may facilitate safe keyhole surgery for cerebral aneurysm clipping. J Neurosurg. 2018;129:883–9.
2. Mori K, Wada K, Otani N, Tomiyama A, Toyooka T, Tomura S, et al. Long-term neurological and radiological results of consecutive 63 unruptured anterior communicating artery aneurysms clipped via lateral supraorbital keyhole minicraniotomy. Oper Neurosurg (Hagerstown). 2018;14:95–103.
3. Toyooka T, Wada K, Otani N, Tomiyama A, Takeuchi S, Tomura S, et al. Potential risks and limited indications of the supraorbital keyhole approach for clipping internal carotid artery aneurysm. World Neurosurg X. 2019;2:100025.
4. Perneczky A, Muller-Forell W, van Lindert E, Fries G. Current strategies in keyhole and endoscope-assisted microneurosurgery. In: Perneczky A, editor. Keyhole concept in neurosurgery. Stuttgart: Thieme Medical; 1999. p. 37–51.

Chapter 16
Repeated Aneurysm Intervention

Vladimír Beneš, Anna Štekláčová, and Ondřej Bradáč

16.1 Introduction

The morbidity and mortality of subarachnoid hemorrhage from ruptured intracranial aneurysm remains high worldwide [1]. According to a meta-analysis of recent epidemiological studies, the morbidity ranges between 8 and 67% and mortality between 8 and 20% [2]. The most effective prevention of aneurysm rupture known today is its complete exclusion from cerebral circulation. The original procedure to accomplish this goal was ligating the artery at the site where aneurysm originated. Nevertheless, with the improvement of neurosurgical techniques over years, occlusion of the aneurysm neck with a microsurgical clip became the gold standard for treatment. Later on, endovascular coiling emerged as less invasive alternative to surgical treatment [3]. One year results of the largest randomized controlled trial comparing clipping and coiling found lower proportion of death and dependency for patients with small ruptured anterior circulation aneurysm in good initial clinical condition who were randomized to endovascular arm [4]. Despite multiple criticisms, the results of this study led to the increased use of endovascular treatment, which in some institutions even surpassed surgery. However, not clinical but radiological results remain the often cited and feared weakness of this newer, less invasive technique.

V. Beneš (✉) · A. Štekláčová · O. Bradáč
Department of Neurosurgery and Neurooncology, Institute of Clinical Neurodisciplines, Charles University and Military University Hospital, Prague, Czech Republic
e-mail: vladimir.benes@uvn.cz

Y. Kato, A. Ansari (eds.), *Cerebrovascular Surgery*, Advances and Technical Standards in Neurosurgery 44, https://doi.org/10.1007/978-3-030-87649-4_16

16.2 Occlusion Rate After Surgical and Endovascular Treatment

Surgical clipping has been traditionally believed to provide definitive and long-term exclusion of aneurysm from intracranial circulation. Nevertheless, some authors argue that consistent data on technical efficacy of this treatment have been lacking over published series [5]. Moreover, the mode of postoperative radiological controls and their timing may not always seem to be stated clearly. Depending on definition and the use of postoperative angiography, the incidence of residual neck after surgery ranges between 3.8 and 18% [6–13]. In the meta-analysis published by Raaymakers et al. [14], 10 of 61 studies reported routinely performed postoperative angiography to verify the occlusion, and the results were stated in five of them. The total number of examined patients was 158, with complete obliteration rate presented to be 93%. Kotowski et al. [15] similarly found that information on occlusion rates was not stated in all examined studies. Still, based on 1969 postoperative examinations available, 91.8% aneurysms were completely occluded, 3.9% had neck remnants, and 4.3% were incompletely occluded. Single center results by Kivisaari et al. [13] presented experience with postoperative angiography in 955 aneurysms treated consecutively by surgery over 3.5-year period. Complete aneurysm occlusion was achieved in 88%, a neck remnant was discovered in 9%, and a fundus remnant was revealed in 3%. The proportion of complete occlusion was higher in unruptured group. In single series by Drake et al. of 1767 vertebrobasilar aneurysms [16], total obliteration was achieved in only 82.5% aneurysms, which probably mirrors the time of the study and technical challenge of surgery in posterior circulation.

Even though, in contrast to surgery, the data on initial occlusion rate after endovascular treatment could be easily accessed at the end of each procedure, this information is not routinely stated in published series either. Moreover, the available data according to some authors indicate, that this younger method would be technically inferior. Indeed, the systematic review published by Naggara et al. [17] revealed that DSA results at the end of the procedure were published in 38 out of 71 studies (3089 UAs), with a complete occlusion or a neck remnant in 2660 (86.1%). Another systematic review published by Ferns et al. [18] evaluated the results of 46 studies (8161 ANs). Complete initial occlusion was reported in 62.3%, near complete occlusion in 29.5% and incomplete occlusion in 8.2%. Prospective multicenter study ATENA of Pierot et al. [19] was designed to evaluate the technical success in endovascular treatment of unruptured aneurysms which were ≤15 mm in size. The study included 649 patients with 1100 aneurysms treated with simple coiling, stent or balloon assistance. Complete aneurysm occlusion was achieved in 59%, a neck remnant was discovered in 21.7%, and residual sac filling in 19.3%. Another study showed that the risk of incomplete occlusion after endovascular intervention is mostly dependent on neck width, size, and shape of aneurysm sac [20].

Complete occlusion rate in ISAT study was achieved in 81% of aneurysms randomized to surgical and 58% randomized to endovascular treatment [21].

16.3 AN Regrowth

Data obtained from several follow-up imaging studies consistently suggest that aneurysm regrowth is more commonly observed in patients who undergo endovascular treatment, as opposed to surgical clipping where this is considered as rather exception.

Meta-analysis published by Spiessberger et al. [22] included 92 articles with 13,723 patients after aneurysm clipping. Pooled annualized incidence rates were 0.13% for recurrence and 0.35% for de novo aneurysm formation. Mean time to recurrence was 12.9 years and mean time to de novo formation was 9.3 years. Recurrent aneurysms were most often seen at the ICA/PCoA, AcoA, and MCA. Three of the analyzed studies reported on remnant growth patterns. David et al. [23] found no growth in 75% of dog-ear remnants and regrowth in 75% of broad-based remnants at a mean follow-up of 4.4 years in 102 patients. Edner and Almquist [24] found a 1% annual enlargement risk for base remnants in 790 patients. Jabbarli et al. [25] found patient age to be a risk factor for remnant growth in a series of 616 patients (the overall proportion of AN remnant regrowth was 6.25%). Tsutsumi et al. presented their long term (mean 9.3 years) follow-up angiography results in 140 patients after clipping [26]. Their data showed that the risk of aneurysm recurrence after complete occlusion was 0.13% per year which was lower than the risk of de novo aneurysm formation (0.89% per year).

As already mentioned, findings presented for endovascular group may be perceived less satisfactory. A systematic review published by Ferns et al. [18] included 46 studies with 8161 coiled aneurysms: reopening occurred in 21.8% at a mean follow-up ranging from 4.7 to 38 months. Another systematic review, presented by Naggara et al. included 22 studies with 1737 unruptured intracranial aneurysms treated by endovascular intervention [17]. The mean follow-up time in studies ranged from 0.4 to 3.2 years and the overall recanalization rate was 24.4%. Interestingly, in the three studies (324 patients) with independent evaluation of DSA results, the overall recanalization rate was significantly higher (34.6%) than it was in remaining 19 studies where the results were self-assessed ($p < 0.001$) [17].

Risk factors for aneurysm recurrence reported in more than one study included larger lumen size (>10 mm), larger aneurysm neck size, and incomplete initial occlusion [18, 27–32]. In order to quantitatively predict the risk of retreatment following endovascular therapy, Ogilvy et al. presented their "Aneurysm Recanalization Stratification Scale" [30]. According to this model, the chance of aneurysm recurrence is stratified based upon aneurysm size (>10 mm vs. ≤10 mm), presence of subarachnoid hemorrhage, presence of intraluminal thrombus, modality of treatment (coils only, stent assistance, or flow diversion), and initial degree of obliteration. Based on these factors, the predicted rate of recurrence can range from 4.9 to 100% [30, 33]. Interestingly, some results suggest that reopening after coiling occurs predominantly within the first year after treatment [15, 29, 34–39] and the long-term risk of reopening would be low in patients with complete or near complete occlusion at 6 month follow-up angiogram [39, 40].

16.4 Rebleeding

As previously stated, the main goal of aneurysm treatment is to prevent its bleeding by aneurysm exclusion from cerebral circulation. Some valuable information regarding protective effect of both treatment methods can be extracted from two studies, namely ISAT (International Subarachnoid Aneurysm Trial) [4, 21, 41, 42] and CARAT (Cerebral Aneurysm Rerupture After Treatment) [27].

The analysis of long-term outcome (mean follow-up 9 years) of 2004 patients randomized in ISAT study was published in 2009 [42]. Data showed that recurrent hemorrhage in the first year after treatment was present in 24 patients, out of which 13 were from previously treated aneurysm (10 by endovascular, 3 by surgery). Besides that the most recent data were published in 2015 [41]. Follow-up was still available in 1003 patients (46.8% of previously randomized) who were observed between 10 and 18.5 years. Recurrent hemorrhage at this point of study was present in 33 cases, out of which 17 were from rupture of previously treated aneurysm (13 by endovascular, 4 by surgery). The cumulative risk of rerupture from previously treated aneurysm in patient after subarachnoid hemorrhage at the end of observation was calculated to be 0.0216 after endovascular intervention and 0.0064 after surgery.

Analysing long term results of CARAT study, authors concluded that the degree of initial occlusion is a strong predictor of repeated rupture [27]. The study included 1010 patients (711 treated by surgery, 299 by endovascular intervention). Cumulative risk of repeated hemorrhage was 1.1% in completely occluded aneurysms, as compared to 2.9% in residual neck filling (91–99% occlusion), 5.9% in aneurysms with larger residual filling (70–90% occlusion), and even 17.9% in case of incomplete occlusion. This trend towards higher risk of bleeding in dependence to lower occlusion rate was similarly observed in endovascular as well as surgical group. Altogether 19 reruptures occurred in 4 years of follow-up. Risk of rebleeding was 3.4% after endovascular intervention and 1.3% after surgery.

Single institution results of 752 patients after clipping for ruptured intracranial aneurysm with 6016 follow-up years were published by Wermer et al. [43]. Authors found that the incidence of recurrence within first 10 years after SAH was 3.2%. Another report on risk of repeated subarachnoid hemorrhage after complete obliteration of cerebral aneurysms was published by Tsutsumi et al. [26], who noted a cumulative risk of SAH from de novo and recurrent aneurysms of 2.2% in 10 years and 9.0% in 20 years. The important fact to mention is that patients in these studies were not routinely screened for recurrent aneurysm between treatment and termination of follow-up. A study of recurrent intracranial aneurysms (ruptured and unruptured) after successful neck clipping by el-Beltragy et al. [44] reported lower incidence of hemorrhage, with only two patients (0.2%) having SAH among 1016 clipped over a 15-year period.

Long-term follow-up data on recurrent hemorrhage after endovascular treatment are scarce - and not too surprising. Previously described surgical series included cases when the aneurysm was treated and subsequent graphical controls were not performed routinely in given intervals for years, thanks to the traditional belief in efficacy of microsurgery. Endovascular, on the other hand, was suspicious from risk of shorter durability from the very beginning, which led to more frequent controls and repeated interventions before the recurrent or bled de novo aneurysms. Only identified single-study information were presented by Schaafsma et al. [45]. This study presented the results of 283 patients followed-up for mean duration of 6.3 years after "adequate" coiling (>90% obliteration) of ruptured intracranial aneurysm. Frequency of recurrent SAH in their series was only 0.4%, which would seem lower than observed in surgical series, nevertheless the selection bias in addition to shorter follow-up period is obvious.

Altogether, the available information imply that the risk of repeated rupture of previously treated aneurysm is generally low after both treatment methods (surgical and endovascular) and is increased in case of incomplete initial occlusion as well as the length of follow-up. Available results further suggest that endovascularly treated patients might be at somehow higher risk of rebleeding from the original aneurysm than patients treated surgically (although the data are limited).

16.5 Retreatment: Indications and Risks

Most experts agree that substantial residual filling (more than 90% of initial size) or aneurysm regrowth are indications for repeated intervention, as they pose (although low) the risk of rupture with potentially negative sequelae [7, 10, 45–47]. Some authors postulate that younger patients are at higher risk to create a larger aneurysm from tiny remnant [10, 25]. In addition, enlarging remnants can produce compressive symptoms from local mass effect [46–48]. Thus, treatment of aneurysm remnants is usually advocated, especially in young patients. The results of ISAT trial at 10 year follow-up showed that retreatment rate was 17.4% for patients randomized to coiling and 3.9% to surgery [21, 28]. Similar results were observed in BRAT study, where the rate of retreatment at 6 year follow-up was 17.4% for coiling and 3.9% for surgery [49].

Nevertheless, repeated interventions pose very specific challenges. Surgical treatment of previously coiled or clipped aneurysm, owing to the formation of arachnoid scars or appearance of foreign material in the form of coils or stents implanted during previous endovascular intervention, may present one of the most difficult procedures in aneurysm surgery [44, 47, 50]. Repeated endovascular procedure, on the other hand, may pose the risk of lower technical feasibility.

Meta-analysis published by Petr et al. [34] focused on the outcome of endovascular treatment of the previously clipped aneurysms. The authors included 27 studies with 271 patients, overall complete occlusion rate was 76.1% with combined procedure-related morbidity/mortality of 4.5%. In another meta-analysis by Muskens et al. [51], the authors calculated pooled prevalence rates for complete occlusion rate and mortality for different treatment and retreatment strategies. Their results showed that surgical retreatment was associated with a higher complete occlusion rate but considerable morbidity and conversely, endovascular retreatment was associated with low mortality but also low complete occlusion rate. Surgery after coiling had a complete occlusion rate of 92.6% with mortality of 5.6%. Coiling after coiling had a pooled complete occlusion rate of 51.3% with mortality of 0.8%. Coiling after surgery had an occlusion rate of 56.1% with mortality of 9.3%. Surgery after surgery had pooled mortality rate of 5.9% and pooled complete occlusion rate could not be calculated because only one study reported their results (88.7%, Drake et al.) [46]. All included studies in both meta-analyses were retrospective.

16.6 Follow-up Controls

General guidelines recommending frequency and length of follow-up after aneurysm treatment are not available. We can still make some suggestions based on published data available.

Regarding surgical treatment, early postoperative catheter angiographic control to verify the quality of aneurysm occlusion should be performed routinely [11, 13]. Good results of intraoperative angiography have also been well documented in present studies [52–54], though the method is not widely available and its clear advantage over postoperative angiography has not yet been proved. Subsequent long-term follow-up imaging should be certainly managed given the risk of aneurysm recurrence and de novo formation [22–26]. The timing of controls should be planned individually, based on the initial occlusion rate, age, and general status of patients. First control after release from hospital should be performed in 12–36 months. In clipped aneurysms, CT angiography is the noninvasive method of choice [55].

After endovascular treatment, a large variety of schemes are used among different departments and different countries [56]. First follow-up control is mostly scheduled 3–6 months after procedure, with further follow-up depending on the patient/aneurysm characteristics. Classical scheme includes 12–24 months period and a midterm follow-up at 3–5 years [57]. Noninvasive imaging modality of choice after endovascular treatment is MR angiography [58]. First year after endovascular intervention is crucial, because most recurrences occur during this period. The ideal frequency of examinations and the length of follow-up is not determined, but more frequent follow-up may be indicated in patients harboring risk factors of recurrence [59, 60].

Despite many advances of noninvasive methods, conventional angiography still remains the gold standard and should be used to resolve any cases of diagnostic uncertainty.

16.7 Future Directions

Recent years meant the evolution of research at molecular level in all fields of neurosurgery, and aneurysms are no exception. Most investigations are focused on aneurysm wall biology. Observational data imply that to ensure permanent and long-term occlusion, the aneurysm wall must be healed and angiographic occlusion after endovascular treatment or surgical clipping does not equate to biological healing [61–65]. Human studies further confirm that half of aneurysms deemed completely occluded on angiography show tiny openings between coils at the neck [61]. The healing after clipping relies on mechanical occlusion, whereas healing after coiling mainly requires the induction of a biological response [66]. During embolization, the aneurysm sac is filled with material which should induce thrombosis and subsequent healing that requires growth of new tissue over the thrombus or organization of the thrombus into fibrous tissue [3]. Nevertheless, some studies revealed that many aneurysm walls lack the smooth muscle cells which are crucial elements in the process of thrombus formation and subsequent aneurysm healing and these aneurysms are thus predisposed to recurrence after endovascular treatment [67–69]. This means that the development of imaging to identify decellularized aneurysm could help identify at risk lesions. To date, we are able to image aneurysm walls by modern MRI techniques [70–72]. Several studies show that gadolinium uptake was more frequently observed in unstable aneurysms and has been associated with major recurrence after embolization [70, 73]. Nevertheless, the exact relation between wall decellularization, MRI findings and pattern of aneurysm recurrence is not fully understood yet. Another approach how molecular findings could help resolve aneurysm recurrence is focus on pharmacological affection of process in aneurysm wall. Similar research is ongoing in unruptured aneurysm management where biological therapy or nonsteroidal anti-inflammatory drugs might be potential future treatment options [74, 75].

16.8 Conclusion

After century of improving technical standards and strategies, the primary goal of aneurysm treatment remains stable: its complete occlusion from cerebral circulation. To date, we have two well established standard treatment modalities, surgical and endovascular, both proved to bring similar clinical benefit for patients. Thus, technical results, namely initial occlusion rate, regrowth and retreatment rate, all appear to be more satisfactory after surgery. On the other hand, the risk of endovascular retreatment does not seem to negate the advantage of initial intervention and appears to be safe even in case of additional treatment after surgery, when risk pending from additional open procedure could be substantial. Nevertheless, the choice of treatment should be individualized, with both neurosurgeon and endovascular neuroradiologist being involved. The postop control should be mandatory and long lasting. CTA and MRA seem to be suitable procedures with angiography being used in any uncertainties. Molecular therapy appears to be potential future strategy, even though its exact role is not clearly understood yet.

16.9 Our Experience

Between January 2000 and December 2019 we treated altogether 2032 aneurysms (769 indicated for clipping, 1263 for endovascular intervention) in 1742 patients and total number of procedures performed was 2167. The proportion of aneurysms that required repeated intervention was 3.5% (27/769) in surgical and 12.6% (159/1263) in endovascular group ($p < 0.001$) (Fig. 16.1a). The reasons for repeated intervention were divided into several subgroups. Most often reason for retreatment in both surgical and endovascular groups was incomplete initial occlusion: 16 aneurysms of initially clipped (2.1%) and 96 aneurysms of initially coiled (7.6%) (Fig. 16.1b). Three aneurysm in surgical and 65 in endovascular group were retreated for regrowth (Fig. 16.2). We observed 9 reruptures after endovascular treatment (6× early, 3× late) and none after surgery.

Illustrative case No. 1: 58-year-old patient with giant left MCA aneurysm indicated for surgical treatment. Clip reconstruction was performed with dysplastic aneurysm base remnant which was treated by additional coiling 7 months after original surgery. AN treatment is illustrated on Fig. 16.3.

Illustrative case No. 2: 34-years old patient with unruptured ophtalmic artery aneurysm was indicated for clipping. The surgeon was not satisfied at the end of the procedure and thus immediate angiography 20 min after surgery was performed. Post-angiography revealed residual filling which was managed by immediate coiling. AN treatment is illustrated on Fig. 16.4.

Illustrative case No. 3: 42-year-old patient with SAH HH 3, WFNS 3, Fisher 4 from ruptured bilobed aneurysm at VA junction. Aneurysm lobe that had ruptured was

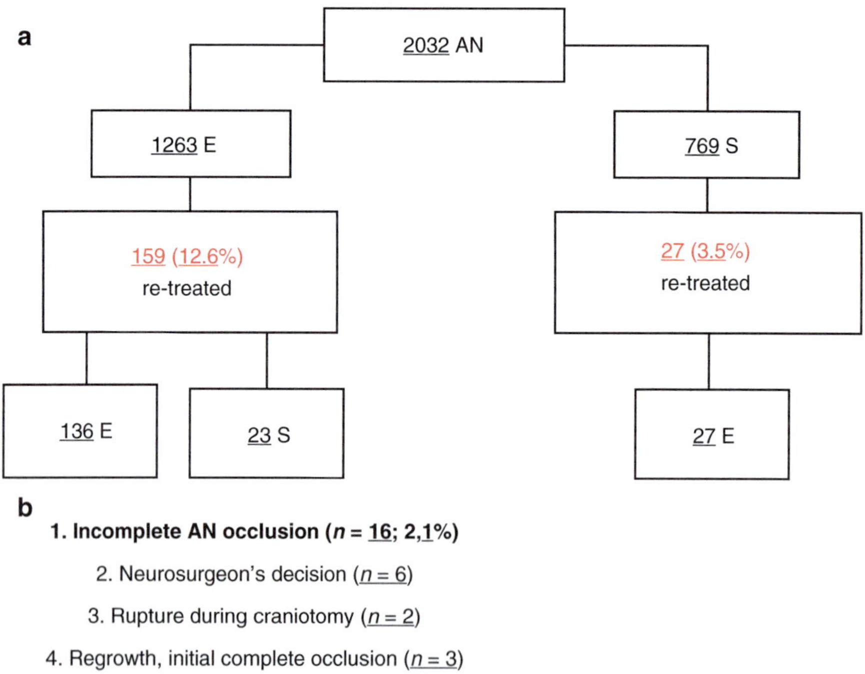

Fig. 16.1 (**a**) Proportion of retreatment according to initial treatment modality. (**b**) Reasons for retreatment in surgical group

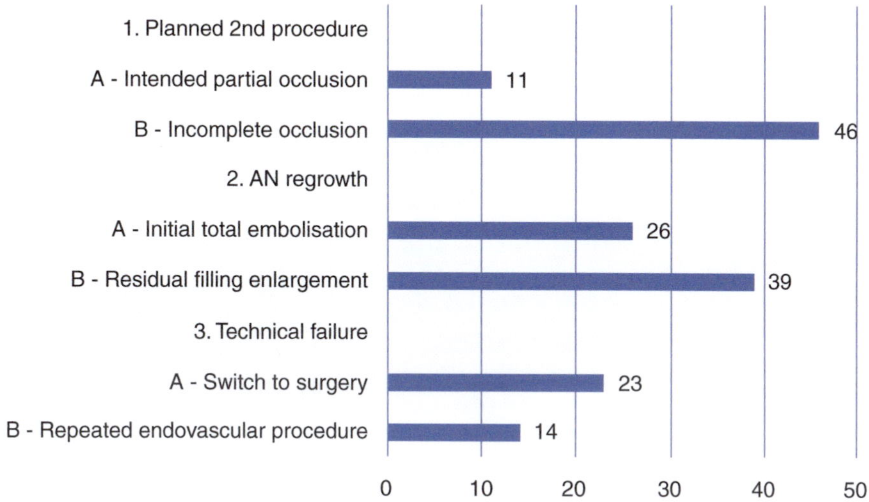

Fig. 16.2 Reasons for retreatment in endovascular group

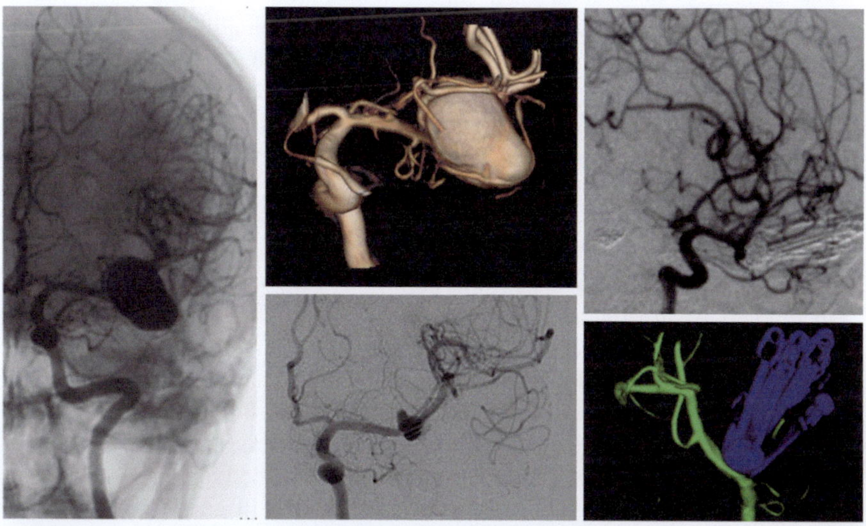

Fig. 16.3 Coiling of residual giant AN filling after clip reconstruction of dysplastic aneurysm base

coiled, second lobe not feasible for endovascular intervention was clipped 3 weeks later. Coiled aneurysm lobe requires additional treatment for regrowth by stent + coils in 183 months after original procedure. AN treatment is illustrated on Fig. 16.5a, b.

Illustrative case No. 4: 48-year-old patient presented with ruptured left ophtalmic artery aneurysm, HH 2, WFNS 1, Fisher 2. The aneurysm was indicated for clipping. During surgery, left optic nerve was identified to be ``smashed flat`` over

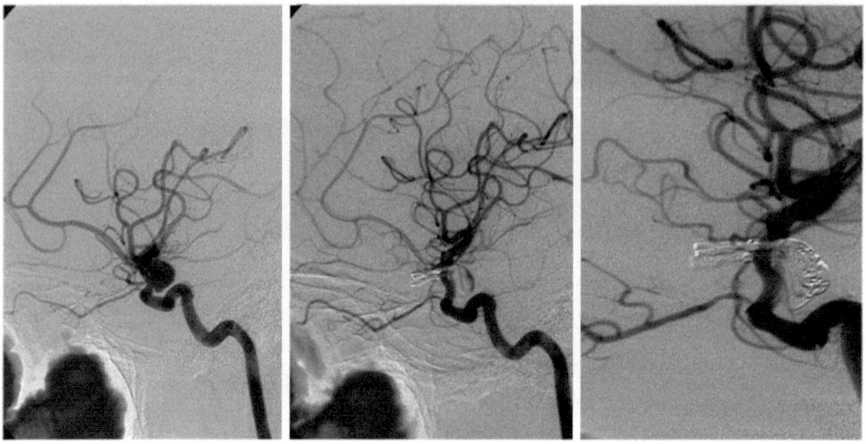

Fig. 16.4 Coiling of residual sac of clipped unruptured ophthalmic artery aneurysm

aneurysm and surgeon deemed further preparation unnecessary hazardous. Under the same anesthesia, patient was transferred to angio ward and aneurysm treated by coiling. AN treatment is illustrated on Fig. 16.6.

Illustrative case No. 5: 73-year-old patient with unruptured fusiform aneurysm at MCA which was successfully clipped. 51 months after treatment, recurrence of aneurysm filling was discovered and treated by additional coiling. AN treatment is illustrated on Fig. 16.7.

Illustrative case No. 6: 37-year-old patient with unruptured aneurysm at anterior communicating artery indicated for endovascular intervention. During the first session, the implantation of stent was performed with planned additional coiling in 1 month. AN treatment is illustrated on Fig. 16.8.

Illustrative case No. 7: 54-year-old male patient with ruptured ACoA aneurysm, HH 5, WFNS 5, Fisher 4. The aneurysm was coiled subtotally in acute phase with additional coiling in 7 days. AN treatment is illustrated on Fig. 16.9.

Illustrative case No. 8: 56-year-old woman with unruptured bilobed aneurysm at carotid artery bifurcation. Planned coiling was performed in two sessions with 6 months interval between procedures. AN treatment is illustrated on Fig. 16.10.

Illustrative case No. 9: 58-year-old patient with unruptured aneurysm at basilar artery bifurcation. The aneurysm was coiled subtotally with residual neck (Raymond class II), in 8 months regrowth was observed and aneurysm was secured by additional coiling. AN treatment is illustrated on Fig. 16.11.

Illustrative case No. 10: 48-year-old male with unruptured aneurysm at ACoA which was coiled with residual filling (Raymond III). At follow-up in 49 months, the coil was found to migrate into distal ACA and AN was treated by stent and coil. AN treatment is illustrated on Fig. 16.12.

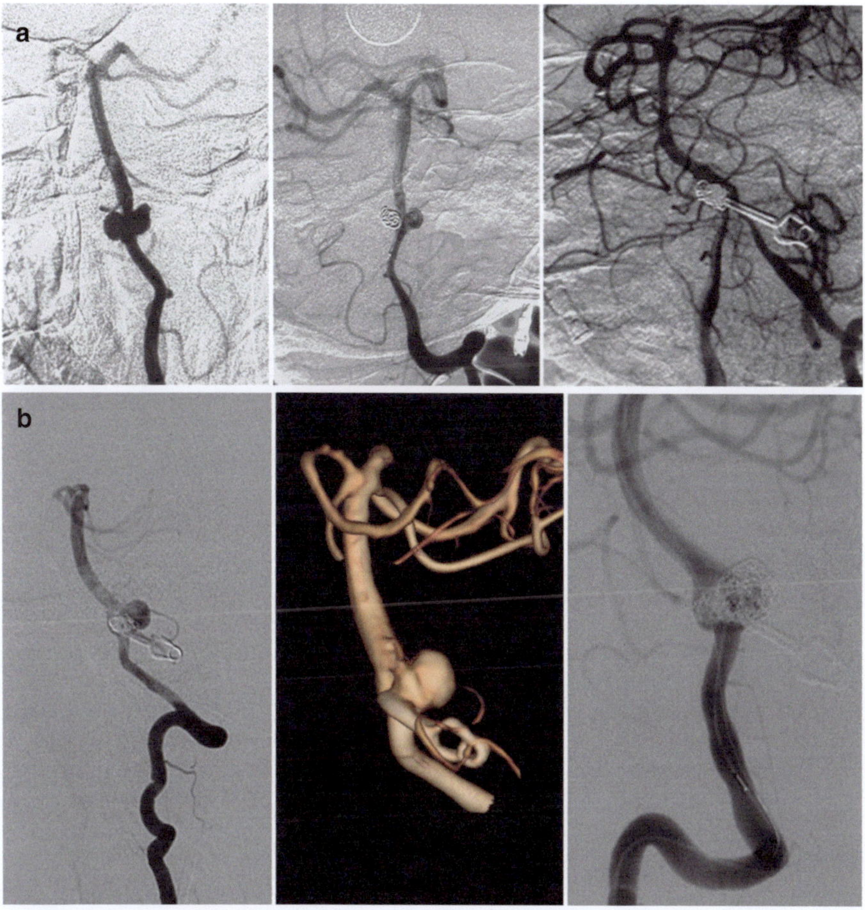

Fig. 16.5 (**a**) Ruptured bilobed aneurysm at VA junction. First lobe was coiled, second clipped. (**b**) Regrowth of coiled lobe and subsequent retreatment by stent+ coils

Illustrative case No. 11: 47-year-old patient presented with subarachnoid hemorrhage HH 1, WFNS 1, Fisher 3. Ruptured AN at PCoA was coiled. 61 months after initial treatment, she presented with recurrent bleeding. Catheter angiography revealed recurrent AN which was treated with additional coiling. AN treatment is illustrated on Fig. 16.13.

Illustrative case No. 12: 60-year-old patient presented with SAH HH 2, WFNS 2, Fisher 4. Ruptured AN at ACoA was treated by stent + coils. Two days after original procedure, neurological state deteriorated. CT revealed recurrent hemorrhage. Catheter angiogram was emergently performed and revealed residual filling at the base of aneurysm and tiny daughter sac, additional coils were implanted. AN treatment is illustrated on Fig. 16.14.

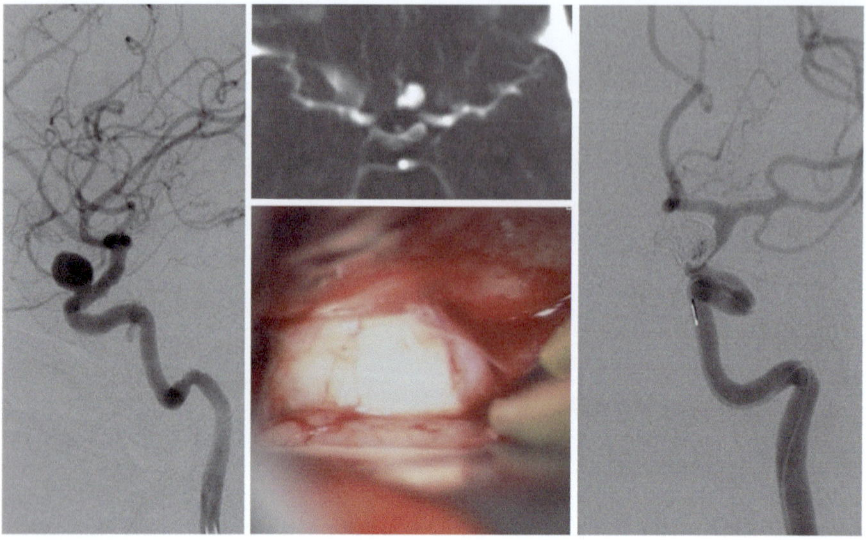

Fig. 16.6 Peroperatively identified conflict between left ophthalmic artery aneurysm and optic nerve

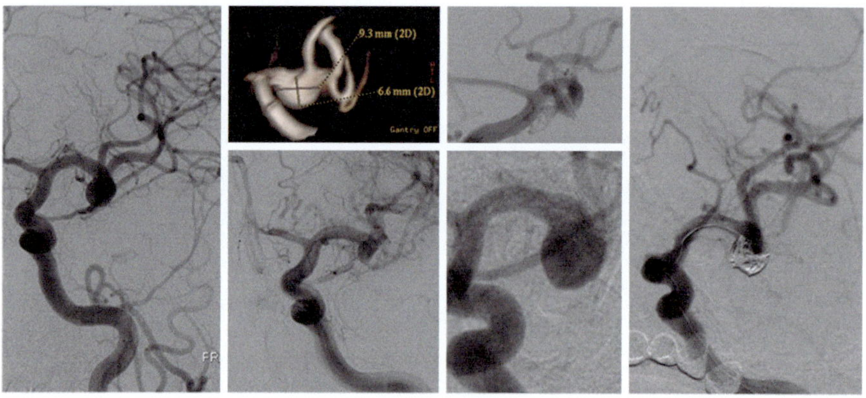

Fig. 16.7 Aneurysm regrowth after successful clipping

Illustrative case No. 13: 87-year-old patient with unruptured AN at PCoA was treated by coiling. 23 months after original procedure, she presented with SAH HH 2, WFNS 2, Fisher 3. Control examination revealed aneurysm regrowth which was treated by additional coils placement. AN treatment is illustrated on Fig. 16.15.

Illustrative case No. 14: 45-year-old patient with SAH from ruptured PCoA aneurysm (HH2, WFNS 1, Fisher 3). AN coiling was performed. Regrowth occurred

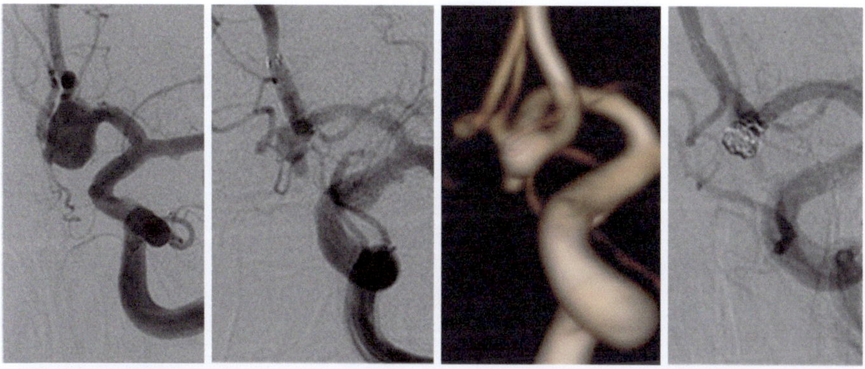

Fig. 16.8 Stent implantation in the first session and additional coiling in 1 month

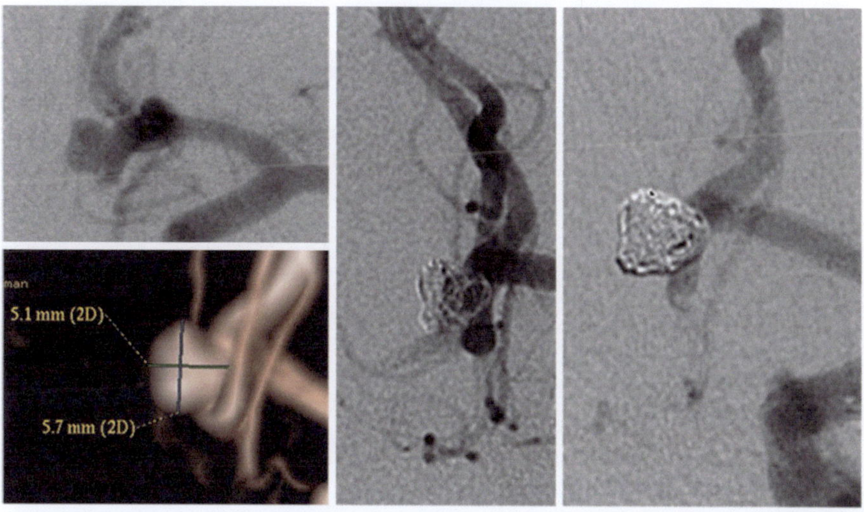

Fig. 16.9 Ruptured AN at ACoA coiled subtotally in acute phase with additional procedure in 7 days

after 3 years. During repeated endovascular intervention, patient developed anaphylactic shock and procedure was terminated prematurely. Subsequently, AN was treated by resection of coiled sac and clip reconstruction. AN treatment is illustrated on Fig. 16.16.

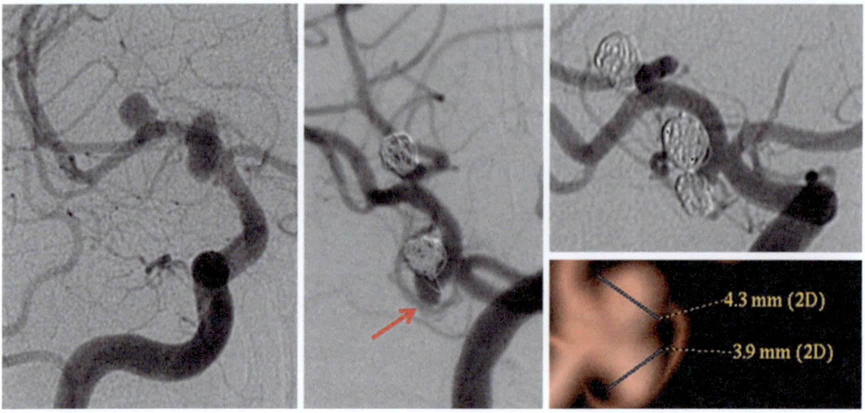

Fig. 16.10 Bilobed aneurysm at carotid artery bifurcation coiled in two sessions

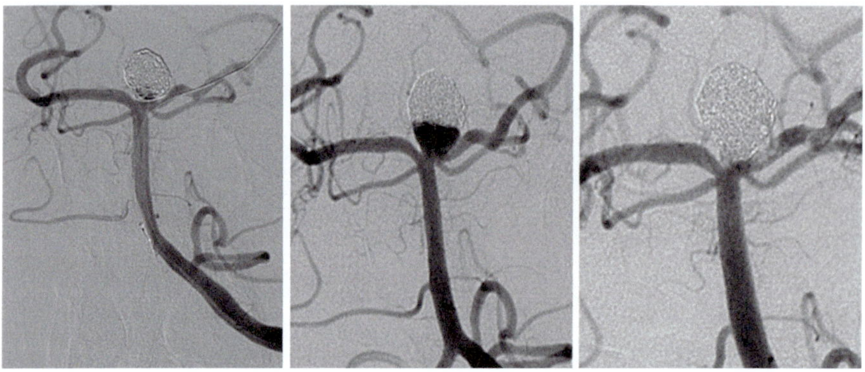

Fig. 16.11 Aneurysm regrowth after initial subtotal occlusion (Raymond class II) and additional coiling

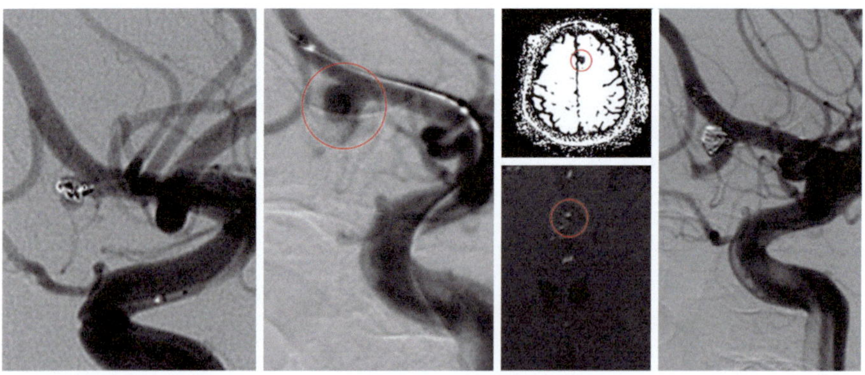

Fig. 16.12 AN recurrence after coil migration and additional intervention (stent + coils) 4 years later

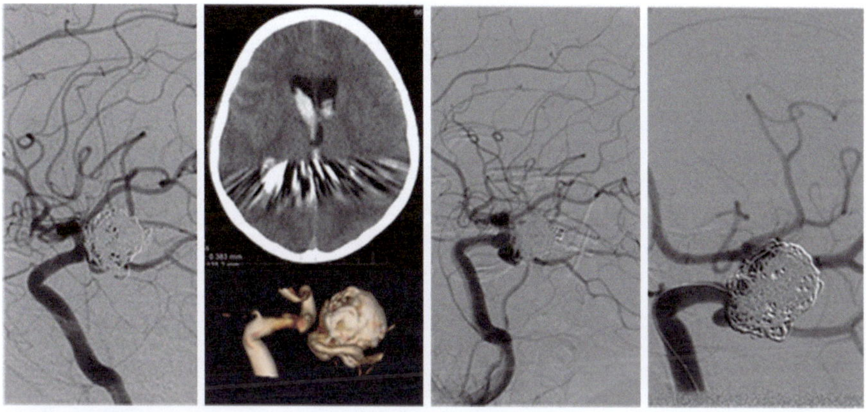

Fig. 16.13 Late (after 5 years) rerupture of previously coiled aneurysm

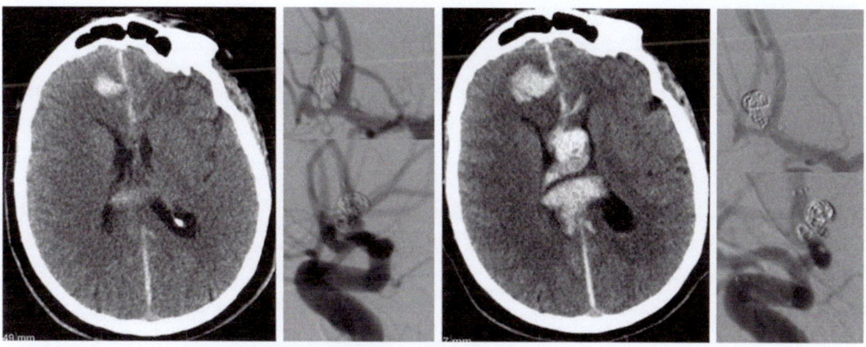

Fig. 16.14 Early (2 days) rerupture of residual neck and daughter sac after stent + coil

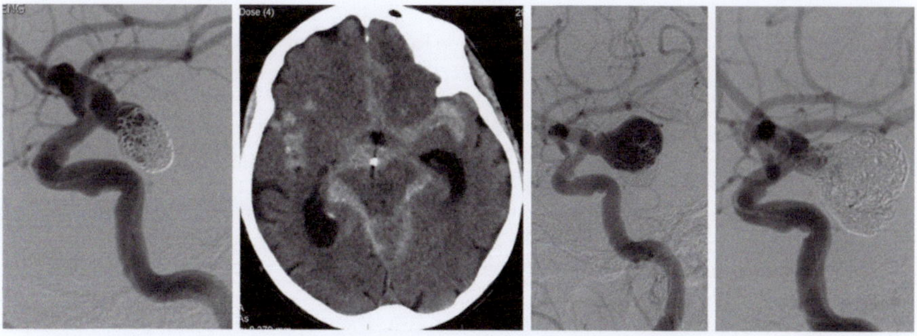

Fig. 16.15 Regrowth and rupture of previously coiled unruptured aneurysm

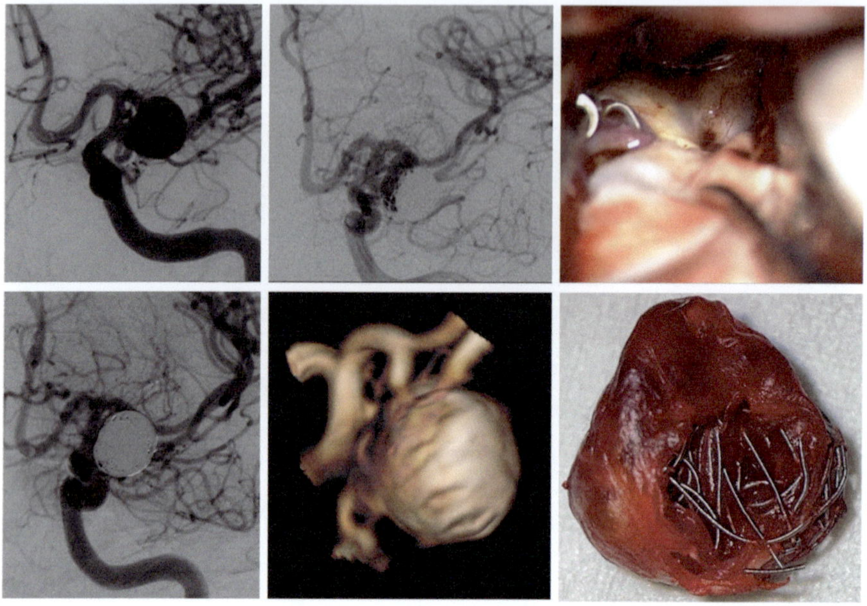

Fig. 16.16 Aneurysm regrowth after coiling treated by AN wall resection and clip reconstruction

Funding Financial support was provided by Grant NV19-04-00270. The sponsor had no role in the design or conduct of this research.

References

1. Feigin VL, Lawes CM, Bennett DA, Barker-Collo SL, Parag V. Worldwide stroke incidence and early case fatality reported in 56 population-based studies: a systematic review. Lancet Neurol. 2009;8(4):355–69.
2. Nieuwkamp DJ, Setz LE, Algra A, Linn FH, de Rooij NK, Rinkel GJ. Changes in case fatality of aneurysmal subarachnoid haemorrhage over time, according to age, sex, and region: a meta-analysis. Lancet Neurol. 2009;8(7):635–42.
3. Marbacher S, Niemela M, Hernesniemi J, Frosen J. Recurrence of endovascularly and microsurgically treated intracranial aneurysms-review of the putative role of aneurysm wall biology. Neurosurg Rev. 2019;42(1):49–58.
4. Molyneux A, Kerr R, Stratton I, Sandercock P, Clarke M, Shrimpton J, et al. International Subarachnoid Aneurysm Trial (ISAT) of neurosurgical clipping versus endovascular coiling in 2143 patients with ruptured intracranial aneurysms: a randomised trial. Lancet. 2002;360(9342):1267–74.
5. Thompson BG, Brown RD Jr, Amin-Hanjani S, Broderick JP, Cockroft KM, Connolly ES Jr, et al. Guidelines for the management of patients with unruptured intracranial aneurysms: a guideline for healthcare professionals from the American Heart Association/American Stroke Association. Stroke. 2015;46(8):2368–400.

6. Drake CG, Allcock JM. Postoperative angiography and the “slipped” clip. J Neurosurg. 1973;39(6):683–9.
7. Feuerberg I, Lindquist C, Lindqvist M, Steiner L. Natural history of postoperative aneurysm rests. J Neurosurg. 1987;66(1):30–4.
8. Hernesniemi J, Vapalahti M, Niskanen M, Tapaninaho A, Kari A, Luukkonen M, et al. One-year outcome in early aneurysm surgery: a 14 years experience. Acta Neurochir. 1993;122(1–2):1–10.
9. Koivisto T, Vanninen R, Hurskainen H, Saari T, Hernesniemi J, Vapalahti M. Outcomes of early endovascular versus surgical treatment of ruptured cerebral aneurysms. A prospective randomized study. Stroke. 2000;31(10):2369–77.
10. Lin T, Fox AJ, Drake CG. Regrowth of aneurysm sacs from residual neck following aneurysm clipping. J Neurosurg. 1989;70(4):556–60.
11. Macdonald RL, Wallace MC, Kestle JR. Role of angiography following aneurysm surgery. J Neurosurg. 1993;79(6):826–32.
12. Sindou M, Acevedo JC, Turjman F. Aneurysmal remnants after microsurgical clipping: classification and results from a prospective angiographic study (in a consecutive series of 305 operated intracranial aneurysms). Acta Neurochir. 1998;140(11):1153–9.
13. Kivisaari RP, Porras M, Ohman J, Siironen J, Ishii K, Hernesniemi J. Routine cerebral angiography after surgery for saccular aneurysms: is it worth it? Neurosurgery. 2004;55(5):1015–24.
14. Raaymakers TW, Rinkel GJ, Limburg M, Algra A. Mortality and morbidity of surgery for unruptured intracranial aneurysms: a meta-analysis. Stroke. 1998;29(8):1531–8.
15. Kotowski M, Naggara O, Darsaut TE, Nolet S, Gevry G, Kouznetsov E, et al. Safety and occlusion rates of surgical treatment of unruptured intracranial aneurysms: a systematic review and meta-analysis of the literature from 1990 to 2011. J Neurol Neurosurg Psychiatry. 2013;84(1):42–8.
16. Drake CG, Peerless SJ, Hernesniemi JA. Surgery of the vertebrobasilar aneurysms-experience on 1767 patients. In: Peerless SJ, Hernesniemi JA, editors. Multiple aneurysms. New York: Springer; 1995. p. 249–55.
17. Naggara ON, White PM, Guilbert F, Roy D, Weill A, Raymond J. Endovascular treatment of intracranial unruptured aneurysms: systematic review and meta-analysis of the literature on safety and efficacy. Radiology. 2010;256(3):887–97.
18. Ferns SP, Sprengers ME, van Rooij WJ, Rinkel GJ, van Rijn JC, Bipat S, et al. Coiling of intracranial aneurysms: a systematic review on initial occlusion and reopening and retreatment rates. Stroke. 2009;40(8):e523–9.
19. Pierot L, Spelle L, Vitry F, Investigators A. Immediate clinical outcome of patients harboring unruptured intracranial aneurysms treated by endovascular approach: results of the ATENA study. Stroke. 2008;39(9):2497–504.
20. Murayama Y, Nien YL, Duckwiler G, Gobin YP, Jahan R, Frazee J, et al. Guglielmi detachable coil embolization of cerebral aneurysms: 11 years’ experience. J Neurosurg. 2003;98(5):959–66.
21. Molyneux AJ, Kerr RS, Yu LM, Clarke M, Sneade M, Yarnold JA, et al. International subarachnoid aneurysm trial (ISAT) of neurosurgical clipping versus endovascular coiling in 2143 patients with ruptured intracranial aneurysms: a randomised comparison of effects on survival, dependency, seizures, rebleeding, subgroups, and aneurysm occlusion. Lancet. 2005;366(9488):809–17.
22. Spiessberger A, Vogt DR, Fandino J, Marbacher S. Formation of intracranial de novo aneurysms and recurrence after neck clipping: a systematic review and meta-analysis. J Neurosurg. 2019;132(2):456–64.
23. David CA, Vishteh AG, Spetzler RF, Lemole M, Lawton MT, Partovi S. Late angiographic follow-up review of surgically treated aneurysms. J Neurosurg. 1999;91(3):396–401.
24. Edner G, Almqvist H. The Stockholm 20-year follow-up of aneurysmal subarachnoid hemorrhage outcome. Neurosurgery. 2007;60(6):1017–23; discussion 23–4.

25. Jabbarli R, Pierscianek D, Wrede K, Dammann P, Schlamann M, Forsting M, et al. Aneurysm remnant after clipping: the risks and consequences. J Neurosurg. 2016;125(5):1249–55.
26. Tsutsumi K, Ueki K, Morita A, Usui M, Kirino T. Risk of aneurysm recurrence in patients with clipped cerebral aneurysms: results of long-term follow-up angiography. Stroke. 2001;32(5):1191–4.
27. Johnston SC, Dowd CF, Higashida RT, Lawton MT, Duckwiler GR, Gress DR, et al. Predictors of rehemorrhage after treatment of ruptured intracranial aneurysms: the Cerebral Aneurysm Rerupture After Treatment (CARAT) study. Stroke. 2008;39(1):120–5.
28. Campi A, Ramzi N, Molyneux AJ, Summers PE, Kerr RS, Sneade M, et al. Retreatment of ruptured cerebral aneurysms in patients randomized by coiling or clipping in the International Subarachnoid Aneurysm Trial (ISAT). Stroke 2007;38(5):1538–44.
29. Raymond J, Guilbert F, Weill A, Georganos SA, Juravsky L, Lambert A, et al. Long-term angiographic recurrences after selective endovascular treatment of aneurysms with detachable coils. Stroke. 2003;34(6):1398–403.
30. Ogilvy CS, Chua MH, Fusco MR, Reddy AS, Thomas AJ. Stratification of recanalization for patients with endovascular treatment of intracranial aneurysms. Neurosurgery. 2015;76(4):390–5; discussion 5.
31. Choi DS, Kim MC, Lee SK, Willinsky RA, Terbrugge KG. Clinical and angiographic long-term follow-up of completely coiled intracranial aneurysms using endovascular technique. J Neurosurg. 2010;112(3):575–81.
32. Ferns SP, Sprengers ME, van Rooij WJ, van Zwam WH, de Kort GA, Velthuis BK, et al. Late reopening of adequately coiled intracranial aneurysms: frequency and risk factors in 400 patients with 440 aneurysms. Stroke. 2011;42(5):1331–7.
33. Ogilvy CS, Chua MH, Fusco MR, Griessenauer CJ, Harrigan MR, Sonig A, et al. Validation of a system to predict recanalization after endovascular treatment of intracranial aneurysms. Neurosurgery. 2015;77(2):168–73; discussion 73–4.
34. Byrne JV, Sohn MJ, Molyneux AJ, Chir B. Five-year experience in using coil embolization for ruptured intracranial aneurysms: outcomes and incidence of late rebleeding. J Neurosurg. 1999;90(4):656–63.
35. Cognard C, Weill A, Spelle L, Piotin M, Castaings L, Rey A, et al. Long-term angiographic follow-up of 169 intracranial berry aneurysms occluded with detachable coils. Radiology. 1999;212(2):348–56.
36. Ries T, Siemonsen S, Thomalla G, Grzyska U, Zeumer H, Fiehler J. Long-term follow-up of cerebral aneurysms after endovascular therapy prediction and outcome of retreatment. AJNR Am J Neuroradiol. 2007;28(9):1755–61.
37. Slob MJ, van Rooij WJ, Sluzewski M. Coil thickness and packing of cerebral aneurysms: a comparative study of two types of coils. AJNR Am J Neuroradiol. 2005;26(4):901–3.
38. Sluzewski M, van Rooij WJ, Beute GN, Nijssen PC. Late rebleeding of ruptured intracranial aneurysms treated with detachable coils. AJNR Am J Neuroradiol. 2005;26(10):2542–9.
39. Sluzewski M, van Rooij WJ, Rinkel GJ, Wijnalda D. Endovascular treatment of ruptured intracranial aneurysms with detachable coils: long-term clinical and serial angiographic results. Radiology. 2003;227(3):720–4.
40. Sprengers ME, Schaafsma J, van Rooij WJ, Sluzewski M, Rinkel GJ, Velthuis BK, et al. Stability of intracranial aneurysms adequately occluded 6 months after coiling: a 3 T MR angiography multicenter long-term follow-up study. AJNR Am J Neuroradiol. 2008;29(9):1768–74.
41. Molyneux AJ, Birks J, Clarke A, Sneade M, Kerr RS. The durability of endovascular coiling versus neurosurgical clipping of ruptured cerebral aneurysms: 18 year follow-up of the UK cohort of the International Subarachnoid Aneurysm Trial (ISAT). Lancet. 2015;385(9969):691–7.
42. Molyneux AJ, Kerr RS, Birks J, Ramzi N, Yarnold J, Sneade M, et al. Risk of recurrent subarachnoid haemorrhage, death, or dependence and standardised mortality ratios after clipping or coiling of an intracranial aneurysm in the International Subarachnoid Aneurysm Trial (ISAT): long-term follow-up. Lancet Neurol. 2009;8(5):427–33.

43. Wermer MJ, Greebe P, Algra A, Rinkel GJ. Incidence of recurrent subarachnoid hemorrhage after clipping for ruptured intracranial aneurysms. Stroke. 2005;36(11):2394–9.
44. Mohamed el-Beltagy M, Muroi C, Roth P, Fandino J, Imhof HG, Yonekawa Y. Recurrent intracranial aneurysms after successful neck clipping. World Neurosurg. 2010;74(4–5):472–7.
45. Schaafsma JD, Sprengers ME, van Rooij WJ, Sluzewski M, Majoie CB, Wermer MJ, et al. Long-term recurrent subarachnoid hemorrhage after adequate coiling versus clipping of ruptured intracranial aneurysms. Stroke. 2009;40(5):1758–63.
46. Drake CG, Friedman AH, Peerless SJ. Failed aneurysm surgery. Reoperation in 115 cases. J Neurosurg. 1984;61(5):848–56.
47. Giannotta SL, Litofsky NS. Reoperative management of intracranial aneurysms. J Neurosurg. 1995;83(3):387–93.
48. Rabinstein AA, Nichols DA. Endovascular coil embolization of cerebral aneurysm remnants after incomplete surgical obliteration. Stroke. 2002;33(7):1809–15.
49. Spetzler RF, McDougall CG, Zabramski JM, Albuquerque FC, Hills NK, Russin JJ, et al. The Barrow Ruptured Aneurysm Trial: 6-year results. J Neurosurg. 2015;123(3):609–17.
50. Kashimura H, Ogasawara K, Kubo Y, Otawara Y, Ogawa A. Microsurgical removal of previously placed aneurysm clips and application of new clips for recurrent cerebral aneurysms. Technical note. J Neurosurg. 2007;107(4):881–3.
51. Muskens IS, Hertgers O, Lycklama ANGJ, Broekman MLD, Moojen WA. Outcomes of retreatment for intracranial aneurysms—a meta-analysis. Neurosurgery. 2019;85(6):750–61.
52. Tang G, Cawley CM, Dion JE, Barrow DL. Intraoperative angiography during aneurysm surgery: a prospective evaluation of efficacy. J Neurosurg. 2002;96(6):993–9.
53. Klopfenstein JD, Spetzler RF, Kim LJ, Feiz-Erfan I, Han PP, Zabramski JM, et al. Comparison of routine and selective use of intraoperative angiography during aneurysm surgery: a prospective assessment. J Neurosurg. 2004;100(2):230–5.
54. Chiang VL, Gailloud P, Murphy KJ, Rigamonti D, Tamargo RJ. Routine intraoperative angiography during aneurysm surgery. J Neurosurg. 2002;96(6):988–92.
55. Wallace RC, Karis JP, Partovi S, Fiorella D. Noninvasive imaging of treated cerebral aneurysms, Part II: CT angiographic follow-up of surgically clipped aneurysms. AJNR Am J Neuroradiol. 2007;28(7):1207–12.
56. Soize S, Gawlitza M, Raoult H, Pierot L. Imaging follow-up of intracranial aneurysms treated by endovascular means: why, when, and how? Stroke. 2016;47(5):1407–12.
57. Lecler A, Raymond J, Rodriguez-Regent C, Al Shareef F, Trystram D, Godon-Hardy S, et al. Intracranial aneurysms: recurrences more than 10 years after endovascular treatment-a prospective cohort study, systematic review, and meta-analysis. Radiology. 2015;277(1):173–80.
58. Ahmed SU, Mocco J, Zhang X, Kelly M, Doshi A, Nael K, et al. MRA versus DSA for the follow-up imaging of intracranial aneurysms treated using endovascular techniques: a meta-analysis. J Neurointerv Surg. 2019;11(10):1009–14.
59. Hope JK, Byrne JV, Molyneux AJ. Factors influencing successful angiographic occlusion of aneurysms treated by coil embolization. AJNR Am J Neuroradiol. 1999;20(3):391–9.
60. Pierot L, Cognard C, Anxionnat R, Ricolfi F, Investigators C. Endovascular treatment of ruptured intracranial aneurysms: factors affecting midterm quality anatomic results: analysis in a prospective, multicenter series of patients (CLARITY). AJNR Am J Neuroradiol. 2012;33(8):1475–80.
61. Bavinzski G, Talazoglu V, Killer M, Richling B, Gruber A, Gross CE, et al. Gross and microscopic histopathological findings in aneurysms of the human brain treated with Guglielmi detachable coils. J Neurosurg. 1999;91(2):284–93.
62. Raymond J, Darsaut T, Salazkin I, Gevry G, Bouzeghrane F. Mechanisms of occlusion and recanalization in canine carotid bifurcation aneurysms embolized with platinum coils: an alternative concept. AJNR Am J Neuroradiol. 2008;29(4):745–52.
63. Reul J, Weis J, Spetzger U, Konert T, Fricke C, Thron A. Long-term angiographic and histopathologic findings in experimental aneurysms of the carotid bifurcation embolized with platinum and tungsten coils. AJNR Am J Neuroradiol. 1997;18(1):35–42.

64. Szikora I, Seifert P, Hanzely Z, Kulcsar Z, Berentei Z, Marosfoi M, et al. Histopathologic evaluation of aneurysms treated with Guglielmi detachable coils or matrix detachable microcoils. AJNR Am J Neuroradiol. 2006;27(2):283–8.
65. Szikora I, Turanyi E, Marosfoi M. Evolution of flow-diverter endothelialization and thrombus organization in giant fusiform aneurysms after flow diversion: a histopathologic study. AJNR Am J Neuroradiol. 2015;36(9):1716–20.
66. Killer-Oberpfalzer M, Aichholzer M, Weis S, Richling B, Jones R, Virmani R, et al. Histological analysis of clipped human intracranial aneurysms and parent arteries with short-term follow-up. Cardiovasc Pathol. 2012;21(4):299–306.
67. Frosen J. Smooth muscle cells and the formation, degeneration, and rupture of saccular intracranial aneurysm wall—a review of current pathophysiological knowledge. Transl Stroke Res. 2014;5(3):347–56.
68. Frosen J, Piippo A, Paetau A, Kangasniemi M, Niemela M, Hernesniemi J, et al. Remodeling of saccular cerebral artery aneurysm wall is associated with rupture: histological analysis of 24 unruptured and 42 ruptured cases. Stroke. 2004;35(10):2287–93.
69. Kataoka K, Taneda M, Asai T, Kinoshita A, Ito M, Kuroda R. Structural fragility and inflammatory response of ruptured cerebral aneurysms. A comparative study between ruptured and unruptured cerebral aneurysms. Stroke. 1999;30(7):1396–401.
70. Edjlali M, Gentric JC, Regent-Rodriguez C, Trystram D, Hassen WB, Lion S, et al. Does aneurysmal wall enhancement on vessel wall MRI help to distinguish stable from unstable intracranial aneurysms? Stroke. 2014;45(12):3704–6.
71. Matouk CC, Mandell DM, Gunel M, Bulsara KR, Malhotra A, Hebert R, et al. Vessel wall magnetic resonance imaging identifies the site of rupture in patients with multiple intracranial aneurysms: proof of principle. Neurosurgery. 2013;72(3):492–6; discussion 6.
72. Nagahata S, Nagahata M, Obara M, Kondo R, Minagawa N, Sato S, et al. Wall enhancement of the intracranial aneurysms revealed by magnetic resonance vessel wall imaging using three-dimensional turbo spin-echo sequence with motion-sensitized driven-equilibrium: a sign of ruptured aneurysm? Clin Neuroradiol. 2016;26(3):277–83.
73. Fanning NF, Willinsky RA, ter Brugge KG. Wall enhancement, edema, and hydrocephalus after endovascular coil occlusion of intradural cerebral aneurysms. J Neurosurg. 2008;108(6):1074–86.
74. Frosen J, Piippo A, Paetau A, Kangasniemi M, Niemela M, Hernesniemi J, et al. Growth factor receptor expression and remodeling of saccular cerebral artery aneurysm walls: implications for biological therapy preventing rupture. Neurosurgery. 2006;58(3):534–41; discussion 41.
75. Fisher CL, Demel SL. Nonsteroidal anti-inflammatory drugs: a potential pharmacological treatment for intracranial aneurysm. Cerebrovasc Dis Extra. 2019;9(1):31–45.

Chapter 17
Management of Wide-Necked Basilar tip Aneurysms

Yuichiro Kikkawa and Hiroki Kurita

17.1 Introduction

Basilar artery aneurysms are difficult to approach surgically because of their deep location [1–4]. Endovascular treatment is the first-line treatment for basilar artery aneurysms, and direct surgery for such lesions is becoming increasingly less common, which limits the experience of surgeons. Despite endovascular treatment being the first-line approach, it is often difficult to treat large wide-necked aneurysms using endovascular treatment alone. Thus, in recent years, surgery and endovascular treatment have been combined for difficult cerebrovascular lesions, also termed hybrid surgery [5–8]. We herein describe our original surgical approach for large wide-necked basilar tip aneurysms.

17.2 Selection of Surgical Approach

The pterional approach, subtemporal approach, and a combination of these approaches are commonly used to treat basilar tip aneurysms [9–13]. The pterional approach has some advantages over the subtemporal approach; for example, with the pterional approach, it is easy to visualize the bilateral P1 portions of the posterior cerebral artery (PCA), superior cerebellar artery, and perforators. In addition,

Y. Kikkawa (✉)
Department of Neurosurgery, Saitama Cardiovascular Respiratory Center, Kumagaya, Japan

H. Kurita
Department of Cerebrovascular Surgery, Saitama Medical University International Medical Center, Hidaka, Japan

Y. Kato, A. Ansari (eds.), *Cerebrovascular Surgery*, Advances and Technical Standards in Neurosurgery 44, https://doi.org/10.1007/978-3-030-87649-4_17

with the pterional approach, there is no need to compress cranial nerves III and IV, and less retraction of the temporal lobe is required.

Despite these advantages, regardless of the space outside, inside, or above the internal carotid artery (ICA), the operative field is narrow and the flexibility of manipulation is limited with the pterional approach. Therefore, it is often necessary to retract the ICA to obtain an adequate operative field. Furthermore, the posterior communicating artery or the posterior clinoid process often obstructs the visual field.

To overcome the limitations of the pterional approach, we use the orbitozygomatic approach to treat basilar tip aneurysms, which combines the pterional approach with orbitozygotomy [14–17]. The orbitozygomatic approach makes it possible to look upward from the skull base to a higher position, increasing the surgical corridor and allowing inspection from different directions [14–17].

Although the orbitozygomatic approach has some advantages, one disadvantage is that it is difficult to visualize the perforators behind the aneurysm with this approach. However, in such cases, the field of view that can be achieved using the subtemporal approach is helpful to visualize the perforators. In addition, we usually use the anterior temporal approach together with the orbitozygomatic approach [18, 19].

When dissecting the Sylvian fissure using the distal Sylvian approach, the temporal lobe can be sufficiently retracted backward by detaching the superficial middle cerebral vein and anterior temporal artery from the temporal lobe and cutting off the arachnoid membrane between the oculomotor nerve and the uncus. This provides a sufficient field of view on the lateral side of the ICA. When sufficient posterior retraction of the temporal lobe cannot be achieved due to the variation in the running pattern of the Sylvian vein, epidural retraction of the temporal lobe using an extradural temporopolar approach is useful [20, 21]. Moreover, the visible range is further expanded by obtaining the mobility of the ICA by removing the anterior clinoid process and incising the distal dural ring of the ICA [22, 23]. Whether it is best to approach from the left or right side is determined by referring to the height and protrusion of the P1 portion of the PCA, the length and running pattern of the ICA, and the direction in which the aneurysm leans.

17.3 Treatment Strategy Using Hybrid Surgery

With large wide-necked basilar tip aneurysms, cerebral infarction sometimes occurs in the area of P1 perforators after surgery, even if the perforator that adheres to the aneurysm neck is carefully detached and preserved during surgery [7]. This may occur because even if the perforator is preserved in the visible range near the aneurysm neck, deformation of the dome by neck clipping may cause kinking in the peripheral part of the perforator that adheres to the dome, leading to perforator circulation failure [7]. Moreover, with large basilar tip aneurysms, it is practically impossible to observe the relationship between bilateral perforators and the aneurysm over the entire length. Dissociation of intraoperative findings and postoperative complications may thus result [7].

For large wide-necked basilar tip aneurysms, we use hybrid surgery in which aneurysm neck plastic clipping and coil embolization are performed simultaneously. We perform partial clipping of the aneurysm neck with preserving perforators to shape the aneurysm such that coil embolization is possible [7]. Just after deforming the aneurysm to a highly curative "side wall-type" using aneurysm neck plastic clipping, intraoperative angiography is performed to confirm the residual aneurysm, followed by coil embolization [7]. Then, total obliteration of the aneurysm is confirmed by intraoperative angiography, and the wound is closed. This method, which only partially deforms the aneurysm without detaching the perforators, may overcome the limitations of direct surgery and contribute to preservation of neurological function [7].

17.4 Case Presentation

In a 70-year-old woman, a basilar tip aneurysm, which was incidentally identified by magnetic resonance angiography performed to investigate the cause of dizziness, increased in size over time. Preoperative angiography revealed a broad-necked aneurysm. It was determined that tight packing would be difficult by coil embolization alone (Fig. 17.1). It was also expected that bilateral perforators would adhere to the dome; thus, we performed hybrid surgery.

After administering general anesthesia, a guiding catheter with a balloon was placed in the basilar artery, followed by craniotomy. After orbitozygomatic osteotomy (Fig. 17.2), the Sylvian fissure was opened and the basilar cistern was observed from the carotid-oculomotor space via the anterior temporal approach (Fig. 17.3). As expected preoperatively, P1 perforators in front of the aneurysm strongly adhered to the dome, and it was difficult to peel off perforators over the entire length. Subsequently, we attempted to decompress the aneurysm and confirm the proximal portion of the P1 perforator under temporary occlusion of the basilar artery using an endovascular procedure, but this could only be partially confirmed (Fig. 17.4). Because strong adhesion between the contralateral perforator and the dome was expected, a fenestrated clip was applied so that the tip of the blade did not exceed the neck on the opposite side. The perforator in front of the aneurysm was preserved using the clip fenestration (Fig. 17.5). Immediately after intraoperative angiography, to confirm that the aneurysm had been deformed into a shape capable of tight packing, endovascular coil embolization was performed (Fig. 17.6). Then, after confirming complete obliteration by intraoperative angiography (Fig. 17.7), the head was closed and surgery was concluded.

After surgery, asymptomatic embolic complications were found in the area of the PCA on magnetic resonance images (Fig. 17.8), but the postoperative course was uneventful, and the patient was discharged from hospital. Delayed complications, such as coil compaction, have not been observed over a 7-year follow-up period.

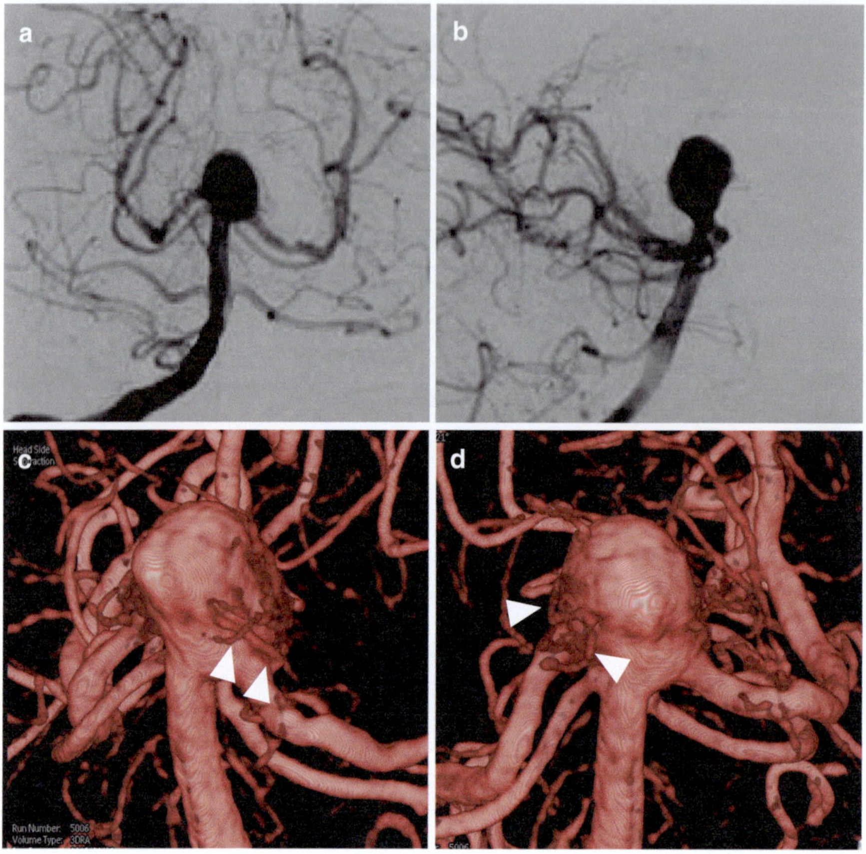

Fig. 17.1 Preoperative images. Anteroposterior (**a**) and lateral (**b**) views on preoperative angiography showing a large wide-necked basilar tip aneurysm. Volume-rendering images from three-dimensional angiography showing the aneurysm from the front *left* side (**c**) and the front *right* side (**d**). *Arrowheads* indicate the P1 perforators

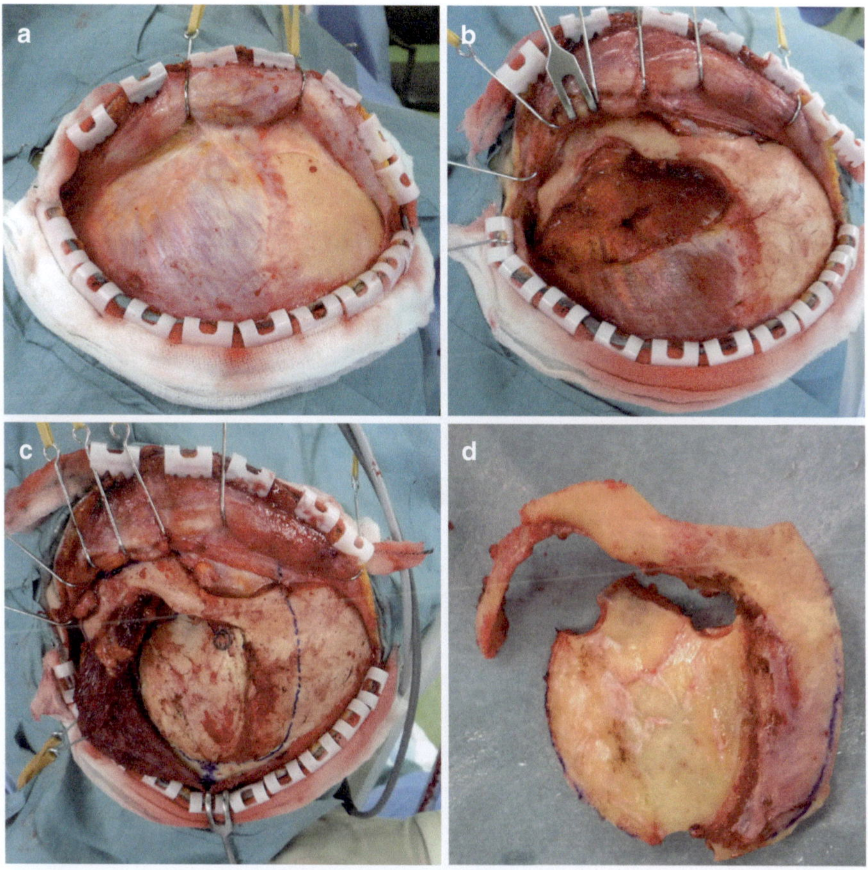

Fig. 17.2 Intraoperative photograph. (**a**) After a semi-coronal skin incision, the superior temporal fascia was fully exposed. (**b**) Interfascial dissection between the superficial layer and the deep layer of the deep temporal fascia was performed to preserve the facial nerve and to expose the zygomatic arch. The supraorbital rim, lateral orbital rim, and zygomatic arch were exposed over the entire length. (**c**) Temporal muscle was retracted posteriorly and a one-piece orbitozygomatic osteotomy was performed along the marked line with three burr holes, including the MacCarty keyhole, a temporal bone burr hole, and a burr hole just above the temporal line. (**d**) A bone flap created by one-piece orbitozygomatic osteotomy is shown

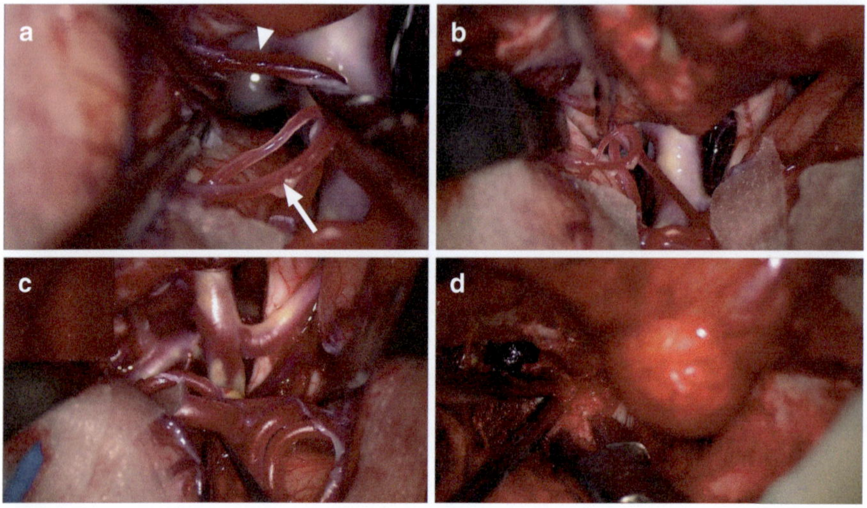

Fig. 17.3 Intraoperative photograph. The distal Sylvian approach was used to open the Sylvian fissure. The anterior temporal approach was performed to sufficiently pull the temporal lobe posteriorly and obtain the visual field from the lateral side of the internal carotid artery. In addition, to achieve internal carotid artery mobility, the anterior clinoid process was removed and a distal dural ring was cut. (**a**) The anterior temporal artery (*arrow*) and the superficial middle cerebral vein (*arrowhead*) were detached from the medial aspect of the temporal lobe to provide space to insert a spatula to retract the temporal lobe. (**b**) After sufficient dissection of the arachnoid membrane between the cerebral tentorium and the uncus, a brain spatula was inserted from below the anterior temporal artery and the superficial middle cerebral vein toward the cerebellar tentorium. (**c**) The frontal and temporal lobes were widely separated after dissection of the Sylvian fissure. The M2 portions of middle cerebral arteries and the anterior temporal artery were detached from the brain surface. The oculomotor nerve (*asterisk*) was observed over the entire length by retracting the temporal lobe posteriorly. (**d**) The anterior clinoid process was completely removed using extradural procedures

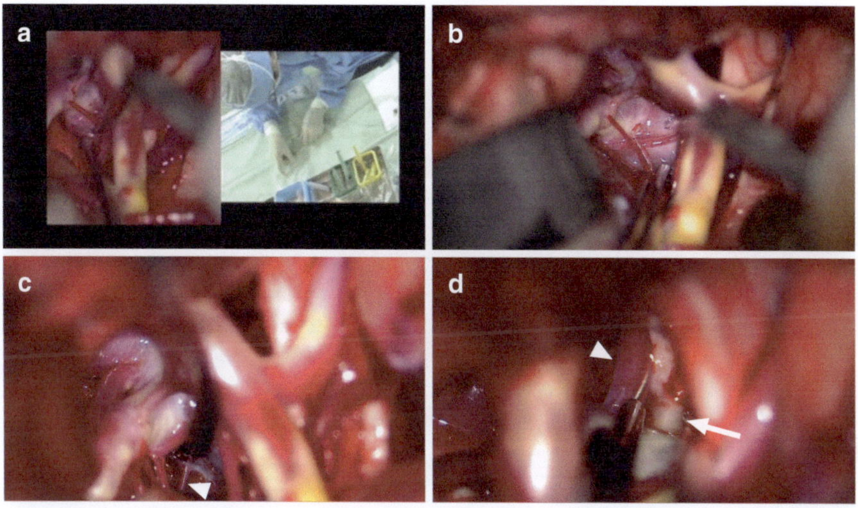

Fig. 17.4 Intraoperative photograph. (**a**) As the aneurysm was exposed, the endovascular team prepared for temporary basilar artery occlusion using a balloon. (**b**) From the carotid-oculomotor space, a perforator on the front side arising from the aneurysm neck was confirmed. (**c**) Under temporary occlusion of the basilar artery, a contralateral perforator arising from the aneurysm neck behind the aneurysm was confirmed (*arrowhead*). The tip of the clip blade was stopped just before the perforator. (**d**) From the optico-carotid space, the contralateral oculomotor nerve (*asterisk*), superior cerebellar artery (*arrowhead*), and posterior cerebral artery (*arrow*) were confirmed. The guidewire in the superior cerebellar artery can be visualized

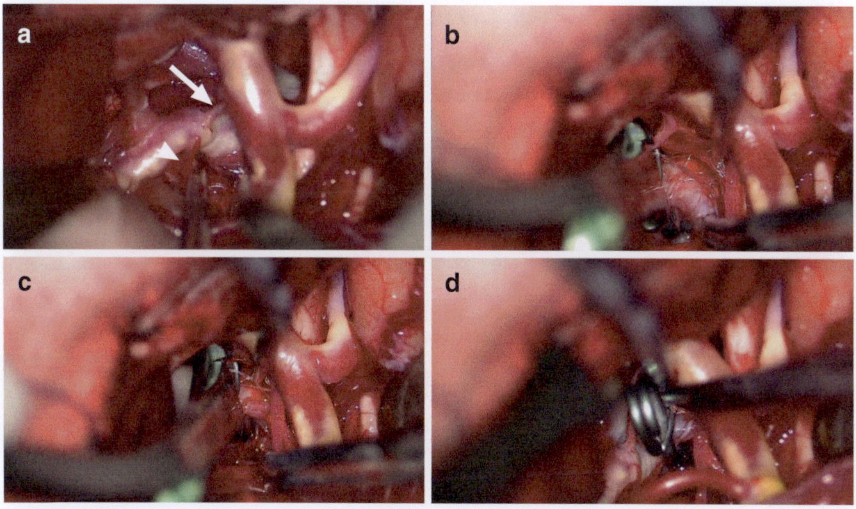

Fig. 17.5 Intraoperative photograph. (**a**) Of the two perforators on the front side of the aneurysm, one was moved outward (*arrowhead*). Then, a space for the clip blade was provided at the neck on the left side of the aneurysm. The *asterisk* and *arrow* indicate the ipsilateral oculomotor nerve and posterior communicating artery, respectively. (**b–d**) From the carotid-oculomotor space, a fenestrated straight clip was applied to preserve another perforator originating from the dome, which adhered to the anterior surface of the aneurysm. The tip of the clip blade was stopped just before the contralateral perforator

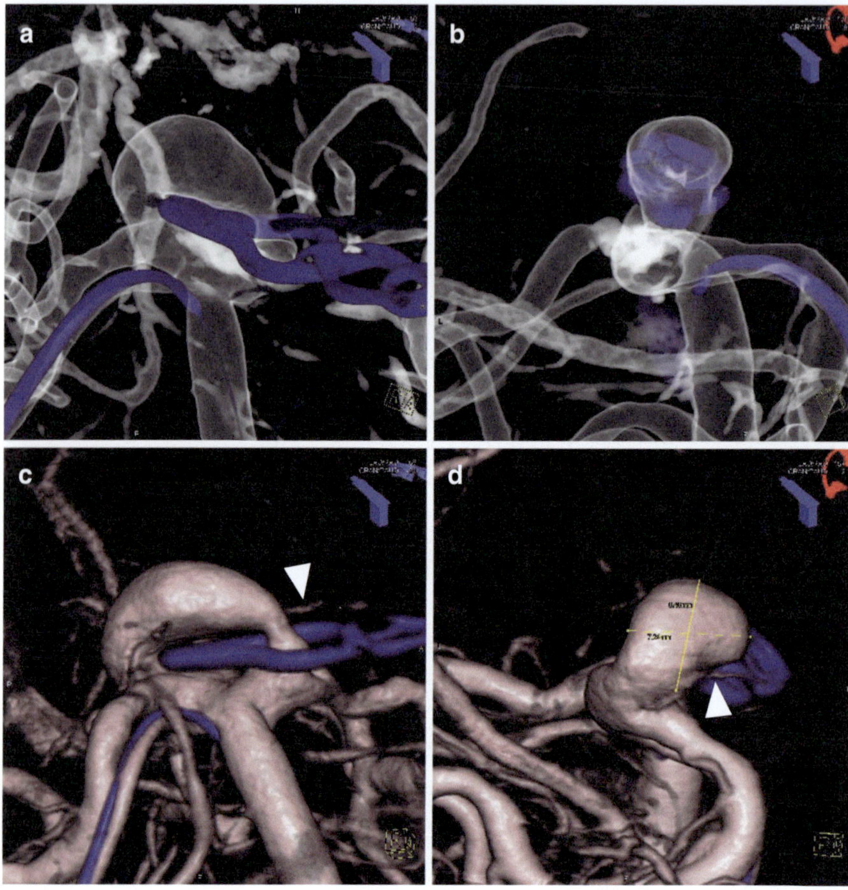

Fig. 17.6 Intraoperative angiogram. Anteroposterior (**a**) and lateral (**b**) views on intraoperative three-dimensional angiography showing dome clipping and aneurysm deformation. Ipsilateral (**c**) and contralateral (**d**) perforators were preserved at the ring of the clip and at the tip of the blade, respectively. The *arrowhead* indicates the perforators

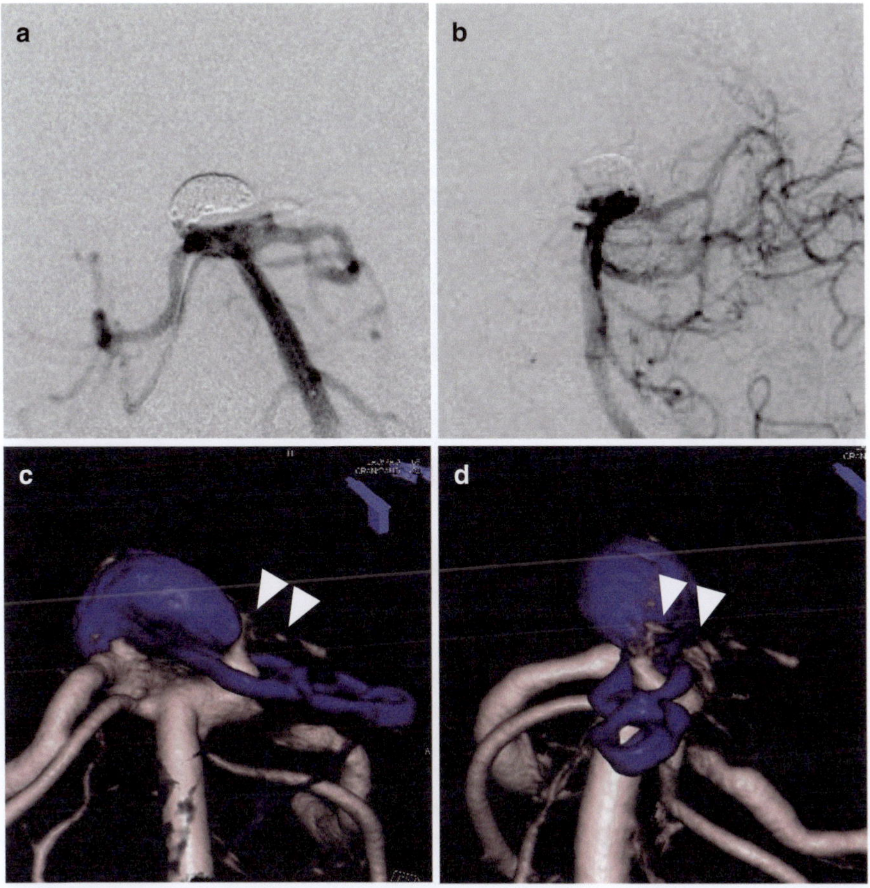

Fig. 17.7 Intraoperative angiogram. Anteroposterior (**a**) and lateral (**b**) views on intraoperative angiography showing complete obliteration of the aneurysm after coil embolization. AP (**a**) and lateral (**b**) views of intraoperative three-dimensional angiography showing dome clipping and aneurysm deformation. (**c**, **d**) The P1 perforator was preserved after coil embolization. Double *arrowheads* indicate the ipsilateral P1 perforator

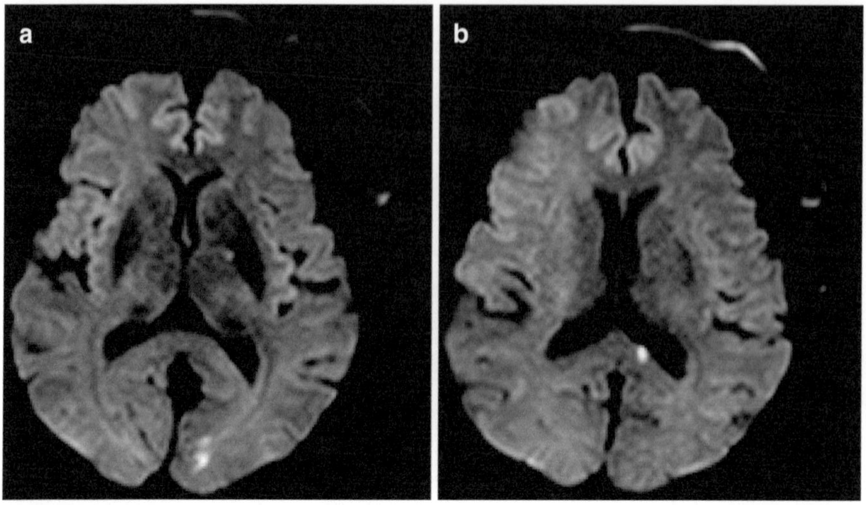

Fig. 17.8 Postoperative diffusion-weighted magnetic resonance image showing small infarctions in the left occipital lobe (**a**) and the splenium of the corpus callosum (**b**)

17.5 Conclusion

While the frequency of direct surgery for basilar tip aneurysms is decreasing, the need for safe and effective surgical treatments for difficult-to-treat aneurysms, including large or wide-necked aneurysms, is likely to continue. Surgeons with extensive experience in direct surgery for basilar aneurysms can exercise surgical judgment based on the experience; however, the number of direct surgeries performed is decreasing, limited surgeons' experience and making it difficult to rely on empirical rules. The orbitozygomatic approach and the anterior temporal approach are considered essential for the treatment of basilar tip aneurysms because these approaches allow the surgical field to be expanded to the maximum achievable. In addition, hybrid surgery, which incorporates the advantages of both endovascular and direct surgery and bypasses the limitations of both, is useful to improve surgical results.

References

1. Krisht AF, Krayenbuhl N, Sercl D, Bikmaz K, Kadri PA. Results of microsurgical clipping of 50 high complexity basilar apex aneurysms. Neurosurgery. 2007;60(2):242–50; discussion 50-2.
2. Krisht AF, Kadri PA. Surgical clipping of complex basilar apex aneurysms: a strategy for successful outcome using the pretemporal transzygomatic transcavernous approach. Neurosurgery. 2005;56(2 Suppl):261–73; discussion -73.
3. Lozier AP, Kim GH, Sciacca RR, Connolly ES Jr, Solomon RA. Microsurgical treatment of basilar apex aneurysms: perioperative and long-term clinical outcome. Neurosurgery. 2004;54(2):286–96; discussion 96-9.

4. Spiessberger A, Strange F, Fandino J, Marbacher S. Microsurgical clipping of basilar apex aneurysms: a systematic historical review of approaches and their results. World Neurosurg. 2018;114:305–16.
5. Choi E, Lee JY, Jeon HJ, Cho BM, Yoon DY. A hybrid operating room for combined surgical and endovascular procedures for cerebrovascular diseases: a clinical experience at a single centre. Br J Neurosurg. 2019;33(5):490–4.
6. Jeon HJ, Lee JY, Cho BM, Yoon DY, Oh SM. Four-year experience using an advanced interdisciplinary hybrid operating room: potentials in treatment of cerebrovascular disease. J Korean Neurosurg Soc. 2019;62(1):35–45.
7. Kurita H, Takeda R, Ikeda T, Kikkawa Y, Fushihara G, Ooigawa H, et al. Hybrid cerebrovascular surgery for complex cerebral aneurysms and arteriovenous malformations. Jpn J Neurosurg (Tokyo). 2015;24(3):173–9.
8. Murayama Y, Arakawa H, Ishibashi T, Kawamura D, Ebara M, Irie K, et al. Combined surgical and endovascular treatment of complex cerebrovascular diseases in the hybrid operating room. J Neurointerv Surg. 2013;5(5):489–93.
9. Bendok BR, Getch CC, Parkinson R, O'Shaughnessy BA, Batjer HH. Extended lateral transsylvian approach for basilar bifurcation aneurysms. Neurosurgery. 2004;55(1):174–8; discussion 8.
10. Drake CG. The treatment of aneurysms of the posterior circulation. Clin Neurosurg. 1979;26:96–144.
11. Hernesniemi J, Ishii K, Niemela M, Kivipelto L, Fujiki M, Shen H. Subtemporal approach to basilar bifurcation aneurysms: advanced technique and clinical experience. Acta Neurochir Suppl. 2005;94:31–8.
12. Samson DS, Hodosh RM, Clark WK. Microsurgical evaluation of the pterional approach to aneurysms of the distal basilar circulation. Neurosurgery. 1978;3(2):135–41.
13. Yasargil MG, Antic J, Laciga R, Jain KK, Hodosh RM, Smith RD. Microsurgical pterional approach to aneurysms of the basilar bifurcation. Surg Neurol. 1976;6(2):83–91.
14. Balasingam V, Noguchi A, McMenomey SO, Delashaw JB Jr. Modified osteoplastic orbitozygomatic craniotomy. Technical note. J Neurosurg. 2005;102(5):940–4.
15. Campero A, Martins C, Socolovsky M, Torino R, Yasuda A, Domitrovic L, et al. Three-piece orbitozygomatic approach. Neurosurgery. 2010;66(Suppl. 1):ons-E119–ons-E20.
16. Chanda A, Nanda A. Anatomical study of the orbitozygomatic transsellar-transcavernous-transclinoidal approach to the basilar artery bifurcation. J Neurosurg. 2002;97(1):151–60.
17. Kurita H, Ooigawa H, Takeda R, Nakajima H, Yoshikawa S, Otsuka M, et al. Clinical application of the orbitozygomatic approach in cerebrovascular surgery. Jpn J Neurosurg (Tokyo). 2012;21(11):842–7.
18. Tanikawa R, Wada H, Ishizaki T, Izumi N, Fujita C, Hashimoto M, et al. Anterior temporal approach for basilar bifurcation aneurysms as a modified distal transsylvian approach. Surg Cerebral Stroke. 1998;26(4):259–64.
19. Wongsuriyanan S, Sriamornrattanakul K. Anterior temporal approach for clipping of ruptured basilar tip aneurysms: surgical techniques and treatment outcomes. Surg Neurol Int. 2020;11:146.
20. Otani N, Toyooka T, Takeuchi S, Tomiyama A, Wada K, Mori K. Modified extradural temporopolar approach with mini-peeling of dura propria for paraclinoid and/or parasellar tumors: operative technique and nuances. Surg Neurol Int. 2017;8:199.
21. Zada G, Day JD, Giannotta SL. The extradural temporopolar approach: a review of indications and operative technique. Neurosurg Focus. 2008;25(6):E3.
22. Coscarella E, Baskaya MK, Morcos JJ. An alternative extradural exposure to the anterior clinoid process: the superior orbital fissure as a surgical corridor. Neurosurgery. 2003;53(1):162–6; discussion 6-7.
23. Sato S, Sato M, Oizumi T, Nishizawa M, Ishikawa M, Inamasu G, et al. Removal of anterior clinoid process for basilar tip aneurysm: clinical and cadaveric analysis. Neurol Res. 2001;23(4):298–303.

Author Index

Y. Kato, A. Ansari (eds.), *Cerebrovascular Surgery*, Advances and Technical Standards in Neurosurgery 44, https://doi.org/10.1007/978-3-030-87649-4

C

G

H

L

M

N

O

Q

R

S

T

Subject Index

Y. Kato, A. Ansari (eds.), *Cerebrovascular Surgery*, Advances and Technical Standards in Neurosurgery 44, https://doi.org/10.1007/978-3-030-87649-4

B

C

MIX
Papier aus verantwortungsvollen Quellen
Paper from responsible sources
FSC® C105338
FSC
www.fsc.org

If you have any concerns about our products,
you can contact us on
ProductSafety@springernature.com

In case Publisher is established outside the EU,
the EU authorized representative is:
Springer Nature Customer Service Center GmbH
Europaplatz 3, 69115 Heidelberg, Germany

Printed by Libri Plureos GmbH
in Hamburg, Germany

Emerging Topics in Statistics and Biostatistics

Emerging Topics in Statistics and Biostatistics (ETSB) showcases research and applications in statistics and biostatistics. It publishes books in statistical and biostatistical theory, applications, and education. Books may be monographs, edited volumes, textbooks and proceedings.

Tze-San Lee

Misclassification in Epidemiology

Springer

Tze-San Lee
Mathematics
Western Illinois University
Lilburn, GA, USA

ISSN 2524-7735 ISSN 2524-7743 (electronic)
Emerging Topics in Statistics and Biostatistics
ISBN 978-3-032-12562-0 ISBN 978-3-032-12563-7 (eBook)
https://doi.org/10.1007/978-3-032-12563-7

This Springer imprint is published by the registered company Springer Nature Switzerland AG
The registered company address is: Gewerbestrasse 11, 6330 Cham, Switzerland

Preface

This book summarizes my research on the misclassification present in a variety of epidemiological studies. Epidemiology has several designs of study, and misclassification appears differently in each of the designs.

After presenting a brief review in Chap. 1: "Introduction," the remainder of this book is divided into six parts: Part I focuses on the misclassification in cross-sectional studies and has one chapter: Chap. 2: "Risk Factor Is Misclassified." Part II concentrates on the misclassification in cohort studies and has three chapters: Chap. 3: "Disease Variable Is Misclassified," Chap. 4: "Estimation of Adjusted Relative Risk," and Chap. 5: "Both Disease and Exposure Variables Are Misclassified." Part III investigates the misclassification in case-control studies and has two chapters: Chap. 6: "One Exposure Variable Is Misclassified" and Chap. 7: "Two Misclassified Exposure Variables." Part IV covers hypothesis testing of no misclassification and has one chapter: Chap. 8: "No Misclassification." Part V addresses the misclassification in contingency tables and has one chapter: Chap. 9: "Misclassification in Two-Way Tables," and Part VI contains two chapters: Chap. 10: "Misclassification in Two Cohort Groups" and Chap. 11: "Latent Class Models for Misclassified Data." Two tables are included in the Appendix. This book could be used as a textbook for graduate students in medical school or for advanced undergraduate students majoring in statistics. It could also be used as a personal reference book for anyone interested in the research of misclassification in epidemiologic studies.

During the investigation and writing of this book, I benefited from the input of my former colleagues and my previous students. I would like to thank them for their suggestions and feedback. The section "Preliminary" is written based on the suggestions made by the book's associate editor and reviewers. I would also like to thank my wife for her understanding and support of my endeavors.

Lilburn, GA, USA Tze-San Lee

Competing Interests The author has no competing interests to declare that are relevant to the content of this manuscript.

Contents

List of Notations

$\tilde{RR}$	Adjusted estimator of RR
BF(D)	Bayes factor of the disease variable D
$B_g(\tilde{\mathfrak{X}}_{RD})$	Bayes factor in favor H_0 against H_1
$\widehat{RR}$	Better relative risk estimator of RR
$\tilde{CIR}$	Bias-adjusted cumulative confidence ratio
$\tilde{R}$	Corrected odds ratio
$CF(p)$	Counterfactual of probability p
$\tilde{\mathfrak{X}}_{RD}$	Estimator of evidence between $\tilde{\varepsilon}^2_{RD}$ and variance $\tilde{\sigma}^2_{\varepsilon_{RD}}$
$\tilde{\varepsilon}_{RD}$	Estimated prevalence difference between cases and controls
$E(\widehat{p})$	Expected value of the estimated value of the prevalence
$Effi(\tilde{p})$	Efficiency of total mean square estimator of $\tilde{p}$
φ	False negative probability
ψ	False positive probability
$\varphi_{ij}^{(k\ell)}$	False negative probability of the joint variables
$\psi_{ij}^{(k\ell)}$	False positive probability of the joint variables
RR^*	Observed relative risk
$\check{R}$	Observed odds ratio
$\check{p}_i$	Observed prevalence rate of the ith group
R	Odds ratio
$Pred_{0-}$	Predictive negative value in the exposure group
$Pred_{0+}$	Predictive positive value in the exposure group
ε_{RD}	Prevalence difference between cases and controls
Se_D	Sensitivity of the disease variable D
Sp_D	Specificity of the disease variable D
Se_E	Sensitivity of the exposure variable E
Sp_E	Specificity of the exposure variable E
B_g	The minimum Bayes factor
$mg(\tilde{\mathfrak{X}}_{RD})$	The posterior marginal probability density function of m_g

$\pi_{ABCDX_{ijk\ell t}}$	The probability of an individual at level (i,j,k,ℓ,t) with respect to the joint variables (A, B, C, D, X)
p_1	True prevalence of case group
p_0	True prevalence of control group
RR	True relative risk

List of Figures

List of Tables

Chapter 1
Introduction

1.1 Preliminary

Although Dr. Gustafson wrote a book titled, *Measurement Error and Misclassification in Statistics and Epidemiology* [4], he used a term "mismeasurement" to combine two scenarios when the explanatory variable is continuous or categorical. However, the method to deal with the categorical data is very different from that of the continuous variable. Moreover, he adopts a Bayesian approach to deal with mismeasurement error in the data. However, this book exclusively deals with the categorical data by non-Bayesian classical statistical methodology. Therefore, this book is entirely different from his book.

The way to collect the epidemiologic data is basically based upon two major categories of study design: observational and experimental studies. In an observational study, the investigator does not intervene but merely observes and assesses the strength of the relationship between the exposure and disease variables. Cohort, cross-sectional, and case-control studies are collectively referred to as observational studies. The definitions and examples are given in detail in Chapter 10 of my other book [5]. To save space, readers are referred to that book.

If asked to identify novel aspects of this book, I would like to start by noting that when the validation data is not available in case-control study, I introduce the idea of providing the counterfactual data modeling to the misclassified data in the main model so that we are able to compute the adjusted relative risk for the problem. See Sect. 6.2 for reference.

A second novel feature of this book is that I apply the Kolmogorov-Smirnov test to test the nondifferential misclassification assumption through the use of Youden's index upon the pair of points sitting on the exposure operating characteristic (EOC) curve. See Sect. 6.6 for details.

A third novel feature of this book is that we augment the misclassification parameter into the null hypothesis and then calculate the Bayes factor for no misclassification errors in a case-control study. Furthermore, we apply the idea of

T.-S. Lee, *Misclassification in Epidemiology*, Emerging Topics in Statistics and Biostatistics, https://doi.org/10.1007/978-3-032-12563-7_1

Bayes factor for testing no misclassification errors for general categorical data. See Sect. 8.2 for illustration.

This book should be accessible to graduate students, practitioners, and researchers in statistics and biostatistics as well as to epidemiologists with a particular interest in quantitative methods.

1.2 Historical Review

The effect of misclassification on the estimation and significance test was first studied by Bross [1]. It was pointed out that the misclassification has a more serious effect on estimation than on significance test. If the same classification system is used in two populations, then misclassification will not affect the validity of the significance test. Yet, misclassification tends to reduce the power of the test.

Suppose that a sample of n individuals is drawn randomly from a population. Let $0 < p < ½$ be the prevalence of a certain disease in the population and $q = 1 - p$ be the rate of non-disease in the population. Let ω_1 and ω_0 be the probability of misclassifying the disease case and non-disease case, respectively. As a result of misclassification, the estimated prevalence $\widehat{p}$ of disease cases will not in general be p as before. Instead, the expected value of $\widehat{p}$ will be [1]

$$E(\widehat{p}) = p(1 - \omega_1) + q\omega_0 = \mathcal{K}p \tag{1.1}$$

where $\mathcal{K} = 1 - \omega_1 + qp^{-1}\omega_0 = p(1 - \omega_1 - \omega_0) + \omega_0$. By Eq. (1.1), the adjusted estimator $\tilde{p}$ $(= \mathcal{K}^{-1}\widehat{p})$ is an unbiased estimator of p.

It can be shown that the variance of $\widehat{p}$ is

$$\sigma^2_{\widehat{p}} = nE(\widehat{p}) \cdot E(\widehat{q}) = npq\mathcal{K}', \tag{1.2}$$

where $E(\widehat{p})\cdot E(\widehat{q}) = [p(1-\omega_1-\omega_0)+\omega_0][q(1-\omega_1-\omega_0)+\omega_1] = pq\left[(1-\omega_1-\omega_0)^2 + \omega_1(1-\omega_1)q^{-1} + \omega_0(1-\omega_0)p^{-1}\right] = pq\mathcal{K}'$.

Remarks

1. If there is no misclassification, i.e., $\omega_1 = \omega_0 = 0$, then $\mathcal{K} = \mathcal{K}' = 1$.
2. If, as will usually be the case, ω_1 and ω_0 are small fractions whose square are negligible, then $\mathcal{K}'$is approximated by $\mathcal{K}''$ as

$$\mathcal{K}'' = 1 + \omega_1(q^{-1} - 2) + \omega_0(p^{-1} - 2). \tag{1.3}$$

3. The bias of $\widehat{p}$ is defined by using Eq. (1.1)

$$\text{Bias}(\widehat{p}) = E(\widehat{p}) - p = \mathcal{K}p - p = (\mathcal{K} - 1)p. \tag{1.4}$$

From Eq. (1.4), $\mathcal{K}$ is a measure of the relative bias. Under the above assumptions, the chief bias will arise from misclassification of the non-disease cases and the bias is getting progressively worse as p gets smaller and smaller. For example, if there is a 2% of misclassification in either ω_1 or ω_0 and the prevalence in the population is 5%, then by using Eq. (1.1)

$$\mathcal{K} = 1 - 0.02 + \left(\frac{0.95}{0.05}\right) \times 0.02 = 1.36.$$

Hence, from Eq. (1.4) the prevalence of the disease cases will be overestimated by 36%.

4. The misclassification not only introduces a bias but also affects the variance of the estimate. The quantity $\mathcal{K}'$ measures the effect of misclassification on the variance of the estimate; however, it is easier to see the effects of misclassification if the approximate quantity $\mathcal{K}''$ of Eq. (1.3) is examined. As p becomes smaller, the variance of $\widehat{p}$ tends to increase. The effect of misclassification of the disease cases is to reduce the variance of $\widehat{p}$. The effect of misclassification of the non-disease cases is to increase the variance and this effect increases as p becomes smaller and smaller. The efficiency of the adjusted $\tilde{p}$ is defined as the variance of the unbiased estimator $\widehat{p}$ divided by the total measure square error of $\tilde{p}$ as

$$Effi(\tilde{p}) = \frac{\sigma^2_{\widehat{p}}}{MSE(\tilde{p})} = \left(\mathcal{K}' + \frac{n(q\omega_0 - p\omega_1)^2}{pq}\right)^{-1}, \tag{1.5}$$

where $\sigma^2_{\widehat{p}} = npq$, and $MSE(\tilde{p}) = \sigma^2_{\tilde{p}} + (bias(\tilde{p}))^2$. Thus, in a sample of n $=100$ with $\omega_1 = \omega_0 = 0.05$ and p $= 0.1$, we have from using Eq. (1.5)

$$Effi(\tilde{p}) = (1.31 + 1.78)^{-1} = 0.3236 \approx 0.32.$$

A 32% efficiency implies that about $\frac{2}{3}$ of the original 100 observations are lost due to misclassification.

Our interest lies in the comparison of samples from two populations G_1 and G_2. Let

$$\breve{d} = \breve{p}_1 - \breve{p}_2 = \frac{x_1}{n_1} - \frac{x_2}{n_2}, \tag{1.6}$$

where $\tilde{p}_1$ and $\tilde{p}_2$ are the estimated prevalence of p_1 and p_2 from G_1 and G_2 with the observed number of x_1 and x_2 diseased cases and their sample size n_1 and n_2, respectively. If the same classification system has been used for G_1 and G_2,that is, the same misclassification probabilities are the same for two populations

($\omega_1 = \omega_2 = \omega$ and $\lambda_1 = \lambda_2 = \lambda$), then the expected value of Eq. (1.6) is under the null hypothesis ($p_1 = p_2 = p$)

$$E\left(\breve{d}\right) = E(\breve{p}_1) - E(\breve{p}_2) = \mathfrak{L}(p_1 - p_2) = 0, \tag{1.7}$$

where $\mathfrak{L}1 - \omega + qp^{-1}\lambda$, regardless whether there is misclassification or not. The variance of $\breve{d}$ under the null hypothesis is

$$\sigma_{\breve{d}}^2 = \frac{\sigma_{x_1}^2}{n_1} + \frac{\sigma_{x_2}^2}{n_2} = \frac{pq\mathfrak{L}'}{n_1} + \frac{pq\mathfrak{L}'}{n_2} = pq\mathfrak{L}'A, \tag{1.8}$$

where $A = n_1{}^{-1} + n_2{}^{-1}$, and $\mathfrak{L}' = (1 - \omega - \lambda)^2 + \omega(1 - \omega)q^{-1} + \lambda(1 - \lambda)p^{-1} - \omega\lambda(pq)^{-1}$.

Remark

Yet, the assumption that the misclassification probabilities are the same for two populations is not realistic in practical applications [2].

If the misclassification is altogether ignored, the unbiased estimated prevalence of p is

$$\breve{p} = \frac{x_1 + x_2}{n_1 + n_2} = \frac{x_1 + x_2}{N},$$

and the unbiased estimated variance of $\breve{d}$ is then given by

$$\breve{\sigma}_{\breve{d}}^2 = \frac{N}{N-1}\breve{p}\breve{q}A. \tag{1.9}$$

When misclassification occurs,

$$E(\breve{p}\breve{q}) = E(\breve{p}(1 - \breve{p})) = E(\breve{p}) - E\left(\breve{p}^2\right). \tag{1.10}$$

But

$$\sigma_{\breve{p}}^2 = \frac{pq\mathfrak{L}'}{N} = E\left(\breve{p}^2\right) - (E(\breve{p}))^2. \tag{1.11}$$

From Eq. (1.11), we solve for $E\left(\breve{p}^2\right)$

$$E\left(\breve{p}^2\right) = \frac{pq\mathfrak{L}'}{N} + \mathcal{K}^2p^2. \tag{1.12}$$

By substituting Eq. (1.12) into Eq. (1.10),

$$E(\breve{p}\breve{q}) = \mathcal{K}p(1 - \mathcal{K}p) - \frac{pq\mathfrak{L}'}{N}. \tag{1.13}$$

By substituting Eq. (1.13) into Eq. (1.9),

$$E\left(\breve{\sigma}_d^2\right) = \frac{N}{N-1}A\left\{\mathcal{K}p(1 - \mathcal{K}p) - \frac{pq\mathfrak{L}'}{N}\right\}. \tag{1.14}$$

While the actual variance is given by Eq. (1.8) and $\mathcal{K}p(1 - \mathcal{K}p) = pq\mathfrak{L}'$, Eq. (1.14) is reduced to

$$E\left(\breve{\sigma}_d^2\right) = pq\mathfrak{L}'A. \tag{1.15}$$

Equation (1.14) implies that $\breve{\sigma}_d^2$ is an unbiased estimate of σ_d^2. This means that the existence of misclassification does not affect the validity of a significance test based on d, and since the ordinary chi-square test is equivalent to a test based on d, it follows that the validity of the chi-square test is also not affected by ignoring misclassification. Although the tests are valid, the power may be drastically reduced [6]. In calculating the power of the test effectively, sample sizes of $(\mathfrak{L}')^{-1}$ times the actual sample sizes should be used. A table of the efficiency $(\mathfrak{L}')^{-1}$ for representative values of ω, λ, and p was obtained [1]. It shows that when the disease case is a rare event, the even small rates of ψ can result in the loss of half of the data. As far as the significance test is concerned, the effect of misclassification of disease cases is not very great, but estimates will be much more seriously affected by this kind of misclassification.

If the misclassification probabilities (ω_i, λ_i), $i = 1, 2$ are different for G_1 and G_2, the expected value of Eq. (1.6) under the null hypothesis is

$$E(d) = (\mathcal{K}_1 - \mathcal{K}_2)p = \omega_2 - \omega_1 + qp^{-1}(\lambda_1 - \lambda_2), \tag{1.16}$$

where $\mathcal{K}_i = 1 - \omega_i + q_i p_i^{-1}\lambda_i$. Unlike Eq. (1.7), Eq. (1.16) is no longer unbiased under the null hypothesis $H_0 : p_1 = p_2$, because it is for equal misclassification rates [4]. Under the assumption of two independent binomial samples, the variance of d is

$$\sigma_d^2 = \sigma_{\tilde{p}_1}^2 + \sigma_{\tilde{p}_2}^2 = \frac{p_1 q_1 \mathcal{K}_1'}{n_1} + \frac{p_2 q_2 \mathcal{K}_2'}{n_2}, \tag{1.17}$$

where $\mathcal{K}_i' = (1 - \omega_i - \lambda_i)^2 + \frac{\omega_i(1-\omega_i)}{q_i} + \frac{\lambda_i(1-\lambda_i)}{p_i} - \frac{\omega_i\lambda_i}{p_i q_i}$. Equation (1.16) shows that the expected bias of d depends both on the prevalence rates in both populations and the misclassification rates. From a limited numerical simulation, it is shown [3] that the difference between λ_1 and λ_2 is more important than that of the false negative rates ω_1 and ω_2 in determining the degree of bias for the range of prevalence considered. It produces severe bias in the estimate of the difference between two prevalence seen in the restricted range of the error rates. Under the alternative hypothesis $H_1 : p_1 \neq p_2$, the expected bias depends similarly on the error rates, and in addition, on the magnitudes of p_1 and p_2.

The aim of this book is to estimate the misclassification rates and to adjust the relative risk due to misclassification in epidemiological studies. In Chap. 2, the relative risk is adjusted on the exposure variable in cross-sectional study. In Chaps. 3, 4, and 5, the adjusted relative risk is derived due to the misclassification on the disease variable in cohort studies, while in Chap. 6, the adjusted odds ratio is obtained due to the misclassification on the exposure variable in case-control studies. A topic on two misclassified exposure variables is covered in Chap. 7. Hypothesis testing of no misclassification errors is given in Chap. 8. The misclassification of two-way table is studied in Chap. 9. The misclassification in other studies is mentioned in Chap. 10. Finally, the misclassified data for latent variables is outlined in Chap. 11.

References

1. Bross, I. (1954). Misclassification in 2 × 2 tables. *Biometrics, 10*, 478–486.
2. Copeland, K. T., Checkoway, H., McMichael, A. J., & Holbrook, R. H. (1977). Bias due to misclassification in the estimation of relative risk. *American Journal of Epidemiology, 105*, 488–495.
3. Goldberg, J. D. (1975). The effects misclassification on the bias in the difference between two populations and the relative odds in the fourfold table. *Journal of the American Statistical Association, 70*, 561–567.
4. Gustafson, P. (2004). *Measurement error and misclassification in statistics and epidemiology*. Chapman & Hall/CRC.
5. Lee, T.-S. (2021). *Medical statistics: A practical approach*. World Scientific Publishing.
6. Rubin, I., Rosenbaum, J., & Cobb, S. (1956). The use of interview data for the detection of association in field studies. *Journal of Chronic Diseases, 4*, 253–266.

Part I
Cross-Sectional Study

Chapter 2
Risk Factor Is Misclassified

Like cohort studies, cross-sectional studies conceptually begin with a population base. But unlike cohort studies, in cross-sectional studies we do not follow individuals over time. Instead, we only look at the prevalence of disease and/or exposure at one moment in time. Cohort studies begin by selecting a population of persons who are at risk for a specific disease or health outcome; cross-sectional studies also differ from cohort studies in the population studied. Cross-sectional studies begin by selecting a sample population and then obtaining data to classify all individuals in the sample as either having or not having the disease outcome. Let D denotes a disease variable (= 1 if an individual has the disease outcome, = 0 otherwise) and E be a risk factor (= 1 if he/she does not have E, = 0 otherwise). The result of distribution of cell frequencies with true classification or being misclassified is given in Table 2.1.

Two measure tools are given as follows. For acute disease studies, the risk $\mathcal{PR}$ (prevalence ratio) defined by [1]

$$\mathcal{PR} = \frac{a/n_1}{b/n_0} \tag{2.1}$$

Is the preferred measure of association, where a, c, n_1, and n_2 are given in Table 2.1. On the other hand, for chronic disease studies or studies of long-lasting risk factors, the prevalence odds ratio ($\mathcal{POR}$) defined by [1]

$$\mathcal{POR} = \frac{ad}{bc} \tag{2.2}$$

is the preferred measure of association.

For the misclassified data in Table 2.1, let the false negative and false positive probabilities of the misclassified exposure status are defined by

T.-S. Lee, *Misclassification in Epidemiology*, Emerging Topics in Statistics and Biostatistics, https://doi.org/10.1007/978-3-032-12563-7_2

Table 2.1 Distribution of cell frequencies with correct classification or with misclassification on the exposure variable

cc	Correct classification			Misclassification	
	D = 1	D = 0		$D = 1$	$D = 0$
E = 1	a	b	$E^* = 1$	a^*	b^*
E = 0	c	d	$E^* = 0$	c^*	d^*
	n_1	n_0		n_1^*	n_0^*

where E^* is the classified surrogate of E

$$\gamma = \Pr(E^* = 0|E = 1), \tag{2.3}$$

and

$$\delta = \Pr(E^* = 1|E = 0). \tag{2.4}$$

The cell frequencies under misclassification may be expressed in terms of the true cell frequencies and the false negative and false positive rate of the classification procedure as follows:

$$a^* \approx E(a^*) = (1 - \gamma) \cdot a + \delta \cdot c, \tag{2.5}$$

$$b^* \approx E(b^*) = (1 - \gamma) \cdot b + \delta \cdot d, \tag{2.6}$$

$$c^* \approx E(c^*) = (1 - \delta) \cdot c + \gamma \cdot a, \tag{2.7}$$

and

$$d^* \approx E(d^*) = (1 - \delta) \cdot d + \gamma \cdot b. \tag{2.8}$$

By using Eq. (2.5) and the cell frequencies given in Table 2.1, the adjusted relative prevalence of Eq. (2.1) is given by

$$\widehat{\mathcal{PR}} = \frac{n_0(a^* - n_1\delta)}{n_1(b^* - n_0\delta)}. \tag{2.9}$$

By using Eqs. (2.5) to (2.8), the adjusted prevalence odds ratio of Eq. (2.2) is given by

$$\widehat{\mathcal{POR}} = \frac{(a^* - n_1\delta)(d^* - n_0\gamma)}{(b^* - n_0\delta)(c^* - n_1\gamma)}. \tag{2.10}$$

Remarks

1. The diagnostic test is well defined if $\gamma + \delta < 1$. The background rate of disease does not appear in Eq. (2.9). In addition, the effect of misclassification of risk factor on $\widehat{\mathcal{POR}}$ depends on the relative and not on the absolute disease rates.
2. The bias of Eq. (2.9) depends δ only. But, as can be seen from Flegal et al. [2], the value of Eq. (2.10) depends on the individual values of γ and δ rather than on their sum unless $\gamma + \delta = 1$.

Table 2.2 The data of true disease status and Pap smear status

Observed risk factor (Pap smear)	True disease status		
	D = 1	D = 0	Total
$E^* = 1$	406	2394	2800
$E^* = 0$	289	1911	2200
Total	695	4305	5000

Example 2.1
Suppose that, in cross-sectional study, the incidence of cervical cancer in 5000 women, classified by marital status and the diagnostic criterion used is the Pap smear which is known as imperfect. Imagine that the observed data are given in Table 2.2 [3].

Find the observed and adjusted relative risk $\mathcal{POR}$ and $\widehat{\mathcal{POR}}$.

Solution
Since cervical cancer is a long-term disease, we have to use the observed prevalence odds ratio Eq. (2.2) and its estimator Eq. (2.10) given respectively by

$$\mathcal{POR} = \frac{406 \cdot 1911}{289 \cdot 2394} = 0.89. \tag{2.11}$$

The validity of the Pap smear test was studied by using biopsy as the validation criterion. Since 4 out of 48 cases proved cervical cancer [4], a pair of the false negative rate and false positive rate was estimated as $\gamma = 0.21$ (= 10/48) and $\delta = 0.19$ (= 9/48). After substituting the above information into Eq. (2.10), the better estimate of the true relative risk is given by using Eq. (2.1)

$$\widehat{\mathcal{POR}} = \frac{(406 - 695 \cdot 0.19)(1911 - 4305 \cdot 0.21)}{(2394 - 4305 \cdot 0.19)(289 - 695 \cdot 0.21)} \approx 1.22 \tag{2.12}$$

Indeed, the value of Eq. (2.12) is much larger than the observed Eq. (2.11).

References

1. Alexander, L. K., Lopes, B., Ricchetti-Masterson, K., & Yeatts, K. B. (2009). *ERIC notebook* (Fundamentals of epidemiology course lectures 2009–2013) (2nd ed.). The University of North Carolina at Chapel Hill.
2. Flegal, K. M., Brownie, C., & Haas, J. D. (1986). The effects of exposure misclassification on estimates of relative risk. *American Journal of Epidemiology, 123*, 736–751.
3. Rogan, W. J., & Gladen, B. (1978). Estimating prevalence from the results of a screening test. *American Journal of Epidemiology, 107*, 71–76.
4. Shy, C. M, Kleinbaum, D. G, Morgenstern, H. (1978). The effect of misclassification of exposure in epidemiological studies of air pollution health effects, *Bulletin of New York Academy of Medicine, 54*: 1155–1165

Part II
Cohort Study

Chapter 3
Disease Variable Is Misclassified

Consider a misclassification on the disease (D) status that occurs in a cohort study, where D = 1 if a subject is diseased, = 0 otherwise; E = 1 if a subject is exposed, = 0 otherwise. The observed findings are given in Table 3.1.

In theory, the observed relative risk ($\widehat{RR}$) is given by

$$\widehat{RR} = \frac{\frac{a}{a+b}}{\frac{c}{c+d}} = \frac{an_0}{cn_1}. \tag{3.1}$$

From Table 3.2, the observed relative risk ($\widehat{RR}$) can be calculated as follows:

$$\widehat{RR} = \frac{a^* n_0}{c^* n_1}. \tag{3.2}$$

The exposed (E = 1) and unexposed (E = 0) subjects from Table 3.1 can be theoretically classified into diseased (D = 1) and disease-free (D = 0) as given in Table 3.3. In this table,

e_1 = number of exposed subjects correctly classified as D = 1;
f_1 = number of exposed subjects incorrectly classified as D = 1;
g_1 = number of exposed subjects incorrectly classified as D = 0;
h_1 = number of exposed subjects correctly classified as D = 0;
e_0 = number of unexposed subjects correctly classified as D = 1;
f_0 = number of unexposed subjects incorrectly classified as D = 1;
g_0 = number of unexposed subjects incorrectly classified as D = 0;
h_0 = number of unexposed subjects correctly classified as D = 0;

Let the false-negative probability (φ_i) and false-positive probability (ψ_i) of the incorrectly classified procedure of the diseased status in the exposed (E = 1) and unexposed (E = 0) be defined by (i = 1, 0)

T.-S. Lee, *Misclassification in Epidemiology*, Emerging Topics in Statistics and Biostatistics, https://doi.org/10.1007/978-3-032-12563-7_3

Table 3.1 Original cell frequencies in a cohort study

		Disease status		
Exposure status		$D = 1$	D = 0	Total
	E = 1	a	b	n_1
	E = 0	c	d	n_0

Table 3.2 Misclassified cell frequencies in a cohort study

		Disease status	
Exposure status		$D^* = 1$	$D^* = 0$
	E = 1	a^*	b^*
	E = 0	c^*	d^*

Table 3.3 Results of misclassification: interrelation between observed and true cell frequencies

	Actual disease status					
	E = 1			E = 0		
Classified disease status	D = 1	D = 0	Total	D = 1	D = 0	Total
$D^* = 1$	e_1	f_1	a^*	e_0	f_0	c^*
$D^* = 0$	g_1	h_1	b^*	g_0	h_0	d^*
Total	a	b	n_1	c	d	n_0

D^* is the misclassified random variable of the diseased status

$$\varphi_i = \Pr(D^* = 1|D = 0, E = i), \tag{3.3}$$

and

$$\psi_i = \Pr(D^* = 0|D = 1, E = i). \tag{3.4}$$

Case 1 Assume that nondifferential misclassification exists between the exposed and unexposed groups, that is

$$\varphi_1 = \varphi_0 \equiv \varphi = \frac{f_1}{b} = \frac{f_0}{d}, \tag{3.5}$$

and

$$\psi_1 = \psi_0 \equiv \psi = \frac{g_1}{a} = \frac{g_0}{b}. \tag{3.6}$$

It then follows that

$$a^* \approx E(a^*) = e_1 + f_1 = (1 - \psi) \cdot a + \varphi \cdot b, \tag{3.7}$$

$$b^* \approx E(b^*) = g_1 + h_1 = \psi \cdot a + (1 - \varphi) \cdot b, \tag{3.8}$$

$$c^* \approx E(c^*) = e_0 + f_0 = (1 - \psi) \cdot c + \varphi \cdot d, \tag{3.9}$$

$$d^* \approx E(d^*) = g_0 + h_0 = \psi \cdot c + (1 - \varphi) \cdot d. \tag{3.10}$$

To find the estimate of the true relative risk, we need only to solve for a and c. By substituting $b = n_1 - a$ into Eq. (3.7) and solving for a

$$a = \frac{a^* - n_1\varphi}{1 - (\varphi + \psi)}, \tag{3.11}$$

where $\varphi + \psi < 1$ and $a^* > n_1\varphi$.

Similarly, we solve, respectively, b, c, and d from Eqs. (3.8), (3.9) and (3.10)

$$b = \frac{b^* - n_1\psi}{1 - (\varphi + \psi)}, \tag{3.12}$$

$$c = \frac{c^* - n_0\varphi}{1 - (\varphi + \psi)}, \tag{3.13}$$

and

$$d = \frac{d^* - n_0\psi}{1 - (\varphi + \psi)}, \tag{3.14}$$

where $\varphi + \psi < 1$, $b^* > n_1$, $c^* > n_0\varphi$, and $d^* > n_0\psi$.

By substituting Eqs. (3.11) and (3.13) into Eq. (3.2), the better estimate ($\widetilde{RR}$) of the adjusted relative risk is given by

$$\widetilde{RR} = \frac{n_0(a^* - n_1\varphi)}{n_1(c^* - n_0\varphi)}. \tag{3.15}$$

Remarks

1. In the calculation of $\widetilde{RR}$, the misclassification probability of ψ is not needed.
2. In cohort studies, the bias is primarily on the false-negative rate and increases with disease rarity [2].

Example 3.1

Suppose that the observed data in a cohort study are given in Table 3.4. Note that the misclassification is nondifferential because the false-negative rate ($\varphi = \frac{8}{40} = \frac{4}{20} = 0.2$) and false positive rate ($\psi = \frac{6}{60} = \frac{8}{80} = 0.1$) are the same for both population A and B.

Find the observed and adjusted relative risk, $\widehat{RR}$ and $\widetilde{RR}$, of the study.

Solution

From Table 3.4, the observed relative risk is obtained by using Eq. (3.1)

Table 3.4 Observed data in a cohort study

	Actual status					
	Population A			Population B		
Classified status	D = 1	D = 0	Total	D = 1	D = 0	Total
$D^* = 1$	32	6	38	16	8	24
$D^* = 0$	8	54	62	4	72	76
Total	40	60	100	20	80	100

$$\widehat{RR} = \frac{38/100}{24/100} = 1.6. \tag{3.16}$$

By substituting $a^* = 38$, $c^* = 24$, $n_1 = n_2 = 100$, $\varphi = 0.2$, and $\psi = 0.1$ into Eq. (3.15),

$$\widetilde{RR} = \frac{100[38 - 100 \cdot 0.2]}{100[24 - 100 \cdot 0.2]} = 4.5. \tag{3.17}$$

Note that the adjusted estimate of Eq. (3.17) is greater than that of Eq. (3.16) as confirmed by the above remark 2.

On the other hand, if the misclassification is differential, we have

From Table 3.3,

$$\varphi_1 = \frac{f_1}{b}; \quad \varphi_0 = \frac{f_0}{d}; \text{and } \psi_1 = \frac{g_1}{a}, \quad \psi_0 = \frac{g_0}{c}. \tag{3.18}$$

It then follows that

$$a^* = a \cdot (1 - \psi_1) + b \cdot \varphi_1, \tag{3.19}$$

$$b^* = a \cdot \psi_1 + b \cdot (1 - \varphi_1), \tag{3.20}$$

$$c^* = c \cdot (1 - \psi_0) + d \cdot \varphi_0, \tag{3.21}$$

$$d^* = c \cdot \psi_0 + d \cdot (1 - \varphi_0). \tag{3.22}$$

Solving Eqs. (3.19) and (3.21), respectively, for a and c,

$$a = \frac{a^* - n_1\varphi_1}{\Delta_1}, \tag{3.23}$$

and

$$c = \frac{c^* - n_0\varphi_0}{\Delta_0}, \tag{3.24}$$

where $\Delta_i = 1 - \varphi_i - \psi_i > 0$, $i = 0, 1$.

By substituting Eqs. (3.23) and (3.24) into Eq. (3.2), the better estimate of the true relative risk is given by

$$\check{RR} = \frac{n_0 \Delta_0 [a^* - n_1 \varphi_1]}{n_1 \Delta_1 [c^* - n_0 \varphi_0]}. \tag{3.25}$$

Remark

Unlike the case of nondifferential misclassification, the ratio of $\check{RR}$ to RR^* could be either greater or less than one.

Example 3.2

Over the 8-year period from 1947 to 1954, 5617 women were studied at the Johns Hopkins Hospital by cervical smear, vaginal smear, and biopsy. An Ayre spatula was employed to obtain the smears by the standard technique. Biopsy specimens were taken from at least each of four quadrants of the cervix at the squamocolumnar junction with a punch biopsy forceps.

Of the total of 5617 women, 4785 had a normal smear and biopsy, while 216 were given a diagnosis of cervical cancer by both smear and biopsy. The incidence of doubtful smears was 376, of false positive smears 124, and of false-negative smears 35, unsatisfactory smears 321, and positive smear correct with negative biopsy incorrect 10 (Table 3.3) [2]. Of the 376 women with doubtful smears, 45 were shown to have cancer in the corresponding biopsy. An additional 77 of the women with doubtful smears was shown histologically to have some degree of basal cell hyperactively that necessitated follow-up studies.

Find the observed and adjusted relative risk, $\widehat{RR}$ and $\widetilde{RR}$, of the study.

Solution

From the given information, we have $g_1 = 216$, $h_1 = 4785$, $g_0 = 45$, $h_0 = 77$. Assume that the misclassification is nondifferential, i.e., $\varphi_1 = \varphi_0 = \varphi$ and $\psi_1 = \psi_0 = \psi$. By substituting the given information into Table 3.3, we have from Eqs. (3.5) and (3.6)

$$\varphi = 0.022 = \frac{f_1}{4785 + f_1}, \tag{3.26}$$

and

$$\psi = 0.006 = \frac{e_1}{216 + e_1}, \tag{3.27}$$

By solving Eqs. (3.26) and (3.27) for e_1 and f_1,

$$e_1 = 13.08 \cong 13, \quad f_1 = 106.3 \cong 106. \tag{3.28}$$

Similarly, we have

$$e_0 = 0.302 \cong 0.3, \quad f_0 = 0.465 \cong 0.47. \tag{3.29}$$

From Table 3.3 and Eqs. (3.28) and (3.29),

$$n_1 = a^* + b^* = 13 + 106 + 4785 + 106 = 5120$$

and

$$n_0 = c^* + d^* = 0.3 + 0.47 + 45 + 77 = 122.77 \cong 123 \tag{3.30}$$

By using Eq. (3.1), the observed relative risk is given

$$\widehat{RR} = \frac{123 \cdot 119}{5120 \cdot 0.77} = 3.71 \approx 3.7. \tag{3.31}$$

One can calculate the adjusted estimate of the true relative risk by using Eq. (3.15)

$$\widetilde{RR} = \frac{123 \cdot [119 - 5120 \cdot 0.022]}{5120 \cdot [0.77 - 123 \cdot 0.022]} = -\frac{787.2}{9728} \approx -0.08. \tag{3.32}$$

Remark
Clearly, from Eq. (3.32), the adjusted relative risk is a negative number indicates that the assumption of nondifferential assumption is inappropriate.

References

1. Bross, I. (1954). Misclassification in 2 × 2 tables. *Biometrics, 10*, 478–486.
2. Nesbitt, R. E. L., & Brack, C. B. (1956). Role of cytology in detection of carcinoma of cervix. *Journal of the American Medical Association, 161*, 183–188.

Chapter 4
Estimation of Adjusted Relative Risk

In epidemiologic studies of risk factors for coronary artery disease, cases are identified by overt manifestation of myocardial ischemia. The diagnostic may be validated by angiographic examination of the coronary arteries in symptomatic subjects. Currently, there is no comparable means for determining the presence or absence of significant atherosclerosis of the coronary arteries in asymptomatic subjects.

If disease frequency is small, the adjusted relative risk may be approximated by a function of the predictive value of a positive classification only.

4.1 Sensitivity and Specificity for the Adjusted Relative Risk

Consider a cohort study in which a dichotomous exposure variable (E) for a given factor is determined for each individual at the start of the study period and a dichotomous disease variable (D) is determined at the end of that period. The true disease-exposure frequencies are given in Table 4.1.

Let π_1 and π_0 be, respectively, denote the true disease incidence (or prevalence) of the exposed (E = 1) and unexposed (E = 0) population. The true relative risk of the exposed to unexposed is

$$RR = \frac{\Pr(D=1|E=1)}{\Pr(D=1|E=0)} = \frac{\Pr(D|E)}{\Pr(D|\overline{E})} = \frac{\pi_1}{\pi_0}, \tag{4.1}$$

where (D, $\overline{D}$) and (E, $\overline{E}$) are the abbreviation of (D = 1, D = 0) and (E = 1, E = 0).

Let the sensitivity (Se) and the specificity (Sp) of the classification procedure be defined by [1]

T.-S. Lee, *Misclassification in Epidemiology*, Emerging Topics in Statistics and Biostatistics, https://doi.org/10.1007/978-3-032-12563-7_4

Table 4.1 Distribution of original disease-exposure frequencies according to exposure and disease status

		Exposure status		
Disease status		E = 1	E = 0	Total
	D = 1	a	b	$a + b$
	D = 0	c	d	$c + d$
	Total	$a + c$	$b + d$	n

Where $n = a + b + c + d$

Table 4.2 Distribution of observed disease-exposure frequencies according to exposure and disease status

	E = 1		E = 0		
Observed disease status	D = 1	D = 0	D = 1	D = 0	Total
$D^* = 1$	a*	b*	e^*	f^*	$e^* + f^*$
$D^* = 0$	c*	d*	g^*	h^*	$g^* + h^*$
Total	a	c	b	d	$b + d$

Where D* and E* are the misclassified surrogates of D and E

$$\begin{aligned} \text{Se} &= \Pr(D^*|D), \text{ and} \\ \text{Sp} &= \Pr\left(\overline{D^*}|\overline{D}\right). \end{aligned} \tag{4.2}$$

Results of misclassified cell frequencies are given in Table 4.2.

Let π_1^* and π_0^* denote, respectively, the observed disease prevalence of the exposed and unexposed samples. It is assumed that the misclassification is nondifferential. Then, the observed relative risk is given by

$$\begin{aligned} RR^* &= \frac{\Pr(D^*=1|E=1)}{\Pr(D^*=1|E=0)} = \frac{Se\pi_1 + (1-Sp)(1-\pi_1)}{Se\pi_0 + (1-Sp)(1-\pi_0)} \\ &= \frac{1 - Sp + RR\pi_0(\nabla - 1)}{Se\pi_0 + (1-Sp)(1-\pi_0)}, \end{aligned} \tag{4.3}$$

where $\nabla = \varphi + \psi$.

Re-expressing Eq. (4.3) in terms of Eq. (4.1),

$$\text{RR} = \frac{\{\widehat{RR} - (1-Sp)/\left[Se\pi_0 + (1-Sp)\left(1-\pi_0\right)\right]\}}{\{1 - (1-Sp)/[Se\pi_0 + (1-Sp)(1-\pi_0)]\}}. \tag{4.4}$$

4.2 Predictive Values for Adjusted Relative Risk

Now the predictive values of a positive test result in the unexposed population are given, respectively, by[1]

$$Pred_{0+} = \Pr\left(D|D^*\overline{E}\right) = \frac{Se\pi_0}{Se\pi_0 + (1 - Sp)(1 - \pi_0)}, \tag{4.5}$$

and

$$1 - Pred_{0+} = \frac{(1 - Sp)(1 - \pi_0)}{Se\pi_0 + (1 - Sp)(1 - \pi_0)}. \tag{4.6}$$

By substituting Eqs. (4.6) into Eq. (4.4), the adjusted relative risk given by

$$\widetilde{RR} = \frac{\widehat{RR} - \left[1 - Pred_{0+}(1 - \pi_0)^{-1}\right]}{1 - (1 - \pi_0)^{-1} Pred_{0+}}, \tag{4.7}$$

is completely defined by the predictive value in the unexposed group only and the observed relative risk this reflects the assumption of nondifferential nature of the misclassification procedure.

Remarks

1. When the disease prevalence is low in the unexposed populations relative to the predictive value of a positive test, then the following approximation is reasonable.

$$1 - (1 - \pi_0)^{-1} Pred_{0+} = 1 - Pred_{0+}.$$

Thus, from Eq. (4.7), we have

$$\widetilde{RR} = Pred_{0+}^{-1}\left(\widehat{RR} - 1 + Pred_{0+}\right). \tag{4.8}$$

2. A general formula for relative bias in the relative risk is derived as follows.

$$Bias\left(\widehat{RR}\right) = \frac{\widetilde{RR} - \widehat{RR}}{\widehat{RR}}. \tag{4.9}$$

By substituting Eq. (4.7) into Eq. (4.9) and simplifying,

$$Bias\left(\widehat{RR}\right) = \frac{\left(\widehat{RR} + 1\right) Pred_{0+}}{1 - \pi_0 - Pred_{0+}}. \tag{4.10}$$

Example 4.1

In a cohort study of 1000 subjects (of whom 500 were smokers) to evaluate the relative risk associated with cigarette smoking and coronary atherosclerosis. The diagnosis of myocardial infarction that was recorded as the underlying cause of death was considered to be indicative of significant coronary artery disease. Subjects

Table 4.3 Distribution of 1000 study subjects according to true and classified coronary atherosclerosis and smoking status

	Actual disease status					
Classified disease status	Smokers			Nonsmokers		
	D = 1	D = 0	Total	D = 1	D = 0	Total
$D^* = 1$	–	–	40	14	6	20
$D^* = 0$	–	–	460	–	–	480
Total	–	–	500	–	–	500

Where "–" indicates that information is either unavailable for these cells or not needed for the computation of $\tilde{RR}$

who died from other causes and those alive at the end of the study were regarded as being free of coronary artery disease. Misclassification would occur by missing those subjects with atherosclerosis who did not die from "probable myocardial infarction" (false-negatives) and by including some cases incorrectly classified as coronary artery disease (false-positives). At the end of the study period, 60 deaths from coronary artery disease were recorded, of whom 20 were nonsmokers. On the postmortem examination of the nonsmokers, 14 were found to have significant atherosclerosis of the coronary arteries. For the adjustment of relative risk, postmortem information on the deaths of smokers is not required. Sufficient information on the behavior of the classification procedure is contained in validation of cases in either one of the exposed or unexposed groups, provided that misclassification is nondifferential as assumed. The results of the study are given in Table 4.3.

(a) Find the adjusted relative risk.
(b) Find the relative bias of $\widehat{RR}$.

Solution

(a) By using Eq. (4.1), the observed relative risk of coronary atherosclerosis for smokers is given by

$$\widehat{RR} = \frac{40/500}{20/500} = 2. \tag{4.11}$$

The predictive value of a positive response (i.e., death recorded due to coronary artery disease) in the nonsmokers is given by

$$Pred_{0+} = \frac{14}{20} = 0.7. \tag{4.12}$$

When one assumes that prevalence of the coronary artery atherosclerosis in the nonsmokers is low relative to the predictive value, the adjusted relative risk is calculated by using Eq. (4.8)

Table 4.4 Distribution of 1000 study subjects according to overt manifestations of coronary artery disease, coronary angiography, and serum cholesterol levels

Overt manifestations of coronary artery disease	Coronary angiography (> 200 mg/dl)			Coronary angiography (≤ 200 mg/dl)		
	D	$\overline{D}$	Total	D	$\overline{D}$	Total
D*	?#	?	75	15	15	30
$\overline{D^*}$	?	?	425	?	?	470
Total	?	?	500	?	?	500

Where "#" indicates that information is either unavailable for these cells or not needed for the computation of $\tilde{RR}$

$$\widetilde{RR} = \frac{2 - 1 + 0.7}{0.7} = 2.43. \tag{4.13}$$

(b) By substituting Eqs. (4.11) and (4.12) into Eq. (4.10), the relative bias of RR^* is given by

$$Bias(RR^*) = \frac{(2+1) \times 0.7}{1 - 0.04 - 0.7} = 8.0769 \approx 8.08. \tag{4.14}$$

Thus, by using Eq. (4.14) the relative bias of $\widehat{RR}$ is 8.08 in the positive direction.

Example 4.2

In a population survey to evaluate the association between serum cholesterol and coronary atherosclerosis, 1000 subjects were screened. Among them, 105 individuals had a history of angina pectoris or nonfatal myocardial infarction. These were classified as cases of coronary artery disease, and the remainder of the subjects as non-cases. Of the 500individuals who had serum cholesterol levels above 220 mg/l, 75 were classified as cases of coronary artery disease. Coronary angiograph was carried out on all classified coronary artery disease cases. In the 30 cases of coronary artery disease in whom serum cholesterol was less than 220 mg/dl, 15 were found to have significant atherosclerosis of the coronary arteries. The results are given in Table 4.4.

Find the adjusted relative risk for those with low coronary angiography.

Solution

From Table 4.4, The observed relative risk of coronary atherosclerosis for those with elevated serum cholesterol is

$$RR^* = \frac{75/500}{30/500} = 2.5. \tag{4.15}$$

The predictive value of a positive response in the unexposed group is given by

$$Pred_{0+} = \frac{15}{30} = 0.5. \tag{4.16}$$

Thus, the adjusted relative risk when one assumes low disease frequency in those with serum cholesterol below 200 mg/dl is given by

$$\widetilde{RR} = \frac{2.5 - 1 + 0.5}{0.5} = 4.0. \tag{4.17}$$

Note that the angiography information in the exposed group was not necessary for adjustment of the relative risk since the misclassification was assumed to be nondifferential.

Reference

1. Green, M. S. (1983). Use of predictive value to adjust relative risk estimates biased by misclassification of outcome status. *American Journal of Epidemiology, 117*, 98–105.

Chapter 5
Both Disease and Exposure Variables Are Misclassified

For example, we might want to compare coronary disease rates among smokers and nonsmokers or among diabetes or nondiabetics [2]. There can be error not only in classifying subjects according to presence of coronary disease but also in classifying subjects according to presence of diabetics (the exposure).

If there were no misclassification errors, Table 5.1 is a descriptive table of the sample:

The observed table allows for the various misclassification errors is given by Table 5.2.

The misclassification matrices of D*|D and E*|E are the conditional probabilities given, respectively, by

$$\mathcal{U} = \left[u_{ij}\right]_{i,j=0,1} = \begin{bmatrix} u_{11} & u_{10} \\ u_{01} & u_{00} \end{bmatrix}, \tag{5.1}$$

and

$$\mathcal{V} = \left[v_{ij}\right]_{i,j=0,1} = \begin{bmatrix} v_{11} & v_{10} \\ v_{01} & v_{00} \end{bmatrix}, \tag{5.2}$$

where u_{ij} and v_{ij} are defined, respectively, by

$$u_{ij} = \Pr(D^* = j|D = i),$$

and

$$v_{ij} = \Pr(E^* = j|E = i).$$

The relationship between the true and observed sample matrix is given by [1].

T.-S. Lee, *Misclassification in Epidemiology*, Emerging Topics in Statistics and Biostatistics, https://doi.org/10.1007/978-3-032-12563-7_5

Table 5.1 No misclassification errors are present

Status	E = 1	E = 0	Total
D = 1	p_{11}	p_{10}	p_{1+}
D = 0	p_{01}	p_{00}	p_{0+}
Total	p_{+1}	p_{+0}	p_{++}

Note, D and E denote the disease and the exposure variables, respectively.

Table 5.2 The observed data that allow for the various misclassification errors

Status	$E^* = 1$	$E^* = 0$	Total
$D^* = 1$	p_{11}^*	p_{10}^*	p_{1+}^*
$D^* = 0$	p_{01}^*	p_{00}^*	p_{0+}^*
Total			

Where D^* and E^* are misclassified variables of D and E, respectively.

$$\mathcal{P}^* = \mathcal{U}^T \mathcal{P} \mathcal{V}, \tag{5.3}$$

where $\mathcal{P}$ and $\mathcal{P}^*$ are given, respectively, by entries in Tables 5.1 and 5.2

$$\mathcal{P} = \begin{bmatrix} p_{11} & p_{10} \\ p_{01} & p_{00} \end{bmatrix},$$

and

$$\mathcal{P}^* = \begin{bmatrix} p_{11}^* & p_{10}^* \\ p_{01}^* & p_{00}^* \end{bmatrix}.$$

Solving for $\mathcal{P}$ from Eq. (5.3), the adjusted prevalence matrix is given by

$$\tilde{\mathcal{P}} = \left(\mathcal{U}^T\right)^{-1} \mathcal{P}^* \mathcal{V}^{-1}, \tag{5.4}$$

where $\mathcal{U}$ and $\mathcal{V}$ are assumed to be nonsingular.

The observed and adjusted prevalence of D with respect to E are given by using entries in Tables 5.1 and 5.2

$$\vec{p} = [p_1 \ p_0]^T = \begin{bmatrix} \frac{p_{11}}{p_{1+}} & \frac{p_{10}}{p_{0+}} \end{bmatrix}^T, \tag{5.5}$$

and

$$\vec{p}^{\,*} = [p_1^* \ p_0^*]^T = \begin{bmatrix} \frac{p_{11}^*}{p_{1+}^*} & \frac{p_{10}^*}{p_{0+}^*} \end{bmatrix}^T, \tag{5.6}$$

Table 5.3 The observed sample data between Hypertension (E^*) and endometrial cancer (D^*)

	$D^* = 1$	$D^* = 0$	Total
$E^* = 1$	0.11	0.07	0.18
$E^* = 0$	0.22	0.6	0.82
Total	0.33	0.67	1.00

while the observed and adjusted relative risk of D, $\widehat{RR}$, and $\tilde{}RR$, with respect to E are similarly defined by using Eqs. (5.5) and (5.6)

$$RR = \frac{p_1}{p_0}, \tag{5.7}$$

and

$$\tilde{}\mathcal{RR} = \frac{p_1^*}{p_0^*}. \tag{5.8}$$

Remark
The sampling errors in Table 5.2 are ignored in setting up Eq. (5.3).

Example 5.1
A study on the natural history of adenocarcinoma of the endometrium was resulted in the following observed sample matrix $\mathcal{P}^*$ given by the following table [1].

The misclassification matrix of hypertension was shown by [3]

$$\mathcal{U} = \begin{bmatrix} 0.9 & 0.1 \\ 0.02 & 0.98 \end{bmatrix}. \tag{5.9}$$

The method of ascertainment of endometrial cancer has a misclassification matrix $\mathcal{V}$ given by [3]

$$\mathcal{V} = \begin{bmatrix} 0.95 & 0.05 \\ 0.02 & 0.98 \end{bmatrix}. \tag{5.10}$$

From Table 5.3, the observed sample matrix of D with respect to E is given by

$$\mathcal{P}^* = \begin{bmatrix} 0.11 & 0.07 \\ 0.22 & 0.6 \end{bmatrix}. \tag{5.11}$$

Since $\det(\mathcal{U}) = 0.88$ and $\det(\mathcal{V}) = 0.93$ are not zero, both the inverse of $\mathcal{U}^T$ and $\mathcal{V}$ exist. Their inverses are given by

$$\left(\mathcal{U}^T\right)^{-1} = \begin{bmatrix} 1.1136 & -0.0227 \\ -0.1136 & 1.0227 \end{bmatrix}, \tag{5.12}$$

and

$$\mathcal{V}^{-1} = \begin{bmatrix} 1.0538 & -0.0538 \\ -0.0215 & 1.0215 \end{bmatrix}. \tag{5.13}$$

By substituting Eqs. (5.11) to (5.13) into Eq. (5.4),

$$\tilde{\mathcal{P}} = \left(\mathcal{U}^T\right)^{-1}\mathcal{P}^*\mathcal{V}^{-1} = \begin{bmatrix} 0.1224 & 0.0594 \\ 0.2109 & 0.6073 \end{bmatrix}$$

By using Eqs. (5.5) and (5.6), the observed and adjusted prevalence of D with respect to E are

$$\vec{p} = \begin{bmatrix} p_1 & p_0 \end{bmatrix}^T = \left[\frac{0.11}{0.11 + 0.22} \quad \frac{0.07}{0.07 + 0.6}\right]^T = \begin{bmatrix} 0.3333 & 0.1045 \end{bmatrix}^T, \tag{5.14}$$

and

$$\tilde{\vec{p}}^* = \left[\frac{0.1224}{0.1224 + 0.2109} \quad \frac{0.0594}{0.0594 + 0.6073}\right]^T = \begin{bmatrix} 0.3673 & 0.0891 \end{bmatrix}^T, \tag{5.15}$$

By substituting Eqs. (5.14) and (5.15) into Eqs. (5.7) and (5.8), the observed and adjusted relative risk are

$$\widehat{RR} = \frac{0.3333}{0.1045} = 3.1895 \approx 3.19. \tag{5.16}$$

and

$$\tilde{RR} = \frac{0.3673}{0.0891} = 4.1223 \approx 4.12. \tag{5.17}$$

Remarks

1. In computing the inverse of Eqs. (5.12) and (5.13), we apply the inverse formula "MINVERSE" provided in the EXCEL spreadsheet.
2. To solve the issue posed in this chapter, there is another approach provided by Gullen et al. (1968) [4].

References

1. Barron, B. A. (1977). The effect of misclassification on the estimation of relative risk. *Biometrics, 33*, 414–418.
2. Cohen, C. J., & Gusberg, S. B. (1975). Screening for endometrial cancer. *Clinical Obstetrics and Gynecology, 8*, 27–40.
3. Gullen, W. H., Bearman, J. E., & Johnson, E. A. (1968). Effects of misclassification in epidemiologic studies. *Public Health Reports (1896–1970), 83*, 914–918.
4. Karvonen, M. J., Telvivo, L. J., & Jarvinem, E. J. (1964). Sphygmonanometer cuff size and the accuracy of indirect measurement of blood pressure. *American Journal of Cardiology, 13*, 688.

Part III
Case-Control Study

Chapter 6
One Exposure Variable Is Misclassified

6.1 Parameter Estimation

6.1.1 True Misclassification Rates Are Given

Assume that a fourfold table in a case-control study is exposed to the risk factor X and the disease factor Y is not misclassified as shown in Table 6.1.

In Table 6.1, p_1 and p_0 denote the true unknown prevalence rate of the cases and controls, respectively.

As a measure of the relative risk in case-control study, the odds ratio is given by

$$R = \frac{p_1 q_0}{p_0 q_1}. \tag{6.1}$$

If the observed X is misclassified, say as X^* as given in Table 6.2, then it is well known that the observed prevalence rate $\widehat{p}_i$ in Table 6.2 is no longer an unbiased estimator for the true unknown prevalence rate p_i in Table 6.1.

Let the misclassification error (false negative and false positive) probability φ_i and ψ_i be defined, respectively, by

$$\varphi_i = \Pr(X^* = 0 | X = 1, Y = i), \tag{6.2}$$

and

$$\psi_i = \Pr(X^* = 1 | X = 0, Y = i). \tag{6.3}$$

In term of the misclassification error probabilities of Eqs. (6.2) and (6.3), it is easily shown [2] (Exercise 6.7-1) that

T.-S. Lee, *Misclassification in Epidemiology*, Emerging Topics in Statistics and Biostatistics, https://doi.org/10.1007/978-3-032-12563-7_6

Table 6.1 The true distribution of the exposure status of the case and control groups

		Group of subjects	
		Y = 1 (cases)	Y = 0 (controls)
True exposure status	X = 1	p_1	p_0
	X = 0	q_1	q_0
Total		1.0	1.0

Where X = 1 if a subject is truly exposed, 0 otherwise, $\sum_{i=0}^{1}(p_i + q_i) = 1$

Table 6.2 The distribution of the misclassified exposure status of the case and control groups

		Group of subjects	
		Y = 1 (cases)	Y = 0 (controls)
Observed exposure status	$X^* = 1$ (present)	$\widehat{p}_1$	$\widehat{p}_0$
	$X^* = 0$ (absent)	$\widehat{q}_1$	$\widehat{q}_0$
	Total	1.0	1.0

Where $X^* = 1$ if a subject is wrongly classified as exposed, 0 otherwise; $\sum_{i=0}^{1}(\widehat{p}_i + \widehat{q}_i) = 1$

$$E(\widehat{p}_i) = p_i \Delta_i + \psi_i. \tag{6.4}$$

where Δ_i is defined by

$$\Delta_i = 1 - \varphi_i - \psi_i. \tag{6.5}$$

Remark
From Eq. (6.4), $\widehat{p}_i$ is never an unbiased estimator of p_i unless the method of classification is perfect, namely, $\varphi_i = \psi_i = 0$, i = 0, 1.

Let n_i denote the sample size of the case and control group in Table 6.2. If $n_i\widehat{p}_i$ is assumed to follow a binomial distribution with mean $n_i[p_i\Delta_i + \psi_i]$, the variance of $\widehat{p}_i$, i = 0, 1 is given by

$$\sigma^2_{\widehat{p}_i} = \frac{(p_i\Delta_i + \psi_i)(q_i\Delta_i + \varphi_i)}{n_i}. \tag{6.6}$$

As a consequence, the estimated odds ratio given by

$$\widehat{R} = \frac{\widehat{p}_1\widehat{q}_0}{\widehat{p}_0\widehat{q}_1}, \tag{6.7}$$

is a biased estimator for the true relative risk R of Eq. (6.1). a corrected odds ratio is thus derived as follows.

By using Eq. (6.4) and an approximation $E(\widehat{p}_i) \approx \widehat{p}_i$, we obtain

$$\widehat{p}_i \approx p_i\Delta_i + \psi_i. \tag{6.8}$$

Solving Eq. (6.8) for p_i, we have the so-called bias-adjusted prevalence estimate

$$\tilde{p}_i \approx \frac{\widehat{p}_i - \psi_i}{\Delta_i}. \tag{6.9}$$

Since $\tilde{p}_i$ of Eq. (6.9) is a probability, it has to be positive. As a result, φ_i, ψ_i and Δ_i have to satisfy the following inequalities for $i = 0, 1$

$$\psi_i < \widehat{p}_i, \tag{6.10}$$

$$\varphi_i < \widehat{q}_i, \tag{6.11}$$

and

$$\varphi_i + \psi_i < 1. \tag{6.12}$$

It is easily shown (Exercise 6.7-2) that Eq. (6.9) is an unbiased estimator of p_i, provided that φ_i and ψ_i are given. Further, the variance of Eq. (6.9) is given by, for $i = 0, 1$

$$\sigma^2_{\tilde{p}_i} = \frac{\sigma^2(\widehat{p}_i)}{\Delta_i^2} = \frac{(p_i\Delta_i + \psi_i)(q_i\Delta_i + \varphi_i)}{n_i\Delta_i^2}. \tag{6.13}$$

After substituting Eq. (6.9) for p_i in Eq. (6.1), the adjusted odds ratio that accounts for the misclassification errors is given by

$$\tilde{R} = \frac{(\widehat{p}_1 - \psi_1)(\widehat{q}_0 - \varphi_0)}{(\widehat{q}_1 - \varphi_1)(\widehat{p}_0 - \psi_0)}. \tag{6.14}$$

The standard error of Eq. (6.14) is obtained indirectly by taking the logarithmic transformation of Eq. (6.14) and using the independence between the sample errors of the cases and the controls [8, 11]. The approximate standard error of $\ln(\tilde{R})$ is given by (Exercise 6.7-3)

$$\sigma_{\ln(\tilde{R})} = \sqrt{\sum\nolimits_{i=0}^{1}\left\{\sigma^2(\widehat{p}_i)\left[\frac{1}{(p_i - \psi_i)^2} + \frac{1}{(q_i - \varphi_i)^2}\right]\right\}}, \tag{6.15}$$

where p_i is the true unknown prevalence rate, $q_i = 1 - p_i$, and Δ_i is given by Eq. (6.5).

Remarks

1. In practical applications, the true unknown p_i and q_i have to be replaced by their estimators $\widehat{p}_i$ and $\widehat{q}_i$ $(= 1 - \widehat{p}_i)$.
2. Equation (6.15) is similar to that of Eq. (19.5) in Rothman-Greenland (1998) [23] except that their expressions are expressed in absolute frequency.
3. By using Eq. (6.1), the bias between the logarithm of $\tilde{R}$ of Eq. (6.14) and R of Eq. (6.1) is given by (Exercise 6.7-3)

$$\text{bias}\left(ln\,\tilde{R}\right) \equiv \ln\left(\frac{\tilde{R}}{R}\right) = \frac{1}{2}\left[\frac{\sigma^2(\widehat{p}_1)(p_1 - q_1)}{(p_1 q_1)^2} + \frac{\sigma^2(\widehat{p}_0)(q_0 - p_0)}{(p_0 q_0)^2}\right] \tag{6.16}$$

Remark

However, when φ_i and ψ_i are unknown and replaced by their estimators $\widehat{\varphi}_i$ and $\widehat{\psi}_i$, Eq. (6.9) becomes

$$\widehat{\tilde{p}}_i = \frac{\widehat{p}_i - \widehat{\psi}_i}{1 - \widehat{\varphi}_i - \widehat{\psi}_i}. \tag{6.17}$$

Since Eq. (6.17) is a function of three random variables, let

$$g(\widehat{p}_i, \widehat{\varphi}_i, \widehat{\psi}_i) = \frac{\widehat{p}_i - \widehat{\psi}_i}{1 - \widehat{\varphi}_i - \widehat{\psi}_i}. \tag{6.18}$$

By using the delta method [1], the approximate variance of Eq. (6.18) is given by i = 0, 1

$$\sigma^2_{\widehat{\tilde{p}}_i} = \left(n_i \Delta_i^2\right)^{-1} \cdot diag\left[(p_i\Delta_i + \psi_i)(q_i\Delta_i + \varphi_i), \frac{\varphi_i\overline{\varphi}_i(\psi_i - p_i)^2}{\Delta_i^2}, \frac{\psi_i\overline{\psi}_i(\varphi_i - q_i)^2}{\Delta_i^2}\right], \tag{6.19}$$

where $\overline{\varphi}_i = 1 - \varphi_i$ and $\overline{\psi}_i = 1 - \psi_i$.

By using the estimator $\widehat{\tilde{p}}_i$ of Eq. (6.17), the 100·(1 − α)% confidence interval for p_i is given by

$$\widehat{\tilde{p}}_i - z_{1-\frac{\alpha}{2}} \cdot \widehat{\sigma}_{\widehat{\tilde{p}}_i} \le p_i \le \widehat{\tilde{p}}_i + z_{1-\frac{\alpha}{2}} \cdot \widehat{\sigma}_{\widehat{\tilde{p}}_i}, \tag{6.20}$$

where $z_{1-\frac{\alpha}{2}}$ is the $100\cdot(1 - \frac{\alpha}{2})$ percentile of the standard normal distribution, and $\widehat{\sigma}_{\widehat{\tilde{p}}_i}$ is given by taking the square root of Eq. (6.19) with replacing the unknown φ_i and ψ_i, with their corresponding estimators of $\widehat{\varphi}_i$ and $\widehat{\psi}_i$.

Similarly, the corrected odds ratio estimator is given by

$$\widehat{\tilde{R}} = \frac{\widehat{\tilde{p}}_1 \widehat{\tilde{q}}_0}{\widehat{\tilde{p}}_0 \widehat{\tilde{q}}_1}, \tag{6.21}$$

where $\widehat{\tilde{p}}_i$ is given by Eq. (6.17), and $\widehat{\tilde{q}}_i = 1 - \widehat{\tilde{p}}_i$. The approximate standard error of $\ln\left(\widehat{\tilde{R}}\right)$ is given by

$$\sigma_{\ln\left(\widehat{\tilde{R}}\right)} = \sqrt{\sum_{i=0}^{1} \left[\frac{\sigma^2_{\widehat{p}_i} + \sigma^2_{\widehat{\psi}_i}}{(\mathrm{p}_i - \psi_i)^2} + \frac{\sigma^2_{\widehat{p}_i} + \sigma^2_{\widehat{\varphi}_i}}{(q_i - \varphi_i)^2} + \frac{2\left(\widehat{\varphi}_i^2 + \widehat{\psi}_i^2\right)}{\Delta_i^2} \right]}. \tag{6.22}$$

In order to use Eqs. (6.21) and (6.22), we need the estimator of the unknown φ and ψ. This issue will be addressed later in Sect. 6.4.

6.1.2 Misclassification Error Rates Are Estimated

Let's now turn our attention to another scenario. Suppose that patients of three type have been assessed for presence or absence of a risk factor Z, where Z = 1 if present; = 0 if absent. There are two clinics A and B. In Clinic A, a sample of n_1 diseased patients ("cases") includes x_1 who report Z = 1, while a sample of n_2 asymptomatic patients ("controls") includes x_2 who report that Z = 1 in a different Clinic B. We suppose that the data have also been collected on a third group of n_3 + n_4 patients who were interviewed in both clinics. Of n_3 patients reporting Z = 1 in Clinic B, y_1 also report having Z = 1 in Clinic A, while of n_4 patients reporting to have Z = 0 in Clinic B, y_2 report having Z = 1 in Clinic A. Assume that the true state to be that reported in Clinic B, so y_2 is the number of false positive results in Clinic A, and $n_3 - y_1$ is the number of false negatives. We wish to estimate the ratio of the disease prevalence among those with Z = 1 to the disease prevalence among those without it, taking into account the unreliable reporting in Clinic A. We do this in terms of true and false positive rates in clinic A, obtained from the data on individuals who have attended both clinics. Let p_1 and p_2 be the probabilities for controls and cases, respectively, that an individual would have reported Z = 1 had that individual being interviewed in Clinic B. Let p_3 and p_4 be the true and false positive rates, respectively, for Clinic A. The four random variables x_1, x_2, y_1, and y_2 are distributed as follows [5]: (Exercise 6.7-4)

$$\begin{aligned} x_1 &\sim \mathit{Binomial}(n_1, \pi_1), \\ x_2 &\sim \mathit{Binomial}(n_2, p_2), \\ y_1 &\sim \mathit{Binomial}(n_3, p_3), \text{ and} \\ y_2 &\sim \mathit{Binomial}(n_4, p_4), \end{aligned} \tag{6.23}$$

where $\pi_1 = p_1 p_3 + (1 - p_1) p_4$.

The likelihood function $\mathcal{L}(p_1, p_2, p_3, p_4)$ is given by the two separate likelihood functions

$$\mathcal{L} = \pi_1{}^{x_1}(1-\pi_1)^{n_1-x_1} \cdot p_2^{x_2}(1-p_2)^{n_2-x_2} p_3^{y_1}(1-p_3)^{n_3-y_1} \cdot p_4^{y_2}(1-p_4)^{n_4-y_2}. \quad (6.24)$$

By taking the partial derivatives of the logarithm of Eq. (6.24),

$$\frac{\partial \ln(\mathcal{L})}{\partial p_1} = \frac{\partial \ln(\mathcal{L})}{\partial \pi_1}\frac{\partial \pi_1}{\partial p_1} = \frac{x_1(p_3-p_4)}{\pi_1} + \frac{(n_1-x_1)(p_4-p_3)}{1-\pi_1}, \quad (6.25)$$

$$\frac{\partial \ln(\mathcal{L})}{\partial p_2} = \frac{x_2}{p_2} - \frac{n_2-x_2}{1-p_2}. \quad (6.26)$$

$$\frac{\partial \ln(\mathcal{L})}{\partial p_3} = \frac{y_1}{p_3} - \frac{n_3-y_1}{1-p_3}, \quad (6.27)$$

$$\frac{\partial \ln(\mathcal{L})}{\partial p_4} = \frac{y_2}{p_4} - \frac{n_4-y_2}{1-p_4}, \quad (6.28)$$

By setting Eqs. (6.26) to (6.28) equal to zero, the maximum likelihood estimator of p_2 p_3, and p_4 gives

$$\widehat{p}_2 = \frac{x_2}{n_2}. \quad (6.29)$$

$$\widehat{p}_3 = \frac{y_1}{n_3}, \quad (6.30)$$

and

$$\widehat{p}_4 = \frac{y_2}{n_4}, \quad (6.31)$$

By substituting Eqs. (6.30) and (6.31) into Eq. (6.25) and setting it equal to zero,

$$\widehat{p}_1 = \frac{x_1 - n_1\widehat{p}_4}{n_1(\widehat{p}_3 - \widehat{p}_4)}, \quad (6.32)$$

provided that $n_1\widehat{p}_4 < x_1$, $\widehat{p}_3 > \widehat{p}_4$. Now the odds ratio $\theta = \frac{p_1 q_2}{p_2 q_1}$ is estimated as

$$\widehat{\theta} = \frac{\widehat{p}_1 \cdot \widehat{q}_2}{\widehat{p}_2 \cdot \widehat{q}_1}, \quad (6.33)$$

where $\widehat{p}_1$ and $\widehat{p}_2$ are given, respectively, by Eqs. (6.32) and (6.29), $\widehat{q}_i = 1 - \widehat{p}_i$.

The estimated variance of the logarithm of Eq. (6.33) is given by [1]

$$\widehat{\sigma}^2_{\ln\left(\widehat{\theta}\right)} = n_{11}^{-1} + n_{12}^{-1} + n_{21}^{-1} + n_{22}^{-1}, \tag{6.34}$$

where $n_{11} = n_1 \cdot \widehat{p}_1$, $n_{12} = n_1 \cdot \widehat{q}_1$, $n_{21} = n_2 \cdot \widehat{p}_2$, and $n_{22} = n_2 \cdot \widehat{q}_2$.

By using the estimator $\widehat{\theta}$ of Eq. (6.33), the 100·(1 − α)% confidence interval for θ is given by

$$\exp\left[\ln\left(\widehat{\theta}\right) - z_{1-\frac{\alpha}{2}}\widehat{\sigma}_{\ln\left(\widehat{\theta}\right)}\right] \le \exp\left[\ln\left(\widehat{\theta}\right) + z_{1-\frac{\alpha}{2}}\widehat{\sigma}_{\ln\left(\widehat{\theta}\right)}\right], \tag{6.35}$$

where $\widehat{\sigma}_{\ln\left(\widehat{\theta}\right)}$ is the square root of Eq. (6.34).

Example 6.1

In an epidemiological study of risk factors in breast cancer, data were available on 236 confirmed cases from a diagnostic clinic and on 2692 asymptomatic controls from screening clinic that sampled the general population [7]. The records were also available 167 women (mostly with benign breast disease and therefore not qualifying for either the case or control groups), who had attended both clinics within a 6-month period. These records showed considerable evidence of bias between clinics. The fact that most of this bias took the form of consistently negative reporting in the diagnostic clinic (Clinic A) indicating that the interviewers in the screening clinic (Clinic B) were more thorough in recording information. Moreover, the staff of the diagnostic clinic were mainly males, whereas the staff of the screening clinic were all female, suggesting the possibility of more candid responses attending the screening clinic. It was therefore decided to regard the screening clinic responses as the correct ones. One of the interesting results of these data is the assessment of the married state. The data for married individuals are given in Table 6.3.

Table 6.3 provides a surprisingly large bias in favor of status being reported as married in the diagnostic clinic; this is probably explained by the fact that women at this clinic were recorded as married 'by default' when the interviewer had not ascertained their married status explicitly. If the data on bias between clinics were ignored, a straightforward relative risk estimation from Table 6.3 would yield a relative risk estimate, associated with married state, of

$$\theta^* = \frac{205 \cdot 674}{31 \cdot 2288} = 1.948032 \approx 1.95. \tag{6.36}$$

By using Eq. (6.36), the 95% confidence interval for θ is given by

$$1.32 \le \theta \le 2.87. \tag{6.37}$$

By substituting the data given in Table 6.3 into Eqs. (6.29) to (6.31),

Table 6.3 Cases and controls of married and unmarried women plus women attending both clinics

Case-control study data			Women attending both clinics		
	Cases	Controls	Clinic A response	Clinic B response	
Married	205	2288		Yes	No
Not married	31	674	Yes	120	18
			No	4	25

$$\begin{aligned}
\widehat{p}_2 &= \frac{2288}{2962} = 0.7725 \approx 0.77,\\
\widehat{p}_3 &= \frac{120}{124} = 0.967742 \approx 0.97,\\
\widehat{p}_4 &= 1 - \text{true negative} = 1 - \frac{25}{43} = 0.4186 \approx 0.42, \text{and}\\
\widehat{p}_1 &= \frac{205 - 236 \cdot 0.42}{236(0.97 - 0.42)} = 0.8182 \approx 0.82.
\end{aligned} \tag{6.38}$$

By substituting Eq. (6.38) into Eq. (6.33),

$$\widehat{\theta} = \frac{0.82 \cdot (1 - 0.77)}{(1 - 0.82) \cdot 0.77} = 1.3607 \approx 1.36. \tag{6.39}$$

By substituting Eq. (6.38) into Eq. (6.34), the variance of Eq. (6.38) is

$$\sigma^2_{\ln\left(\widehat{\theta}\right)} = (236 \cdot 0.82)^{-1} + (236 \cdot 0.18)^{-1} + (2962 \cdot 0.77)^{-1} + (2962 \cdot 0.23)^{-1} = 0.1918. \tag{6.40}$$

By substituting Eqs. (6.38) and (6.39) into Eq. (6.35),

$$\exp\left[\ln(1.36) - 1.96 \cdot \sqrt{0.1918}\right] \leq \theta \leq \exp\left[\ln(1.36) + 1.96 \cdot \sqrt{0.1918}, \text{or}\, 0.37 \leq \theta \leq 4.89.\right. \tag{6.41}$$

From Eqs. (6.37) and (6.41), we find that the tendency for women to be recorded as married in in the diagnostic clinic when they would not be so in the screening clinic is after being adjusted for the misclassification rates.

Remarks

1. The only assumption made in the analysis is that the probability of a positive response in the "case" environment, conditional on the response in the "control" environment, is the same in the population of cases as in the population of those attending both clinics. There seems having no obvious reason to doubt it, even though no data are available to check this assumption.

2. Obviously, the use of this bias-corrected method is not limited to the situation where the procedures used for the controls are the reliable ones. Little alteration is required to use the method when the procedures of the cases' clinic are more reliable.

6.2 Comparison of Two Prevalence Rates

Let us consider a comparison of two true prevalence rates between the cases and the controls when the sample data are misclassified. The following three pairs of hypotheses are set up:

$$\begin{aligned}&\text{Case i} \quad H_0 : p_1 = p_0 \text{ versus } H_1 : p_1 \neq p_0;\\&\text{Case ii} \quad H_0 : p_1 = p_0 \text{ versus } H_1 : p_1 \geq p_0;\\&\text{Case iii} \quad H_0 : p_1 = p_0 \text{ versus } H_1 : p_1 \leq p_0.\end{aligned} \tag{6.42}$$

Suppose that the sample data is wrongly classified as given in Table 6.2. By letting the difference between p_1 and p_0 be defined by

$$d = p_1 - p_0. \tag{6.43}$$

The unbiased estimator of d is given by

$$\widehat{d} = \widehat{p}_1 - \widehat{p}_0. \tag{6.44}$$

Definition 6.1
A misclassification is said to be nondifferential if the misclassification error rates are the same for both cases and controls, that is, $\varphi_1 = \varphi_0 = \varphi$ and $\psi_1 = \psi_0 = \psi$; otherwise, it is said to be differential.

If the misclassification is nondifferential, the result follows.

Theorem 6.1
If the misclassification is nondifferential in which $\varphi + \psi < 1$, then the expected value of the difference between classical prevalence estimates are biased toward the null value in the hypothesis testing.

Proof
By using the fact that $\varphi_1 = \varphi_0 = \varphi$ and $\psi_1 = \psi_0 = \psi$, we have by applying Eq. (6.45)

$$E(\widehat{p}_1 - \widehat{p}_0) = (1 - \varphi - \psi)(p_1 - p_0). \tag{6.45}$$

Since $\varphi + \psi < 1$, it follows from Eq. (6.45) that on the average the difference between classical prevalence estimate is always less than that of the true prevalence rate.

Remark

The expected value of the difference between bias-adjusted prevalence estimates is exactly equal to that of the true unknown prevalence rate, provided that the misclassification error probabilities are given.

The variance of $\widehat{d}$ is given by

$$\sigma^2_{\widehat{d}} = \sum\nolimits_{i=0}^{1} \sigma^2_{\widehat{p_i}} = \sum\nolimits_{i=0}^{1} \frac{\sigma^2_{\widehat{p_i}}}{\Delta_i^2}, \tag{6.46}$$

where Δ_i and $\sigma^2_{\widehat{p_i}}$ and are given, respectively, by Eqs. (6.5) and (6.6). The testing statistic for Eq. (6.42) is given by

$$z_{\widehat{d}} = \frac{\widehat{d}}{\sigma_{\widehat{d}}}, \tag{6.47}$$

where $\widehat{d}$ is given by Eq. (6.44) and $\sigma_{\widehat{d}}$ is the positive square root of Eq. (6.46).

If the misclassification is nondifferential, the decision rule for testing Eq. (6.42) is given as follows.

Decision Rule (DR) 6.1

For all three tests below, the significance level is α.

(i) A two-tailed test for Case i of Eq. (6.42) is to reject H_0 if the computed $z_{\widehat{d}}$ of Eq. (6.47) is greater than $z_{1-\frac{\alpha}{2}}$ or less than

$$z_{\frac{\alpha}{2}}. \tag{6.48}$$

(ii) A right-tailed test for Case ii of Eq. (6.42) is to reject H_0 if the computed $z_{\widehat{d}}$ of Eq. (6.47) is greater than

$$z_{1-\frac{\alpha}{2}}. \tag{6.49}$$

(iii) A left-tailed test for Case iii of Eq. (6.42) is to reject H_0 if the computed $z_{\widehat{d}}$ of Eq. (6.47) is less than

$$z_{\frac{\alpha}{2}}. \tag{6.50}$$

Remarks

1. If the sample sizes for the cases and the controls are large enough ($n_i \geq 30$), the sampling distribution of Eq. (6.47) is a standard normal distribution, provided that φ_i and ψ_i are known. Otherwise, they have to be replaced, respectively, by their estimators $\widehat{\varphi}_i$ and $\widehat{\psi}_i$. If the classification method is the diagnostic test, $\widehat{\varphi}_i = 1 - Se$ and $\widehat{\psi}_i = 1 - Sp$, where *Se* and *Sp* are the sensitivity and specificity of the diagnostic test.
2. If the sample sizes are small ($n_i < 30$), the sampling distribution of Eq. (6.47) is a t-distribution with the appropriate degree of freedom.

Example 6.2

A study of the validity of statement concerning the circumcision status was conducted because of an interest in epidemiological studies of the cancer of cervix in which the lack of circumcision was suggested as being etiological importance. This possibility is illustrated with data reported by Wynder [27] in his study on the relationship of circumcision to cancer of the cervix. The effect of misclassification on inferences was stimulated by the results of a study made on a consecutive series of 192 male patients admitted to the Roswell Park Memorial Institute was concerned with a Table 6.4 comparison of their statements concerning their circumcision status and physical examination findings [6] (Table 6.4).

Since the probabilities of the diagonal entries given in Table 6.4 are not one, it is obvious that the data are somewhat misclassified. It is reasonable to assume that the data of examination findings are accurate without errors, but the data of patient's statement are misclassified. Thus, the probabilities of misclassification, the rates of false negative (φ) and false positive (ψ), can be estimated from Table 6.4 as

$$\widehat{\varphi} = 1 - \textit{sensitivity} = 1 - \frac{37}{84} = 0.5595 \approx 0.56, \tag{6.51}$$

and

$$\widehat{\psi} = 1 - \textit{specificity} = 1 - \frac{89}{108} = 0.1759 \approx 0.18, \tag{6.52}$$

where the sampling errors are ignored in Eqs. (6.51) and (6.52).

Table 6.4 Comparison of patients' statements with examination findings concerning their circumcision status

	Patients' statements		
Examination findings	Circumcised	Not circumcised	Total
Circumcised	37	47	84
Not circumcised	19	89	108
Total	56	136	192

On the other hand, the status of circumcised and uncircumcised husbands as stated by wife (Wynder's data [27]) among patients with and without cancer of the cervix is collected as given in Table 6.5.

The observed prevalence rates of circumcision between cases and controls in Table 6.5 are given by

$$\widehat{p}_1 = \frac{5}{100} = 0.05, \tag{6.53}$$

and

$$\widehat{p}_0 = \frac{14}{100} = 0.14. \tag{6.54}$$

By calculating the difference between cases and controls,

$$\widehat{d} = 0.05 - 0.14 = -0.09. \tag{6.55}$$

Also, the variance of $\widehat{d}$ is obtained as

$$\sigma_{\widehat{d}}^2 = \sigma_{\widehat{p}_1}^2 + \sigma_{\widehat{p}_0}^2 = \frac{\widehat{p}_1 \widehat{q}_1}{n_1} + \frac{\widehat{p}_0 \widehat{q}_0}{n_0} = \frac{0.05 \cdot 0.95}{100} + \frac{0.14 \cdot 0.86}{100} = 0.00168. \tag{6.56}$$

By substituting Eqs. (6.55) and (6.56) into Eq. (6.47),

$$z_{\widehat{d}} = -\frac{0.09}{\sqrt{0.00168}} = -2.19643 \approx -2.20. \tag{6.57}$$

Since Eq. (6.57) is significant at the level of 0.05 by using Appendix Table A.1, the prevalence of cases is significantly less than that of controls.

Suppose that the data of Table 6.5 is misclassified, we need to check the validity of the calculated false negative and false positive rates of Eqs. (6.51) and (6.52). Unfortunately, the adjusted prevalence rate is not applicable to this data of Table 6.5 because the values of Eqs (6.51) and (6.52) are no less than the values of Eqs. (6.53) and (6.54).

Nevertheless, we can try to calculate the misclassification probabilities by applying the counterfactual true frequencies to Table 6.5. Let $\{N_{ij(k)}\}$ denote the kth

Table 6.5 The observed data of circumcised and uncircumcised husbands with (cases) and without (controls) the cancer of cervix as stated by wife

	Cases	Controls	Total
Circumcised	5	14	19
Uncircumcised	95	86	181
Total	100	100	200

counterfactual true frequencies corresponding to the observed frequencies $\{n_{ij}\}$ in Table 6.5. Then, the false negative and false positive probability can be calculated as for j = 0, 1

$$\varphi_{j(k)} = \frac{| N_{11(k)} - n_{11} |}{n_{+j}}, \tag{6.58}$$

and

$$\psi_{j(k)} = \frac{| N_{01(k)} - n_{01} |}{n_{+j}}. \tag{6.59}$$

The values of $\{\varphi_{j(k)}, \psi_{j(k)}\}$ are given in Table 6.6.

After checking the validity of the values $\{\varphi_{j(k)}, \psi_{j(k)}\}$, all counterfactual true frequencies for cases and controls are feasible.

We can apply Eq. (6.9) to obtain the bias-adjusted prevalence for cases and controls, respectively. Thus, by calculating the values of

$$\tilde{p}_{1(k)} = \frac{\widehat{p}_1 - \psi_{1(k)}}{\Delta_{1(k)}} \text{ and } \tilde{p}_{0(k)} = \frac{\widehat{p}_0 - \psi_{0(k)}}{\Delta_{0(k)}}, \tag{6.60}$$

where $\tilde{q}_{j(k)} = 1 - \tilde{p}_{j(k)}$, j = 1, 0. They are given in Table 6.7.

From Table 6.7, there are 4 possible bias-adjusted prevalence rates for cases and 13 possible bias-adjusted prevalence rates for controls. As all possible combinations, there are 52 bias-adjusted difference between cases and controls which are defined as.

Table 6.6 The values of $\varphi_{j(k)}, \psi_{j(k)}$ for cases and controls

k	$N_{11(k)}$	$N_{10(k)}$	$N_{01(k)}$	$N_{00(k)}$	φ_{1k}	$\psi_{1(k)}$	$\varphi_{0(k)}$	ψ_{0k}
1	4	96	13	87	0.01	0.01	0.01	0.01
2	3	97	12	88	0.02	0.02	0.02	0.02
3	2	98	11	89	0.03	0.03	0.03	0.03
4	1	99	10	90	0.04	0.04	0.04	0.04
5			9	91			0.05	0.05
6			8	92			0.06	0.06
7			7	93			0.07	0.07
8			6	94			0.08	0.08
9			5	95			0.09	0.09
10			4	96			0.1	0.1
11			3	97			0.11	0.11
12			2	98			0.12	0.12
13			1	99			0.13	0.13

Table 6.7 The values of $\Delta_{j(k)}$ and $\tilde{p}_{j(k)}$

k	$\Delta_{1(k)}$	$\Delta_{0(k)}$	$\tilde{p}_{1(k)}$	$\tilde{p}_{0(k)}$
1	0.98	0.98	0.04	0.13
2	0.96	0.96	0.03	0.13
3	0.94	0.94	0.02	0.12
4	0.92	0.92	0.01	0.11
5		0.9		0.1
6		0.88		0.09
7		0.86		0.08
8		0.84		0.07
9		0.82		0.06
10		0.8		0.05
11		0.78		0.04
12		0.76		0.03
13		0.74		0.01

Table 6.8 The values of $\tilde{d}_{\ell(k)}$ and $z_{\tilde{d}_{\ell(k)}}$

k	$\tilde{d}_{1(k)}$	$\tilde{d}_{2(k)}$	$\tilde{d}_{3(k)}$	$\tilde{d}_{4(k)}$	$z_{\tilde{d}_{1(k)}}$	$z_{\tilde{d}_{2(k)}}$	$z_{\tilde{d}_{3(k)}}$	$z_{\tilde{d}_{4(k)}}$
1	−0.09	−0.10	−0.11	−0.12	−0.23	−0.26	−0.29	−0.33
2	−0.08	−0.09	−0.10	−0.11	−0.21	−0.24	−0.28	−0.31
3	−0.08	−0.09	−0.10	−0.11	−0.19	−0.22	−0.26	−0.29
4	−0.07	−0.08	−0.09	−0.10	−0.17	−0.20	−0.24	−0.27
5	−0.06	−0.07	−0.08	−0.09	−0.15	−0.18	−0.21	−0.25
6	−0.05	−0.06	−0.07	−0.08	−0.13	−0.16	−0.19	−0.23
7	−0.04	−0.05	−0.06	−0.07	−0.11	−0.14	−0.17	−0.21
8	−0.03	−0.04	−0.05	−0.06	−0.08	−0.11	−0.15	−0.19
9	−0.02	−0.03	−0.04	−0.05	−0.06	−0.09	−0.12	−0.16
10	−0.01	−0.02	−0.03	−0.04	−0.03	−0.06	−0.09	−0.13
11	0.002	−0.01	−0.02	−0.03	0.01	−0.02	−0.06	−0.10
12	0.02	0.01	−0.01	−0.02	0.05	0.02	−0.02	−0.06
13	0.03	0.02	0.01	−0.002	0.11	0.07	0.04	−0.01

$$\tilde{d}_{\ell(k)} = \tilde{p}_{1(\ell)} - \tilde{p}_{0(k)}, \ell = 1, 2, 3, 4, \mathrm{k} = 1, 2, \ldots, 13. \tag{6.61}$$

The variance of Eq. (6.61) can be calculated accordingly. The values of Eq. (6.61) and the corresponding value of $z_{\tilde{d}_{\ell(k)}}$ are given in Table 6.8.

Since none of the $z_{\tilde{d}_{\ell(k)}}$ are significant, the conclusion drawn from the data without misclassification is likely to be incorrect.

Remark

As was pointed out in Newell [22], the observed prevalence rates must be in the range of $\varphi = 0.18$ and $1 - \widehat{\psi} = 0.44$. But neither $\widehat{p}_1 = 0.05$ nor $\widehat{p}_0 = 0.14$ are in the above range. Hence, Wynder's data (Table 6.5) are inconsistent with that of Table 6.4. As a result, Diamond-Lilienfeld [6] perpetuate an error in the analysis of false negatives and false positives.

6.3 McNemar's Test

McNemar's test [20] was proposed in 1947 for a comparison of two correlated proportions or percentages. Assume that for a population there exists a dichotomous disease variable D with two levels D_1 and D_2 and a causal factor C with two levels C_1 and C_2 and covariate X with J levels $X_1, X_2, \ldots,$ and X_J. A random sample of size n (case group) is selected from a population that has the disease. Another sample of size n (control group) is taken randomly and independently from the population free of the disease D. In the control group, each individual is selected to match on his covariate value with an individual in the case group. At the end, a sample of n independent matched pairs is obtained in all.

The data from such a design is presented in Table 6.9, in which a, b, c, d and n_{11}, n_{12}, n_{21}, n_{22} represent the sample and the population absolute frequencies (positive integers), respectively, and n the sample grand total defined by.

$$\mathrm{n} = \mathrm{a} + \mathrm{b} + \mathrm{c} + \mathrm{d}. \tag{6.62}$$

The joint probability responses in Table 6.9 are described as follows:

$$\pi_{11} = \Pr([C_1|D_1] \cap [C_1|D_2]) = \frac{n_{11}}{N}, \tag{6.63}$$

$$\pi_{12} = \Pr([C_1|D_1] \cap [C_2|D_2]) = \frac{n_{12}}{N}, \tag{6.64}$$

$$\pi_{21} = \Pr([C_2|D_1] \cap [C_1|D_2]) = \frac{n_{21}}{N}, \tag{6.65}$$

$$\pi_{22} = \Pr([C_2|D_1] \cap [C_2|D_2]) = \frac{n_{22}}{N}, \tag{6.66}$$

where N is the grand total population frequency, that is,

Table 6.9 The comparison data of two correlated proportions

	D_2 (controls)		
D_1 (cases)	*C_1 (present)*	*C_2 (absent)*	Total
C_1 (present)	a (n_{11})	b (n_{12})	a + b (n_{1+})
C_2 (absent)	c (n_{21})	d (n_{22})	c + d (n_{2+})
Total	a + c (n_{+1})	b + d (n_{+2})	n (N)

$$N = \sum_{i,j=1}^{2} n_{ij}. \tag{6.67}$$

If we let

$$\omega_{ij} = \Pr(C_1|D_i X_j), \tag{6.68}$$

and

$$\eta_j = \Pr(X_j|D_1), \tag{6.69}$$

it follows that

$$\pi_{11} = \sum_{j=1}^{J} \omega_{1j}\omega_{2j}\eta_j, \tag{6.70}$$

$$\pi_{12} = \sum_{j=1}^{J} \omega_{1j}(1 - \omega_{2j})\eta_j, \tag{6.71}$$

$$\pi_{21} = \sum_{j=1}^{J} (1 - \omega_{1j})\omega_{2j}\eta_j, \tag{6.72}$$

$$\pi_{22} = \sum_{j=1}^{J} (1 - \omega_{1j})(1 - \omega_{2j})\eta_j, \tag{6.73}$$

where ω_{ij} and η_j are given, respectively, by Eqs. (6.68) and (6.69). Thus, if j = 1, 2, . . ., J

$$\frac{\omega_{1j}(1 - \omega_{2j})}{(1 - \omega_{1j})\omega_{2j}} \tag{6.74}$$

is constant over j, say equal to a common θ, we have from Eqs. (6.71) and (6.72)

$$\theta = \frac{\pi_{12}}{\pi_{21}}. \tag{6.75}$$

Remark

Equation (6.75) closely approximates the relative risk, provided that the disease is rare [3].

Assume that Eqs. (6.63) to (6.66) are the parameters of a multinomial distribution. The maximum likelihood estimators for θ, $\widehat{\pi}_{11}$, $\widehat{\pi}_{12}$, $\widehat{\pi}_{21}$, and $\widehat{\pi}_{22}$ are given, respectively, by [4]

$$\widehat{\theta} = \frac{b}{c}, \tag{6.76}$$

$$\widehat{\pi}_{11} \equiv \frac{\widehat{n}_{11}}{n} = \frac{a}{n}, \tag{6.77}$$

$$\widehat{\pi}_{12} \equiv \frac{\widehat{n}_{12}}{n} = \frac{b}{n}, \tag{6.78}$$

$$\widehat{\pi}_{21} \equiv \frac{\widehat{n}_{21}}{n} = \frac{c}{n}, \tag{6.79}$$

$$\widehat{\pi}_{22} \equiv \frac{\widehat{n}_{22}}{n} = \frac{d}{n}, \tag{6.80}$$

and the asymptotic variance of Eq. (6.76) is given by

$$\sigma^2\left(\widehat{\theta}\right) = \frac{n_{12}(n_{12} + n_{21})}{n_{21}^3}. \tag{6.81}$$

If we wish to test the hypotheses

$$H_0 : \pi_{1+} = \pi_{+1} \text{ versus } H_1 : \pi_{1+} > \pi_{+1}, \tag{6.82}$$

where $\pi_{1+} = \pi_{11} + \pi_{12}$ and $\pi_{+1} = \pi_{11} + \pi_{21}$. The maximum likelihood estimators for π_{1+} and π_{+1} are given, respectively, by

$$\widehat{\pi}_{1+} = \frac{a+b}{n} \text{ and } \widehat{\pi}_{+1} = \frac{a+c}{n}. \tag{6.83}$$

As a result, the difference between π_{1+} and π_{+1} is estimated by applying Eq. (6.83)

$$\widehat{\pi}_{1+} - \widehat{\pi}_{+1} = \frac{b-c}{n}. \tag{6.84}$$

The standard error of Eq. (6.84) is given by

$$\sigma(\widehat{\pi}_{1+} - \widehat{\pi}_{+1}) = \frac{\sqrt{b+c}}{n}. \tag{6.85}$$

The square of the ratio of Eqs. (6.84) to (6.85) with a correction for continuity yields the McNemar's chi-squared test

$$\widehat{\chi}^2_{McN} = \left\{ \frac{|\widehat{\pi}_{1+} - \widehat{\pi}_{+1}| - n^{-1}}{\sigma(\widehat{\pi}_{1+} - \widehat{\pi}_{+1})} \right\}^2 = \frac{(|b-c|-1)^2}{b+c}, \tag{6.86}$$

which is used to test for the statistical significance of $\pi_{1+} - \pi_{+1}$.

Remark

In large samples, the value of Eq. (6.76) may be referred to the table of chi-squared distribution with one degree of freedom [15].

Suppose that Table 6.9 is misclassified. Let C^* be the surrogate classification variable for C. Let φ_i and ψ_i, i = 1 2, be the false negative and false positive probabilities for classifying the exposure status among samples from cases and controls, respectively, that is,

$$\varphi_i = \Pr(C^* = C_2 | C = C_1; D = D_i), \tag{6.87}$$

and

$$\psi_i = \Pr(C^* = C_1 | C = C_2; D = D_i). \tag{6.88}$$

Then, the expected value of those sample frequencies in Table 6.9 are given, respectively, by

$$E(a) = (1-\varphi_1)(1-\varphi_2)n_{11} + (1-\varphi_1)\psi_2 n_{12} + \psi_1(1-\phi_2)n_{21} + \psi_1\psi_2 n_{22}, \tag{6.89}$$

$$E(b) = \varphi_2(1-\varphi_1)n_{11} + (1-\varphi_1)(1-\psi_2)n_{12} + \psi_1\phi_2 n_{21} + \psi_1(1-\psi_2)n_{22}, \tag{6.90}$$

$$E(c) = \varphi_1(1-\varphi_2)n_{11} + \varphi_1\psi_2 n_{12} + (1-\psi_1)(1-\phi_2)n_{21} + (1-\psi_1)\psi_2 n_{22}, \tag{6.91}$$

$$E(d) = \varphi_1\varphi_2 n_{11} + \varphi_1(1-\psi_2)n_{12} + (1-\psi_1)\phi_2 n_{21} + (1-\psi_1) \times (1-\psi_2)n_{22}, \tag{6.92}$$

By replacing the expected value of the left-hand side of Eqs. (6.89) to (6.92) with their observed sample frequencies and solve for the unknown true population frequencies n_{ij}, we obtain the bias-adjusted estimators $\tilde{n}_{ij}$ that accounts for the misclassification bias have to satisfy

$$W\tilde{\vec{n}} = \hat{\vec{n}}, \tag{6.93}$$

where $\hat{\vec{n}} = (a, b, c, d)^T$, $\tilde{\vec{n}}$ and the misclassification matrix W are given, respectively, by

$$\tilde{\vec{n}} = (\tilde{n}_{11}, \tilde{n}_{12}, \tilde{n}_{21}, \tilde{n}_{22})^T, \tag{6.94}$$

and the misclassification matrix W is given by

$$W = \begin{bmatrix} (1-\varphi_1)(1-\varphi_2) & (1-\varphi_1)\psi_2 & \psi_1(1-\varphi_2) & \psi_1\psi_2 \\ \varphi_2(1-\varphi_1) & (1-\varphi_1)(1-\psi_2) & \psi_1\varphi_2 & \psi_1(1-\psi_2) \\ \varphi_1(1-\varphi_2) & \varphi_1\psi_2 & (1-\psi_1)(1-\varphi_2) & \psi_2(1-\psi_1) \\ \varphi_1\varphi_2 & \varphi_1(1-\psi_2) & (1-\psi_1)\varphi_2 & (1-\psi_1)(1-\psi_2) \end{bmatrix} \tag{6.95}$$

It is easily shown (Exercise 6.7-5) that

$$\det(\mathrm{W}) = (\Delta_1\Delta_2)^2, \tag{6.96}$$

where Δ_i, i = 1, 2, is defined by Eq. (6.5).

Thus, W of Eq. (6.95) is invertible if Eq. (6.96) is positive, that is, for i = 1, 2

$$\varphi_i + \psi_i < 1. \tag{6.97}$$

If Eq. (6.97) holds, we have after solving Eq. (6.93)

$$\tilde{n}_{11} = \frac{(1-\psi_1)(1-\psi_2)a - (1-\psi_1)\psi_2 b - (1-\psi_2)\psi_1 c + \psi_1\psi_2 d}{\Delta_1\Delta_2} \tag{6.98}$$

$$\tilde{n}_{12} = \frac{-(1-\psi_1)\varphi_2 a + (1-\psi_1)(1-\varphi_2)b + \psi_1\varphi_2 c - \psi_1(1-\varphi_2)d}{\Delta_1\Delta_2} \tag{6.99}$$

$$\tilde{n}_{21} = \frac{-\varphi_1(1-\psi_2)a + \varphi_1\psi_2 b + (1-\varphi_1)(1-\psi_2)c - (1-\varphi_1)\psi_2 d}{\Delta_1\Delta_2} \tag{6.100}$$

$$\tilde{n}_{22} = \frac{\psi_1\varphi_2 a - \varphi_1(1-\varphi_2)b - (1-\varphi_1)\varphi_2 c + (1-\varphi_1)(1-\varphi_2)d}{\Delta_1\Delta_2} \tag{6.101}$$

In order that the numerator of Eqs. (6.98) to (6.101) be positive, sufficient conditions are needed to be imposed on φ_i and ψ_i as follows:

$$(1-\psi_1)(1-\psi_2)a + \psi_1\psi_2 d > (1-\psi_1)\psi_2 b + (1-\psi_2)\psi_1 c \tag{6.102}$$

$$(1-\psi_1)(1-\varphi_2)b + \psi_1\varphi_2 c > (1-\psi_1)\varphi_2 a + \psi_1(1-\varphi_2)d \tag{6.103}$$

$$\varphi_1\psi_2 b + (1-\varphi_1)(1-\psi_2)c > \varphi_1(1-\psi_2)a + (1-\varphi_1)\psi_2 d \tag{6.104}$$

$$\psi_1\varphi_2 a + (1-\varphi_1)(1-\varphi_2)d > \varphi_1(1-\varphi_2)b + (1-\varphi_1)\varphi_2 c \tag{6.105}$$

Pairs of (φ_i, ψ_i), $i = 1, 2$ are said to be admissible if Eqs. (6.97) and (6.102) to (6.105) are satisfied. Eqs. (6.98) to (6.101) are said to be plausible if all $\tilde{n}_{ij}$ are positive, provided that Eq. (6.97) is satisfied.

Remarks

1. For plausible bias-adjusted cell counts of Eqs. (6.98) to (6.101), it is easily shown (Exercise 6.7-5) that they are unbiased for the true unknown $\{n_{ij}\}$, $i, j = 1, 2$.
2. In practical applications, we do not have to check if the constraints of Eqs. (6.102) to (6.105) are satisfied in order to determine the admissibility of φ_i and ψ_i. As long as Eq. (6.97) is satisfied, we proceed to calculate the bias-adjusted cell count

estimators of Eqs. (6.98) to (6.101). If all of $\tilde{n}_{ij}$ are positive, Eqs. (6.102) to (6.105) are automatically satisfied. Otherwise, pairs of φ_i and ψ_i are inadmissible and thus they should be discarded (See Example 6.3).
3. For one to m-paired design, the bias-adjusted cell count estimators were considered in Lee [15].

Now to account for the misclassification errors, a bias-adjusted MeNemar's test is given by

$$\tilde{\chi}^2_{McN} = \frac{(|\tilde{n}_{12} - \tilde{n}_{21}| - 1)^2}{\tilde{n}_{12} + \tilde{n}_{21}}, \qquad (6.106)$$

where $\tilde{n}_{12}$ and $\tilde{n}_{21}$ are given, respectively, by Eqs. (6.99) and (6.100). Similarly, the bias-adjusted odds ratio that accounts for misclassification errors is given by

$$\tilde{\theta} = \frac{\tilde{n}_{12}}{\tilde{n}_{21}} = \frac{-(1-\psi_1)\varphi_2 a + (1-\psi_1)(1-\varphi_2)b + \psi_1\varphi_2 c - \psi_1(1-\varphi_2)d}{-\varphi_1(1-\psi_2)a + \varphi_1\psi_2 b + (1-\varphi_1)(1-\psi_2)c - (1-\varphi_1)\psi_2 d} \qquad (6.107)$$

By using the delta method, the asymptotic variance of the logarithm of Eq. (6.107) is given by [12]

$$\sigma^2\left(\ln\left(\tilde{\theta}\right)\right) = \frac{1}{B_1^2 B_2^2}\{A_{11}^2\sigma^2(\widehat{\epsilon}_{11}) + A_{12}^2\sigma^2(\widehat{\epsilon}_{12}) + A_{21}^2\sigma^2(\widehat{\epsilon}_{21}) + A_{22}^2\sigma^2(\widehat{\epsilon}_{22})$$

$$+2A_{11}A_{12}cov(\widehat{\epsilon}_{11},\widehat{\epsilon}_{12}) + 2A_{11}A_{21}cov(\widehat{\epsilon}_{11},\widehat{\varepsilon}_{21})$$

$$+2A_{11}A_{22}cov(\widehat{\epsilon}_{11},\widehat{\epsilon}_{22})$$

$$+2A_{12}A_{21}cov(\widehat{\epsilon}_{12},\widehat{\epsilon}_{21})$$

$$+2A_{12}A_{22}cov(\widehat{\epsilon}_{12},\widehat{\epsilon}_{22}) + 2A_{21}A_{22}cov(\widehat{\epsilon}_{21},\widehat{\epsilon}_{22}), \qquad (6.108)$$

where $\widehat{\epsilon}_{ij}$ is defined by Eq. (6.119) in Appendix 6.3A and the covariance of $\widehat{\epsilon}_{ij}$ is given by

$$\widehat{cov}\left(\vec{\epsilon}\right) = n^{-3}\begin{bmatrix} n_{11}(n-n_{11}) & -n_{12}n_{11} & -n_{21}n_{11} & -n_{22}n_{11} \\ -n_{11}n_{12} & n_{12}(n-n_{12}) & -n_{21}n_{12} & -n_{22}n_{12} \\ -n_{11}n_{21} & -n_{12}n_{21} & n_{21}(n-n_{21}) & -n_{22}n_{21} \\ -n_{11}n_{22} & -n_{12}n_{22} & -n_{21}n_{22} & n_{22}(n-n_{22}) \end{bmatrix}, \qquad (6.109)$$

A_{ij} and B_j are defined, respectively, by

$$A_{11} = \varphi_1(1-\psi_1)\Delta_2 n_{12} - \varphi_2\psi_2\Delta_1 n_{21} + (\varphi_2\psi_2\Delta_1 - \varphi_1\psi_1\Delta_2)n_{22} \quad (6.110)$$

$$A_{12} = -\varphi_1(1-\psi_1)\Delta_2 n_{11} + [\Delta_1\Delta_2 - \varphi_1\varphi_2\Delta_2 - \psi_1\psi_2\Delta_1]n_{21} + (1-\varphi_2)\psi_2\Delta_1 n_{22} \quad (6.111)$$

$$A_{21} = \varphi_2\psi_2\Delta_1 n_{11} - (\Delta_1\Delta_2 + \varphi_1\psi_1\Delta_2 + \varphi_2\psi_2\Delta_1)n_{12} - (1-\varphi_1)\psi_1\Delta_2 n_{22} \quad (6.112)$$

$$A_{22} = [\varphi_1\psi_1 - \varphi_2\psi_2 - \varphi_1\varphi_2(\psi_2-\psi_1) + \psi_1\psi_2(\varphi_2-\varphi_1)]n_{11} + (1-\varphi_2)\psi_2\Delta_1 n_{12} - (1-\varphi_1)\psi_1\Delta_2 n_{21} \quad (6.113)$$

$$B_1 = -(1-\psi_1)\varphi_2 n_{11} + (1-\psi_1)(1-\varphi_2)n_{12} + \psi_1\varphi_2 n_{21} - \psi_1(1-\varphi_2)n_{22} \quad (6.114)$$

$$B_2 = -\varphi_1(1-\psi_2)n_{11} + \varphi_1\psi_2 n_{12} + (1-\varphi_1)(1-\psi_2)n_{21} - (1-\varphi_1)\psi_2 n_{22} \quad (6.115)$$

Remarks

1. The derivation of Eq. (6.108) is given in Appendix 6.3A.
2. In practical applications, all the unknown n_{ij} in Eqs. (6.108) to (6.115) are substituted by Eqs. (6.98) to (6.101).

   Using Eqs. (6.108) to (6.115), the 100%·(1 − α) confidence interval (LCL, UCL) for the true θ is given as follows: (0 < α < 1)

$$(\text{LCL}, \text{UCL}) = \exp\left\{ \ln(\tilde{\theta}) \pm z_{1-\alpha} \cdot \sqrt{\sigma(\ln(\tilde{\theta}))} \right\}. \quad (6.116)$$

Example 6.3

In a study on the etiological factor for the acute myocardial infarction (AMI) disease among Navajo Indians, Coulehan et al. [5] employed a 1:1 matched-pair case-control studies. For each AMI patient identified, a comparison patient with gallbladder (GB) disease was selected from those who were discharged with a diagnosis of cholelithiasis or cholecystitis. The comparison patient was matched for age, sex, and hospital. Then, the relative risk of the causal factors: hypertension, diabetes, smoking, alcohol abuse, nontraditional employment, and stroke were calculated. They concluded hypertension and diabetes were more frequently seen in the AMI patients than in the GB patients.

For illustration, I only used the data for diabetes. Previous diagnosis of diabetes for 144 matched-pairs of AMI and GB patients among Navajo Indians that is given in Table 6.10.

If the observed data in Table 6.10 were not misclassified, we obtain from using Eqs. (6.76) and (6.81), the estimated crude odds ratio with its 95% confidence interval as: $\widehat{\theta} = 2.31$ ($95\%CI$: $1.25 - 4.54$). Also, the value of McNemar's test by using Eq. (6.86) is $\widehat{\chi}^2_{McN} = 7.55$ (p-value = 0.006).

Table 6.10 The data of matched pairs of AMI and GB patients

	Controls (D_2:GB)		
Cases (D_1:AMI)	Diabetes	No diabetes	Total
Diabetes	9	37	46
No diabetes	16	82	98
Total	25	119	144

Table 6.11 Five possible true counterfactual entries when n_{+1} and n_{+2} are fixed

Model	n_{11}^*	n_{22}^*	n_{+1}	n_{+2}	φ_2	ψ_2
1	8	83	25	119	0.04	0.008
2	7	84	25	119	0.08	0.017
3	6	85	25	119	0.12	0.025
4	5	86	25	119	0.16	0.034
5	4	87	25	119	0.020	0.042

Table 6.12 Five possible true counterfactual entries when n_{1+} and n_{2+} are fixed

Model	n_{11}^*	n_{22}^*	n_{1+}	n_{2+}	φ_1	ψ_1
1	8	83	46	98	0.022	0.01
2	7	84	46	98	0.044	0.02
3	6	85	46	98	0.065	0.031
4	5	86	46	98	0.087	0.041
5	4	87	46	98	0.109	0.051

But, if the observed data in Table 6.10 were misclassified, we need to use the bias-adjusted McNemar's test (Eq. (6.106)) and the bias-adjusted odds ratio (Eq. (6.107)). Since no validation sample was available, I will take a counterfactual approach to calculate the unknown misclassification error probabilities φ_i and ψ_i.

With the fixed observed marginal totals, n_{1+}=a + b = 46, n_{2+}=b + d = 98, n_{+1}=a + c = 25, n_{+2}=b + d = 119, five possible true counterfactual entries n_{11}^* and n_{22}^* are given in columns 2 to 3 of Tables 6.11 and 6.12 when the column marginal totals n_{+1} and n_{+2} are fixed. The false negative and false positive error probabilities are estimated from the following formula

$$\begin{aligned} \varphi_2 &= \frac{|\, n_{11}^* - a \,|}{n_{+1}} \text{ and } \psi_2 = \frac{|\, n_{22}^* - d \,|}{n_{+2}} \text{ or} \\ \varphi_1 &= \frac{|\, n_{11}^* - a \,|}{n_{1+}} \text{ and } \psi_1 = \frac{|\, n_{22}^* - d \,|}{n_{2+}}. \end{aligned} \tag{6.117}$$

According to Eq. (6.117), φ_i or ψ_i are calculated in columns 6 to 9 of Tables 6.11 and 6.12.

By examining the admissibility of bias-adjusted entries $\tilde{n}_{12}$ and $\tilde{n}_{21}$ in Table 6.13, we find that model 5 is inadmissible because the estimated values of $\tilde{n}_{21} = -5.35$ is not positive. Hence, model 5 must be deleted.

By substituting $\widehat{\vec{n}} = (9, 37, 16, 82)^T$ into Eq. (6.109),

Table 6.13 The values of A_{ij} and B_j

Model	A_{11}	A_{12}	A_{21}	A_{22}	B_1	B_2
1	0.76	−14.3	−34.9	0.13	34.0	14.7
2	1.44	−12.6	−32.8	0.25	31.1	13.4
3	2.045	−11.1	−30.7	0.34	28.4	12.1
4	2.56	−9.64	−28.7	0.42	25.7	11.0

Table 6.14 The bias-adjusted entries of the case-control table, their adjusted odds ratio, and the adjusted McNemar's test

Model	$\tilde{n}_{12}$	$\tilde{n}_{21}$	$\sigma\left(\ln\left(\tilde{\theta}\right)\right)$	$\tilde{\theta}$ (95% C.I.)	$\tilde{\chi}^2_{McN}$
1	36.91	15.91	0.0019	2.32 (2.31–2.33)	7.57
2	36.81	15.82	0.0022	2.33 (2.32–2.34)	7.60
3	36.70	15.70	0.0024	2.34 (2.33–2.35)	7.63
4	36.57	15.57	0.0028	2.35 (2.34–2.36)	7.67

$$\hat{\Sigma} = \begin{bmatrix} 0.0004 & -0.0001 & -4.8\cdot10^{-5} & -0.0003 \\ -0.0001 & 0.0013 & 0.0001 & 0.0001 \\ -4.8\cdot10^{-5} & -0.0001 & 0.0007 & -0.0004 \\ -0.0003 & -0.0001 & -0.0004 & 0.0017 \end{bmatrix}, \tag{6.118}$$

By substituting the values of (φ_i, ψ_i) in Tables 6.11 and 6.12 into Eqs. (6.110) to (6.115), the values of A_{ij} and B_j, i, j = 1, 2, are given in the following table.

By substituting the values in Table 6.13 into Eq. (6.108), the values of $\sigma\left(\ln\left(\tilde{\theta}\right)\right)$ for the four counterfactual models are given by the fourth column in Table 6.14. The values of the bias-adjusted odds ratio and McNemar's test given by the fifth and the sixth column of Table 6.14 are calculated accordingly by using Eqs. (6.106) and (6.107).

The bias-adjusted odds ratio deviates very little from the classical odds ratio when the misclassification error probabilities φ_i and ψ_i are small. The 95% confidence interval for $\tilde{\theta}$ are calculated by applying Eq. (6.116) with the substitution of $\tilde{n}_{ij}$ for the unknown n_{ij} in Eqs. (6.108) to (6.115). Similarly, the bias-adjusted McNemar's statistics deviates very little from the classical one ($\widehat{\chi}^2_{McN} = 7.55$) for models 1–4.

Remark

The way to calculate the misclassification probabilities of the counterfactual models in my papers published earlier is not very accurate. The correct way is given by Eq. (6.117) in this example.

Appendix 6.3A

First, for i, j = 1, 2 define

$$\varepsilon_{ij} \equiv \widehat{n}_{ij} - n_{ij}, \tag{6.119}$$

where $\widehat{n}_{ij}$ is defined by

$$\widehat{\vec{n}} = (\widehat{n}_{11}, \widehat{n}_{12}, \widehat{n}_{21}, \widehat{n}_{22})^T = (a, b, c, d)^T. \tag{6.120}$$

Let

$$\vec{\varepsilon} = (\varepsilon_{11}, \varepsilon_{12}, \varepsilon_{21}, \varepsilon_{22})^T. \tag{6.121}$$

By the properties of multinomial distribution, it is easily shown that

$$E\left(\vec{\varepsilon}\right) = 0 \text{ and } \sigma^2_{\vec{\varepsilon}} = \Sigma, \tag{6.122}$$

where Σ is given by

$$\Sigma = cov\left(\hat{\vec{n}}\right) = \frac{1}{n^3}\begin{bmatrix} n_{11}\bar{n}_{11} & -n_{12}n_{11} & -n_{21}n_{11} & -n_{22}n_{11} \\ -n_{11}n_{12} & n_{12}\bar{n}_{12} & -n_{21}n_{12} & -n_{22}n_{12} \\ -n_{11}n_{21} & -n_{12}n_{21} & n_{21}\bar{n}_{21} & -n_{22}n_{21} \\ -n_{11}n_{22} & -n_{12}n_{22} & -n_{21}n_{22} & n_{22}\bar{n}_{22} \end{bmatrix}. \tag{6.123}$$

Next, define

$$\vartheta = \frac{-(1-\psi_1)\varphi_2 n_{11} + (1-\psi_1)(1-\varphi_2)n_{12} + \psi_1\varphi_2 n_{21} - \psi_1(1-\varphi_2)n_{22}}{-\varphi_1(1-\psi_2)n_{11} + \varphi_1\psi_2 n_{12} + (1-\varphi_1)(1-\psi_2)n_{21} - (1-\varphi_1)\psi_2 n_{22}}. \tag{6.124}$$

Thus, we have

$$\begin{aligned}
\ln(\tilde{\theta}) - \ln(\vartheta) &= \ln\left[\frac{-(1-\psi_1)\varphi_2\widehat{n}_{11} + (1-\psi_1)(1-\varphi_2)\widehat{n}_{12} + \psi_1\varphi_2\widehat{n}_{21} - \psi_1(1-\varphi_2)\widehat{n}_{22}}{-(1-\psi_1)\varphi_2 n_{11} + (1-\psi_1)(1-\varphi_2)n_{12} + \psi_1\varphi_2 n_{21} - \psi_1(1-\varphi_2)n_{22}}\right] \\
&- \ln\left[\frac{-\varphi_1(1-\psi_2)\widehat{n}_{11} + \varphi_1\psi_2\widehat{n}_{12} + (1-\varphi_1)(1-\psi_2)\widehat{n}_{21} - (1-\varphi_1)\psi_2\widehat{n}_{22}}{-\varphi_1(1-\psi_2)n_{11} + \varphi_1\psi_2 n_{12} + (1-\varphi_1)(1-\psi_2)n_{21} - (1-\varphi_1)\psi_2 n_{22}}\right], \\
&= \ln\left[1 + \frac{-(1-\psi_1)\varphi_2\varepsilon_{11} + (1-\psi_1)(1-\varphi_2)\varepsilon_{12} + \psi_1\varphi_2\varepsilon_{21} - \psi_1(1-\varphi_2)\varepsilon_{22}}{-(1-\psi_1)\varphi_2 n_{11} + (1-\psi_1)(1-\varphi_2)n_{12} + \psi_1\varphi_2 n_{21} - \psi_1(1-\varphi_2)n_{22}}\right] \\
&- \ln\left[1 + \frac{-\varphi_1(1-\psi_2)\varepsilon_{11} + \varphi_1\psi_2\varepsilon_{12} + (1-\varphi_1)(1-\psi_2)\varepsilon_{21} - (1-\varphi_1)\psi_2\varepsilon_{22}}{-\varphi_1(1-\psi_2)n_{11} + \varphi_1\psi_2 n_{12} + (1-\varphi_1)(1-\psi_2)n_{21} - (1-\varphi_1)\psi_2 n_{22}}\right] \\
&\approx \frac{-(1-\psi_1)\varphi_2\varepsilon_{11} + (1-\psi_1)(1-\varphi_2)\varepsilon_{12} + \psi_1\varphi_2\varepsilon_{21} - \psi_1(1-\varphi_2)\varepsilon_{22}}{B_1} \\
&- \frac{-\varphi_1(1-\psi_2)\varepsilon_{11} + \varphi_1\psi_2\varepsilon_{12} + (1-\varphi_1)(1-\psi_2)\varepsilon_{21} - (1-\varphi_1)\psi_2\varepsilon_{22}}{B_2}
\end{aligned}$$

$$= \frac{A_{11}\varepsilon_{11} - A_{12}\varepsilon_{12} - A_{21}\varepsilon_{21} + A_{22}\varepsilon_{22}}{B_1 B_2}, \tag{6.125}$$

where A_{ij} and B_j, i, j = 1, 2, are defined, respectively, by Eqs. (6.110) to (6.115), and $\Sigma = [\varepsilon_{ij}]_{i,\ j\ =\ 1,\ 2}$ is given by Eq. (6.109). By using the fact that $\sigma^2\left(\ln\left(\tilde{\theta}\right)\right) = E\left\{\left[\ln\left(\tilde{\theta}\right) - \ln(\vartheta)\right]^2\right\}$ and because $E\left[\ln\left(\tilde{\theta}\right) - \ln(\vartheta)\right] = 0$, Eqs. (6.110) to (6.115) follows immediately after taking the expected value of the square of Eq. (6.125).

6.4 Estimation of Misclassification Error Rates

In Sects. 6.1 and 6.2, the misclassification error probabilities are unknown and have to be estimated. There are at least two ways to estimate them. It depends whether the validation subsample is available or not. Without the validation subsample, we can use the counterfactual approach to estimate them. In this section, we assume that internal validation subsample in addition to the main study is available as given in Table 6.15. Assume that we have a case-control study where Y (= 0, 1) denotes disease variable and X^*(= 0, 1) denotes the surrogate (misclassified) exposure variable.

We assume no misclassification on sampling with Y. Together with main study data, there are three types of validation study, namely, internal, external and joint X, X^* [19]. Here a joint validation study with a gold-standard exposure variable X (= 0, 1) is used to randomly select a subset of the participants from within the main study. Now for i = 0, 1define the disease prevalence rate as

$$p_i = \Pr(X = 1|Y = i), \tag{6.126}$$

and the misclassified disease prevalence rate as

$$p_i^* = \Pr(X^* = 1|Y = i). \tag{6.127}$$

The odds ratio of Eq. (6.1) is of main interest. Finally, define the misclassification error probabilities as Eqs. (6.2) and (6.3), respectively, and define for $i = 0$.

Table 6.15 The sample data of the main study and validation study

	Main study			Validation study			
				Y = 1		Y = 0	
	Y = 1	Y = 0		X = 1	X = 0	X = 1	X = 0
$X^* = 1$	n_{11}	n_{10}	$X^* = 1$	n_{12}	n_{13}	n_{02}	n_{03}
$X^* = 0$	n_{01}	n_{00}	$X^* = 0$	n_{14}	n_{15}	n_{04}	n_{05}

Where X is the true exposure variable, $X^*$is the surrogate (misclassified) variable, and Y represents the disease variable defined as 1 if the subject is a case; 0 if a control

6.4.1 The Indirect Method

The design yields six possible types of observations for both cases and controls, the observed data yield n_{ij} subjects of each respective type ($i = 0, 1; j = 0, \ldots, 5$). The likelihood of $\pi = (p_1, p_0, \varphi_1, \varphi_0, \psi_1, \psi_0)^T$ (ignoring constant terms) is

$$L(\pi)=\prod_{i=0}^{1}\{[(1-\varphi_i)p_i+\psi_i q_i]^{n_{i1}}[\varphi_i p_i+(1-\psi_i)q_i]^{n_{i0}}[(1-\varphi_i)p_i]^{n_{i2}}[\psi_i q_i]^{n_{i3}}[\varphi_i p_i]^{n_{i4}}[(1-\psi_i)q_i]^{n_{i5}}\}, \tag{6.128}$$

where $q_i = 1 - p_i$.

By setting partial derivatives of the logarithm of (6.128) with respect to the parameter π equal to zero, we have for $i = 1, 2$

$$\begin{aligned}\frac{\partial \ln(L(\pi))}{\partial p_i} &= \frac{\Delta_i n_{i1}}{\Delta_i p_i + \psi_i} - \frac{\Delta_i n_{i0}}{1-\psi_i-\Delta_i p_i} + \frac{n_{i2}+n_{i4}}{p_i} - \frac{n_{i3}+n_{i5}}{1-p_i} = 0,\\ \frac{\partial \ln(L(\pi))}{\partial \varphi_i} &= -\frac{p_i n_{i1}}{\Delta_i p_i + \psi_i} + \frac{p_i n_{i0}}{1-\psi_i-\Delta_i p_i} - \frac{n_{i2}}{1-\varphi_i} + \frac{n_{i4}}{\varphi_i} = 0,\\ \frac{\partial \ln(L(\pi))}{\partial \psi_i} &= \frac{(1-p_i)n_{i1}}{\Delta_i p_i + \psi_i} - \frac{(1-p_i)n_{i0}}{1-\psi_i-\Delta_i p_i} - \frac{n_{i3}}{\psi_i} - \frac{n_{i5}}{1-\psi_i} = 0,\end{aligned} \tag{6.129}$$

where Δ_i is given by Eq. (6.5).

Equation (6.129) is a nonlinear equation in the parameters π. Hence, the maximum likelihood estimators for π that satisfy Eq. (6.129) do not have a closed form solution. Let us try to simplify them algebraically and then solve by applying the Newton-Raphson method iteratively.

By moving the third and the fourth terms in all three equations of Eq. (6.129) to the right side of the equation and adding them one by one, we have

$$\frac{\Delta_i[n_{i1}-(n_{i1}+n_{i0})(\Delta_i p_i+\psi_i)]}{(\Delta_i p_i+\psi_i)(1-\psi_i-\Delta_i p_i)} = \frac{p_i\cdot\sum_{j=2}^{5} n_{ij}-(n_{i2}+n_{i4})}{(1-p_i)p_i}, \tag{6.130}$$

$$\frac{p_i[(n_{i1}+n_{i0})(\Delta_i p_i+\psi_i)-n_{i1}]}{(\Delta_i p_i+\psi_i)(1-\psi_i-\Delta_i p_i)} = \frac{(n_{i2}+n_{i4})\varphi_i-n_{i4}}{(1-\varphi_i)\varphi_i}, \tag{6.131}$$

$$\frac{(1-p_i)[n_{i1}-(n_{i1}+n_{i0})\psi_i-(n_{i1}+n_{i0})\theta_i p_i]}{(\Delta_i p_i+\psi_i)(1-\psi_i-\Delta_i p_i)} = \frac{(n_{i5}-n_{i3})\psi_i+n_{i3}}{(1-\psi_i)\psi_i}. \tag{6.132}$$

Dividing Eq. (6.130) by Eq. (6.131) and simplifying it,

$$-\frac{\Delta_i}{p_i} = \frac{\left[\mathrm{p}_i\cdot\sum_{j=2}^{5} n_{ij}-(n_{i2}+n_{i4})\right]\varphi_i(1-\varphi_i)}{p_i(1-p_i)[\varphi_i(n_{i2}+n_{i4})-n_{i4}]}, \tag{6.133}$$

Dividing Eq. (6.131) by Eq. (6.132) and simplifying it,

$$-\frac{p_i}{1-p_i}=\frac{[(n_{i2}+n_{i4})\varphi_i-n_{i4}](1-\psi_i)\psi_i}{[(n_{i3}+(n_{i5}-n_{i3})\psi_i](1-\varphi_i)\varphi_i]}. \tag{6.134}$$

By solving p_i from both Eqs. (6.133) and (6.134) separately and making them equal as a nonlinear function in (φ_i, ψ_i),

$$g_i(\varphi_i,\psi_i)=\left\{-\psi_i+\frac{\varphi_i(1-\varphi_i)[n_{i3}+(n_{i5}-n_{i3})\psi_i]}{(1-\psi_i)[n_{i4}-\varphi_i(n_{i2}+n_{i4})]}\right\}^{-1}$$
$$-\frac{n_{i2}+n_{i4}}{(\varphi_i^{-1}-1)\left(1+\sum_{j=2}^{5}n_{ij}\right)-\psi_i}. \tag{6.135}$$

Equation (6.135) are two nonlinear functions in two pair variables (φ_i, ψ_i), i = 0, 1. Since it is not easy to apply an iterative Newton-Raphson's method to solve Eqs. (6.135) for the roots, we instead use the method of function evaluation to find the roots $\breve{\varphi}_i$ and $\breve{\psi}_i$ as shown in Example 6.4. After solving the roots $(\breve{\varphi}_i,\breve{\psi}_i)$ from Eq. (6.135), we substituting them into the expression of $\tilde{p}_i$ given either by solving Eq. (6.133)

$$\tilde{p}_{i(I)}=\frac{\varphi_i\psi_i(n_{i2}+n_{i4})}{(1+\breve{n}_i)(1-\varphi_i)-\psi_i}, \tag{6.136}$$

where $\breve{n}_i=\sum_{j=2}^{5}n_{ij}$, or by solving Eq. (6.134)

$$\tilde{p}_{i(I)}=-\left(1+\frac{\varphi_i(1-\varphi_i)[n_{i3}+(n_{i5}-n_{i3})\psi_i}{\psi_i(1-\psi_i)[\varphi_i(n_{i2}+n_{i4})-n_{i4}]}\right)^{-1}, \tag{6.137}$$

where the subscript (I) refers as the indirect method to be compared with the direct method in Sect. 6.4.2.

The asymptotic variance of $(\tilde{p}_{i(I)},\tilde{\varphi}_i,\tilde{\psi}_i)$is given by [18]

$$\Sigma_{i(I)}=-\begin{bmatrix}\frac{\partial^2\ln L(\pi)}{\partial p_i^2} & \frac{\partial^2 lnL(\pi)}{\partial\varphi_i\partial p_i} & \frac{\partial^2 lnL(\pi)}{\partial\psi_i\partial p_i}\\ \frac{\partial^2 lnL(\pi)}{\partial p_i\partial\varphi_i} & \frac{\partial^2\ln L(\pi)}{\partial\varphi_i^2} & \frac{\partial^2 lnL(\pi)}{\partial\psi_i\partial\varphi_i}\\ \frac{\partial^2 lnL(\pi)}{\partial p_i\partial\psi_i} & \frac{\partial^2 lnL(\pi)}{\partial\varphi_i\partial\psi_i} & \frac{\partial^2\ln L(\pi)}{\partial\psi_i^2}\end{bmatrix}^{-1}, \tag{6.138}$$

where the entries in Eq. (6.138) are given, respectively, by

$$\frac{\partial^2 lnL(\pi)}{\partial p_i^2} = -\frac{\Delta_i^2 n_{i1}}{(\Delta_i p_i + \psi_i)^2} - \frac{\Delta_i^2 n_{i0}}{[1-(\Delta_i p_i + \psi_i)]^2} - \frac{n_{i2}}{p_i^2} - \frac{n_{i3}}{(1-p_i)^2} - \frac{n_{i4}}{p_i^2} - \frac{n_{i5}}{(1-p_i)^2},$$

$$\frac{\partial^2 lnL(\pi)}{\partial \varphi_i \partial p_i} = \frac{\Delta_i p_i n_{i1}}{(\Delta_i p_i + \psi_i)^2} + \frac{\Delta_i p_i n_{i0}}{[1-(\Delta_i p_i + \psi_i)]^2},$$

$$\frac{\partial^2 lnL(\pi)}{\partial \psi_i \partial p_i} = \frac{\Delta_i (1-p_i) n_{i1}}{(\Delta_i p_i + \psi_i)^2} - \frac{\Delta_i (1-p_i) n_{i0}}{[1-(\Delta_i p_i + \psi_i)]^2},$$

$$\frac{\partial^2 lnL(\pi)}{\partial^2 \varphi_i^2} = \frac{n_{i1} p_i^2}{(\Delta_i p_i + \psi_i)^2} - \frac{n_{i0} p_i^2}{[1-(\Delta_i p_i + \psi_i)]^2} - \frac{n_{i2}}{(1-\varphi_i)^2} - \frac{n_{i4}}{\varphi_i^2},$$

$$\frac{\partial^2 \ln \mathrm{L}(\pi)}{\partial \psi_i \partial \varphi_i} = -\frac{p_i (1-p_i) n_{i1}}{(\Delta_i p_i + \psi_i)^2} + \frac{p_i (1-p_i) n_{i0}}{[1-(\Delta_i p_i + \psi_i)]^2},$$

$$\frac{\partial^2 lnL(\pi)}{\partial^2 \psi_i^2} = -\frac{(1-p_i)^2 n_{i1}}{(\Delta_i p_i + \psi_i)^2} + \frac{(1-p_i)^2 n_{i0}}{[1-(\Delta_i p_i + \psi_i)]^2} + \frac{n_{i3}}{\psi_i^2} - \frac{n_{i5}}{(1-\psi_i)^2},$$

$$\frac{\partial^2 lnL(\pi)}{\partial p_i \partial \varphi_i} = \frac{\partial^2 lnL(\pi)}{\partial \varphi_i \partial p_i},$$

$$\frac{\partial^2 lnL(\pi)}{\partial p_i \partial \psi_i} = \frac{\partial^2 lnL(\pi)}{\partial \psi_i \partial p_i},$$

$$\frac{\partial^2 lnL(\pi)}{\partial \varphi_i \partial \psi_i} = \frac{\partial^2 lnL(\pi)}{\partial \psi_i \partial \varphi_i}.$$

By using the estimator $\breve{\tilde{p}}_i$ of eq. (6.136) with (φ_i, ψ_i) being replaced by $(\breve{\varphi}_i, \breve{\psi}_i)$, the $100(1-\alpha)\%$ confidence interval for $p_{i(I)}$ is given by

$$\breve{\tilde{p}}_i - z_{1-\frac{\alpha}{2}} \cdot \breve{\sigma}_{\breve{\tilde{p}}_i} \leq p_{i(I)} \leq \breve{\tilde{p}}_i + z_{1-\frac{\alpha}{2}} \cdot \breve{\sigma}_{\breve{\tilde{p}}_i}, \tag{6.139}$$

where $z_{1-\frac{\alpha}{2}}$ is the $100(1-\alpha)$ percentile of the standard normal, distribution, and $\breve{\sigma}_{\breve{\tilde{p}}_i}$ is obtained by taking the square root of the first diagonal entry of Eq. (6.138) with replacing the unknown $(p_{i(I)}, \varphi_i, \psi_i)$ with their corresponding estimators $(\breve{\tilde{p}}_i, \breve{\varphi}_i, \breve{\psi}_i)$.

The estimators of Eq. (6.1) are given, respectively, by

$$\widehat{R}_{(I)} = \frac{\widehat{\tilde{p}}_{1(I)} \widehat{\tilde{q}}_{0(I)}}{\widehat{\tilde{p}}_{0(I)} \widehat{\tilde{q}}_{1(I)}}, \tag{6.140}$$

where $\widehat{\widehat{p}}_{i(I)}$, i = 0, 1 are given, respectively, by Eq. (6.136) with φ_i and ψ_i replaced by its estimators $\widehat{\varphi}_i$ and $\widehat{\psi}_i$ from the data of the validation study in Table 6.15, and $\widehat{\widehat{q}}_i = 1 - \widehat{\widehat{p}}_i$.

By taking the natural logarithm of Eq. (6.136),

$$\ln\left(\widehat{\widehat{p}}_{i(I)}\right) = \ln[\widehat{\varphi}_i\widehat{\psi}_i(n_{i2}+n_{i4})] - \ln\left[\left(1+\sum_{j=2}^{5} n_{ij}\right)(1-\widehat{\varphi}_i)-\widehat{\psi}_i\right] = \ln(n_{i2}+n_{i4}) + \ln\widehat{\varphi}_i + \ln\widehat{\psi}_i - \ln\left[\left(1+\sum_{j=2}^{5} n_{ij}\right)(1-\widehat{\varphi}_i)-\widehat{\psi}_i\right], \tag{6.141}$$

where $\widehat{\varphi}_i$ and $\widehat{\psi}_i$ are estimated from the data of validation study. Thus, the expected value of the false negative probability is

$$\mu_{\widehat{\psi}_1} \equiv E(\widehat{\psi}_1) = 1 - E\left(\widehat{Se}_1\right) = 1 - \frac{n_{04}+n_{05}}{n_{02}+n_{03}+n_{04}+n_{05}} = \frac{n_{02}+n_{03}}{\breve{n}_0}, \tag{6.142}$$

where $\widehat{Se}_1$ denotes the estimated specificity of the classification procedure in the validation study of Table 6.15, and $\breve{n}_0 = \sum_{j=2}^{5} n_{0j}$.

Again, the expected value of the false positive probability is

$$\mu_{\widehat{\psi}_1} \equiv E(\widehat{\psi}_1) = 1 - E\left(\widehat{Se}_1\right) = 1 - \frac{n_{12}+n_{13}}{n_{12}+n_{13}+n_{14}+n_{15}} = \frac{n_{14}+n_{15}}{\breve{n}_1}, \tag{6.143}$$

where $\widehat{Se}_1$ denotes the sensitivity of the classification procedure in the validation study of Table 6.15, and $\breve{n}_1 = \sum_{j=2}^{5} n_{1j}$.

It is easily shown that $\mu_{\widehat{\varphi}_0} = \mu_{\widehat{\psi}_1}$ and $\mu_{\widehat{\psi}_0} = \mu_{\widehat{\varphi}_1}$.

Furthermore, the variance of $\widehat{\varphi}_i$ is given by

$$\sigma^2_{\widehat{\varphi}_i} = \sigma^2_{\widehat{Sp}_i} = \frac{\widehat{Sp}_i\left(1-\widehat{Sp}_{i)}\right.}{\breve{n}^2_{1-i}}, \tag{6.144}$$

and the variance of $\breve{\psi}_i$ is given by

$$\sigma^2_{\widehat{\psi}_i} = \sigma^2_{\widehat{Se}_i} = \frac{\widehat{Se}_i\left(1-\widehat{Se}_i\right)}{\breve{n}^2_i}. \tag{6.145}$$

From the following derivation of the variance of a logarithm of a random variable, I use the formula: $\sigma^2_{lnX} = \frac{\sigma^2_X}{\mu^2_X}$ (p. 248 in Bland [2]). By finding the variance of Eq. (6.141) with the substitution of Eqs. (6.142) to (6.145),

$$\sigma^2_{ln\,\widehat{\tilde{p}}_{i(I)}} = \sigma^2_{ln\,\widehat{\varphi}_i} + \sigma^2_{ln\,\widehat{\psi}_i} + \sigma^2_{ln[(1+\breve{n}_i)(1-\widehat{\varphi}_i)-\widehat{\psi}_i]} = \frac{\sigma^2_{\widehat{\varphi}_i}}{\mu^2_{\widehat{\varphi}_i}} + \frac{\sigma^2_{\widehat{\psi}_i}}{\mu^2_{\widehat{\psi}_i}} + \frac{\sigma^2_{\ln\{(1+\breve{n}_i)(1-\widehat{\varphi}_i)-\widehat{\psi}_i}}{\mu^2_{\ln[(1+\breve{n}_i)(1-\widehat{\varphi}_i)-\widehat{\psi}_i]}}. \tag{6.146}$$

By substituting Eqs. (6.142) to (6.145) into Eq. (6.146),

$$\sigma^2_{ln\,\widehat{\tilde{p}}_{1(I)}} = \frac{n_{04}+n_{05}}{\breve{n}_0^2(n_{02}+n_{03})} + \frac{n_{14}+n_{15}}{\breve{n}_1^2(n_{12}+n_{13})} + \frac{\breve{n}_1^4(1+\breve{n}_1)^2(n_{02}+n_{03})(n_{04}+n_{05})+\breve{n}_0^4(n_{12}+n_{13})(n_{14}+n_{15})}{[\breve{n}_1^2(1+\breve{n}_1)(n_{04}+n_{05})-\breve{n}_0^2(n_{14}+n_{15})]^2}, \tag{6.147}$$

$$\sigma^2_{ln\,\widehat{\tilde{p}}_{0(I)}} = \frac{n_{12}+n_{13}}{\breve{n}_1^2(n_{14}+n_{15})} + \frac{n_{02}+n_{03}}{\breve{n}_0^2(n_{04}+n_{05})} + \frac{\breve{n}_0^4(1+\breve{n}_0)^2(n_{12}+n_{13})(n_{14}+n_{15})+\breve{n}_1^4(n_{02}+n_{03})(n_{04}+n_{05})}{[\breve{n}_0^2(1+\breve{n}_0)(n_{14}+n_{15})-\breve{n}_1^2(n_{02}+n_{03})]^2}, \tag{6.148}$$

By using the relationship of $ln\,\widehat{\tilde{q}}_i = \ln(1-\widehat{\tilde{p}}_i) = \ln\{[(1+\breve{n}_i)(1-\widehat{\varphi}_i)-\widehat{\psi}_i]-(n_{i2}+n_{i4})\widehat{\varphi}_i\widehat{\psi}_i\} - \ln\ [(1+\breve{n}_i)(1-\widehat{\varphi}_i)-\widehat{\psi}_i$,

$$\begin{aligned}\sigma^2_{ln\,\widehat{\tilde{q}}_{1(I)}} &= \sigma^2_{\ln\{[(1+\breve{n}_1)(1-\widehat{\varphi}_1)-\widehat{\psi}_1]-(n_{12}+n_{14})\widehat{\varphi}_1\widehat{\psi}_1\}} + \sigma^2_{\ln[(1+\breve{n}_1)(1-\widehat{\varphi}_1)-\widehat{\psi}_1]} \\ &= \frac{\sigma^2_{\{[(1+\breve{n}_1)(1-\widehat{\varphi}_1)-\widehat{\psi}_1]-(n_{12}+n_{14})\widehat{\varphi}_1\widehat{\psi}_1\}}}{\mu^2_{\{[(1+\breve{n}_1)(1-\widehat{\varphi}_1)-\widehat{\psi}_1]-(n_{12}+n_{14})\widehat{\varphi}_1\widehat{\psi}_1\}}} + \frac{\sigma^2_{[(1+\breve{n}_1)(1-\widehat{\varphi}_1)-\widehat{\psi}_1]}}{\mu^2_{[(1+\breve{n}_1)(1-\widehat{\varphi}_1)-\widehat{\psi}_1]}} \\ &= \frac{(n_{02}+n_{03})(n_{04}+n_{05})\{[(1+\breve{n}_1^2)\breve{n}_1^4+(n_{12}+n_{14})^2(n_{12}+n_{13})(n_{14}+n_{15})]+\breve{n}_0^4(n_{12}+n_{13})(n_{14}+n_{15})\}}{\breve{n}_0^2\breve{n}_1^2\{[\breve{n}_1(1+\breve{n}_1)-\breve{n}_0](n_{04}+n_{05})-(n_{12}+n_{14})(n_{02}+n_{03})(n_{14}+n_{15})]^2} \\ &\quad + \frac{\breve{n}_1^4(n_{02}+n_{03})(n_{04}+n_{05})+\breve{n}_0^4(n_{12}+n_{13})(n_{14}+n_{15})}{\breve{n}_0^2\breve{n}_1^2[\breve{n}_1(1+\breve{n}_1)(n_{04}+n_{05})-\breve{n}_0(n_{14}+n_{15})]^2},\end{aligned} \tag{6.149}$$

and

$$\begin{aligned}\sigma^2_{ln\,\widehat{\tilde{q}}_{0(I)}} &= \frac{(1+\breve{n}_0)^2\sigma^2_{\widehat{\varphi}_0}+\sigma^2_{\widehat{\psi}}+(n_{02}+n_{04})^2\sigma^2_{\widehat{\varphi}}\sigma^2_{\widehat{\psi}}}{[(1+\breve{n}_0)(1-\mu_{\widehat{\varphi}_0})-\mu_{\widehat{\psi}_0}-(n_{02}+n_{04})\mu_{\widehat{\varphi}_0}\mu_{\widehat{\psi}_0}]^2} + \frac{(1+\breve{n}_0)^2\sigma^2_{\widehat{\varphi}_0}+\sigma^2_{\widehat{\psi}_0}}{[(1+\breve{n}_0)(1-\mu_{\widehat{\varphi}_0})-\mu_{\widehat{\psi}_0}]^2} \\ &= \frac{(n_{12}+n_{13})(n_{14}+n_{15})\{[\breve{n}_0^4(1+\breve{n}_0)^2+(n_{02}+n_{04})^2(n_{02}+n_{03})(n_{04}+n_{05})\}+\breve{n}_1^4(n_{02}+n_{03})(n_{04}+n_{05})\}}{\breve{n}_0^2\breve{n}_1^2\{(n_{14}+n_{15})[\breve{n}_0(1+\breve{n}_0)-(n_{02}+n_{04})(n_{02}+n_{03})]-\breve{n}_1(n_{02}+n_{03})\}^2} \\ &\quad + \frac{\breve{n}_0^4(1+\breve{n}_0)^2(n_{12}+n_{13})(n_{14}+n_{15})+\breve{n}_1^4(n_{02}+n_{03})(n_{04}+n_{05})}{\breve{n}_0^2\breve{n}_1^2[\breve{n}_0(1+\breve{n}_0)(n_{12}+n_{13})-\breve{n}_1(n_{02}+n_{03})]^2}.\end{aligned} \tag{6.150}$$

To find the variance of the natural logarithm of Eq. (6.140), we substitute Eqs. (6.147) to (6.150) into the following

$$\sigma^2_{\ln \widehat{R}_{(I)}} = \sigma^2_{\ln \widehat{\tilde{p}_1}} + \sigma^2_{\ln \widehat{\tilde{p}_0}} + \sigma^2_{\ln \widehat{\tilde{q}_1}} + \sigma^2_{\ln \widehat{\tilde{q}_0}}. \tag{6.151}$$

By using the natural logarithmic estimator of Eq. (6.140), the 100·(1 − α)% confidence interval for R is given by

$$\exp\left[\ln\left(\widehat{R}_{(I)}\right) - z_{1-\frac{\alpha}{2}} \cdot \widehat{\sigma}_{\ln\left(\widehat{R}_{(I)}\right)}\right] \le R \le \exp\left[\ln\left(\widehat{R}_{(I)}\right) + z_{1-\frac{\alpha}{2}} \cdot \widehat{\sigma}_{\ln\left(\widehat{R}_{(I)}\right)}\right], \tag{6.152}$$

where $\widehat{\sigma}_{\ln\left(\widehat{R}_{(I)}\right)}$ is obtained as the square root of Eq. (6.151) with a replacement of $\sigma_{\ln \widehat{\tilde{p}_{i(I)}}}$ and $\sigma_{\ln \widehat{\tilde{q}_{i(I)}}}$ by their corresponding estimators of Eqs. (6.147) to (6.150).

6.4.2 The Direct Method

On the other hand, define the predictive positive and negative rate as

$$\omega_i = \Pr(X = 1 | X^* = 1, Y = i), \tag{6.153}$$

and

$$\gamma_i = \Pr(X = 0 | X^* = 0, Y = i). \tag{6.154}$$

When ω_i and γ_i, are assumed to be unknown, let us obtain their estimators in terms of the alternative parameterization in p_i^*, ω_i and γ_i. The likelihood function of $\vec{\pi}^* = \left(p_1^*, p_0^*, \omega_1, \omega_0, \gamma_1, \gamma_0\right)^T$ is

$$\ell(\pi^*) = \prod_{i=0}^{1} \{ (p_i^*)^{n_{i1}} + (1-p_i^*)^{n_{i0}} + (\omega_i p_i^*)^{n_{i2}} + [(1-\omega_i)p_i^*]^{n_{i3}} + [(1-\gamma_i)(1-p_i^*)]^{n_{i4}} + [\gamma_i(1-p_i^*)]^{n_{i5}} \}, \tag{6.155}$$

where ω_i and γ_i are given by Eqs. (6.153) and (6.154), p_i^* is the prevalence of the disease when the ω_i and γ_i are used to set up the likelihood of $\vec{\pi}^*$.

By setting partial derivatives of the logarithm of (6.155) with respect to the parameter π^* equal to zero, we have for $i = 1, 2$

$$\begin{aligned}
\frac{\partial \ln(\ell(\pi^*))}{\partial p_i^*} &= \frac{\sum_{j=1}^{3} n_{ij}}{p_i^*} - \frac{\sum_{j=0,4,5} n_{ij}}{1-p_i^*} = 0,\\
\frac{\partial \ln(\ell(\pi^*))}{\partial \omega_i} &= \frac{n_{i2}}{\omega_i} - \frac{n_{i3}}{1-\omega_i} = 0,\\
\frac{\partial \ln(\ell(\pi^*))}{\partial \gamma_i} &= -\frac{n_{i4}}{1-\gamma_i} + \frac{n_{i5}}{\gamma_i} = 0.
\end{aligned} \tag{6.156}$$

By solving Eq. (6.156) the maximum likelihood estimators for π^* are given by

$$\widehat{p}_{i(D)}^* = \frac{\sum_{j=1}^{3} n_{ij}}{\breve{n}_i^*}, \tag{6.157}$$

$$\breve{\omega}_i = \frac{n_{i2}}{\sum_{j=2}^{3} n_{ij}}, \tag{6.158}$$

$$\breve{\gamma}_i = \frac{n_{i5}}{\sum_{j=4}^{5} n_{ij}}, \tag{6.159}$$

where $\breve{n}_i^* = \sum_{j=0}^{5} n_{ij}$, i = 0, 1.

The asymptotic variance of $\vec{\theta}_{(D)} = \left(p_i^*, \omega_i, \gamma_i\right)^T$ is given by [18]

$$\Sigma_{i(D)} = -diag\left[\frac{\partial^2 \ell}{\partial p_i^{*2}}, \frac{\partial^2 \ell}{\partial {\omega_i}^2}, \frac{\partial^2 \ell}{\partial {\gamma_i}^2}\right]^{-1}, \tag{6.160}$$

where

$$\frac{\partial^2 \ell\left(\vec{\theta}_{(D)}\right)}{\partial p_i^{*2}} = -\left(\sum_{j=1}^{3} n_{ij}\right)\left[\frac{1}{p_i^{*2}} + \frac{1}{\left(1-p_i^*\right)^2}\right]$$

$$\frac{\partial^2 \ell\left(\vec{\theta}_{(D)}\right)}{\partial {\omega_i}^2} = -\left[\frac{n_{i2}}{\omega_i^2} + \frac{n_{i3}}{\left(1-\omega_i\right)^2}\right]$$

and

$$\frac{\partial^2 \ell\left(\vec{\theta}_{(D)}\right)}{\partial {\gamma_i}^2} = -\left[\frac{n_{i4}}{\left(1-\gamma_i\right)^2} + \frac{n_{i5}}{\gamma_i^2}\right],$$

By using the estimator $\widehat{p}_{i(D)}^*$ the 100·(1 − α)% confidence interval for p_i is given by

$$\widehat{p}^*_{i(D)} - z_{1-\frac{\alpha}{2}} \cdot \sigma_{\widehat{p}_{i(D)}} \le p_i \le \widehat{p}^*_{i(D)} + z_{1-\frac{\alpha}{2}} \cdot \sigma_{\widehat{p}_{i(D)}}, \tag{6.161}$$

where $z_{1-\frac{\alpha}{2}}$ is the $100 \cdot (1-\frac{\alpha}{2})$ percentile of the standard normal distribution, and $\sigma_{\widehat{p}_{i(D)}}$ is given by taking the square root of the first diagonal entry of Eq. (6.160) with replacing the unknown p_i^* with its corresponding estimator of Eq. (6.157).

The maximum likelihood estimators of Eq. (6.1) are given, respectively, by

$$\widehat{R}_{(D)} = \frac{\widehat{p}^*_{1(D)}\widehat{q}^*_{0(D)}}{\widehat{p}^*_{0(D)}\widehat{q}^*_{1(D)}}, \tag{6.162}$$

where $\widehat{p}^*_{i(D)}$, i = 0, 1, is given, respectively, by Eq. (6.157), and $\widehat{q}^*_{i(D)} = 1 - \widehat{p}^*_{i(D)}$.

The variance of the logarithm of $\ln\widehat{R}_{(D)}$ is given by

$$\sigma^2_{\ln\widehat{R}_{(D)}} = \sum\nolimits_{i=0}^{1}\left(\sigma^2_{ln\,\widehat{p}_{i(D)}} + \sigma^2_{ln\,\widehat{q}_{i(D)}}\right), \tag{6.163}$$

where $\sigma^2_{ln\,\widehat{p}_{i(D)}}$ and $\sigma^2_{ln\,\widehat{q}_{i(D)}}$ are given by

$$\sigma^2_{ln\,\widehat{p}_{i(D)}} = \frac{\sigma^2_{\widehat{p}_{i(D)}}}{\mu^2_{\widehat{p}_{i(D)}}} = \frac{\left\{\sum_{j=1}^{3} n_{ij}\left[\left(\widehat{p}^*_{i(D)}\right)^{-2} + \left(1 - \widehat{p}^*_{i(D)}\right)^{-2}\right]\right\}^{-1}}{\left(\breve{n}_i^*\right)^{-1}\sum_{j=1}^{3} n_{ij}}$$

$$= \left[\left(\breve{n}_i^*\right)^2\sum\nolimits_{j=1}^{3} n_{ij}\right]^{-1}\left[\left(\sum\nolimits_{j=1}^{3} n_{ij}\right)^{-2} + \left(\sum\nolimits_{j=0,4}^{5} n_{ij}\right)^{-2}\right]^{-1},$$

and

$$\sigma^2_{ln\,\widehat{q}_{i(D)}} = \left[\sum\nolimits_{j=1}^{3} n_{ij}\right]^{-3}\left[\left(\sum\nolimits_{j=1}^{3} n_{ij}\right)^{-2} + \left(\sum\nolimits_{j=0,4}^{5} n_{ij}\right)^{-2}\right]^{-1}.$$

By using the estimator of Eq. (6.136) or Eq. (6.157), the 100·(1 – α)% confidence interval for R is given by for $k = D$ or I

$$\exp\left[\ln\left(\widehat{R}_{(k)}\right) - z_{1-\frac{\alpha}{2}} \cdot \widehat{\sigma}_{\ln\left(\widehat{R}_{(k)}\right)}\right] \le R \le \exp\left[\ln\left(\widehat{R}_{(k)}\right) + z_{1-\frac{\alpha}{2}} \cdot \widehat{\sigma}_{\ln\left(\widehat{R}_{(k)}\right)}\right], \tag{6.164}$$

where $\widehat{\sigma}_{\ln(\widehat{R}_{(k)})}$ is obtained as the square root of Eq. (6.163) with a replacement of $p_{i(k)}$ and $\sigma_{ln\,\widehat{p}_{i(k)}}$ by their corresponding estimators of Eqs. (6.136) (or Eq. (6.157)) and Eqs. (6.151) (or (6.163)).

Remark
A different derivation of the direct (D) versus indirect (I) methods was proposed by Marshall [19].

Example 6.4
In a case-control study of sudden infant death syndrome (SIDS), a validation study was used to investigate the association of maternal exposure to the use of antibiotics during woman's pregnancy [12]. The error-prone measurement $X^*$was an interview response, while the "true" exposure X was derived from medical records. The validation studies were joint X^*, X designs done as sub-study of primary study and resulted in Table 6.16.

(a) Estimate the true prevalence p_1 and p_0 with 95% confidence interval of women who has and has no SIDS by the maximum likelihood direct and indirect method;
(b) Is there any positive association between the prevalence of the SIDS and the use antibiotics during woman's pregnancy?

Solution
(a) (A) Indirect method
By solving Eq. (6.135) for φ_i and ψ_i with the method of function evaluation, we have from the following table:

φ_1	ψ_1	$g_1(\varphi_1, \psi_1)$	φ_0	ψ_0	$g_0(\varphi_0, \psi_0)$
0.3	0.3	0.523522	0.3	0.3	0.230248
0.4	0.4	−0.308388	0.4	0.4	−0.0723
0.355	0.355	−0.023020	0.365	0.365	0.005224
0.3528	0.3513	−0.005877	0.366517	0.366178	0.001544
0.351855	0.350855	0.001438	0.366517	0.366178	0.001543

where $g_i(\varphi_i, \psi_i)$ is given by Eq. (6.135).

$$\breve{\varphi}_1 = 0.3518556, \breve{\psi}_1 = 0.3508554, \tag{6.165}$$

and

Table 6.16 The case-control data of the main study and validation study of sudden infant death symdrome

	Interview data			Medical record			
				Y = 1		Y = 0	
	Y = 1	Y = 0		X = 1	X = 0	X = 1	X = 0
$X^* = 1$	173	134	$X^* = 1$	29	22	21	12
$X^* = 0$	602	663	$X^* = 0$	17	143	16	168

$X^* = 1$ if she used the antibiotics; = 0 if not used; Y = 1 if she had a SIDS, = 0 if she did not have a SIDS

$$\breve{\varphi}_0 = 0.3665174, \breve{\psi}_0 = 0.3661783. \tag{6.166}$$

By substituting Eqs. (6.165) and (6.166) into Eq. (6.136),

$$\breve{p}_{1(I)} = 0.041433649 \approx 0.0414, \tag{6.167}$$

and

$$\breve{p}_{0(I)} = 0.036054 \approx 0.0361. \tag{6.168}$$

By substituting Eqs. (6.165) to (6.168) into Eq. (6.138),

$$\begin{aligned}\Sigma_{1(I)} &= -\begin{bmatrix} -26750.58 & 20.23 & 279.62 \\ 20.23 & -204.66 & -38.97 \\ 279.62 & -38.97 & 1647.19 \end{bmatrix}^{-1} \\ &= \begin{bmatrix} 3.7\cdot 10^{-5} & 4.8\cdot 10^{-6} & 0.000257 \\ 4.8\cdot 10^{-6} & 0.0049 & 0.0001 \\ -5.9\cdot 10^{-6} & 0.0001 & -0.0006 \end{bmatrix},\end{aligned} \tag{6.169}$$

and

$$\begin{aligned}\Sigma_{0(I)} &= -\begin{bmatrix} -28730.3 & 49.18 & 125.05 \\ 49.18 & -170.8 & 76.86 \\ 125.05 & 76.86 & 4413.3 \end{bmatrix}^{-1} \\ &= \begin{bmatrix} 3.4\cdot 10^{-5} & 9.6\cdot 10^{-6} & -9.7\cdot 10^{-6} \\ 9.6\cdot 10^{-6} & 0.0058 & -8.5\cdot 10^{-5} \\ -9.7\cdot 10^{-7} & -8.5\cdot 10^{-5} & -0.0002 \end{bmatrix}.\end{aligned} \tag{6.170}$$

From Eqs. (6.169) and (6.170),

$$\sigma^2_{\breve{p}_{1(I)}} = 3.7\cdot 10^{-5}, \tag{6.171}$$

and

$$\sigma^2_{\breve{p}_{0(I)}} = 3.4\cdot 10^{-5}. \tag{6.172}$$

By substituting Eqs. (6.167) and (6.168) into Eq. (6.139), the 95% confidence intervals for $p_{i(k)}$ are given, respectively, by

$$
\begin{aligned}
&0.0414 - 1.96 \cdot \sqrt{3.7 \cdot 10^{-5}} \le p_{1(I)} \le 0.0414 + 1.96 \cdot \sqrt{3.7 \cdot 10^{-5}},\\
&\text{or } 0.03 \le p_{1(I)} \le 0.05,\\
&0.0361 - 1.96 \cdot \sqrt{3.4 \cdot 10^{-5}} \le p_{0(I)} \le 0.0361 + 1.96 \cdot \sqrt{3.4 \cdot 10^{-5}},\\
&\text{or } 0.02 \le p_{0(I)} \le 0.05.
\end{aligned}
\tag{6.173}
$$

(B) Direct method
By substituting the data in Table 6.16 into Eqs. (6.157) to (6.159),

$$
\begin{aligned}
\widehat{p}^*_{1(D)} &= \frac{173 + 29 + 22}{134 + 173 + 29 + 22 + 17 + 143} = 0.571429 \approx 0.57,\\
\widehat{p}^*_{0(D)} &= \frac{602 + 17 + 143}{663 + 602 + 17 + 143 + 16 + 168} = 0.428475 \approx 0.43,\\
\breve{\omega}_{1(D)} &= \frac{29}{29 + 22} = 0.568627 \approx 0.59,\\
\breve{\omega}_{0(D)} &= \frac{17}{17 + 43} = 0.283333 \approx 0.28,\\
\breve{\gamma}_{1(D)} &= \frac{12}{21 + 12} = 0.363636 \approx 0.36, \text{and}\\
\breve{\gamma}_{0(D)} &= \frac{168}{16 + 168} = 0.913044 \approx 0.91.
\end{aligned}
\tag{6.174}
$$

From Eq. (6.160),

$$
\begin{aligned}
\Sigma^*_{1(D)} &= diag < 1905.6, 207.9, 170.5 > ,\\
\Sigma^*_{0(D)} &= diag < 5401.9, 142.6, 2317.5 > ,
\end{aligned}
$$

and

$$
\begin{aligned}
\Sigma^{*(-1)}_{1(D)} &= diag < 0.0005, 0.0048, 0.0059 > ,\\
\Sigma^{*(-1)}_{0(D)} &= diag < 0.0002, 0.007, 0.0004 > .
\end{aligned}
$$

By substituting Eq. (6.174) into Eq. (6.161), the 95% confidence interval for

$$
\begin{aligned}
&0.57 - 1.96 \cdot \sqrt{0.0005} \le p_{1(D)} \le 0.57 + 1.96 \cdot \sqrt{0.0005},\\
&\text{or } 0.53 \le p_{1(D)} \le 0.86,\\
&0.43 - 1.96 \cdot \sqrt{0.0002} \le p_{0(D)} \le 0.43 + 1.96 \cdot \sqrt{0.0002},\\
&\text{or } 0.40 \le p_{0(D)} \le 0.46.
\end{aligned}
$$

(b) By substituting Eqs. (6.167), (6.168), and (6.174) into Eq. (6.162), the maximum likelihood estimators of $R_{(k)}$, k = I, or D, are given, respectively, by

$$\begin{aligned} R_{(I)} &= \frac{0.0414 \cdot (1 - 0.0361)}{0.0361 \cdot (1 - 0.0414)} = 1.1557 \approx 1.16, \text{and} \\ R_{(D)} &= \frac{0.57 \cdot (1 - 0.43)}{0.43 \cdot (1 - 0.57)} = 1.7572 \approx 1.76. \end{aligned} \tag{6.175}$$

By substituting Eqs. (6.167), (6.168), (6.171), and (6.172) into Eq. (6.151) and Eq. (6.163), the variance of the logarithm of Eq. (6.175) are given by

$$\begin{aligned} \sigma^2_{\ln(\breve{R}_{(I)})} &= 0.1845 + 1.5021 + 6.7 \cdot 10^{-10} + 0.0002 = 1.6873, \text{and} \\ \sigma^2_{\ln(\breve{R}_{(D)})} &= 0.0007 + 0.0002 + 0.0016 + 0.0013 = 0.0038. \end{aligned} \tag{6.176}$$

By substituting Eq. (6.176) into Eqs. (6.152) and (6.164), the 95% confidence interval for $R_{(k)}$, k = I or D, are given, respectively, by

$$\begin{aligned} &\exp\left[\ln(1.16) - 1.96 \cdot \sqrt{1.6873}\right] \le R_{(I)} \le \exp\left[\ln(1.16) + 1.96 \cdot \sqrt{1.6873}\right], \\ &\text{or } 0.09 \le R_{(I)} \le 14.7 \text{ and} \\ &\exp\left[\ln(1.76) - 1.96 \cdot \sqrt{0.0038}\right] \le R_{(D)} \le \exp\left[\ln(1.76) + 1.96 \cdot \sqrt{0.0038}\right], \\ &\text{or } 1.71 \le R_{(D)} \le 1.80. \end{aligned} \tag{6.177}$$

From Eq. (6.177), the odds ratio by using the misclassification error rate φ_i and ψ_i is insignificant, whereas that by using the predictive positive and negative values are significant. Hence, the direct method is more powerful to indicate that there is positive association between the prevalence of the SIDS and the use antibiotics during woman's pregnancy.

6.4.3 Method of Double Sampling

In some situations, it is reasonable to assume that there are two measuring devices to classify sampling units into one of two categories, denoted by 0 and 1, respectively. The true device is an expensive procedure which makes no mistakes, whereas the fallible device is relatively inexpensive but tends to misclassify units. One such application is a medical survey where the fallible procedure is an interview of the respondent, whereas the true procedure is a physician's diagnosis which will be the correct procedure.

	$\dot{D}$	$\ddot{D}$
$\dot{E}$	a (I)	b (II)
$\ddot{E}$	c (III)	d (IV)

Fig. 6.1 The double sampling scheme. Where "(.)" denote for either (A) or (B), $m_{i+(.)} = m_{i0(.)} + m_{i1(.)}$, $m_{+j(.)} = m_{0j(.)} + m_{1j(.)}$, i, j = 0, 1, and $m_{(.)} = \sum_{i=0}^{1} m_{i+(.)} = \sum_{j=0}^{1} m_{+j(.)}$, $p_1 =$ Pr (T = 1), and $p_2 =$ Pr (F = 1)

Let population A and B denote, respectively, the cases and the controls. If a sample of $m_{(.)}$ units is drawn from either population in which the subscript (.) denotes either population A or B, we could use either the true classifier only, which is expensive, or the fallible classifier only, which may produce misleading results. A double sampling scheme is a compromise between these two extremes. This scheme is described below [25]:

(i) A subsample of $m_{(.)}$ units is drawn from the main sample of $M_{(.)}$ units and each of these $m_{(.)}$ units are classified by both measuring devices.
(ii) The remaining $M_{(.)} - m_{(.)}$ units are classified only by the fallible classifier. (Fig. 6.1).

Assume that the random variables of $m_{11(.)}$, $m_{10(.)}$, $m_{01(.)}$, and $m_{00(.)}$ are multinomially distributed. The likelihood $L(p)$ is given by [25]:

$$L_{(.)} = \pi_{1(.)}{}^{m_{11(.)}} \left(1 - \pi_{1(.)}\right)^{m_{01(.)}} \pi_{2(.)}{}^{m_{10(.)}} \left(1 - \pi_{2(.)}\right)^{m_{00(.)}} p_{2(.)}^{m_{1+(.)}+x_{(.)}} q_{2(.)}^{m_{0+(.)}+y_{(.)}}, \quad (6.178)$$

where $\pi_{1(.)} = \left(1 - \varphi_{(.)}\right) p_{1(.)} p_{2(.)}^{-1}$, $\pi_{2(.)} = \varphi_{(.)} p_{1(.)} q_{2(.)}^{-1}$ $\varphi_{(.)} =$ Pr $(F_{(.)} = 0 | T_{(.)} = 1)$ and $\psi_{(.)} =$ Pr $(F_{(.)} = 1 | T_{(.)} = 0)$ are two misclassification error probabilities for either population, and $q_{i(.)} = 1 - p_{i(.)}$.

By taking derivative of the logarithm of Eq. (6.178) with respect to π_1, π_2, and p_2,

$$\begin{aligned} \frac{\partial \ln\left(L_{(.)}\right)}{\partial \pi_{1(.)}} &= \frac{m_{11(.)}}{\pi_{1(.)}} - \frac{m_{01(.)}}{1 - \pi_{1(.)}} = 0, \\ \text{or } \widehat{\pi}_{1(.)} &= \frac{m_{11(.)}}{m_{+1(.)}}; \end{aligned} \quad (6.179)$$

$$\begin{aligned} \frac{\partial \ln\left(L_{(.)}\right)}{\partial \pi_{2(.)}} &= \frac{m_{10(.)}}{\pi_{2(.)}} - \frac{m_{00(.)}}{1 - \pi_{2(.)}} = 0, \\ \text{or } \widehat{\pi}_{2(.)} &= \frac{m_{10(.)}}{m_{+0(.)}} \end{aligned} \quad (6.180)$$

$$\frac{\partial \ln\left(L_{(.)}\right)}{\partial p_{2(.)}} = \frac{\left(m_{1+(.)} + x_{(.)}\right)}{p_{2(.)}} - \frac{\left(m_{0+(.)} + y_{(.)}\right)}{1 - p_{2(.)}} = 0, \tag{6.181}$$
$$\text{or } \widehat{p}_{2(\cdot)} = \frac{m_{1+(.)} + x}{M}.$$

By using the relationship between $\pi_{i(.)}$ and $p_{i(.)}$, the maximum likelihood estimator of the true unknown prevalence $p_{1(.)} = \Pr\left(T_{(.)} = 1\right)$ is given by (Exercise 6.7-10)

$$\widehat{p}_{1(.)} = \frac{m_{11(.)}\left(m_{1+(.)} + x_{(.)}\right)}{m_{1+(.)}M_{(.)}} + \frac{m_{01(.)}\left(m_{0+(.)} + y_{(.)}\right)}{m_{0+(.)}M_{(.)}}, \tag{6.182}$$

$$\widehat{\varphi}_{(.)} = \frac{m_{01(.)}\left(m_{0+(.)} + y_{(.)}\right)}{\widehat{p}_{1(.)}m_{0+(.)}M_{(.)}}, \tag{6.183}$$

and

$$\widehat{\psi}_{(.)} = \frac{m_{10(.)}\left(m_{1+(.)} + x_{(.)}\right)}{\left(1 - \widehat{p}_{1(.)}\right)m_{1+(.)}M_{(.)}}. \tag{6.184}$$

Remarks

1. Equation (6.182) is undefined when either $m_{+1(.)}$ or $m_{0\,+\,(.)}$ equals zero. It can be shown that the probability of this event is $p_{2(.)}^{m_{(.)}} + \left(1 - p_{2(.)}\right)^{m_{(.)}}$. Thus, the probability of undefined estimate of $p_{1(.)}$ is small unless $m_{(.)}$ is small and $p_{2(.)}$ is close to 0 or 1.
2. This contingency can be avoided by the following stratified modification of the double sampling scheme presented earlier in this section:

   (i) Obtain the fallible classification for all $M_{(.)}$ units in the sample in either population A or B. Let $v_{(.)}$ equal the number of units classified in category 1.
   (ii) Take a stratified subsample of $m_{(.)} = m_{1\,+\,(.)} + m_{0\,+\,(.)}$ units of which $m_{1+(.)} = \frac{m_{(.)}\cdot v_{(.)}}{M_{(.)}}$ is taken from $v_{(.)}$ "category 1" units and $m_{0\,+\,(.)}$ units are taken from $M_{(.)} - v_{(.)}$ "category 0" units.

   To obtain the asymptotic variance of Eq. (6.182), we need the following two lemmas.

Lemma 6.1
Let $\widehat{\pi}_{1(.)}$, $\widehat{\pi}_{2(.)}$, and $\widehat{p}_{2(.)}$ be given, respectively, by Eqs. (6.179) to (6.181). Then asymptotically as $m_{(.)} \to \infty$ and $M_{(.)} \to \infty$ such that $\frac{m_{(.)}}{M_{(.)}} \to f > 0$:

$$\sigma^2_{\widehat{\pi}_{1(.)}} = \pi_{1(.)} \frac{\left(1 - \pi_{1(.)}\right)}{m_{(.)}p_{2(.)}}, \tag{6.185}$$

$$\sigma^2_{\widehat{\pi}_{2(.)}} = \frac{\pi_{2(.)}\left(1 - \pi_{2(.)}\right)}{m_{(.)}\left(1 - p_{2(.)}\right)}, \tag{6.186}$$

$$\sigma^2_{\widehat{p}_{2(.)}} = \frac{p_{2(.)}\left(1 - p_{2(.)}\right)}{M_{(.)}}, \tag{6.187}$$

and

$$cov\left(\widehat{\pi}_{1(.)}, \widehat{\pi}_{2(.)}\right) = cov\left(\widehat{\pi}_{1(.)}, \widehat{p}_{2(.)}\right) = cov\left(\widehat{\pi}_{2(.)}, \widehat{p}_{2(.)}\right) = 0. \tag{6.188}$$

Proof

The variance–covariance matrix Σ of $\left(\widehat{\pi}_{1(.)}, \widehat{\pi}_{2(.)}, \widehat{p}_{2(.)}\right)$ is the negative of the expected value of the inverse of information matrix

$$\Sigma^{-1} = -E\left(\left[\begin{array}{ccc} \frac{\partial^2 lnL}{\partial \pi_{1(.)}^2} & \frac{\partial^2 lnL}{\partial \pi_{2(.)}\partial \pi_{1(.)}} & \frac{\partial^2 lnL}{\partial p_{2(.)}\partial \pi_{1(.)}} \\ \frac{\partial^2 lnL}{\partial \pi_{1(.)}\partial \pi_{2(.)}} & \frac{\partial^2 lnL}{\partial \pi_{2(.)}^2} & \frac{\partial^2 lnL}{\partial p_{2(.)}\partial \pi_{2(.)}} \\ \frac{\partial^2 lnL}{\partial \pi_{1(.)}\partial p_{2(.)}} & \frac{\partial^2 lnL}{\partial \pi_{2(.)}\partial p_{2(.)}} & \frac{\partial^2 lnL}{\partial p_{2(.)}^2} \end{array}\right]\Bigg|_{\substack{\pi_{1(.)}=\widehat{\pi}_{1(.)} \\ \pi_{2(.)}=\widehat{\pi}_{2(.)} \\ p_{2(.)}=\widehat{p}_{2(.)}}}\right)$$

$$= \begin{bmatrix} \frac{m_{(.)}p_{2(.)}}{\pi_{1(.)}\left(1 - \pi_{1(.)}\right)} & 0 & 0 \\ 0 & \frac{m_{(.)}\left(1 - p_{2(.)}\right)}{\pi_{2(.)}\left(1 - \pi_{2(.)}\right)} & 0 \\ 0 & 0 & \frac{M_{(.)}}{p_{2(.)}\left(1 - p_{2(.)}\right)} \end{bmatrix}. \tag{6.189}$$

The proof is done by taking the inverse of Eq. (6.189).

Lemma 6.2

Let $\pi_{1(.)}$, $\pi_{2(.)}$, and $p_{2(.)}$ be defined as before. Then the following identities hold:

(i) $p_{1(.)}\varphi_{(.)}(1-\varphi_{(.)}) + q_{1(.)}\psi_{(.)}(1-\psi_{(.)}) = p_{2(.)}q_{2(.)} - p_{1(.)}q_{1(.)}(1-\varphi_{(.)}-\psi_{(.)})^2$;
(ii) $\pi_{1(.)}\left(1-\pi_{1(.)}\right)p_{2(.)} + \pi_{2(.)}$

$$\left(1-\pi_{2(.)}\right)\left(1-p_{2(.)}\right) = p_{1(.)}q_{1(.)}\left[1-\frac{p_{1(.)}q_{1(.)}\left(1-\varphi_{(.)}-\psi_{(.)}\right)^2}{p_{2(.)}q_{2(.)}}\right]$$

;

(iii) $\left(\pi_{1(.)}-\pi_{2(.)}\right)^2 p_{2(.)}q_{2(.)} = \frac{\left[p_{1(.)}q_{1(.)}\left(1-\varphi_{(.)}-\psi_{(.)}\right)\right]^2}{p_{2(.)}q_{2(.)}}$;

where $q_{i(.)} = 1 - p_{i(.)}$, i = 1, 2.

It can be proved by straightforward substitution (Exercise 6.7-11).

The asymptotic variance of $\widehat{p}_{1(.)}$ is given in the following theorem.

Theorem 6.2
Let $\widehat{\pi}_{1(.)}$, $\widehat{\pi}_{2(.)}$, and $\widehat{p}_{2(.)}$ be the corresponding maximum likelihood estimators given, respectively, by Eqs. (6.179) to (6.181). Then asymptotically as $m_{(.)} \to \infty$ and $M_{(.)} \to \infty$ such that $\frac{m_{(.)}}{M_{(.)}} \to f > 0$:

$$\sigma^2_{\widehat{p}_{1(.)}} = \frac{p_{1(.)}q_{1(.)}}{m_{(.)}}\left[1-\frac{\left(1-\varphi_{(.)}-\psi_{(.)}\right)^2 p_{1(.)}q_{1(.)}}{p_{2(.)}q_{2(.)}}\right] + \frac{\left[\left(1-\varphi_{(.)}-\psi_{(.)}\right)p_{1(.)}q_{1(.)}\right]^2}{M_{(.)}p_{2(.)}q_{2(.)}} \tag{6.190}$$

where $q_{i(.)} = 1 - p_{i(.)}$, I = 1, 2.

Proof
Since

$$p_1 = \pi_1 p_2 + \pi_2(1-p_2), \tag{6.191}$$

we have

$$\frac{\partial p_1}{\partial \pi_1} = p_2,\ \frac{\partial p_1}{\partial \pi_2} = 1 - p_2, \text{ and } \frac{\partial p_1}{\partial p_2} = \pi_1 - \pi_2. \tag{6.192}$$

By applying the delta method [1],

$$\sigma_{\widehat{p_1}}^2 = \sigma_{\widehat{\pi_1}}^2 \left(\frac{\partial p_1}{\partial \pi_1}\right)^2 + \sigma_{\widehat{\pi_2}}^2 \left(\frac{\partial p_1}{\partial \pi_2}\right)^2 + \sigma_{\widehat{p_2}}^2 \left(\frac{\partial p_1}{\partial p_2}\right)^2. \tag{6.193}$$

After substituting both Eq. (6.192) and Lemma 6.2 into Eq. (6.193), Eq. (6.190) follows.

If a more reliable fallible measuring device were used, we would expect the resulting estimate of p_1 to be better. In other words, we would expect that the variance of $\widehat{p}_1$ is a decreasing function of the reliability of the fallible measuring device. Here we define a measure of reliability and study its relationship with Eq. (6.190).

Let T and F be the true and fallible classifications on a single sampling unit. The joint distribution of T and F is given by Fig. 6.1. The coefficient of reliability is defined as the square of the correlation coefficient between T and F:

$$\mathcal{K}_{(.)} = \rho^2\left(T_{(.)}, F_{(.)}\right) = \left[\frac{cov\left(T_{(.)}, F_{(.)}\right)}{\sigma_{T(.)}\sigma_{F(.)}}\right]^2. \tag{6.194}$$

It can be shown that Eq. (6.194) is given by (Exercise 6.7-12)

$$\mathcal{K}_{(.)} = \frac{\left(1 - \varphi_{(.)} - \psi_{(.)}\right)^2 p_{1(.)} q_{1(.)}}{p_{2(.)} q_{2(.)}}. \tag{6.195}$$

By substituting Eq. (6.195) into Eq. (6.190),

$$\sigma_{\widehat{p_{1(.)}}}^2 = \frac{p_{1(.)} q_{1(.)}}{m_{(.)}} \left(1 - \mathcal{K}_{(.)}\right) + \frac{p_{1(.)} q_{1(.)}}{M_{(.)}} \mathcal{K}_{(.)}. \tag{6.196}$$

Remarks

1. Equation (6.196) is a weighted average of the variance of a binomial estimate of $p_{1(.)}$ based on $m_{(.)}$ true measurements and that of a binomial estimate of $p_{1(.)}$ based on $M_{(.)}$ true measurements.
2. When $\mathcal{K}_{(.)} = 0$, the variance of $\widehat{p}_{1(.)}$ that is attained by using the double sampling scheme is no better than that of a binomial estimate of $p_{1(.)}$ based on $m_{(.)}$ true measurements.
3. When $\mathcal{K}_{(\cdot)} = 1$, this implies that the fallible measurement is just as good as the true measurement, because by using $M_{(.)}$ fallible measurement, we obtain the same precision as a binomial estimate of $p_{1(.)}$ based on $M_{(.)}$ true measurements.
4. Equation (6.196) implies that it is a decreasing function of the reliability of $\mathcal{K}_{(.)}$.

Furthermore, the 100·(1 − α)% confidence interval for $p_{1(.)}$ is given by

$$\widehat{p}_{1(.)} - z_{1-\frac{\alpha}{2}} \cdot \widehat{\sigma}_{\widehat{p}_{1(.)}} \le p_{1(.)} \le \widehat{p}_{1(.)} + z_{1-\frac{\alpha}{2}} \cdot \widehat{\sigma}_{\widehat{p}_{1(.)}}. \quad (6.197)$$

where $z_{1-\frac{\alpha}{2}}$ is the $100 \cdot (1-\frac{\alpha}{2})^{\text{th}}$ percentile of the standard normal distribution Z, $\widehat{\sigma}_{\widehat{p}_{1(.)}}$ is the square root of Eq. (6.196) with all the unknown parameters being replaced by their maximum likelihood estimators, and $\widehat{p}_{1(.)}$ is given by Eq. (6.182).

The estimator of the odds ratio R between cases and controls is given by

$$\widehat{R} = \frac{\widehat{p}_{1(1)}\widehat{q}_{1(2)}}{\widehat{q}_{1(1)}\widehat{p}_{1(2)}}, \quad (6.198)$$

where $\widehat{p}_{1(1)}$ and $\widehat{p}_{1(2)}$ are the maximum likelihood estimators of the prevalence of cases and controls, respectively, and $\widehat{q}_{i(.)} = 1 - \widehat{p}_{i(.)}$, i = 1, 2. The asymptotic variance of the logarithm of Eq. (6.198) is given by

$$\sigma^2_{\ln\widehat{R}} = \sigma^2_{\widehat{p}_{1(1)}}\left[\frac{1}{p^2_{1(1)}} + \frac{1}{q^2_{1(1)}}\right] + \sigma^2_{\widehat{p}_{1(2)}}\left[\frac{1}{p^2_{1(2)}} + \frac{1}{q^2_{1(2)}}\right]. \quad (6.199)$$

The $100 \cdot (1-\alpha)\%$ confidence interval for R is given by

$$Exp\left(\ln\widehat{R} - z_{1-\frac{\alpha}{2}} \cdot \widehat{\sigma}_{\ln\widehat{R}}\right) \le R \le Exp\left(\ln\widehat{R} + z_{1-\frac{\alpha}{2}} \cdot \widehat{\sigma}_{\ln\widehat{R}}\right), \quad (6.200)$$

where $\widehat{\sigma}_{\ln\widehat{R}}$ is the square root of Eq. (6.199) with all the unknown parameters being replaced by their maximum likelihood estimators, and $\widehat{R}$ is given by Eq. (6.198).

Example 6.5

Let cases and controls be denoted, respectively, as population 1 and 2. Let X and X^* be the true and fallible exposure measurement, respectively. Assume that the data of SIDS study in Example 6.4 were collected by using the double sampling scheme. Then, Table 6.16 can be rewritten as Table 6.17.

(a) Find the prevalence estimate of women who were exposed to using drugs during pregnancy for cases and controls and its 95% confidence intervals, respectively, by using the double sampling scheme.
(b) Find the estimate of odds ratio between cases and controls.

Solution

(a) From Table 6.17, $m_{11(1)} = 29$, $m_{10(1)} = 22$, $m_{01(1)} = 17$, $m_{00(1)} = 143$, $x_{(1)} = 173$, $m_{(1)} = 211$, and $M_{(1)} = 211 + 775 = 986$. By substituting these values into Eqs. (6.182) to (6.184), (6.181), and (6.195)

$$\widehat{p}_{1(1)} = \frac{(51+173)\cdot 29}{986\cdot 51} + \frac{(160+602)\cdot 17}{986\cdot 160} = 0.211293 \approx 0.21. \quad (6.201)$$

$$\widehat{\varphi}_{(1)} = \frac{(160+602)\cdot 17}{0.211\cdot 986\cdot 160} = 0.388617 \approx 0.389. \quad (6.202)$$

$$\widehat{\psi}_{(1)} = \frac{22\cdot(51+173)}{(1-0.211)\cdot 51\cdot 986} = 0.124253 \approx 0.124 \quad (6.203)$$

$$\widehat{p}_{2(1)} = \frac{51+173}{986} = 0.227181 \approx 0.227. \quad (6.204)$$

$$\widehat{\mathcal{K}}_{(1)} = \frac{0.211\cdot(1-0.211)\cdot(1-0.389-0.124)^2}{0.227\cdot(1-0.227)} = 0.225238 \approx 0.23. \quad (6.205)$$

$$\begin{aligned} \widehat{\sigma}^2_{\widehat{p}_{1(1)}} &= [0.211\cdot(1-0.211)]\cdot\left(\frac{1-0.225}{211}+\frac{0.225}{1014}\right) = 0.0006, \text{or} \\ \widehat{\sigma}_{\widehat{p}_{1(1)}} &= \sqrt{0.0006} = 0.02449 \approx 0.024. \end{aligned} \quad (6.206)$$

The 95% confidence interval for $p_{1(1)}$ is given by

$$\begin{aligned} &0.21 - 1.96\cdot 0.024 \le p_{1(1)} \le 0.21 + 1.96\cdot 0.024, \text{or} \\ &0.16 \le p_{1(1)} \le 0.26. \end{aligned} \quad (6.207)$$

The maximum likelihood estimator of $p_{1(1)}$ is given by Eq. (6.201) with its associated 95% confidence interval given by Eq. (6.207).

Table 6.17 The rewritten of the data in Table 6.16

	Medical record (cases)		**Total**
	$X = 1$	$X = 0$	
$X^* = 1$	29	22	51
$X^* = 0$	17	143	160
Total	46	160	211
Interview data (cases)	173	602	775

and

	Medical record (controls)		**Total**
	$X = 1$	$X = 0$	
$X^* = 1$	21	12	33
$X^* = 0$	16	168	184
Total	37	180	217
Interview data (controls)	134	663	797

Similarly, from Table 6.17, $m_{11(2)} = 21$, $m_{10(2)} = 12$, $m_{01(2)} = 16$, $m_{00(2)} = 168$, $x_{(2)} = 134$, $m_{(2)} = 217$, and $M_{(2)} = 217 + 797 = 1014$. By substituting these values into Eqs. (6.182) to (6.184), (6.181), and (6.195)

$$\widehat{p}_{1(2)} = \frac{(33+134)\cdot 21}{1014\cdot 33} + \frac{(184+663)\cdot 16}{1014\cdot 184} = 0.177441 \approx 0.18. \tag{6.208}$$

$$\widehat{\varphi}_{(2)} = \frac{(184+663)\cdot 16}{0.177\cdot 1014\cdot 184} = 0.40935 \approx 0.41. \tag{6.209}$$

$$\widehat{\psi}_{(2)} = \frac{12\cdot(33+134)}{(1-0.177)\cdot 33\cdot 1014} = 0.072808 \approx 0.07. \tag{6.210}$$

$$\widehat{p}_{2(2)} = \frac{33+134}{1014} = 0.164694 \approx 0.16 \tag{6.211}$$

$$\widehat{\mathcal{K}}_{(2)} = \frac{0.177\cdot(1-0.177)\cdot(1-0.409-0.073)^2}{0.165\cdot(1-0.165)} = 0.284506 \approx 0.28. \tag{6.212}$$

$$\begin{aligned} \widehat{\sigma}^2_{\widehat{p}_{1(2)}} &= [0.18\cdot(1-0.18)]\cdot\left(\frac{1-0.28}{217} + \frac{0.28}{1014}\right) = 0.0005 \text{ or,} \\ \widehat{\sigma}_{\widehat{p}_{1(2)}} &= \sqrt{0.0005} = 0.02236 \approx 0.02. \end{aligned} \tag{6.213}$$

The 95% confidence interval for $p_{1(2)}$ is given by

$$\begin{aligned} &0.18 - 1.96\cdot 0.02 \le p_{1(2)} \le 0.18 + 1.96\cdot 0.02, \text{or} \\ &0.14 \le p_{1(2)} \le 0.22. \end{aligned} \tag{6.214}$$

The maximum likelihood estimator of $p_{1(2)}$ is given by Eq. (6.208) with its associated 95% confidence interval given by Eq. (6.214).

(b) By substituting Eqs. (6.201) and (6.208) into Eq. (6.198),

$$\widehat{R} = \frac{0.21\cdot(1-0.18)}{0.18\cdot(1-0.21)} = 1.21097 \approx 1.21. \tag{6.215}$$

The asymptotic variance of $ln\,\widehat{R}$ is obtained by using Eq. (6.199)

$$\begin{aligned} &\widehat{\sigma}^2_{ln\,\widehat{R}} = 0.0006\cdot\left(\frac{1}{0.21^2} + \frac{1}{0.79^2}\right) + 0.0005\cdot\left(\frac{1}{0.18^2} + \frac{1}{0.82^2}\right) = 0.03, \\ &\text{or } \widehat{\sigma}_{ln\,\widehat{R}} = 0.173205 \approx 0.17 \end{aligned} \tag{6.216}$$

By substituting Eqs. (6.215) and (6.216) into Eq. (6.200),

$$Exp(\ln(1.21) - 1.96 \cdot 0.17) \leq R \leq Exp(\ln(1.21 + 1.96 \cdot 0.17).\text{or } 0.87 \leq \mathrm{R} \leq 1.69 \quad (6.217)$$

The maximum likelihood estimator of R is given by Eq. (6.215) and its 95% confidence interval is given by Eq. (6.217).

Remarks

1. Note that the original sampling plan for the SIDS data is by applying the double sampling scheme. I use this data set is for the convenience of an illustration only.
2. To find the optimal sample size for $m_{(.)}$ and $M_{(.)}$, two problems, (i) fixed cost and (ii) fixed variance, were considered in Tenenbein [25].

6.5 Nondifferential But Dependent Misclassification

In this section, I would like to discuss the bias in the odds ratio when both exposure and disease misclassification errors are nondifferential but dependent. This case is biologically plausible to occur if information on exposure and outcome is based on subjective data from the same source in questionnaire studies. The threshold for reporting indicators of exposure and outcome is likely to vary from subject to subject for biological or social reasons. Let D and E denote, respectively, the dichotomous disease and exposure variables in a certain population. Let $\dot{D}$ and $\dot{E}$ be the respective categories of high but $\ddot{D}$ and $\ddot{E}$ low threshold of D and E. Thus, $\dot{D}, \dot{E}$ and $\ddot{D}, \ddot{E}$ partition the region into four categories I-IV (Fig. 6.2), where a-d represents the true frequency of subjects in each of the four categories.

For each of the four true categories, suppose that the misclassification is possible into the other three categories. The resulting misclassification will be denoted, respectively, by the surrogate variables D^* and E^*in which $\dot{D}^*, \dot{E}^*$ and $\ddot{D}^*, \ddot{E}^*$ are respective presence and absence of D^* and E^*. Assume that misclassification of subjects exists and an interaction also exists in the four categories in Fig. 6.2. The probabilities of the 12 possible misclassification errors are expressed as:

		True classifier ($T_{(.)}$)			
		1	0		
Fallible classifier ($F_{(.)}$)	1	$m_{11(.)}$	$m_{10(.)}$	$m_{1+(.)}$	$x_{(.)}$
	0	$m_{01(.)}$	$m_{00(.)}$	$m_{0+(.)}$	$y_{(.)}$
		$m_{+0(.)}$	$m_{+1(.)}$	$m_{(.)}$	$M_{(.)} - m_{(.)}$

Fig. 6.2 Nondifferential but dependent misclassification

$$
\begin{aligned}
\Pr\left(\ddot{D}^*\dot{E}^*|\dot{D}\dot{E}\right) &= \varepsilon_{12},\\
\Pr\left(\dot{D}^*\ddot{E}^*|\dot{D}\dot{E}\right) &= \varepsilon_{13},\\
\Pr\left(\ddot{D}^*\ddot{E}^*|\dot{D}\dot{E}\right) &= \varepsilon_{14},\\
\Pr\left(\dot{D}^*\dot{E}^*|\ddot{D}\dot{E}\right) &= \varepsilon_{21},\\
\Pr\left(\dot{D}^*\ddot{E}^*|\ddot{D}\dot{E}\right) &= \varepsilon_{23},\\
\Pr\left(\ddot{D}^*\ddot{E}^*|\ddot{D}\dot{E}\right) &= \varepsilon_{24},\\
\Pr\left(\dot{D}^*\dot{E}^*|\dot{D}\ddot{E}\right) &= \varepsilon_{31},\\
\Pr\left(\dot{D}^*\dot{E}^*|\dot{D}\ddot{E}\right) &= \varepsilon_{31},\\
\Pr\left(\ddot{D}^*\dot{E}^*|\dot{D}\ddot{E}\right) &= \varepsilon_{32},\\
\Pr\left(\ddot{D}^*\ddot{E}^*|\dot{D}\ddot{E}\right) &= \varepsilon_{34},\\
\Pr\left(\dot{D}^*\dot{E}^*|\ddot{D}\ddot{E}\right) &= \varepsilon_{41},\\
\Pr\left(\ddot{D}^*\dot{E}^*|\ddot{D}\ddot{E}\right) &= \varepsilon_{42}, \text{ and}\\
\Pr\left(\dot{D}^*\ddot{E}^*|\ddot{D}\ddot{E}\right) &= \varepsilon_{43}.
\end{aligned}
\tag{6.218}
$$

The misclassified frequencies a^*, b^*, c^*, and d^* can be expressed as functions of the true frequencies and the 12 misclassification probabilities ε_{ij}:

$$a^* = (1 - \varepsilon_{12} - \varepsilon_{13} - \varepsilon_{14})a + \varepsilon_{21}b + \varepsilon_{31}c + \varepsilon_{41}d, \tag{6.219}$$

$$b^* = \varepsilon_{12}a + (1 - \varepsilon_{21} - \varepsilon_{23} - \varepsilon_{24})b + \varepsilon_{32}c + \varepsilon_{42}d, \tag{6.220}$$

$$c^* = \varepsilon_{13}a + \varepsilon_{23}b + (1 - \varepsilon_{31} - \varepsilon_{32} - \varepsilon_{34})c + \varepsilon_{43}d, \tag{6.221}$$

$$d^* = \varepsilon_{14}a + \varepsilon_{24}b + \varepsilon_{34}c + (1 - \varepsilon_{41} - \varepsilon_{42} - \varepsilon_{43})d. \tag{6.222}$$

From Fig. 6.2, the true prevalence of exposure (p_E) and disease (p_D) are given, respectively, by

$$p_E = \frac{a+c}{a+b+c+d}, \tag{6.223}$$

and

$$p_D = \frac{a+b}{a+b+c+d}. \tag{6.224}$$

Solving the true frequencies c and d from Eqs. (6.223) and (6.224) in terms of a, b, p_D, and p_E,

$$c = a\left[\frac{p_E - p_D}{p_D} + \frac{b}{a}\left(\frac{p_E}{p_D}\right)\right], \tag{6.225}$$

and

$$d = a\left[\frac{1 - p_E}{p_D} + \frac{b}{a}\left(\frac{1 - p_D - p_E}{p_D}\right)\right]. \tag{6.226}$$

By substituting Eqs. (6.225) and (6.226) into Eqs. (6.219) to (6.222),

$$a^* = \frac{a}{p_D}\left\{\varepsilon_{41} + [1 - (\varepsilon_{12} + \varepsilon_{13} + \varepsilon_{14} + \varepsilon_{31})]p_D + (\varepsilon_{31} - \varepsilon_{41})p_E + \frac{b}{a}[\varepsilon_{41} + p_D(\varepsilon_{21} - \varepsilon_{41}) + p_E(\varepsilon_{31} - \varepsilon_{41})]\right\}, \tag{6.227}$$

$$b^* = \frac{a}{p_D}\left\{\varepsilon_{42} + p_D(\varepsilon_{12} - \varepsilon_{32}) + p_E(\varepsilon_{32} - \varepsilon_{42}) + \frac{b}{a}p_D[1 - (\varepsilon_{21} + \varepsilon_{23} + \varepsilon_{24} + \varepsilon_{42})]\right\}, \tag{6.228}$$

$$\begin{aligned} c^* = \frac{a}{p_D}\Big\{&\varepsilon_{43} + p_D(\varepsilon_{13} + \varepsilon_{31} + \varepsilon_{32} + \varepsilon_{34} + \varepsilon_{43} - 1) + p_E[1 - (\varepsilon_{31} + \varepsilon_{32} + \varepsilon_{34} + \varepsilon_{43})] \\ &+ \frac{b}{a}[\varepsilon_{43} + p_D(\varepsilon_{23} - \varepsilon_{43}) + p_E(1 - \varepsilon_{31} - \varepsilon_{32} - \varepsilon_{34} - \varepsilon_{43})]\Big\}, \end{aligned} \tag{6.229}$$

$$d^* = \frac{a}{p_D}\left\{p_D(\varepsilon_{14} - \varepsilon_{34}) + p_E\varepsilon_{34} + \frac{b}{a}[1 - \varepsilon_{41} - \varepsilon_{42} - \varepsilon_{43} - p_D(1 - \varepsilon_{24} - \varepsilon_{41} - \varepsilon_{42} - \varepsilon_{43}) - p_E(1 - \varepsilon_{41} - \varepsilon_{42} - \varepsilon_{43} - \varepsilon_{34})]\right\}, \tag{6.230}$$

The observed odds ratio (R^*) is expressed as a function of true exposure and outcome prevalence (p_D, p_E), the true odds ratio ($\mathrm{R} = \frac{ad}{bc}$) and the 12 misclassification probabilities (ε_{12} to ε_{43}) using Eqs. (6.227) to (6.230):

$$R^* = \frac{a^* d^*}{b^* c^*} = \frac{a^{**} d^{**}}{b^{**} c^{**}}, \tag{6.231}$$

where a^{**}, b^{**}, c^{**}, and d^{**} are obtained by dividing a^*, b^*, c^*, and d^*, respectively, with $\frac{a}{p_D}$.

By substituting Eqs. (6.225) and (6.226) into the true odds ratio R and solving for $\frac{b}{a}$,

$$\frac{b}{a} = \frac{-[(1+R)p_D + (1+R)p_E + 1] + \sqrt{p_D^2(R^2 + 6\mathrm{R} + 1) + 1 + [p_E(1-R) + 1]^2 + 2(1-R)(1+p_E)}}{2Rp_D}. \tag{6.232}$$

Remark

Equation (6.232) is different from Eq. (6.209) in Kristensen [14] because an algebraic computational error occurred in Eq. (6.209).

Now suppose that an equal proportion ε of low- and high-threshold subjects distributed uniformly among the four categories of exposure and disease is assumed

(Fig. 6.2). It is further assumed that ε×a high-threshold subjects from category I ($\dot{D}\dot{E}$) are misclassified into category (IV) ($\ddot{D}^*\ddot{E}^*$), whereas ε × d low-threshold subjects from category IV ($\ddot{D}\ddot{E}$) are misclassified as category I ($\dot{D}^*\dot{E}^*$). Subjects from category III ($\dot{D}\ddot{E}$) that have low threshold (ε × c) are misclassified into category I ($\dot{D}^*\dot{E}^*$), whereas the ε × c subjects with high-threshold are misclassified as category IV ($\ddot{D}^*\ddot{E}^*$). Subjects from category III ($\ddot{D}\dot{E}$) with a high and low threshold are misclassified as category IV ($\ddot{D}^*\ddot{E}^*$) and I ($\dot{D}^*\dot{E}^*$), respectively. The ε × a subjects with a low threshold in category I ($\dot{D}\dot{E}$) and the ε × d subjects with a high threshold in category IV ($\ddot{D}\ddot{E}$) are not misclassified. This relation can be expressed as:

$$\begin{aligned} \varepsilon_{14} = \varepsilon_{21} = \varepsilon_{24} = \varepsilon_{31} = \varepsilon_{34} = \varepsilon_{41} = \varepsilon, \text{ and} \\ \varepsilon_{12} = \varepsilon_{13} = \varepsilon_{23} = \varepsilon_{32} = \varepsilon_{42} = \varepsilon_{43} = 0. \end{aligned} \tag{6.233}$$

Under the above assumption of Eq. (6.233), it results in nondifferential misclassification, since sensitivity (ζ) and specificity (η) of one variable is the same in different levels of the other variable: $\zeta_{\dot{D}^*\dot{E}^*|\dot{D}\dot{E}} = \zeta_{\ddot{D}^*\dot{E}^*|\ddot{D}\dot{E}} = 1 - \varepsilon$, $\eta_{\dot{D}^*\ddot{E}^*|\dot{D}\ddot{E}} = \eta_{\ddot{D}^*\ddot{E}^*|\ddot{D}\ddot{E}} = 1 - \varepsilon$.

For a specific case when the true odds ratio is unity, Eq. (6.232) becomes

$$\frac{b}{a} = \frac{1 + 2p_D + \sqrt{2(4p_D^2 + 1)}}{2p_D}. \tag{6.234}$$

In this scenario, the observed odds ratio of Eq. (6.231) reduces to

$$R^* = \frac{\mathcal{U}}{\mathcal{V}}, \tag{6.235}$$

where $\mathcal{U}$ and $\mathcal{V}$ are given by

$$\mathcal{U} = \left[\varepsilon + p_D(1 - 2\varepsilon) + \frac{b}{a}\varepsilon\right]\left\{\varepsilon p_E + \frac{b}{a}[1 - \varepsilon - (p_D + p_E)(1 - 2\varepsilon)]\right\},$$

$$\mathcal{V} = \frac{b}{a}p_D(1 - 2\varepsilon)^2\left[p_E\left(1 + \frac{b}{a}\right) - p_D\right],$$

and $\frac{b}{a}$ is given by Eq. (6.234).

Example 6.6

This example is based on a survey among elevator installers in Norway [14]. One aim was to investigate the association between cumulative exposure to solvents and indicators of neuropsychiatric disturbances among the installers.

A questionnaire mailed to a 40% random sample (n = 348) of all former and present members of the Norwegian Elevator Workers' union was answered by

Table 6.18 The data of the symptom score of elevator installers

	Exposure category		
Symptom score	High	Low/moderate	Total
High	6	20	26
Low	8	201	209
Total	14	221	235

Table 6.19 The outcome data of 23,500 subjects under exposure category

	Outcome category	
Exposure category	$\dot{D}$	$\ddot{D}$
$\dot{E}$	85	838
$\ddot{E}$	2092	20,485

235 subjects (71%). Some of the questions referred to task involving use of solvents when installing and maintaining the elevators. Participants were asked to assess historic levels of exposure, partly on the basis of perceived discomfort at work (feeling of drunkenness, fatigue). The 16-question neuropsychiatric symptom score served as outcome variable. One investigator coded the exposure, whereas another coded all other variable.

Twenty-six subjects (11.1%) reported a high symptom score (> 6 symptoms). The odds for high symptom scores were higher among worker with a high cumulative exposure to solvents compared with workers with low or medium exposure (Table 6.18). The risk estimate did not change substantially in the multivariate analysis.

Assume that there are 23,500 subjects with the data given in Table 6.19. We obtain that the prevalence of exposure is

$$p_E = \frac{85 + 838}{23,500} \approx 0.04, \tag{6.236}$$

and the prevalence of outcome is

$$p_D = \frac{85 + 2,092}{23,500} \approx 0.09. \tag{6.237}$$

Table 6.19 provides a hypothetical data that is chosen so that the true odds ratio is

$$R = \frac{85 \cdot 20,485}{838 \cdot 2,092} = 0.993229 \approx 1. \tag{6.238}$$

Therefore, there is no association between exposure and outcome shown by Eq. (6.238).

Let 2.2% of this group have a low-threshold level and 2.2% have a high-threshold level for reporting exposure and outcome that are uniformly distributed among the four categories in Fig. 6.2. The resulting bias is then given by

$$\varepsilon = 0.022. \tag{6.239}$$

By using Eq. (6.234) to compute the value of $\frac{b}{a}$

$$\frac{b}{a} = \frac{1 - 2 \cdot 0.09 + \sqrt{2 \cdot (1 + 4 \cdot 0.09^2)}}{2 \cdot 0.09} = 16.27. \tag{6.240}$$

By substituting Eqs. (6.236), (6.237), (6.239), and (6.240) into Eq. (6.235), the observed estimate of the odds ratio is

$$R^* = \frac{0.571033}{0.070195} = 8.08888 = 8.1. \tag{6.241}$$

This seemingly modest misclassification has a dramatic effect on the odds ratio that is biased away from true unity to an observed estimate of 8.1 given by Eq. (6.241). In fact, the resulting frequencies from this hypothetic example are identical to the observed frequencies in the elevator installer study (Table 6.18), except that all numbers are 100 times higher.

The observed odds ratio of Table 6.18 is

$$\widehat{R} = \frac{6 \cdot 201}{20 \cdot 8} = 7.5375 \approx 7.5. \tag{6.242}$$

Therefore, in theory, a similar misclassification, caused by inter-subject variation in the threshold of exposure and outcome recognition, might explain the observed strong association shown by Eq. (6.242) in the elevator installer study.

Remarks

1. The presented misclassification (Eq. (6.233)) is only one choice out of several possibilities of the general case. Different types of dependent misclassification will result in varying magnitude and direction of the bias and may not invariably produce positive bias 7.1 (= 8.1 − 1). The most plausible scenario is probably a mixture of nondifferential but dependent misclassification.
2. There is increasing interest in the use of biological markers as indicators of both exposure and outcome. One potential problem is concerned with fluctuation in reliability for exposure and outcome parameters over the different occasions of sampling and analysis. Several sources of such variation are plausible in field studies, for example, impaired standardization of calibration, sampling, or analysis procedures, due to differences in external conditions. The result could be dependent errors [14].
3. Dependent errors are logically avoided by using separate sources for collecting information on exposure and outcome, respectively.

Appendix 6.5A
For i, j = 1, 2 define

$$\widehat{\epsilon}_{ij} \equiv \widehat{n}_{ij} - n_{ij}, \tag{6.243}$$

where $\widehat{n}_{ij}$ is defined by Eq. (6.93). Let

$$\vec{\epsilon} = (\epsilon_{11}, \epsilon_{12}, \epsilon_{21}, \epsilon_{22})^T \tag{6.244}$$

By the properties of multinomial distribution, it is easily shown that

$$E\left(\vec{\epsilon}\right) = 0 \text{ and } \sigma^2\left(\vec{\epsilon}\right) = \Sigma, \tag{6.245}$$

where $\Sigma = \text{cov}\left(\vec{\epsilon}\right)$ is given by (6.109). Now define

$$\dot{\theta} = \frac{-(1-\psi_1)\varphi_2 n_{11} + (1-\psi_1)(1-\varphi_2)n_{12} + \psi_1\varphi_2 n_{21} - \psi_1(1-\varphi_2)n_{22}}{-\varphi_1(1-\psi_2)n_{11} + \varphi_1\psi_2 n_{12} + (1-\varphi_1)(1-\psi_2)n_{21} - (1-\varphi_1)\psi_2 n_{22}} \tag{6.246}$$

Thus, we have

$$\begin{aligned}
\ln(\tilde{\theta}) - \ln(\dot{\theta}) &= \ln\left[\frac{-(1-\psi_1)\varphi_2\widehat{n}_{11} + (1-\psi_1)(1-\varphi_2)\widehat{n}_{12} + \psi_1\varphi_2\widehat{n}_{21} - \psi_1(1-\varphi_2)\widehat{n}_{22}}{-(1-\psi_1)\varphi_2 n_{11} + (1-\psi_1)(1-\varphi_2)n_{12} + \psi_1\varphi_2 n_{21} - \psi_1(1-\varphi_2)n_{22}}\right] \\
&- \ln\left[\frac{-\varphi_1(1-\psi_2)\widehat{n}_{11} + \varphi_1\psi_2\widehat{n}_{12} + (1-\varphi_1)(1-\psi_2)\widehat{n}_{21} - (1-\varphi_1)\psi_2\widehat{n}_{22}}{-\varphi_1(1-\psi_2)n_{11} + \varphi_1\psi_2 n_{12} + (1-\varphi_1)(1-\psi_2)n_{21} - (1-\varphi_1)\psi_2 n_{22}}\right] \\
&= \ln\left[1 + \frac{-(1-\psi_1)\varphi_2\widehat{\epsilon}_{11} + (1-\psi_1)(1-\varphi_2)\widehat{\epsilon}_{12} + \psi_1\varphi_2\widehat{\epsilon}_{21} - \psi_1(1-\varphi_2)\widehat{\epsilon}_{22}}{B_1}\right] \\
&- \ln\left[1 + \frac{-\varphi_1(1-\psi_2)\widehat{\epsilon}_{11} + \varphi_1\psi_2\widehat{\epsilon}_{12} + (1-\varphi_1)(1-\psi_2)\widehat{\epsilon}_{21} - (1-\varphi_1)\psi_2\widehat{\epsilon}_{22}}{B_2}\right] \\
&\approx \frac{-(1-\psi_1)\varphi_2\widehat{\epsilon}_{11} + (1-\psi_1)(1-\varphi_2)\widehat{\epsilon}_{12} + \psi_1\varphi_2\widehat{\epsilon}_{21} - \psi_1(1-\varphi_2)\widehat{\epsilon}_{22}}{B_1} \\
&- \frac{-\varphi_1(1-\psi_2)\widehat{\epsilon}_{11} + \varphi_1\psi_2\widehat{\epsilon}_{12} + (1-\varphi_1)(1-\psi_2)\widehat{\epsilon}_{21} - (1-\varphi_1)\psi_2\widehat{\epsilon}_{22}}{B_2} \\
&= \frac{A_{11}\widehat{\epsilon}_{11} + A_{12}\widehat{\epsilon}_{12} + A_{21}\widehat{\epsilon}_{21} + A_{22}\widehat{\epsilon}_{22}}{B_1 B_2}
\end{aligned} \tag{6.247}$$

where A_{ij} and B_j, i, j = 1, 2 are defined, respectively, by Eqs. (6.110) to (6.115). By using the fact that $\sigma^2(\ln(\tilde{\theta})) = E\left[\left\{\ln(\tilde{\theta}) - \ln(\dot{\theta})\right\}^2\right]$, because of

$E\left[\ln\left(\tilde{\theta}\right) - \ln\left(\dot{\theta}\right)\right] = 0$, Eq. (6.108) follows immediately after taking the expected value of the square of Eq. (6.247).

6.6 Testing Nondifferential Misclassification

One of the issues regarding misclassification in case-control studies is whether the misclassification error rates are the same for both cases and controls [26]. At present, a common practice is to assume that the rates are the same. This is the so-called the nondifferential misclassification (NDMC) assumption. Many nice theoretical results are found under this assumption. For instance, in a 2×2 case-control study, the adjusted odds ratio is always biased toward the value of the null hypothesis if the misclassification error rates are assumed to be non-differentia [3, 11]. However, it is intuitively clear that the NDMC assumption may not be valid in many practical applications. In this section, two methods are presented for testing the validity of the NDMC assumption.

First, we need to develop the theory of exposure operating characteristic curve. The idea of exposure operating characteristic (EOC) curve is parallel to that the receiver operating characteristic (ROC) curve used in medical diagnostic test [28]. Suppose that the collected data for a case-control study is arranged as given in Table 6.20. Assume that Table 6.20 is possibly misclassified. Evidently, we are able to construct the counterfactual true table from the misclassified observed table [9]. The random variable E concerning the exposure condition of the subjects in Table 6.21 is correctly classified, whereas E^* in Table 6.20 is the misclassified surrogate of E.

Let the number of misclassified subjects between true and misclassified cell frequencies be defined by

Table 6.20 The observed cell frequencies in a 2×2 case-control study

	Subject Group	
Classified exposure status	Y = 1 (Cases)	Y = 0 (Controls)
$E^* = 1$ (exposed)	n_{11}	n_{10}
$E^* = 0$ (unexposed)	n_{01}	n_{00}
Total	n_{+1}	n_{+0}

Table 6.21 The kth counterfactual true cell frequencies in a 2×2 case-control study

	Subject Group	
Classified exposure status	Y = 1 (Cases)	Y = 0 (Controls)
E = 1 (exposed)	$N_{11(k)}$	$N_{10(k)}$
E = 0 (unexposed)	$N_{01(k)}$	$N_{00(k)}$
Total	$N_{+1(k)} = n_{+1}$	$N_{+0(k)} = n_{+0}$

$$m_{i(k)}^{(j)} = N_{ij(k)} - n_{ij} \tag{6.248}$$

where n_{ij} and N_{ij} are given in Tables 6.20 and 6.21, respectively. Although N_{ij} are not known in advance, we can let $m_{i(k)}^{(j)}$ to be assigned first as whatever we are pleased. Note that the column marginal totals in Table 6.21 are fixed as the same as that of Table 6.20.

The observed cell frequency $\{n_{ij}\}$ is said to be under-misclassified if $m_{i(k)}^{(j)} > 0$; otherwise, it is said to be over-misclassified. Thus, the false negative and false positive probabilities are defined for cases and controls by

$$\begin{aligned}
\varphi\left(m_{1(k)}^{(1)}\right) &= \Pr(E^* = 0|E = 1; D = 1) = \frac{| m_{1(k)}^{(1)} |}{n_{+1}}, \\
\psi\left(m_{0(k)}^{(1)}\right) &= \Pr(E^* = 1|E = 0; D = 1) = \frac{| m_{0(k)}^{(1)} |}{n_{+1}}, \text{ and} \\
\varphi\left(m_{1(k)}^{(0)}\right) &= \Pr(E^* = 0|E = 1; D = 0) = \frac{| m_{1(k)}^{(0)} |}{n_{+0}}, \\
\psi\left(m_{0(k)}^{(0)}\right) &= \Pr(E^* = 1|E = 0; D = 0) = \frac{| m_{0(k)}^{(0)} |}{n_{+0}}.
\end{aligned} \tag{6.249}$$

Note that not all $\varphi\left(m_{i(k)}^{(j)}\right)$ and/or $\psi\left(m_{i(k)}^{(j)}\right)$ defined by Eq. (6.249) are feasible for all possible kth counterfactual models. They are required to satisfy the three constraints given by

$$\varphi\left(m_{i(k)}^{(j)}\right) + \psi\left(m_{i(k)}^{(j)}\right) < 1, \tag{6.250}$$

$$\varphi\left(m_{ik}^{(j)}\right) < 1, \tag{6.251}$$

and

$$\psi\left(m_{i(k)}^{(j)}\right) < 1. \tag{6.252}$$

By varying the values of $m_{i(k)}^{(j)}$, we obtain many feasible pairs of false negative and false positive probabilities. A plot of all feasible pairs of the points $\left(\varphi\left(m_{i(k)}^{(j)}\right), 1 - \psi\left(m_{i(k)}^{(j)}\right)\right)$ is said to be the EOC curve for cases or controls depending on j = 1 or 0.

In terms of the EOC curve, a test on the NDMC is given by

$$H_0 : EOC_1 = EOC_0 \text{ versus } H_1 : EOC_1 \neq EOC_0. \tag{6.253}$$

There are at least two ways to test Eq. (6.253). One way is to use a summary defined by Eq. 6.254,

$$\theta = \text{AUC (Eq (5) in Lee [19])} \tag{6.254}$$

The use of AUC is widely applied in testing whether two ROC curves associated with the disease or healthy populations are the same [13]. The other way is to use the Kolmogorov-Smirnov test (Eq. (6.264)) [17] on the bivariate data specified by the pairs of false negative and false positive probabilities.

In terms of the Youden's index, here two nonparametric methods for testing Eq. (6.253) are summarized as follows.

Method A: The Wilcoxon-Mann-Whiney (WMW) Test [17]
For each point lying on the EOC_i curve, define the Youden's index (YI) as [28]

$$YI\left(P^{(i)}\right) = 1 - \varphi\left(P^{(i)}\right) - \psi\left(P^{(i)}\right), \tag{6.255}$$

where $P^{(i)}$ is the point lying on the EOC_i curves, i = 0, 1.

Let $P_j^{(1)}$ and $Q_k^{(0)}$ be the points lying on the empirical EOC_i curves for i = 1 (cases) and 0 (controls), respectively. Define

$$U_{jk} = 1 \text{ if } YI\left(P_j^{(1)}\right) > YI\left(Q_k^{(0)}\right); = 0 \text{ otherwise (assuming no ties)}. \tag{6.256}$$

With Eq. (6.256) the null and alternative hypotheses of Eq. (6.253) are replaced by

$$H_0^* : \theta = 0.5 \text{ versus } H_1^* : \theta < 0.5. \tag{6.257}$$

An unbiased estimator for θ of Eq. (5.6-7) is given by [21]

$$\hat{\theta} = \frac{1}{m_0 m_1} \sum_{j=1}^{m_1} \sum_{k=1}^{m_0} U_{jk} \tag{6.258}$$

where U_{jk} are defined by Eq. (6.256) and its variance is given by

$$\sigma^2\left(\hat{\theta}\right) = \frac{\theta(1-\theta)}{M}, \tag{6.259}$$

where M is given by

$$M = \frac{m_0 m_1}{(m_0 - 1)\delta_1 + (m_1 - 1)\delta_2 + 1},$$

and for $\ell = 1, 2$

$$\delta_\ell = \frac{\theta_\ell - \theta^2}{\theta(1 - \theta)},$$
$$\theta_1 = \Pr\left(U_{ij}U_{kj} = 1\right), i \neq k,$$
$$\theta_2 = \Pr\left(U_{ij}U_{ik} = 1\right), j \neq k.$$

Note that the estimators for θ_1, θ_2 δ_ℓ, and M are

$$\begin{aligned}
\widehat{\theta}_1 &= \sum\nolimits_{i=1}^{m_0} \sum\nolimits_{j=1}^{m_1} \sum\nolimits_{k \neq i}^{m_0} \frac{U_{ij}U_{kj}}{m_0 m_1 (m_0 - 1)}, \\
\widehat{\theta}_2 &= \sum\nolimits_{i=1}^{m_0} \sum\nolimits_{j=1}^{m_1} \sum\nolimits_{k \neq j}^{m_1} \frac{U_{ij}U_{ik}}{m_0 \mathrm{m}_1 (m_1 - 1)}, \\
\tilde{\theta}^2 &= \frac{m_0 m_1 \widehat{\theta}^2 - (m_0 - 1)\widehat{\theta}_1 - (m_1 - 1)\widehat{\theta}_2 - \widehat{\theta}}{(m_0 - 1)(m_1 - 1)}, \\
\tilde{\delta}_\ell &= \frac{\left| \widehat{\theta}_\ell - \tilde{\theta}^2 \right|}{\widehat{\theta} - \tilde{\theta}^2}, \text{ and} \\
\tilde{M} &= \frac{m_0 m_1 (m_0 - 1)(m_1 - 1)}{m_1 (m_0 - 1)\left[(m_0 - 1)\tilde{\delta}_1 + 1\right] + m_0 (m_1 - 1)\left[(m_1 - 1)\tilde{\delta}_2 + 1\right]}.
\end{aligned} \tag{6.260}$$

Consequently, an estimator of $\sigma^2\left(\widehat{\theta}\right)$ is given by

$$\widehat{\sigma}^2\left(\widehat{\theta}\right) = \frac{\widehat{\theta}\left(1 - \widehat{\theta}\right)}{\tilde{M}}. \tag{6.261}$$

Hence, a standard normal z_θ-statistic for testing Eq. (6.257) is given by

$$z_\theta = \frac{\widehat{\theta} - 0.5}{\widehat{\sigma}\left(\widehat{\theta}\right)}. \tag{6.262}$$

Method B: The Kolmogorov-Smirnov Test

Let S_{m_1} and T_{m_0} be the sample cumulative distribution function of Youden's index (Eq. (6.255)) associated with the number of points lying on the EOC curves for cases and controls, respectively, where S_{m_1} and T_{m_0} are defined, respectively, as

$$S_{m_1}(t) = \begin{cases} 0, t < YI\left(P^{(1)}\right)_{(1)} \\ \dfrac{k}{m_1}, YI\left(P^{(1)}\right)_{(k)} \le t \le YI\left(P^{(1)}\right)_{(k+1)} \end{cases}, \tag{6.263}$$

and

$$T_{m_0} = \begin{cases} 0, t < YI\left(Q^{(0)}\right)_1 \\ \dfrac{k}{m_0}, YI\left(Q^{(0)}\right)_{(k)} \le t \le YI\left(Q^{(0)}\right)_{(k+1)}, \\ 1, t \ge YI\left(Q^{(0)}\right)_{(m_0)} \end{cases} \tag{6.264}$$

where $YI(P^{(1)})_{(i)}$, i = 1, 2, . . ., m_1 and $YI(Q^{(0)})_{(j)}$, j = 1, 2, . . ., m_0 points are lying on the EOC curves for cases and controls, respectively.

The Kolmogorov-Smirnov test is based on the statistic $K_{m_0 m_1}$ defined by

$$K_{m_0 m_1} = sup_t |S_{m_1} - T_{m_0}|, \tag{6.265}$$

A decision rule for testing Eq. (6.253) is given as follows.

Decision Rule 6.2 (The Kolmogorov-Smirnov Test [16]))
Reject H_0 of Eq. (6.253) at the level of significance α if the observed number $K_{m_0 m_1}$ of Eq. (6.265) is larger than the two-tailed critical value K_a, where a is the probability of type I error [16]. Otherwise, do not reject H_0.

Example 6.7
The data given in Table 6.22 are taken from a study of deaths caused by landslides that occurred in the State of Chuuk, Federated States of Micronesia, in which a case-control study was used to identify the risk factors [24]. A case was defined to be a person who died as a result of landslides. Proxies were the surviving villagers who were able to provide information for the decedents or persons in the control group who were too young to answer questions. Because proxies were used to obtain information on the questions asked in the survey, misclassification was possibly occurred. For an illustration, a table was taken from their study regarding whether a person saw natural warning signs (Table 6.22). If a person did not see natural warning signs, E (exposure) = 1; otherwise, E = 0.

Assume that the observed table (Table 6.20) is misclassified, the counterfactual true table is able to be constructed as follows. By taking cases (D = 1) as an example,

Table 6.22 Survey data: whether a person was inside or outside the house or buildings for cases (deaths) and controls

Exposure factor	D = 1 (cases)	D = 0 (controls)	Total
E = 1 (inside)	23	22	45
E = 0 (outside)	18	30	48
Total	41	52	91

Table 6.23 17 Counterfactual true frequencies and the corresponding false negative and false positive probabilities for cases

Model k	$N_{01(k)}$	$N_{11(k)}$	$\varphi_{1(k)}$	$\psi_{1(k)}$
1	17	24	0.0244	0.0244
2	16	25	0.0488	0.0488
3	15	26	0.0732	0.0732
4	14	27	0.0976	0.0976
5	13	28	0.1220	0.1220
6	12	29	0.1463	0.1463
7	11	30	0.1707	0.1707
8	10	31	0.1951	0.1951
9	9	32	0.2195	0.2195
10	8	33	0.2439	0.2439
11	7	34	0.2683	0.2683
12	6	35	0.2927	0.2927
13	5	36	0.3171	0.3171
14	4	37	0.3415	0.3415
15	3	38	0.3659	0.3659
16	2	39	0.3902	0.3902
17	1	40	0.4146	0.4146

there are 17 possible under-misclassifying true tables for cases as shown in Table 6.23. Similarly, there are 21 counterfactual true tables for controls in Table 6.24. All counterfactual true tables are feasible.

As a result, $m_1 = 17$ and $m_0 = 21$. All feasible $(\varphi_{0(k)}, 1 - \psi_{0(k)})$ and $(\varphi_{1(k)}, 1 - \psi_{1(k)})$ pairs are plotted as shown as the EOC curves shown in Fig. 6.3.

From the result of Table 6.25, both $z_\theta = -0.21$ and $K_{m_1,m_0} = 0.056$ are not significant (see Note 2 in Table 6.25). Because the testing results of both WMW and Kolmogorov-Smirnov methods are not significant, H_0 of Eq. (6.253) is not rejected at the level of significance 0.05. Hence the null hypothesis is not rejected, that is, the assumption of a nondifferential misclassification with respect to being inside or outside the house or buildings for cases and controls in the Chuuk landslide data is accepted.

Remarks

1. The calculation of the false negative and false positive probabilities is not accurate in Lee [16].
2. The EOC curve is intrinsically different from that of the ROC curve. The ROC curve is used to judge the accuracy of a diagnostic test on the individual's disease status, while the EOC curve is concerned with the correct classification of the subject's exposure condition.
3. Unlike the ROC curve that is a single continuous curve, the EOC curve is comprised of discrete points. Furthermore, the ROC curve is strictly increasing, whereas the EOC curve is monotonically decreasing.
4. The Kolmogorov-Smirnov method is preferred to the WMW method because it is possible that two EOC curves are different, but they have the same area.

Table 6.24 21 counterfactual true frequencies and the corresponding false negative and false positive probabilities for controls

Model k	$N_{10(k)}$	$N_{00(k)}$	$\psi_{0(k)}$	$\varphi_{0(k)}$
1	21	31	0.0192	0.0192
2	20	32	0.0385	0.0385
3	19	33	0.0577	0.0577
4	18	34	0.0769	0.0769
5	17	35	0.0962	0.0962
6	16	36	0.1154	0.1154
7	15	37	0.1346	0.1346
8	14	38	0.1538	0.1538
9	13	39	0.1731	0.1731
10	12	40	0.1923	0.1923
11	11	41	0.2115	0.2115
12	10	42	0.2308	0.2308
13	9	43	0.25	0.25
14	8	44	0.2692	0.2692
15	7	45	0.2885	0.2885
16	6	46	0.3077	0.3077
17	5	47	0.3269	0.3269
18	4	48	0.3462	0.3462
19	3	49	0.3654	0.3654
20	2	50	0.3846	0.3846
21	1	51	0.4038	0.4038

Table 6.25 Results of applying the WMW and Kolmogorov-Smirnov methods

WMW method				Kolmogorov-Smirnov method	
m_0	21	$\tilde{\delta}_1$	0.3286	m_0	21
m_1	17	$\tilde{\delta}_2$	0.3710	m_1	17
$\widehat{\theta}_1$	0.1474	$\tilde{M}$	25	K_{m_1,m_0}	0.056
$\widehat{\theta}_2$	0.1368	$\widehat{\theta}$	0.479	$K_{0.05;\,9}$	0.43
$\tilde{\theta}^2$	0.2403	$\widehat{\sigma}\left(\widehat{\theta}\right)$	0.1		
		z_θ	−0.21		

Notes. [1]The critical value of $K_{0.05;\,9}$ in Table 6.25 is obtained by the approximation of using that of Kolmogorov-Smirnov's one-sample statistic $N = \frac{m_1 m_0}{m_1 + m_0} = 9.43 \approx 9$ in Gibbon's book [10] and Appendix Table A.2

[2]All the values in Table 6.25 are computed by applying Eqs. (6.262) and (6.265) with Appendix Tables A.1 and A.2, respectively

6.7 Exercises

1. Show that Eq. (6.4) holds.
2. Show that Eq. (6.13) is an unbiased estimator of the exposure prevalence p_i, namely, $E(\tilde{p}_i) = p_i$.

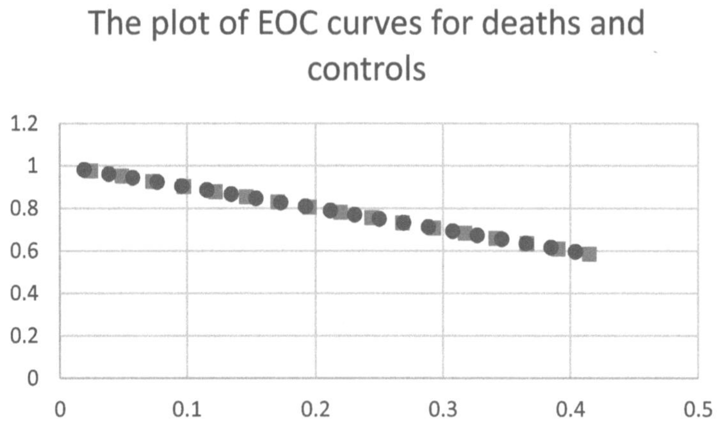

Fig. 6.3 The EOC curves for cases versus controls

3. Show that Eq. (6.16) holds.
4. Show that in Eq. (6.23) $\pi_1 = p_1p_3 + (1 - p_1)p_4$ holds.
5. Show that Eq. (6.96) holds.
6. Show that Eqs. (6.98) to (6.101) hold.
7. Show that Eq. (6.17) holds.
8. Show that Eqs. (6.153) and (6.154) hold.
9. Show that Eq. (6.184) holds.
10. Show that the identities in Lemma 6.2 hold.
11. Show that Eq. (6.195) holds.

References

1. Agresti, A. (2002). *Categorical data analysis* (2nd ed.). Wiley.
2. Bland, M. (1995). *An introduction to medical statistics*. Oxford University Press.
3. Bross, I. (1954). Misclassification in 2 × 2 tables. *Biometrics, 10*, 478–486.
4. Cornfield, J. (1956). A statistical problem arising from retrospective studies. In *Proceedings of the 3rd Berkeley symposium on mathematical Statistics and Probability* (pp. 135–148). University of California Press.
5. Coulean, J. L., Lerner, G., Helzlsouer, K., et al. (1986). Acute myocardial infarction among Navajo Indians, 1976-83. *American Journal of Public Health, 76*, 412–414.
6. Diamond, E. L., & Lilienfeld, A. M. (1962). Effects of errors in classification and diagnosis in various types of epidemiological studies. *American Journal of Public Health, 52*, 1137–1144.
7. Duffy, S. W., Roberts, M. M., & Elton, R. A. (1983). Risk factors for breast cancer: Relevance to screening. *Journal of Epidemiology and Community Health, 37*, 127–137.
8. Elton, R. A., & Duffy, S. W. (1983). Correcting for the effect of misclassification bias in a case-control study using data from two different questionnaires. *Biometrics, 39*, 659–663.
9. Epstude, K., & Rose, N. J. (2008). The functional theory of counterfactual thinking. *Personnel Social and Psychological Review, 12*, 168–192.
10. Gibbon, J. D. (1971). *Nonparametric statistical inference*. McGraw Hill Book Company.

11. Goldberg, J. D. (1975). The effect of misclassification on the bias in the difference between proportions and the relative odds in the fourfold table. *Journal of the American Statistical Association, 70*, 561–567.
12. Greenland, S. (1988). Statistical uncertainty due to misclassification: Implications for validation substudies. *Journal of Clinical Epidemiology, 41*, 1167–1174.
13. Hanley, J. A., & McNeil, B. J. (1982). The meaning and use of the area under a receiver operating characteristic (ROC) curve. *Radiology, 143*, 29–36.
14. Kristensen, P. (1992). Bias from nondifferential but dependent misclassification of exposure and outcome. *Epidemiology, 3*(210), 215.
15. Lee, T.-S. (2010). Bias-adjusted McNemar's test for misclassified data. *Journal of Probability and Statistical Science, 8*, 69–83.
16. Lee, T.-S. (2013). Testing the assumption of non-differential misclassification in case-control studies. *Journal of Modern Applied Statistical Methods, 12*, 211–230.
17. Lee, T.-S. (2021). *Medical statistics: A practical approach*. Scientific Publishing Company.
18. Lehmann, E. L. (1986). *Theory of estimation* (2nd ed.). Wiley.
19. Marshall, R. J. (1990). Validation study methods for estimating exposure proportions and odds ratios with misclassified data. *Journal of Clinical Epidemiology, 43*, 941–947.
20. McNemar, Q. (1947). Note on the sampling error of the difference between correlated proportions or percentages. *Psychometrika, 12*, 153–157.
21. Mee, R. W. (1990). Confidence intervals for probabilities and tolerance regions based on a generalization of the Mann-Whiney statistic. *Journal of the American Statistical Association, 85*, 793–800.
22. Newell, D. J. (1962). Errors in the interpretation of errors in epidemiology. *American Journal of Public Health, 52*, 1925–1928.
23. Rothman, K. J., & Greenland, S. (1998). *Modern epidemiology* (2nd ed.). Lippincott, Williams & Wilkins.
24. Sanchez, C., Lee, T. S., Young, S., et al. (2009). Risk factors for mortality during 2002 landslides in the State of Chuuk, Federated States of Micronesia. *Journal of Disaster, 33*, 705–720.
25. Tenenbein, A. (1970). A double sampling scheme for estimating from binomial data with misclassifications. *Journal of the American Statistical Association, 65*, 1350–1361.
26. Walker, S. D., & Irwig, L. M. (1988). Estimation of test error rates, disease prevalence and relative risk from misclassified data: A review. *Journal of Clinical Epidemiology, 41*, 923–937.
27. Wynder, E. L., Cornfield, J., Shroff, P. D., & Doraiswami, K. R. (1954). A study of environmental factors in carcinoma of the cervix. *American Journal of Obstetrics & Gynecology, 68*, 1016–1052.
28. Zhou, X.-H., McClish, D. K., & Obuchowski, N. A. (2002). *Statistical methods in diagnostic medicine*. Wiley.

Chapter 7
Two Misclassified Exposure Variables

7.1 Two Jointly Misclassified Variables

In this section, we consider the joint misclassification of two random variables in a general context.

Let X and Y be two dichotomous random variables (1 if present; 0 otherwise) that may represent two traits of interest in a target population in an epidemiologic study (Table 7.1). The joint probabilities for four possible true states are defined as follows:

$$\pi_{11} = \Pr(X = 1, Y = 1), \tag{7.1}$$

$$\pi_{10} = \Pr(X = 1, Y = 0), \tag{7.2}$$

$$\pi_{01} = \Pr(X = 0, Y = 1), \tag{7.3}$$

$$\pi_{00} = \Pr(X = 0, Y = 0), \tag{7.4}$$

where $\{\pi_{ij}\}$, i, j = 0, 1 satisfy the following constraint of total probability:

$$\sum\nolimits_{i,j=0}^{1} \pi_{ij} = 1, 0 < \pi_{ij} < 1. \tag{7.5}$$

The joint probabilities $\{\pi_{ij}\}$, i, j = 0, 1 between X and Y of Eqs. (7.1) to (7.4) are summarized in a 2 × 2 contingency table (Table 7.1). Assume that a simple multinomial sample of size n is collected from the target population through a cross sectional design and classify jointly by surrogate variables X^* and Y^* as given in Table 7.2.

T.-S. Lee, *Misclassification in Epidemiology*, Emerging Topics in Statistics and Biostatistics, https://doi.org/10.1007/978-3-032-12563-7_7

Table 7.1 The data for the true state of X and Y

	True state of Y	
True state of X	Y = 1 (Yes)	Y = 0 (No)
X = 1 (Yes)	π_{11}	π_{10}
X = 0 (No)	π_{01}	π_{00}

Table 7.2 The misclassified data of X^* and Y^*

	Classified state of Y^*	
Classified state of X^*	$Y^* = 1$ (Yes)	$Y^* = 0$ (No)
$X^* = 1$ (Yes)	n_{11}	n_{10}
$X^* = 0$ (No)	n_{01}	n_{00}

For all possible classifications of X* and Y* in the actual study population, we define 4 correctly classified and 12 misclassified error probabilities, conditioned on the true X and Y, as follows:

$$\delta_{11}^{[11]} = \Pr(X^* = 1, Y^* = 1 | X = 1, Y = 1), \tag{7.6}$$

$$\delta_{10}^{[10]} = \Pr(X^* = 1, Y^* = 0 | X = 1, Y = 0), \tag{7.7}$$

$$\delta_{01}^{[01]} = \Pr(X^* = 0, Y^* = 1 | X = 0, Y = 1), \tag{7.8}$$

$$\delta_{00}^{[00]} = \Pr(X^* = 0, Y^* = 0 | X = 0, Y = 0), \tag{7.9}$$

$$\delta_{11}^{[10]} = \Pr(X^* = 1, Y^* = 0 | X = 1, Y = 1), \tag{7.10}$$

$$\delta_{11}^{[01]} = \Pr(X^* = 0, Y^* = 1 | X = 1, Y = 1), \tag{7.11}$$

$$\delta_{11}^{[00]} = \Pr(X^* = 0, Y^* = 0 | X = 1, Y = 1), \tag{7.12}$$

$$\delta_{10}^{[11]} = \Pr(X^* = 1, Y^* = 1 | X = 1, Y = 0), \tag{7.13}$$

$$\delta_{10}^{[01]} = \Pr(X^* = 0, Y^* = 1 | X = 1, Y = 0), \tag{7.14}$$

$$\delta_{10}^{[00]} = \Pr(X^* = 0, Y^* = 0 | X = 1, Y = 0), \tag{7.15}$$

$$\delta_{01}^{[11]} = \Pr(X^* = 1, Y^* = 1 | X = 0, Y = 1), \tag{7.16}$$

$$\delta_{01}^{[10]} = \Pr(X^* = 1, Y^* = 0 | X = 0, Y = 1), \tag{7.17}$$

$$\delta_{01}^{[00]} = \Pr(X^* = 0, Y^* = 0 | X = 0, Y = 1), \tag{7.18}$$

$$\delta_{00}^{[11]} = \Pr(X^* = 1, Y^* = 1 | X = 0, Y = 0), \tag{7.19}$$

$$\delta_{00}^{[10]} = \Pr(X^* = 1, Y^* = 0 | X = 0, Y = 0), \tag{7.20}$$

$$\delta_{00}^{[01]} = \Pr(X^* = 0, Y^* = 1 | X = 0, Y = 0), \tag{7.21}$$

where $\left\{\delta_{k\ell}^{[ij]}\right\}$ for k, $\ell = 0$, 1 are required to satisfy the following constraints:

$$\sum_{i,j=0}^{1} \delta_{k\ell}^{[ij]} = 1, 0 < \delta_{k\ell}^{[ij]} < 1. \tag{7.22}$$

Because of the constraints of Eq. (7.22), only 12 out of 16 jointly classified probabilities of Eqs. (7.6) to (7.21) are regarded as independent parameters. Through this context, we use Eqs. (7.10) to (7.21) as independent parameters for further development.

Furthermore, assume that there is no confounding or selection bias that are hidden in the collected data. If no misclassification errors are present in either X* or Y*, the observed sample given by

$$\widehat{\pi}_{ij} = \frac{n_{ij}}{n}, \mathrm{i,j} = 0, 1 \text{ with } n = \sum_{i,j=0}^{1} n_{ij}, n_{ij} > 0. \tag{7.23}$$

are unbiased estimators for the true unknown π_{ij} in Table 7.1 and the variance-covariance matrix of $\overrightarrow{\widehat{\pi}}$ is given by [2]

$$\sigma^2\left(\overrightarrow{\widehat{\pi}}\right) = \frac{1}{n} \cdot \begin{bmatrix} \pi_{11}\overline{\pi}_{11} & -\pi_{11}\pi_{10} & -\pi_{11}\pi_{01} & -\pi_{11}\pi_{00} \\ -\pi_{11}\pi_{10} & \pi_{10}\overline{\pi}_{10} & -\pi_{10}\pi_{01} & -\pi_{10}\pi_{00} \\ -\pi_{11}\pi_{01} & -\pi_{10}\pi_{01} & \pi_{01}\overline{\pi}_{01} & -\pi_{01}\pi_{00} \\ -\pi_{11}\pi_{00} & -\pi_{10}\pi_{00} & -\pi_{01}\pi_{00} & \pi_{00}\overline{\pi}_{00} \end{bmatrix}, \tag{7.24}$$

where $\overline{\pi}_{ij} = 1 - \pi_{ij}$, and $\overrightarrow{\widehat{\pi}}$ is defined by

$$\overrightarrow{\widehat{\pi}} = \left[\widehat{\pi}_{11}, \widehat{\pi}_{10}, \widehat{\pi}_{01}, \widehat{\pi}_{00}\right]^T. \tag{7.25}$$

If both X and Y are misclassified, Eq. (7.23) is no longer unbiased and its expected value are corrected by

$$E(\widehat{\pi}_{11}) = \left(1 - \delta_{11}^{[10]} - \delta_{11}^{[01]} - \delta_{11}^{[00]}\right)\pi_{11} + \delta_{10}^{[11]}\pi_{10} + \delta_{01}^{[11]}\pi_{01} + \delta_{00}^{[11]}\pi_{00}, \tag{7.26}$$

$$E(\widehat{\pi}_{10}) = \delta_{11}^{[10]}\pi_{11} + \left(1 - \delta_{10}^{[11]} - \delta_{10}^{[01]} - \delta_{10}^{[00]}\right)\pi_{10} + \delta_{01}^{[10]}\pi_{01} + \delta_{00}^{[10]}\pi_{00}, \tag{7.27}$$

$$E(\widehat{\pi}_{01}) = \delta_{11}^{[01]}\pi_{10} + \delta_{10}^{[01]}\pi_{10} + \left(1 - \delta_{01}^{[11]} - \delta_{01}^{[10]} - \delta_{01}^{[00]}\right)\pi_{01} + \delta_{00}^{[01]}\pi_{00}, \tag{7.28}$$

$$E(\widehat{\pi}_{00}) = \delta_{11}^{[00]}\pi_{11} + \delta_{10}^{[00]}\pi_{10} + \delta_{01}^{[00]}\pi_{01} + \left(1 - \delta_{00}^{[11]} - \delta_{00}^{[10]} - \delta_{00}^{[01]}\right)\pi_{00}, \tag{7.29}$$

By replacing the left side of Eqs. (7.26) to (7.29) to equal to $\pi_{ij}$and solve for the unknown π_{ij}, we define the bias-adjusted estimators $\widetilde{\pi}_{ij}$, which account for the misclassification bias for the true unknown π_{ij} in Table 7.1 by

$$\overrightarrow{\widetilde{\pi}} = \mathcal{W}^{-1}\overrightarrow{\widehat{\pi}}, \tag{7.30}$$

where $\overrightarrow{\widehat{\pi}}$ is given by Eq. (7.23), $\mathcal{W}^{-1}$ is the inverse of $\mathcal{W}$, $\overrightarrow{\widetilde{\pi}}$ and are given by

$$\overrightarrow{\tilde{\pi}} = \left[\tilde{\pi}_{11}, \tilde{\pi}_{10}, \tilde{\pi}_{01}, \tilde{\pi}_{00}\right]^T, \tag{7.31}$$

and $\mathcal{W}$ is the coefficient matrix of π_{ij} in Eqs. (7.26) to (7.29). Because in many practical applications, it is very rare that both variables are simultaneously misclassified across the diagonal cells, we assume that $\delta_{11}^{[00]} = \delta_{10}^{[01]} = \delta_{01}^{10} = \delta_{00}^{[11]} = 0$. Also, because the total sample size is fixed, we have $\delta_{11}^{[10]} = \delta_{11}^{[01]}$, $\delta_{10}^{[11]} = \delta_{10}^{[00]}$, $\delta_{01}^{[11]} = \delta_{01}^{[00]}$, and $\delta_{00}^{[10]} = \delta_{00}^{[01]}$. Under these conditions, a closed form for the inverse $\mathcal{V}$ of $\mathcal{W}$ is given by

$$\mathcal{V} \equiv \mathcal{W}^{-1} = \left[v_{jk}\right]_{j,k=1}^{4}, \tag{7.32}$$

where $\left\{v_{jk}\right\}_{j,k=1}^{4}$ are given by

$$\begin{aligned}
&v_{11} \\
&= \mathcal{D}^{-1}\left\{\left(1-2\delta_{01}^{[11]}\right)\left[1-2\left(\delta_{10}^{[11]}+\delta_{00}^{[10]}\right)+3\delta_{10}^{[11]}\delta_{00}^{[10]}\right]-\delta_{01}^{[11]}\delta_{00}^{[10]}\left(1-2\delta_{10}^{[11]}\right)\right\},
\end{aligned}$$

$$v_{12} = -\mathcal{D}^{-1}\delta_{10}^{[11]}\left[1-2\left(\delta_{01}^{[11]}+\delta_{00}^{[10]}\right)\right]+4\delta_{01}^{[11]}\delta_{00}^{[10]},$$

$$v_{13} = -\mathcal{D}^{-1}\delta_{01}^{[11]}\left[1-2\left(\delta_{10}^{[11]}+\delta_{00}^{[10]}\right)\right]+4\delta_{10}^{[11]}\delta_{00}^{[10]},$$

$$v_{14} = \mathcal{D}^{-1}\delta_{00}^{[10]}\left(\delta_{10}^{[11]}+\delta_{01}^{[11]}-4\delta_{10}^{[11]}\delta_{01}^{[11]}\right),$$

$$v_{21} = -\mathcal{D}^{-1}\delta_{11}^{[10]}\left[1-2\left(\delta_{01}^{[11]}+\delta_{00}^{[10]}\right)+4\delta_{01}^{[11]}\delta_{00}^{[10]}\right],$$

$$\begin{aligned}
&v_{22} \\
&= \mathcal{D}^{-1}\left\{\left(1-2\delta_{00}^{[10]}\right)\left[1-2\left(\delta_{11}^{[10]}+\delta_{01}^{[11]}\right)+3\delta_{11}^{[10]}\delta_{01}^{[11]}\right]-\delta_{01}^{[11]}\delta_{00}^{[10]}\left(1-2\delta_{11}^{[10]}\right)\right\},
\end{aligned}$$

$$v_{23} = \mathcal{D}^{-1}\delta_{01}^{[11]}\left(\delta_{11}^{[10]}+\delta_{00}^{[10]}-4\delta_{11}^{[10]}\delta_{00}^{[10]}\right),$$

$$v_{24} = -\mathcal{D}^{-1}\delta_{00}^{[10]}\left[1-2\left(\delta_{11}^{[10]}+\delta_{01}^{[11]}\right)+4\delta_{11}^{[10]}\delta_{01}^{[11]}\right],$$

$$v_{31} = -\mathcal{D}^{-1}\delta_{11}^{[10]}\left[1-2\left(\delta_{10}^{[11]}+\delta_{00}^{[10]}\right)+4\delta_{10}^{[11]}\delta_{00}^{[10]}\right],$$

$$v_{32} = \mathcal{D}^{-1}\delta_{10}^{[11]}\left(\delta_{11}^{[10]}+\delta_{00}^{[10]}-4\delta_{11}^{[10]}\delta_{00}^{[10]}\right),$$

$$\begin{aligned}
&v_{33} \\
&= \mathcal{D}^{-1}\left\{\left(1-2\delta_{00}^{[10]}\right)\left[1-2\left(\delta_{11}^{[10]}+\delta_{10}^{[11]}\right)+3\delta_{11}^{[10]}\delta_{10}^{[11]}\right]-\delta_{10}^{[11]}\delta_{00}^{[10]}\left(1-2\delta_{11}^{[10]}\right)\right\},
\end{aligned}$$

$$v_{34} = -\mathcal{D}^{-1}\delta_{00}^{[10]}\left[1-2\left(\delta_{11}^{[10]}+\delta_{10}^{[11]}\right)+4\delta_{11}^{[10]}\delta_{10}^{[11]}\right],$$

$$v_{41} = \mathcal{D}^{-1}\delta_{11}^{[10]}\left(\delta_{10}^{[11]}+\delta_{01}^{[11]}-4\delta_{10}^{[11]}\delta_{01}^{[11]}\right),$$

$$v_{42} = -\mathcal{D}^{-1}\delta_{10}^{[11]}\left[1-2\left(\delta_{11}^{[10]}+\delta_{01}^{[11]}\right)+4\delta_{11}^{[10]}\delta_{01}^{[11]}\right],$$

$$v_{43} = -\mathcal{D}^{-1}\delta_{01}^{[11]}\left[1-2\left(\delta_{11}^{[10]}+\delta_{10}^{[11]}\right)+4\delta_{11}^{[10]}\delta_{10}^{[11]}\right],$$

$$\begin{aligned} v_{44} \\ &= \mathcal{D}^{-1}\left\{\left(1-2\delta_{01}^{[11]}\right)\left[1-2\left(\delta_{11}^{[10]}+\delta_{10}^{[11]}\right)+3\delta_{11}^{[10]}\delta_{10}^{[11]}\right]-\delta_{11}^{[10]}\delta_{01}^{[11]}\left(1-2\delta_{10}^{[11]}\right)\right\}, \end{aligned}$$

$$\begin{aligned} \mathcal{D} \equiv \det(\mathcal{W}) &= 1-2\left(\delta_{11}^{[10]}+\delta_{10}^{[11]}+\delta_{01}^{[11]}+\delta_{00}^{[10]}\right)+\delta_{11}^{[10]}\delta_{10}^{[11]}\left(3-2\delta_{01}^{[11]}\right) \\ &+ \delta_{01}^{[11]}\left[\left(\delta_{11}^{[10]}+2\delta_{10}^{[11]}\right)\left(1-\delta_{00}^{[10]}\right)+2\left(\delta_{11}^{[10]}+\delta_{10}^{[11]}-\delta_{11}^{[10]}\delta_{10}^{[11]}\right)\right] \\ &+ \delta_{00}^{[10]}\left[\left(2\delta_{11}^{[10]}+\delta_{10}^{[11]}\right)\left(1-2\delta_{01}^{[11]}\right)+2\left(\delta_{11}^{[10]}+\delta_{10}^{[11]}\right)+3\left(\delta_{01}^{[11]}-\delta_{11}^{[10]}\delta_{10}^{[11]}\right)\right], \end{aligned}$$

The misclassification error probabilities $\left\{\delta_{k\ell}^{[ij]}\right\}_{i,j,k,\ell=0}^{1}$ are said to be feasible if the determinant of $\mathcal{W}$ is positive. Furthermore, Eq. (7.30) is said to be admissible if for feasible $\left\{\delta_{k\ell}^{[ij]}\right\}$, i, j, k, $\ell = 0$, 1 we have $\sum_{i,j=0}^{1}\tilde{\pi}_{ij} = 1, 0 < \tilde{\pi}_{ij} < 1$.

From Eq. (7.30), the bias-adjusted estimators of $\{\pi_{ij}\}$ are given by

$$\tilde{\pi}_{11} = v_{11}\widehat{\pi}_{11} + v_{12}\widehat{\pi}_{10} + v_{13}\widehat{\pi}_{01} + v_{14}\widehat{\pi}_{00}, \tag{7.33}$$

$$\tilde{\pi}_{10} = v_{21}\widehat{\pi}_{11} + v_{22}\widehat{\pi}_{10} + v_{23}\widehat{\pi}_{01} + v_{24}\widehat{\pi}_{00}, \tag{7.34}$$

$$\tilde{\pi}_{01} = v_{31}\widehat{\pi}_{11} + v_{32}\widehat{\pi}_{10} + v_{33}\widehat{\pi}_{01} + v_{34}\widehat{\pi}_{00}, \tag{7.35}$$

$$\tilde{\pi}_{00} = v_{41}\widehat{\pi}_{11} + v_{42}\widehat{\pi}_{10} + v_{43}\widehat{\pi}_{01} + v_{44}\widehat{\pi}_{00}, \tag{7.36}$$

where $\left\{v_{jk}\right\}, j, k = 1, 2, 3, 4$ are the entries of $\mathcal{V}$ of Eq. (7.32).

In the analysis of contingency table [21], two random variables X and Y are said to have a zero first-order (or no) interaction if the cross-product ratio θ defined by

$$\theta = \frac{\pi_{11}\pi_{00}}{\pi_{10}\pi_{01}}, \tag{7.37}$$

equals one. Clearly, the naïve estimator of Eq. (7.37) is given by

$$\widehat{\theta} = \frac{\widehat{\pi}_{11}\widehat{\pi}_{00}}{\widehat{\pi}_{10}\widehat{\pi}_{01}}, \tag{7.38}$$

where $\{\widehat{\pi}_{ij}\}$, i, j = 0, 1 are given by Eq. (7.23). The asymptotic standard error of the natural logarithm of Eq. (7.38) is given by

$$s.e.\left(\ln\left(\widehat{\theta}\right)\right)=\sqrt{n^{-1}\left(\pi_{11}^{-1}+\pi_{10}^{-1}+\pi_{01}^{-1}+\pi_{00}^{-1}\right)}. \tag{7.39}$$

The 100(1 − α)% confidence interval for Eq. (7.37) is

$$\exp\left(\ln\left(\widehat{\theta}\right)\right)-z_{1-\frac{\alpha}{2}}\cdot s.e.\left(\ln\left(\widehat{\theta}\right)\right)\leq\theta\leq\exp\left(\ln\left(\widehat{\theta}\right)\right)+z_{1-\frac{\alpha}{2}}\cdot s.e.\left(\ln\left(\widehat{\theta}\right)\right), \tag{7.40}$$

where $z_{1-\frac{\alpha}{2}}$ is the 100(1 − α/2)th percentile of a standard normal distribution [21].

If both X and Y are misclassified, a bias-adjusted cross-product ratio (BACPR) for Eq. (7.37) is given by

$$\tilde{\theta}=\frac{\tilde{\pi}_{11}\tilde{\pi}_{00}}{\tilde{\pi}_{10}\tilde{\pi}_{01}}, \tag{7.41}$$

where $\{\tilde{\pi}_{ij}\}$, i, j = 0, 1 are given by Eqs. (7.33) to (7.36). A BACPR of Eq. (7.41) is said to be admissible if $0<\tilde{\theta}<+\infty$, where $\{\tilde{\pi}_{ij}\}_{i,j=0}^{1}$ of Eqs. (7.33) to (7.36) are admissible.

By applying the delta method [2], the asymptotic standard error of the natural logarithm of Eq. (7.40) is given by

$$s.e.\left(\ln\left(\tilde{\theta}\right)\right)=\sqrt{n^{-1}\left(v_{11}\pi_{11}^{-1}+v_{22}\pi_{10}^{-1}+v_{33}\pi_{01}^{-1}+v_{44}\pi_{00}^{-1}\right)}, \tag{7.42}$$

where $\{v_{ii}\}$, i = 1, 2, 3, 4 are the diagonal entries of $\mathcal{V}$ of Eq. (7.32).

Based on the asymptotic large sample theory, the sampling distribution of

$$z=\frac{\ln\left(\tilde{\theta}\right)}{s.e.\left(\ln\left(\tilde{\theta}\right)\right)\Big|_{\vec{\pi}=\vec{\tilde{\pi}}}}, \tag{7.43}$$

follows a standard normal distribution. The 100(1 − α)% confidence interval for Eq. (7.37) is

$$\exp\left(\ln\left(\tilde{\theta}\right)\right)-z_{1-\frac{\alpha}{2}}\cdot s.e.\left(\ln\left(\tilde{\theta}\right)\right)\leq\theta\leq\exp\left(\ln\left(\tilde{\theta}\right)\right)+z_{1-\frac{\alpha}{2}}\cdot s.e.\left(\ln\left(\tilde{\theta}\right)\right), \tag{7.44}$$

where $z_{1-\frac{\alpha}{2}}$ is the 100(1 − α/2)th percentile of a standard normal distribution.

Remark

When two variables are independently misclassified is not considered in this book, it was covered in Barron [5] or Kleinbaum et al. [18].

Let $\left\{n_{k\ell}^{[ij]}\right\}$ be the observed data where $\sum_{k,\ell=1}^{0} n_{k\ell}^{[ij]} = n$. Calculate the joint misclassification errors, we take the approach of using counterfactual frequency $\{N_{k\ell}^{[ij]}\}$ in which $\sum_{k,\ell=1}^{0} N_{k\ell}^{[ij]} = n$ such that for i, j = 0, 1

$$\delta_{k\ell}^{[ij]} = \frac{|N_{k\ell}^{[ij]} - n_{k\ell}^{[ij]}|}{n}. \tag{7.45}$$

Example 7.1

Placentals were collected in a maternity hospital. Abnormalities of pregnancies were noted and then a small sample of tissues was taken from each placental and used as a culture medium. In the original observations, there were several degrees of growth but these have been grouped together into two categories, "growing" and "poor/no growth." Let X represents the growth of placental (=1 if good growth; otherwise = 0 if poor/no growth;) and Y denote the type of mother's delivery (= 1 if no cesarean section; = 0 otherwise). The data in Table 7.3 are taken from Table 2 [7].

If there are no misclassification errors in Table 7.3, the naïve estimator of the cross-product ratio is obtained by applying Eq. (7.38) $\widehat{\theta} = \frac{47 \cdot 14}{48 \cdot 31} = 0.44$. The 95% confidence interval is given by applying Eq. (7.40).

$$1.07 \le \theta \le 4.78. \tag{7.46}$$

Since Eq. (7.46) exclude the value of one, X and Y have a nonzero first-order interaction.

Now, let us assume that X and Y are jointly misclassified across the row and the column cells in Table 7.1. We would like to test if there is no interaction between X and Y. Before we are able to do so, we need to calculate the misclassification error probabilities. Here we apply an idea of constructing the true counterfactual (CF) table from the observed table. Since the observed table is misclassified from the true table, the true table is merely a counterfactual (CF) to the observed table. To find the true counterfactual model from the observed model, we have constructed some (eight) CF models given in the first four columns of Table 7.4. First of all, we need to assume that a CF true table is obtained from the observed table by misclassifying its cells frequencies by one, two, three, four, and five subjects accordingly. For example, CF true model 1 is obtained from Table 7.3 by over-

Table 7.3 The placental growth under the condition whether a woman has cesarean section

	X = 1 (good growth)	X = 0 (poor/no growth)
Y = 1 (no cesarean section)	47	48
Y = 0 (cesarean section)	31	14

Table 7.4 The data of counterfacture true model

CF true model	$\tilde{n}_{11}$	$\tilde{n}_{10}$	$\tilde{n}_{01}$	$\tilde{n}_{00}$	$\delta_{11}^{[10]} = \delta_{11}^{[01]} = \delta_{11}^{[00]}$	$\delta_{10}^{[11]} = \delta_{10}^{[01]} = \delta_{10}^{[00]}$	$\delta_{01}^{[11]} = \delta_{01}^{[10]} = \delta_{01}^{[00]}$	$\delta_{00}^{[11]} = \delta_{00}^{[10]} = \delta_{00}^{[01]}$
1	48	47	30	15	0.0071	0.0071	0.0071	0.0071
2	49	46	29	16	0.0143	0.0143	0.0143	0.0143
3	50	45	28	17	0.0214	0.0214	0.0214	0.0214
4	51	44	27	18	0.0286	0.0286	0.0286	0.0286
5	52	43	26	19	0.0357	0.0357	0.0357	0.0357
6	53	42	25	20	0.0429	0.0429	0.0429	0.0429
7	54	41	24	21	0.05	0.05	0.05	0.05
8	55	40	23	22	0.0571	0.0571	0.0571	0.0571

misclassifying one subject from n_{11}, under-misclassifying one subject into n_{10}, under-misclassifying one subject into n_{01}, and over-misclassifying one subject from n_{00}. Similarly, CF true model 8 is obtained from Table 7.3 by over-misclassifying eight subjects into n_{11}, under-misclassifying eight subjects from n_{10}, under-misclassifying eight subjects from n_{01}, and over-misclassifying eight subjects into n_{00}.

Furthermore, we assume that the misclassification error probabilities are equal likely from any cell to the other three cells. Consequently, the calculated misclassification error probabilities are given in columns 6 to 9 in Table 7.4. For example, for CF true table 1, the value of $\delta_{11}^{[10]} = \delta_{11}^{[01]} = \delta_{11}^{[00]}$ is computed as

$$\delta_{11}^{[10]} = \frac{|48 - 47|}{140} = 0.007142 \approx 0.0071.$$

For CF true table 10, we have

$$\delta_{11}^{[10]} = \frac{|55 - 47|}{140} = 0.057142 \approx 0.0571.$$

By substituting the values of the misclassification error probabilities into the coefficients of the right side of Eqs. (7.26) to (7.29), we have the misclassification matrices for CF true models 1 to 10 in Table 7.3. To save space, we only list misclassification matrices $\mathcal{W}$ and its inverse $\mathcal{V}$ for two counterfactual models 1 and 8 in Table 7.5.

By computing the naïve estimator of $\widehat{\pi}_{ij}$ substituting the entries of $\mathcal{V}$ in Table 7.5 into Eqs. (7.33) to (7.36), the values of $\{\tilde{\pi}_{ij}\}$, i, j = 0, 1 and $\tilde{\theta}$ for CF true tables are given in Table 7.6.

For the eight CF true models, the estimated BACPR vary from 0.42 to 1.37 which are very different from $\widehat{\theta} = 0.44$ of the observed table.

To calculate the 95% confidence interval from the misclassified data, we need to compute the standard errors of the natural logarithm of the BACPR estimators by applying Eq. (7.42) that are given in Table 7.7.

Table 7.5 Misclassification matrices $\mathcal{W}$ and its inverses for two counterfactual true models 1 and 8

CF true table	$\mathcal{W}$				$\mathcal{V}$			
1	0.979	0.007	0.007	0.007	1.022	−0.007	−0.007	−0.007
	0.007	0.979	0.007	0.007	−0.007	1.022	−0.007	−0.007
	0.007	0.007	0.979	0.007	−0.007	−0.007	1.022	−0.007
	0.007	0.007	0.007	0.979	−0.007	−0.007	−0.007	1.022
8	0.829	0.057	0.057	0.057	1.222	−0.074	−0.074	−0.074
	0.057	0.829	0.057	0.057	−0.074	1.222	−0.074	−0.074
	0.057	0.057	0.829	0.057	−0.074	−0.074	1.222	−0.074
	0.057	0.057	0.057	0.829	−0.074	−0.074	−0.074	1.222

Table 7.6 The estimated BACPR for the eight CF true models

CF true table	$\overrightarrow{\widehat{\pi}}^T$	$\overrightarrow{\tilde{\pi}}^T$	$\tilde{\theta}$
1	[0.336, 0.343, 0.221, 0.1]	[0.338, 0.346, 0.221, 0.1]	0.42
2	[0.35, 0.329, 0.207, 0.114]	[0.356, 0.333, 0.205, 0.106]	0.55
3	[0.357, 0.321, 0.2, 0.121]	[0.367, 0.328, 0.195, 0.109]	0.63
4	[0.364, 0.314, 0.193, 0.128]	[0.379, 0.323, 0.186, 0.113]	0.72
5	[0.371, 0.307, 0.186, 0.134]	[0.392, 0.317, 0.175, 0.117]	0.82
6	[0.379, 0.3, 0.179, 0.143]	[0.405, 0.310, 0.164, 0.121]	0.96
7	[0.386, 0.293, 0.171, 0.15]	[0.420, 0.304, 0.152, 0.125]	1.13
8	[0.393, 0.286, 0.164, 0.157]	[0.435, 0.296, 0.139, 0.130]	1.37

Table 7.7 The 95% C. I. for eight CF true models

CF true model	v_{11}	v_{22}	v_{33}	v_{44}	$s.e.\left(\ln\left(\tilde{\theta}\right)\right)$	95% C. I. for θ
1	1.022	1.022	1.022	1.022	0.390	[0.20, 0.91]
2	1.045	1.045	1.045	1.045	0.388	[0.26, 1.18]
3	1.07	1.07	1.07	1.07	0.391	[0.29, 1.35]
4	1.097	1.097	1.097	1.097	0.40	[0.33, 1.55]
5	1.125	1.125	1.125	1.125	0.401	[0.38, 1.81]
6	1.155	1.155	1.155	1.155	0.336	[0.50, 1.86]
7	1.188	1.188	1.188	1.188	0.415	[0.51, 2.57]
8	1.222	1.222	1.222	1.222	0.424	[0.60, 3.15]

The values of 95%confidence interval in Table 7.7 are obtained by substituting the values of $\tilde{\theta}$ in column 4 of Table 7.6 and that of $s.e.\left(\ln\left(\tilde{\theta}\right)\right)$ in column 6 of Table 7.7 into Eq. (7.42). From the data values of 95% confidence interval for θ in column 7 of Table 7.7, all CF true tables except model 1 do not have a nonzero first-order interaction which are contradicted to the conclusion of the data without misclassification.

Remarks

1. To test if the data in Table 7.3 are misclassified, we need to find its Bayes factor by applying the idea in Sect. 8.3.
2. The computation of the inverse matrix $\mathcal{V}$ is facilitated by using the formula "MINVERSE" available in the Microsoft EXCEL.

7.2 A Case-Control Study with Two Jointly Misclassified Exposure Variables

Consider a case-control study with two exposure factors. Let X and Y be two dichotomous exposure variables (1 if yes; 0 otherwise), and D denotes the disease variable (1 if cases; 0 if controls). Under the multinomial sampling plan a simple

Table 7.8 The collected data for two jointly misclassified Surrogate variables X^* and Y^* in a case-control study

	D = 1 (Cases)			D = 0 (Controls)	
	$Y^*=1$	$Y^*=0$		$Y^*=1$	$Y^*=0$
$X^*=1$	n_{111}	n_{101}	$X^*=1$	n_{110}	n_{100}
$X^*=0$	n_{011}	n_{001}	$X^*=0$	n_{010}	n_{000}
Sample size	$n_{[1]}$			$n_{[0]}$	

Note that in Table 7.8, $n_{[k]}=\sum_{i,j=0}^{1} n_{ijk}$ for k = 0, 1

random sample of size $n_{[1]}$ and $n_{[0]}$ are selected, respectively, with respect to X and Y from the case and control groups. Furthermore, assume that instead of being classified by X and Y the collected data are jointly classified by two surrogate variables X^* and Y^*, respectively. Let n_{ijk} in Table 7.8 denote the observation with the indices i, j, and k corresponding respectively to the variables X, Y and D. As a result, for fixed k $\{n_{ijk}\}$ are assumed to follow a multinomial distribution with cell $\{\pi_{ijk}\}$ and the fixed sample size $n_{[k]}$.

For all possible classifications of X^* and Y^*, we define 4 correctly classified and 12 misclassified error conditional probabilities, conditioned on that X and Y are known, as follows: for fixed k (= 0 or 1) and i', j', i, j = 0, 1

$$\delta_{i'j'(k)}^{[ij]}=\Pr(X^*=i, Y^*=j|X=i', Y=j'; D=k) \tag{7.47}$$

where $\left\{\delta_{i'j'(k)}^{[ij]}\right\}$, i', j' = 0, 1 are required to satisfy the following identities

$$\sum_{i,j=0}^{1} n_{i'j'(k)}^{[ij]}=1, \quad 0\le n_{i'j'(k)}^{[ij]}\le 1. \tag{7.48}$$

Because of the constraint of Eq. (7.48), only 12 out of 16 conditional probabilities are regarded as independent parameters for fixed k. Throughout this section, we will use 12 misclassified error probabilities as independent parameters for cases and controls separately. A misclassification is said to be nondifferential if the misclassification error probabilities are equal one another for case and control groups; it is said to be differential otherwise. In this section only the differential misclassification is considered. Furthermore, it is assumed that there is no confounding or selection bias hidden in the collected data. If the data given in Table 7.8 are not misclassified in X* and Y*, the classical estimators of π_{ijk} for fixed k given by.

$$\widehat{\pi}_{ijk}=\frac{n_{ijk}}{n_{[k]}}, \text{i, j}=0, 1 \tag{7.49}$$

are shown to be unbiased for the true unknown π_{ijk} and the variance-covariance matrix $\Sigma_{[k]}$ of $\widehat{\vec{\pi}}_{[k]}$ is given in Agresti [2].

$$\Sigma_{[k]}=\left[\sigma_{ijk}\right]_{i,j=1}^{4}=\begin{bmatrix}\pi_{11k}\overline{\pi}_{11k} & -\pi_{11k}\pi_{10k} & -\pi_{11k}\pi_{01k} & -\pi_{11k}\pi_{00k}\\ -\pi_{11k}\pi_{10k} & \pi_{10k}\overline{\pi}_{10k} & -\pi_{10k}\pi_{01k} & -\pi_{10k}\pi_{00k}\\ -\pi_{11k}\pi_{01k} & -\pi_{10k}\pi_{01k} & \pi_{01k}\overline{\pi}_{01k} & -\pi_{01k}\pi_{00k}\\ -\pi_{11k}\pi_{00k} & -\pi_{10k}\pi_{00k} & -\pi_{01k}\pi_{00k} & \pi_{00k}\overline{\pi}_{00k}\end{bmatrix}, \tag{7.50}$$

where $\overline{\pi}_{ijk}=1-\pi_{ijk}$.

However, if both X* and Y* are misclassified, Eq. (7.49) are no longer unbiased and its expected value are corrected by for fixed k

$$E\left(\widehat{\vec{\pi}}_{[k]}\right)=\mathcal{W}_{[k]}\vec{\pi}_{[k]}, \tag{7.51}$$

where the column vectors $\widehat{\vec{\pi}}_{[k]}$, $\vec{\pi}_{[k]}$, and the misclassification matrix $\mathcal{W}_{[k]}$ are given, respectively, by

$$\widehat{\vec{\pi}}_{[k]}=\left[\widehat{\pi}_{11k},\widehat{\pi}_{10k},\widehat{\pi}_{01k},\widehat{\pi}_{00k}\right]^{T}, \tag{7.52}$$

$$\vec{\pi}_{[k]}=\left[\pi_{11k},\pi_{10k},\pi_{01k},\pi_{00k}\right]^{T}, \tag{7.53}$$

and

$$\mathcal{W}_{[k]}=\begin{bmatrix}\overline{\delta}_{11(k)}^{[11]} & \delta_{10(k)}^{[11]} & \delta_{01(k)}^{[11]} & \delta_{00(k)}^{[11]}\\ \delta_{11(k)}^{[10]} & \overline{\delta}_{10(k)}^{[10]} & \delta_{01(k)}^{[10]} & \delta_{00(k)}^{[10]}\\ \delta_{11(k)}^{[01]} & \delta_{10(k)}^{[01]} & \overline{\delta}_{01(k)}^{[01]} & \delta_{00(k)}^{[01]}\\ \delta_{11(k)}^{[00]} & \delta_{10(k)}^{[00]} & \delta_{01(k)}^{[00]} & \overline{\delta}_{00(k)}^{[00]}\end{bmatrix}, \tag{7.54}$$

where $\overline{\delta}_{11(k)}^{[11]}=1-\delta_{10(k)}^{[11]}-\delta_{01(k)}^{[11]}-\delta_{00(k)}^{[11]}$, $\overline{\delta}_{10(k)}^{[10]}$, $\overline{\delta}_{01(k)}^{[01]}$, and $\overline{\delta}_{00(k)}^{[00]}$ are defined similarly.

By replacing the left side of Eq. (7.51) by Eq. (7.49), we solve for the unknown $\vec{\pi}_{[k]}$ as

$$\tilde{\vec{\pi}}_{[k]}=\mathcal{W}_{[k]}^{-1}\widehat{\vec{\pi}}_{[k]}, \tag{7.55}$$

which is accounted for the misclassification bias being called the bias-adjusted cell proportion (BACP) estimator, and $\mathcal{W}_{[k]}^{-1}$ is the inverse of $\mathcal{W}_{[k]}$. Also, the bias-adjusted cell frequency (BACF) estimators are defined by $\tilde{\vec{n}}_{[k]}=n_{[k]}\tilde{\vec{\pi}}_{[k]}$. The misclassification error probability $\left\{\delta_{i'j'(k)}^{[ij]}\right\}$ is able to be computed by applying the concept of "counterfactual" as was done in Sect. 7.1.

Although it is possible to find a closed form formula for $\mathcal{W}_{[k]}^{-1}$, it is easier to solve Eq. (7.55) directly as a system of linear equations. Incidentally, a set of misclassification error probabilities $\left\{\delta^{[ij]}_{i'j'(k)}\right\}$, for i', j' = 0, 1 is said to be feasible if all $\left\{\delta^{[ij]}_{i'j'(k)}\right\}$, for i', j' = 0, 1 satisfying Eq. (7.48) and det($\mathcal{W}_{[k]}$), the determinant of $\mathcal{W}_{[k]}$, is nonzero for any given set of $\delta^{[ij]}_{i'j'(k)}$. Furthermore, a set of feasible $\left\{\delta^{[ij]}_{i'j'(k)}\right\}$ for i', j' = 0, 1 is said to be admissible if, for a set of $\left\{\delta^{[ij]}_{i'j'(k)}\right\}$, we have $0 < \tilde{\pi}_{ijk} < 1$ and $\sum_{i,j=0}^{1} \tilde{\pi}_{ijk} = 1$ for fixed k and all i, j, i', j' = 0, 1.

In a case-control study having two exposure variables, the classical notion of odds ratio is no longer applicable [7]. Instead, we need to focus on the issue: if these two exposure factors confer their risks independently or in some interaction fashion. Three possible definitions for interaction, one additive and two multiplicative, are considered in Darroach-Borkent [9]. Here we only adopt two of them, one additive and the other multiplicative. Two exposure variables X and Y are said to have no 2-way additive (or multiplicative) interaction if for fixed k (= 0 or 1) $\theta^{[k]}_{add\_2way} = 0$ (or $\theta^{[k]}_{mult\_2way} = 1$), where $\theta^{[k]}_{add\_2way}$ and $\theta^{[k]}_{mult\_2way}$ are defined, respectively, by

$$\theta^{[k]}_{add\_2way} \equiv \pi_{11k} - \pi_{10k} - \pi_{01k} + \pi_{00k}, \tag{7.56}$$

and

$$\theta^{[k]}_{mult\_2way} = \frac{\pi_{11k}\pi_{00k}}{\pi_{10k}\pi_{01k}}. \tag{7.57}$$

For three variables D, X, and Y, they are said to have no 3-way additive (or multiplicative) interaction Barlett [4] or Bhapkar-Koch [6, 12] if $\theta_{add\_3way} = 0$, $\left(\text{or } \theta_{mult_{3way}} = 1\right)$, where

$$\theta_{add\_3way} \equiv \theta^{[1]}_{add_{2way}} - \theta^{[0]}_{add_{2way}} = \pi_{111} + \pi_{100} + \pi_{010} + \pi_{001} - \pi_{110} - \pi_{000} - \pi_{101} - \pi_{011}, \tag{7.58}$$

or

$$\theta_{mult\_3way} \equiv \frac{\theta^{[1]}_{mult_{2way}}}{\theta^{[0]}_{mult_{2way}}} = \frac{\pi_{111}\pi_{001}\pi_{100}\pi_{010}}{\pi_{101}\pi_{011}\pi_{110}\pi_{000}}. \tag{7.59}$$

Clearly, the naive point estimators for $\theta^{[k]}_{add\_2way}$, $\theta^{[k]}_{mult\_2way}$, $\theta_{add\ \_\ 3way}$, and $\theta_{mult\ \_\ 3way}$ are given, respectively, by

$$\widehat{\theta}^{[k]}_{add\_2way} = \widehat{\pi}_{11k} - \widehat{\pi}_{10k} - \widehat{\pi}_{01k} + \widehat{\pi}_{00k}, \tag{7.60}$$

$$\widehat{\theta}^{[k]}_{mult\_2way} = \frac{\widehat{\pi}_{11k}\widehat{\pi}_{00k}}{\widehat{\pi}_{10k}\widehat{\pi}_{01k}}, \tag{7.61}$$

$$\widehat{\theta}_{add\_3way} = \widehat{\pi}_{111} + \widehat{\pi}_{100} + \widehat{\pi}_{010} + \widehat{\pi}_{001} - \widehat{\pi}_{110} - \widehat{\pi}_{000} - \widehat{\pi}_{101} - \widehat{\pi}_{011}, \tag{7.62}$$

and

$$\widehat{\theta}_{mult\_3way} = \frac{\widehat{\pi}_{111}\widehat{\pi}_{001}\widehat{\pi}_{100}\widehat{\pi}_{010}}{\widehat{\pi}_{101}\widehat{\pi}_{011}\widehat{\pi}_{110}\widehat{\pi}_{000}}, \tag{7.63}$$

where $\{\widehat{\pi}_{ijk}\}$, i, j = 0, 1 are given, respectively, by Eq. (7.49). The asymptotic standard error of Eqs. (7.60) to (7.63) is given, respectively, by

$$s.e.\left(\widehat{\theta}^{[k]}_{add\_2way}\right) = \sqrt{n_{[k]}^{-1}\sum\nolimits_{i,j=0}^{1}\pi_{ijk}\bar{\pi}_{ijk} + 2(\pi_{11k}\pi_{10k} + \pi_{11k}\pi_{01k} - \pi_{11k}\pi_{00k} - \pi_{10k}\pi_{01k} + \pi_{10k}\pi_{00k} + \pi_{01k}\pi_{00k})}, \tag{7.64}$$

$$s.e.\left(\ln\left(\widehat{\theta}^{[k]}_{mult\_2way}\right)\right) = \sqrt{n_{[k]}^{-1}\left(\pi_{11k}^{-1} + \pi_{10k}^{-1} + \pi_{01k}^{-1} + \pi_{00k}^{-1}\right)}, \tag{7.65}$$

$$s.e.\left(\widehat{\theta}_{add\_3way}\right) = \sqrt{\sum\nolimits_{k=0}^{1}\sigma^2\left(\widehat{\theta}^{[k]}_{add\_2way}\right)}, \tag{7.66}$$

and

$$s.e.\left(\ln\left(\widehat{\theta}_{mult\_3way}\right)\right) = \sqrt{\sum\nolimits_{k=0}^{1} n_{[k]}^{-1}\left(\pi_{11k}^{-1} + \pi_{10k}^{-1} + \pi_{01k}^{-1} + \pi_{00k}^{-1}\right)}. \tag{7.67}$$

The details of derivation of Eqs. (7.64) to (7.67) are given in the appendix.

If both X* and Y* are jointly misclassified, the bias-adjusted estimators for $\theta^{[k]}_{add\_2way}$, $\theta^{[k]}_{mult\_2way}$, θ_{add_3way}, and θ_{mult_3way} are given, respectively, by

$$\tilde{\theta}^{[k]}_{add\_2way} = \tilde{\pi}_{11k} - \tilde{\pi}_{10k} - \tilde{\pi}_{01k} + \tilde{\pi}_{00k} \tag{7.68}$$

$$\tilde{\theta}^{[k]}_{mult\_2way} = \frac{\tilde{\pi}_{11k}\tilde{\pi}_{00k}}{\tilde{\pi}_{10k}\tilde{\pi}_{01k}}, \tag{7.69}$$

$$\tilde{\theta}_{add\_3way} = \tilde{\pi}_{111} + \tilde{\pi}_{100} + \tilde{\pi}_{010} + \tilde{\pi}_{001} - \tilde{\pi}_{110} - \tilde{\pi}_{000} - \tilde{\pi}_{101} - \tilde{\pi}_{011}, \tag{7.70}$$

$$\tilde{\theta}_{mult\_3way} = \frac{\tilde{\pi}_{111}\tilde{\pi}_{001}\tilde{\pi}_{100}\tilde{\pi}_{010}}{\tilde{\pi}_{101}\tilde{\pi}_{011}\tilde{\pi}_{110}\tilde{\pi}_{000}}, \tag{7.71}$$

where $\{\tilde{\pi}_{ijk}\}$, i, j, k = 0, 1 are given by Eq. (7.55). The BACP $\{\tilde{\pi}_{ijk}\}$ (or BACF $\tilde{n}_{ijk}$), i, j, k = 0, 1 of Eq. (7.55) are said to be plausible if for all admissible $\left\{\delta^{[ij]}_{i'j'(k)}\right\}$ we have $0<\tilde{\pi}_{ijk}<1$ (or $\tilde{n}_{ijk}>0$) in which $\sum_{i,j=0}^{1}\tilde{\pi}_{ijk}$ (or $\sum_{i,j=0}^{1}\tilde{n}_{ijk}=n_{[0]}+n_{[1]}$) for fixed k.

By conditioning on that the values of $\delta_{i'j'(k)}^{[ij]}$ are known and applying Lemma 2.3.1 in Anderson [3] or the delta method in Agresti [2], the asymptotic standard error of Eqs. (7.68) to (7.71) are given, respectively, by

$$s.e.\left(\tilde{\theta}_{add\_2way}^{[k]}\right)=\sqrt{\sum_{i=1}^{4}u_{iik}-2(u_{12k}+u_{13k}+u_{24k}+u_{34k}-u_{14k}-u_{23k})}, \tag{7.72}$$

$$s.e.\left(\ln\left(\tilde{\theta}_{mult\_2way}^{[k]}\right)\right)=\sqrt{n_{[k]}^{-1}\left(\tilde{\pi}_{11k}^{-1}+\tilde{\pi}_{10k}^{-1}+\tilde{\pi}_{01k}^{-1}+\tilde{\pi}_{00k}^{-1}\right)}, \tag{7.73}$$

$$s.e.\left(\tilde{\theta}_{add\_3way}\right)=\sqrt{\sum_{k=0}^{1}\sigma^2\left(\tilde{\theta}_{add\_2way}^{[k]}\right)}, \tag{7.74}$$

and

$$s.e.\left(\ln\left(\theta_{mult\_3way}\right)\right)=\sqrt{\sum_{k=0}^{1}n_{[k]}^{-1}\sigma^2\left(\ln\left(\ddot{\theta}_{mult\_2way}^{[k]}\right)\right)}, \tag{7.75}$$

where $\{u_{ijk}\}$ in Eq. (7.72) are given by Eq. (7.84) in the appendix, and the details of derivation of Eqs. (7.72) to (7.75).

are also given in the appendix. Based on the asymptotic large sample theory, the sampling distribution of the testing statistics for all the above estimates (Eqs. (7.60) to (7.63) or (7.68) to (7.71)) can be shown to follow a standard normal distribution. Therefore, the 100·(1 − α)% confidence interval (0 < α < 1) for any θ is given for no multiplicative interaction by

$$\begin{aligned}&\exp\left(\ln\left(\tilde{\theta}_{mult}\right)\right)-z_{1-\frac{\alpha}{2}}\\&\cdot s.e.\left(\ln\left(\tilde{\theta}_{mult}\right)\le\theta\le\exp\left(\ln\left(\tilde{\theta}_{mult}\right)\right)+z_{1-\frac{\alpha}{2}}\cdot s.e.\left(\ln\left(\tilde{\theta}_{mult}\right)\right),\right.\end{aligned} \tag{7.76}$$

or for no additive interaction by

$$\tilde{\theta}_{add}-z_{1-\frac{\alpha}{2}}\cdot s.e.\left(\tilde{\theta}_{add}\right)\le\theta\le\tilde{\theta}_{add}-z_{1-\frac{\alpha}{2}}\cdot s.e.\left(\tilde{\theta}_{add}\right), \tag{7.77}$$

where $z_{1-\frac{\alpha}{2}}$ is the $100\cdot\left(1-\frac{\alpha}{2}\right)$th percentile of the standard normal distribution.

Example 7.2
The data is taken from Gardner-Munford [10, 15]. Lung tissues from 120 cases dying of mesothelioma cancer and from 135 controls dying from other causes were examined under electron microscope. The lung samples were examined for the presence of two asbestos fiber types, chrysotile and amphibole. Here the random variable D represents whether a subject died of mesothelioma (= 1 if yes; 0 if the subject was a control), while X (= 1 if yes; 0 if no) and Y (= 1; 0 if no) denote,

Table 7.9 The data of miners dying from lung cancer (cases) and from other causes who were exposed two-type asbestos fibers of chrysotile and amphibole

		Cases		Controls	
		Amphibole (Y^*)			
		1	0	1	0
Chrysotile (X^*)	1	47	27	6	35
	0	37	9	24	70
Sample size		120		135	

Where X^* and Y^* are surrogate variables for X and Y

respectively, the asbestos fiber of chrysotile and amphibole that were found in the lung (Table 7.9).

If there is no joint misclassification between X^* and Y^*, the crude point estimators for the 2-way interaction are estimated by using Eqs. (7.49), (7.60) to (7.63), and (7.72) to (7.75) as $\widehat{\theta}^{[1]}_{add\_2way} = -0.067$ (p-value $=$ 0.23), $\widehat{\theta}^{[1]}_{mult\_2way} = 0.42$ (p-value $=$ 0.026) for cases, while $\widehat{\theta}^{[0]}_{add\_2way} = 0.126$ (p-value $=$ 0.07), $\widehat{\theta}^{[0]}_{mult\_2way} = 0.5$ (p-value $=$ 0.08) for controls. Also, $\widehat{\theta}_{add\_3way} = 0.193$ (p-value $=$ 0.06) and $\widehat{\theta}_{mult\_3way} = 0.85$ (p-value $=$ 0.4). For the 2-way interaction, an inference based on the p-value is tentatively drawn that there is no additive interaction between X and Y for both cases and controls. However, there is a 2_way multiplicative interaction for cases, but not for controls. For the 3_way interaction, there is neither additive nor multiplicative interaction.

Assume that X* and Y* are jointly misclassified, we need to compute the joint misclassification error probabilities $\left\{\delta^{[ij]}_{i'j'(k)}\right\}$ for i′, j′ $=$ 0, 1 from applying the notion of "counterfactual (CF)" true tables like what we did in Sect. 7.1.

By using the observed cell frequencies in Table 7.9, we obtain the cell frequencies for the CF true table for cases and controls by either under- or over-misclassifying the observed cell frequency in cells (1,1) and (0,0) accordingly. The cell frequencies in cells (1, 0) and (0, 1) are obtained by subtracting the cell frequencies in cells (1,1) and (0, 0) from the fixed marginal column totals. The resulting CF true tables for cases and controls are given respectively by Tables 7.10 and 7.11. Here we assume that the misclassification error probabilities are designated equal likely.

For k $=$ 0, 1, we proceed to compute the BACF $\{\tilde{n}_{ij(k)}\}$ for cases and controls separately. For all ten feasible $\left\{\delta^{[ij]}_{i'j'(k)}\right\}$ for i′, j′ $=$ 0, 1 in Tables 7.10 and 7.11, we solve the matrix equation of Eq. (7.55) for the BACP $\vec{\tilde{\pi}}_{[k]}$ and then for the BACF $\vec{\tilde{n}}_{[k]}$ obtained by multiplying $\vec{\tilde{\pi}}_{[k]}$ by the fixed sample size $n_{[k]}$ (Table 7.12).

By using Eqs. (7.68) to (7.71) and (7.72) to (7.75), we are able to compute all the bias-adjusted estimates for 2-way or 3-way additive/multiplicative interaction parameters (Tables 7.13a and 7.13b). Based on the p-values in Table 7.13, all CF true tables have no 2-way additive interaction but have a nonzero 2-way multiplicative interaction for all CF true tables for cases. Similarly, for controls all CF true

Table 7.10 The joint misclassification error probabilities of five CF true models

CF true table	$[n_{111}, n_{101}, n_{011}, n_{001}]$	$\left[\delta^{[11]}_{11(1)}, \delta^{[10]}_{11(1)} = \delta^{[01]}_{11(1)} = \delta^{[00]}_{11(1)}, \delta^{[10]}_{10(1)}, \delta^{[11]}_{10(1)} = \delta^{[01]}_{10(1)} = \delta^{[00]}_{10(1)}, \delta^{[11]}_{01(1)}, \delta^{[11]}_{01(1)}, = \delta^{[10]}_{01(1)} = \delta^{[00]}_{01(1)}, \delta^{[00]}_{00(1)}, \delta^{[11]}_{00(1)} = \delta^{[10]}_{00(1)} = \delta^{[01]}_{00(1)}\right]$	$\mathcal{D}^*$
1	[42, 32, 42, 4]	[0.88, 0.04, 0.88, 0.04, 0.88, 0.04, 0.88, 0.04]	0.58
2	[43, 31, 41, 5]	[0.91, 0.03, 0.91, 0.03,0.91, 0.03, 0.91, 0.03]	0.65
3	[44, 30, 40, 6]	[0.93, 0.02, 0.93, 0.02, 0.93, 0.02, 0.93, 0.02]	0.73
4	[45, 29, 39, 7]	[0.96, 0.01, 0.96,0.01, 0.96, 0.01, 0.96, 0.01]	0.81
5	[46, 28, 38, 8]	[0.98, 0.007,0.98, 0.007, 0.98, 0.007, 0.98, 0.007]	0.90

*$\mathcal{D} = \det(\mathcal{W}_{[1]})$

Table 7.11 The joint misclassification error probabilities for five CF true models under the assumption that probabilities are designated equal likely

CF true table	$[n_{110}, n_{100}, n_{010}, n_{000}]$	$\left[\delta^{[11]}_{11(0)}, \delta^{[10]}_{11(0)} = \delta^{[01]}_{11(0)} = \delta^{[00]}_{11(0)}, \delta^{[10]}_{10(0)}, \delta^{[11]}_{10(0)} = \delta^{[01]}_{10(0)} = \delta^{[00]}_{10(0)}, \delta^{[11]}_{01(0)}, \delta^{[11]}_{01(0)}, = \delta^{[10]}_{01(0)} = \delta^{[00]}_{01(0)}, \delta^{[00]}_{00(0)}, \delta^{[11]}_{00(0)} = \delta^{[10]}_{00(0)} = \delta^{[01]}_{00(0)}\right]$	$\mathcal{D}^*$
1	[1, 40, 29, 65]	[0.89, 0.04, 0.89, 0.04, 0.89, 0.04, 0.89, 0.04]	0.62
2	[2, 39, 28, 66]	[0.91, 0.03, 0.91, 0.03, 0.91, 0.03, 0.91, 0.03]	0.68
3	[3, 38, 27, 67]	[0.93, 0.02, 0.93, 0.02, 0.93, 0.02, 0.93, 0.02]	0.76
4	[4, 37, 26, 68]	[0.96, 0.01, 0.96, 0.01, 0.96, 0.01, 0.96, 0.01]	0.83
5	[5, 36, 25, 69]	[0.98, 0.007, 0.98, 0.007, 0.98, 0.007, 0.98, 0.007]	0.91

$^*\mathcal{D} = \det(\mathcal{W}_{[0]})$

Table 7.12 The BACF frequencies for all five CF true models

CF true table	$[\tilde{n}_{111}, \tilde{n}_{101}, \tilde{n}_{011}, \tilde{n}_{001}]^T$ (Cases)	$[\tilde{n}_{110}, \tilde{n}_{100}, \tilde{n}_{010}, \tilde{n}_{000}]^T$ (Controls)
1	[50.4, 26.4., 38.4, 4.8]	[1.2, 35.2, 22.3, 76.3]
2	[49.6, 26.5, 38.1, 5.8]	[2.3, 35.2, 22.7, 74.9]
3	[48.9, 26.7, 37.8, 6.7]	[3.3, 35.1, 23.0, 73.5]
4	[48.2, 26.8, 37.5, 7.5]	[4.3, 35.1, 23.4, 72.3]
5	[47.6, 26.9, 37.2, 8.3]	[5.2, 35.0, 23.7, 71.1]

Table 7.13 Bias-adjusted estimates for 2-way additive/multiplicative interaction

CF true model	$\tilde{\theta}^{[1]}_{add\_2way}$ (p-value)	$\tilde{\theta}^{[1]}_{mult_{2way}}$ (p-value)	$\tilde{\theta}^{[0]}_{add_{2way}}$ (p-value)	$\tilde{\theta}^{[0]}_{mult\_2way}$ (p-value)
1	−0.08 (0.23)	0.24 (0.07)	0.15 (0.07)	0.11 (0.01)
2	−0.08 (0.20)	0.28 (0.09)	0.14 (0.07)	0.21 (0.01)
3	−0.07 (0.23)	0.32 (0.10)	0.14(0.08)	0.30 (0.03)
4	−0.07 (0.20)	0.36 (0.12)	0.13 (0.07)	0.37 (0.04)
5	−0.07 (0.23)	0.39 (0.13)	0.13 (0.07)	0.44 (0.06)

Table 7.14 Bias-adjusted estimates for 3-way additive/multiplicative interaction

CF true model (Cases, Controls)	$\tilde{\theta}_{add\_3way}$ (p-value)	$\tilde{\theta}_{mult\_3way}$ (p-value)
(1)	−0.22 (0.06)	2.09 (0.0)
(2)	−0.22 (0.04)	1.33 ($8.0 \cdot 10^{-5}$)
(3)	−0.21 (0.07)	1.08 (0.13)
(4)	−0.21 (0.049)	0.96 (0.27)
(5)	−0.20 (0.06)	0.89 (0.03)

tables have no 2-Way additive interaction, but have a nonzero 2-way multiplicative interaction.

To compute the 3-way additive/multiplicative interaction for a combination of (cases, controls) CF true tables, respectively, their values are given in Table 7.14. Only two combinations of (2,2) and (4,4) have a nonzero 3-way additive interaction as shown by their p-values, whereas three combinations of (1,1), (2,2) and (5,5) have a nonzero 3-way multiplicative interaction.

Remarks

1. The inherent feature of the data for cases is intrinsically different from that for controls. The proportion of subjects in cases exposed to both types of asbestos is not low (0.39 = 47/120), whereas that exposed to none of the two types of asbestos is low (0.08 = 9/120). In contrast, the proportion of subjects in controls

exposed to both types of asbestos is low (0.04 = 6/135), whereas that exposed to none of the two types of asbestos is not low (0.52 = 70/135). For additional discussions on this data set, see Acheson-Gardner [1].

2. Our 3-way additive interaction parameter (Eq. (7.58)) is different from that used in Gardner-Munford [10, 15]. We notice that the 2-way additive/multiplicative interaction parameters are unable to be defined by the GM's approach. Further our definition does not need the rare disease assumption; hence they are more universally applicable than the GM's.
3. Our definition for additive/multiplicative interaction follow from the statistical viewpoint rather than from the epidemiological perspective [21, 22]. Eqs. (7.56) and (7.57) do have an epidemiological interpretation. It defines an exact balance between the amounts of synergistic and parallel action in population who are exposed to both exposure factors. In fact, Eq. (7.57) is a necessary, but not sufficient condition for the immunity model [12].
4. Because the only unknown parameters in Eqs. (7.72) to (7.75) are misclassification error probabilities and we apply the theory of CF true table to compute the misclassification error probability, there is no need to provide the estimated standard error of the bias-adjusted estimators of either 2-way or 3-way additive or multiplicative interaction.

Appendix 7.2A

Equation (7.60) can be written in the inner product form of two vectors

$$\widehat{\theta}^{[k]}_{add\_2way} = \vec{c}^{\,T} \widehat{\vec{\pi}}_{[k]}, \tag{7.78}$$

where $\vec{c}$ is defined by

$$\vec{c} = [1, -1, -1, 1]^T. \tag{7.79}$$

By using Lemma 2.3.1 in Anderson [3], we have

$$\begin{aligned}\sigma^2\left(\widehat{\theta}^{[k]}_{add_{2way}}\right) &= \vec{c}^{\,T}\,\Sigma_{\{k\}}\,\vec{c} = \sum\nolimits_{i=1}^{4} \sigma_{iik} \\ &- 2(\sigma_{12k} + \sigma_{13k} - \sigma_{14k} - \sigma_{23k} + \sigma_{24k} + \sigma_{34k}).\end{aligned} \tag{7.80}$$

Equation (7.60) follows immediately from Eqs. (7.80) and (7.50).

The derivation of Eq. (7.69) is exactly the same as Eq. (3.1) in Agresti [2]. By applying the independence between cases and controls to Eq. (7.68), we have

$$\sigma^2\left(\widehat{\theta}_{add\_3way}\right) = \sum\nolimits_{k=0}^{1} \sigma^2\left(\widehat{\theta}^{[k]}_{add\_2way}\right). \tag{7.81}$$

Equation (7.70) follows directly from Eqs. (7.81) and (7.68). Similarly, Eq. (7.71) follows directly from applying the independence between cases and controls to Eq. (7.69).

Let $\vec{v}^{\,T}_{ik}$ be the ith row of the matrix $\mathcal{W}^{-1}_{[k]}$. Thus, we have

$$\tilde{\vec{\pi}}_{[k]} = \mathcal{W}^{-1}_{[k]}\widehat{\vec{\pi}}_{[k]} == \left[\vec{v}^{\,T}_{[1]k}\widehat{\vec{\pi}}_{[k]}, \vec{v}^{\,T}_{[2]k}\widehat{\vec{\pi}}_{[k]}, \vec{v}^{\,T}_{[3]k}\widehat{\vec{\pi}}_{[k]}, \vec{v}^{\,T}_{[4]k}\widehat{\vec{\pi}}_{[k]}\right]^T. \tag{7.82}$$

Let the matrix $\mathcal{U}$ be defined by

$$\mathcal{U} = \left[u_{ijk}\right]^4_{i,j=1} \equiv \mathcal{W}^{-1}_{[k]}\Sigma_{[k]}\left(\mathcal{W}^{-1}_{[k]}\right)^T. \tag{7.83}$$

Again, by applying Lemma 2.3.1 in Anderson [3] on Eq. (7.82), we have

$$\sigma^2\left(\tilde{\theta}^{[k]}_{add\_2way}\right) = \vec{c}^{\,T}\mathcal{W}^{-1}_{[k]}\Sigma_{[k]}\left(\mathcal{W}^{-1}_{[k]}\right)^T\vec{c}. \tag{7.84}$$

Equation (7.72) follows directly from Eqs. (7.78), (7.83), and (7.84). Since $\tilde{\vec{\pi}}_{[k]}$ is required to be admissible, this implies that $\mathcal{W}^{-1}_{[k]}$ has to be positive definite. Consequently, the value of Eq. (7.84) must be positive.

Let

$$g(\vec{\pi}_{[k]}) = \left[\ln\left(\vec{v}^{\,T}_{[1]k}\vec{\pi}_{[k]}\right), \ln\left(\vec{v}^{\,T}_{[2]k}\vec{\pi}_{[k]}\right), \ln\left(\vec{v}^{\,T}_{[3]k}\vec{\pi}_{[k]}\right), \ln\left(\vec{v}^{\,T}_{[4]k}\vec{\pi}_{[k]}\right)\right]^T,$$

where $\vec{\pi}_{[k]} = [\pi_{11k}, \pi_{10k}, \pi_{01k}, \pi_{00k}]^T$. Thus,

$$\frac{\partial g}{\partial \vec{\pi}_{[k]}} = \left(\mathcal{W}^{-1}_{[k]}\right)^T\left[diag\left(\vec{\pi}^{\,*}_{[k]}\right)\right]^{-1}, \tag{7.85}$$

where $\vec{\pi}^{\,*}_{[k]} = \mathcal{W}^{-1}_{[k]}\vec{\pi}_{[k]}$, and $diag\left(\vec{\pi}^{\,*}_{[k]}\right)$ is a diagonal matrix with the entries of $\vec{\pi}^{\,*}_{[k]}$ as the diagonal entries. Then, we have by applying the delta method [2]

$$\sigma^2\left(\ln\left(\tilde{\theta}^{[k]}_{mult_{2way}}\right)\right) = n^{-1}_{[k]}\left\{\vec{c}^{\,T}\left(\mathcal{W}^{-1}_{[k]}\right)^T\Sigma^*_{[k]}\mathcal{W}^{-1}_{[k]}\vec{c}\right\}, \tag{7.86}$$

where $\Sigma^*_{[k]}$ is given by

$$\Sigma^*_{[k]} = \left[\sigma^*_{ij}\right]^4_{i,j=1} = \begin{bmatrix} \frac{\pi_{11k}\overline{\pi}_{11k}}{\pi^{*2}_{11k}} & -\frac{\pi_{11k}\pi_{10k}}{\pi^*_{11k}\pi^*_{10k}} & -\frac{\pi_{11k}\pi_{01k}}{\pi^*_{11k}\pi^*_{01k}} & -\frac{\pi_{11k}\pi_{00k}}{\pi^*_{11k}\pi^*_{00k}} \\ -\frac{\pi_{11k}\pi_{10k}}{\pi^*_{11k}\pi^*_{10k}} & \frac{\pi_{10k}\overline{\pi}_{10k}}{\pi^{*2}_{10k}} & -\frac{\pi_{10k}\pi_{01k}}{\pi^*_{10k}\pi^*_{01k}} & -\frac{\pi_{10k}\pi_{00k}}{\pi^*_{10k}\pi^*_{00k}} \\ -\frac{\pi_{11k}\pi_{01k}}{\pi^*_{11k}\pi^*_{01k}} & -\frac{\pi_{10k}\pi_{01k}}{\pi^*_{10k}\pi^*_{01k}} & \frac{\pi_{01k}\overline{\pi}_{01k}}{\pi^{*2}_{01k}} & -\frac{\pi_{01k}\pi_{00k}}{\pi^*_{01k}\pi^*_{00k}} \\ -\frac{\pi_{11k}\pi_{00k}}{\pi^*_{11k}\pi^*_{00k}} & -\frac{\pi_{10k}\pi_{00k}}{\pi^*_{10k}\pi^*_{00k}} & -\frac{\pi_{01k}\pi_{00k}}{\pi^*_{01k}\pi^*_{00k}} & \frac{\pi_{00k}\overline{\pi}_{00k}}{\pi^{*2}_{00k}} \end{bmatrix}.$$

After a simplification of Eq. (7.86), we have

$$\sigma^2\left(\ln\left(\tilde{\theta}^{[k]}_{mult_{2way}}\right)\right) = n^{-1}_{[k]}\left[\sum\nolimits_{i=1}^4 b_{ii} - 2(b_{12} + b_{13} + b_{24} + b_{34} - b_{14} - b_{23})\right], \tag{7.87}$$

where $\{b_{ij}\}$, i, j = 1, 2, 3, 4 are given by a symmetric matrix $B = \left[b_{ij}\right]^4_{i,j=1} = \left(\mathcal{W}^{-1}_{[k]}\right)^T \Sigma^*_{[k]} \mathcal{W}^{-1}_{[k]}$. Eq. (7.73) follows directly from Eq. (7.87). Eqs. (7.74) and (7.75) follows directly by applying the independence between cases and controls to Eqs. (7.72) and (7.73).

7.3 Misclassified Exposure and Confounding Factors

Let D, E, and C be three dichotomous variables, in which D denotes the subject's disease variable (= 1 if present, 0 otherwise), E the subject's exposure variable (= 1 if exposed, 0 otherwise), and C the extraneous (a suspected confounding) variable (= 1 if present, 0 otherwise). Assume that a simple random sampling scheme is used to collect the data of size n which are then cross-classified into Table 7.15 in which E^* and C^* are imperfect surrogate variables for E and C.

For fixed i, the crude cell proportion estimators are given by

$$\widehat{p}_{ijk} = \frac{n_{ijk}}{n_{[i]}}, \tag{7.88}$$

where $n_{[i]} \equiv n_{i++} = n_{i11} + n_{i10} + n_{i01} + n_{i00}$. We assume that Eq. (7.88) follows a multinomial distribution with parameters $n_{[i]}$ and p_{ijk}. For fixed i, the variance-covariance matrix of $\{\widehat{p}_{ijk}\}$ is given by

Table 7.15 The data collected by a simple random sampling

		$C^* = 1$	$C^* = 0$	Total
D = 1 (cases)	$E^* = 1$	n_{111}	n_{110}	n_{11+}
	$E^* = 0$	n_{101}	n_{100}	n_{10+}
	Total	n_{1+1}	n_{1+0}	n_{1++}
D = 0 (controls)	$E^* = 1$	n_{011}	n_{010}	n_{01+}
	$E^* = 0$	n_{001}	n_{000}	n_{00+}
		n_{0+1}	n_{0+0}	n_{0++}

Where $\sum_{i,j,k=0}^{1} n_{ijk} = 1$, the subscript "+" denotes the partial sum of either column or row

$$\Sigma_{[i]} = \left[\sigma_{(i)jk}\right]_{j,k=1}^{4} = n_{[i]} \cdot \begin{bmatrix} p_{i11}\bar{p}_{i11} & -p_{i11}p_{i10} & -p_{i11}p_{i01} & -p_{i11}p_{i00} \\ -p_{i11}p_{i10} & p_{i10}\bar{p}_{i10} & -p_{i10}p_{i01} & -p_{i10}p_{i00} \\ -p_{i11}p_{i01} & -p_{i01}p_{i10} & p_{i01}\bar{p}_{i01} & -p_{i01}p_{i00} \\ -p_{i11}p_{i00} & -p_{i00}p_{i10} & -p_{i00}p_{i01} & p_{i00}\bar{p}_{i00} \end{bmatrix}. \quad (7.89)$$

To measure the effect of the exposure and the extraneous C, calculate, respectively, from Table 7.15, the following estimates for the exposure odds ratio of E unstratified and stratified by C

$$\widehat{R}_E = \frac{n_{11+}n_{00+}}{n_{10+}n_{01+}}, \quad (7.90)$$

$$\widehat{R}_{E|C=1} = \frac{n_{111}n_{001}}{n_{101}n_{011}}, \quad (7.91)$$

and

$$\widehat{R}_{E|C=0} = \frac{n_{110}n_{000}}{n_{100}n_{010}}. \quad (7.92)$$

In addition, the Mantel-Haenszel summary odds ratio is given by [22]

$$\widehat{R}_{E|MH} = \frac{n_{111}n_{001}n_{++1}^{-1} + n_{110}n_{000}n_{++0}^{-1}}{n_{101}n_{011}n_{++1}^{-1} + n_{100}n_{010}n_{++0}^{-1}}. \quad (7.93)$$

Now let the ratios of odds ratios be defined, respectively, by

$$\widehat{\psi}_{E|C} = \frac{\widehat{R}_{E|MH}}{\widehat{R}_E}, \quad (7.94)$$

and

$$\widehat{\psi}_{homo} = \frac{\widehat{R}_{E\,|\,C=1}}{\widehat{R}_{E\,|\,C=0}}, \tag{7.95}$$

where "homo" in the subscript of Eq. (7.95) means the word "homogeneous." If the estimated value of $\widehat{\psi}_{E\,|\,C}$ is greater or less than 10% of the null value of unity, the extraneous variable C is said to be a confounder. Two strata are said to be heterogeneous if the estimated value of $\widehat{\psi}_{homo}$ is significantly different from the null value of unity; otherwise, it is said to be homogeneous.

Let $R_{[i]mult\,|\,EC}$ and $R_{mult\,|\,DEC}$ denote, respectively, the first- and second-order multiplicative interaction between E and C or among D, E and C. Then the estimates of these ratios are given, respectively, by

$$\widehat{R}_{[i]mult\,|\,EC} = \frac{n_{i11}n_{i00}}{n_{i10}n_{i01}}, \tag{7.96}$$

and

$$\widehat{R}_{mult\,|\,DEC} = \frac{n_{111}n_{010}n_{100}n_{010}}{n_{101}n_{011}n_{110}n_{000}}. \tag{7.97}$$

Two variables E and C are said to have a nonzero first-order multiplicative interaction if the estimated value of Eq. (7.96) is significantly from the null value of unity; otherwise, there is no first-order multiplicative interaction between E and C. Three variables D, E, and C are said to have a nonzero second-order multiplicative interaction if the estimated value of Eq. (7.97) is significantly different from the null value of unity; otherwise, there is no second-order multiplicative interaction among D, E, and C. The extraneous variable C is said to be an effect modifier if either the estimated value of Eqs. (7.95) or (7.97) are significantly different from the null value of unity; otherwise, C is not an effect modifier. Let R_C be a measure of the strength of confounding by the extraneous variable C [23]

$$\widehat{R}_C = \frac{n_{110}n_{101}n_{100}^{-1} + n_{010}n_{001}n_{000}^{-1}}{n_{10+}n_{01+}}. \tag{7.98}$$

Remark

Show that Eqs. (7.95) and (7.97) are equal. (Exercise 7.5-1).

Assume that D is not misclassified, while E and C are jointly misclassified. There are two scenarios between E and C that have to be considered separately.

Scenario I The classification errors between E and C are independent.

For this scenario, each cell misclassification error probability is obtained as the product of the corresponding two row/column marginal misclassification error probabilities. The false positive and false negative probabilities for Y = E or C are defined as follows:

$$\gamma_{Y[i]} = \Pr(Y^* = 0 | Y = 1; D = i), \tag{7.99}$$

and

$$\eta_{Y[i]} = \Pr(Y^* = 1 | Y = 0; D = i). \tag{7.100}$$

For $i = 1, 0$ let

$$\vec{p}_{[i]} = [p_{i11}, p_{i10}, p_{i01}, p_{i00}]^T, \tag{7.101}$$

$$\widehat{\vec{p}}_{[i]} = [\widehat{p}_{i11}, \widehat{p}_{i10}, \widehat{p}_{i01}, \widehat{p}_{i00}]^T. \tag{7.102}$$

Thus, for i = 0, 1, we have by using Eqs. (7.99) and (7.100)

$$E\left(\widehat{\vec{p}}_{[i]}\right) = \mathcal{W}_{I[i]} \vec{p}_{[i]}, \tag{7.103}$$

where the misclassification matrix $\mathcal{W}_{I[i]}$ is given by Barron [5] or Tzonou et al. [21].

$$\begin{aligned} \mathcal{W}_{I[i]} &= [\beth_{I[ijk]}] \\ &= \begin{bmatrix} \left(1-\gamma_{E[i]}\right)\left(1-\gamma_{C[i]}\right) & \left(1-\gamma_{E[i]}\right)\eta_{C[i]} & \left(1-\gamma_{C[i]}\right)\eta_{E[i]} & \eta_{E[i]}\eta_{C[i]} \\ \left(1-\gamma_{E[i]}\right)\gamma_{C[i]} & \left(1-\gamma_{E[i]}\right)\left(1-\eta_{C[i]}\right) & \eta_{E[i]}\gamma_{C[i]} & \eta_{E[i]}\left(1-\eta_{C[i]}\right) \\ \gamma_{E[i]}\left(1-\gamma_{C[i]}\right) & \gamma_{E[i]}\eta_{C[i]} & \left(1-\eta_{E[i]}\right)\left(1-\gamma_{C[i]}\right) & \left(1-\eta_{E[i]}\right)\eta_{C[i]} \\ \gamma_{E[i]}\gamma_{C[i]} & \gamma_{E[i]}\left(1-\eta_{C[i]}\right) & \left(1-\eta_{E[i]}\right)\gamma_{C[i]} & \left(1-\eta_{E[i]}\right)\left(1-\eta_{C[i]}\right) \end{bmatrix} \end{aligned} \tag{7.104}$$

By conditioning on that $\gamma_{Y[i]}$ and $\eta_{Y[i]}$ for Y = E or C are known, the bias-adjusted cell probability estimator (BACP) is then defined by

$$\tilde{\vec{p}}_{I[i]} = \mathcal{W}_{I[i]}^{-1} \widehat{\vec{p}}_{[i]}, \tag{7.105}$$

where the inverse $\mathcal{V}_{I[i]}$ of $\mathcal{W}_{I[i]}$ is given by

$$\begin{aligned} \mathcal{V}_{I[i]} &\equiv \mathcal{W}_{I[i]}^{-1} \\ &= \frac{1}{\ddagger} \cdot \begin{bmatrix} \left(1-\eta_{E[i]}\right)\left(1-\eta_{C[i]}\right) & -\gamma_{C[i]}\left(1-\eta_{E[i]}\right) & -\gamma_{E[i]}\left(1-\eta_{C[i]}\right) & \gamma_{E[i]}\gamma_{C[i]} \\ -\eta_{C[i]}\left(1-\eta_{E[i]}\right) & \left(1-\gamma_{C[i]}\right)\left(1-\eta_{E[i]}\right) & \gamma_{E[i]}\eta_{C[i]} & -\gamma_{E[i]}\left(1-\gamma_{C[i]}\right) \\ -\eta_{E[i]}\left(1-\eta_{C[i]}\right) & \eta_{E[i]}\gamma_{C[i]} & \left(1-\gamma_{E[i]}\right)\left(1-\eta_{C[i]}\right) & -\gamma_{C[i]}\left(1-\gamma_{E[i]}\right) \\ \eta_{E[i]}\eta_{C[i]} & -\eta_{E[i]}\left(1-\gamma_{C[i]}\right) & -\eta_{C[i]}\left(1-\gamma_{E[i]}\right) & \left(1-\gamma_{E[i]}\right)\left(1-\gamma_{C[i]}\right) \end{bmatrix} \\ &= \mathcal{D}_{I[i]} \end{aligned} \tag{7.106}$$

where $\mathcal{D}_{I[i]} \equiv \det\left(\mathcal{W}_{I[i]}\right) = \left[\left(1 - \gamma_{E[i]} - \eta_{E[i]}\right)\left(1 - \gamma_{C[i]} - \eta_{C[i]}\right)\right]^2$. In order for $\mathcal{W}_{I[i]}$ to be invertible, the following constraints on the false positive and false negative rates for both E and C are imposed:

$$\gamma_{E[i]} + \eta_{E[i]} < 1 \text{ and } \gamma_{C[i]} + \eta_{C[i]} < 1 \tag{7.107}$$

Scenario II The classification errors of E and C are not independent.

For this scenario, there are 4 correctly classified and 12 misclassified conditional probabilities of E^* and C^* defined by: for fixed j′, k′, j, k = 0, 1

$$\delta_{j'k'[i]}^{jk} = \Pr(E^* = j, C^* = k | E = j', C = k'; D = i), \tag{7.108}$$

where $\left\{\delta_{j'k'[i]}^{jk}\right\}$ for j′, k′ = 0, 1 are required to satisfy

$$\sum\nolimits_{j,k=0}^{1} \delta_{j'k'[i]}^{jk} = 1, 0 \le \delta_{j'k'[i]}^{jk} \le 1 \tag{7.109}$$

Because the misclassification can go equally likely from one cell to another three cells, we assume that they are all equal to one another, that is, $\zeta_{1[i]} \equiv \delta_{11[i]}^{10} = \delta_{11[i]}^{01} = \delta_{11[i]}^{00}$, $\zeta_{2[i]} \equiv \delta_{10[i]}^{11} = \delta_{10[i]}^{01} = \delta_{10[i]}^{00}$, $\zeta_{3[i]} \equiv \delta_{01[i]}^{11} = \delta_{01[i]}^{10} = \delta_{01[i]}^{00}$, $\zeta_{4[i]} = \delta_{00[i]}^{11} = \delta_{00[i]}^{10} = \delta_{00[i]}^{01}$. The misclassification matrix is given by

$$\mathcal{W}_{II[i]} = \begin{bmatrix} \overline{\zeta}_{1[i]} & \zeta_{1[i]} & \zeta_{1[i]} & \zeta_{1[i]} \\ \zeta_{2[i]} & \overline{\zeta}_{2[i]} & \zeta_{2[i]} & \zeta_{2[i]} \\ \zeta_{3[i]} & \zeta_{3[i]} & \overline{\zeta}_{3[i]} & \zeta_{3[i]} \\ \zeta_{4[i]} & \zeta_{4[i]} & \zeta_{4[i]} & \overline{\zeta}_{4[i]} \end{bmatrix}, \tag{7.110}$$

where $\overline{\zeta}_{j[i]} = 1 - 3\zeta_{j[i]}$, j = 1, 2, 3, 4. Further, the inverse $\mathcal{V}_{II[i]}$ of $\mathcal{W}_{II[i]}$ is given by

$$\mathcal{V}_{II[i]} \equiv \mathcal{W}_{II[i]}^{-1} = \mathcal{D}_{II[i]}^{-\frac{1}{3}} \cdot \begin{bmatrix} 1 - \zeta_{1[i]} - 2\zeta_{2[i]} & -\zeta_{1[i]} & -\zeta_{1[i]} & -\zeta_{1[i]} \\ -\zeta_{2[i]} & 1 - \zeta_{2[i]} - 2\zeta_{4[i]} & -\zeta_{2[i]} & -\zeta_{2[i]} \\ -\zeta_{3[i]} & -\zeta_{3[i]} & 1 - 2\zeta_{1[i]} - \zeta_{3[i]} & -\zeta_{3[i]} \\ -\zeta_{4[i]} & -\zeta_{4[i]} & -\zeta_{4[i]} & 1 - 2\zeta_{3[i]} - \zeta_{4[i]} \end{bmatrix}, \tag{7.111}$$

where $\mathcal{D}_{II[i]} \equiv \det\left(\mathcal{W}_{II[i]}\right) = \left(1 - \zeta_{1[i]} - \zeta_{2[i]} - \zeta_{3[i]} - \zeta_{4[i]}\right)^3$.

For this scenario, the BACP estimator is given by

$$\tilde{\vec{p}}_{II[i]} = \mathcal{W}_{II[i]}^{-1} \widehat{\vec{p}}_{[i]} = \mathcal{V}_{II[i]} \widehat{\vec{p}}_{[i]}. \tag{7.112}$$

The misclassification error probabilities ((γ_Y, η_Y) or $(\zeta_{1[i]}, \zeta_{2[i]}, \zeta_{3[i]}, \zeta_{4[i]})$) are sad to be feasible if the misclassification matrix ($\mathcal{W}_{I[i]}$ *or* $\mathcal{W}_{II[i]}$) is nonsingular. The BACP estimator (Eqs. (7.105) or (7.112)) if each component of its vector is nonnegative and their sum equals the total probability one. From Eq. (7.105) and for j, k = 0, 1 we define

$$\tilde{n}_{ijk} = n_{[i]} \cdot n_{ijk}. \tag{7.113}$$

By substituting Eqs. (7.105) or (7.112) into Eqs. (7.90) to (7.98), we obtain the corresponding bias-adjusted estimates $\tilde{R}_E$, $\tilde{R}_{E\,|\,C=1}$, $\tilde{R}_{E\,|\,C=0}$, $\tilde{R}_{E\,|\,MH}$, $\tilde{\psi}_E$, $\tilde{\psi}_{homo}$, $\tilde{R}_{[i]mut\,|\,EC}$, $\tilde{R}_{mult\,|\,DEC}$, and $\tilde{R}_C$.

Example 7.3

The data in Table 7.16 are taken from Crane [11]. A case-control study was conducted to examine the hypothesis that fenoterol by metered dose inhaler increases the risk of death in patients with asthma. Cases were drawn from the National Asthma Mortality Survey which identified all asthma deaths in New Zealand from August 1981 to July 1983. Of the 271 asthma deaths identified in the survey, 125 occurred in patients aged 5–45 years, and these formed in the case group. For each case, four controls matched for to which the Cases themselves would have been admitted, had they survived. Controls were obtained for the 124 out of the 125 cases. Seven cases were subsequently excluded because they died after admission to hospitals. Therefore, the analysis pertains to the 117 cases and 468 matched controls.

In terms of symbols, the disease, exposure and extraneous variables are given as follows:

D = asthma death (= 1 if outpatient dies, 0 if hospitalized controls),
E = use of prescribed fenoterol (= 1 if yes, 0 if no),
C = use of corticosteroid (= 1 if used, 0 if not used).

If the data are not misclassified, the crude estimators with its 95% confidence interval (CI) are obtained (Table 7.17) from Eqs. (7.90) to (7.98) and (7.114) to (7.118) in the appendix.

Table 7.16 The data of asthma death in patients inhaled by fenoterol and corresponding to four controls

D = 1 (cases)		$C^* = 1$	$C^* = 0$	Total
	$E^* = 1$	26	34	60
	$E^* = 0$	7	50	57
	Total	33	84	117
D = 0 (controls)	$E^* = 1$	38	151	189
	$E^* = 0$	66	213	279
	Total	104	364	468

Table 7.17 The estimated value of Eqs. (7.90) to (7.98) with its 95% confidence interval

A crude estimator	Estimated value	95% CI
$\widehat{R}_E$	1.55	[1.50, 1.61]
$\widehat{R}_{E\mid C=1}$	6.45	[2.89, 7.06]
$\widehat{R}_{E\mid C=0}$	0.96	[0.94, 0.97]
$\widehat{R}_{E\mid MH}$	1.53	[1.44, 1.62]
$\widehat{\psi}_{E\mid C}$	0.98	[0.64, 1.52]
$\widehat{\psi}_{homo}$	6.73	[4.26, 10.6]
$\widehat{R}_{[1]mult\mid EC}$	5.46	[5.45, 5.47]
$\widehat{R}_{[0]mult\mid EC}$	0.81	[0.812, 0.813]
$\widehat{R}_{mult\mid DEC}$	6.73	[6.29, 7.18]
$\widehat{R}_C$	0.21	[0.205, 0.215]

As was pointed out by O'Donnel et al. [24] who reviewed the data for the group allegedly at higher risk, some of 20 such fatal cases that were recorded by Crane [11] might not use prescribed fenoterol as reported by the general practitioner. In 7 of the 18 cases, the beta-agonist in use immediately before death was not or might not have been fenoterol. Hence the data used by Crane [11] are likely to be misclassified.

Assume that the data are indeed misclassified. The proposed bias-adjusted estimator can be applied. Before using Eqs. (7.105) or (7.112), we need to know the misclassification error probabilities. Here we apply the idea of finding the counterfactual (CF) true table from the observed misclassified table. (Exercise 7.5-2) (Tables 7.18 and 7.19).

All five CF true models are admissible for both cases and controls.

After getting all possible combinations from admissible CF true models under scenario I (or scenario II) for cases and controls, the best bias-adjusted values of Eqs. (7.90) to (7.98) are computed for all five combinations (Tables 7.20 or 7.21).

The value of $\tilde{R}_E$ under scenario I or II is exactly the same for all CF models as that of $\widehat{R}_E$, because the marginal totals of all counterfactual models are the same as that of the observed table. The effect of joint misclassification of the exposure and confounding for cases and controls varies. It depends on which measure is used. The values of $\tilde{R}_{E\mid C=1}$, $\tilde{\psi}_{homo}$ $\tilde{R}_{[1]mult\mid EC}$ and $\tilde{R}_{mult\mid DEC}$ are much smaller under either scenario than that of the corresponding crude estimators $\widehat{R}_{E\mid C=1}$, $\widehat{\psi}_{homo}$ $\widehat{R}_{[1]mult\mid EC}$ and $\widehat{R}_{mult\mid DEC}$. The larger the misclassification error probabilities, the smaller their values are. The effect of joint misclassification of E and C on the measure of $R_{E\mid C=0}$, $R_{E\mid MH}$, $R_{[0]mult\mid EC}$ and $\psi_{E\mid C}$ is negligible. Lastly, the 95% confidence interval for $\tilde{R}_{E\mid C=0}$ and $\tilde{\psi}_{homo}$ are much wider under scenario II than under scenario I.

Although the extraneous variable C (the use of corticosteroid) is not judged as a confounder by the value of $\widehat{\psi}_{E\mid C}=0.98$, it was considered as a confounder as shown by indication [25] or by association with the death and the exposure [23] or by not being equally distributed (lack of comparability) in the category of the exposure

Table 7.18 The odds ratio for five CF true frequency models under two scenarios for cases

CF true model	$[n_{111}, n_{110}, n_{101}, n_{100}]$	Scenario I $[\gamma_{E[1]}, \zeta_{E[1]}, \gamma_{C[1]}, \zeta_{C[1]}]$	$\vec{\tilde{p}}_{I[1]}$	Scenario II $[\zeta_{1[1]}, \zeta_{2[1]}, \zeta_{3[1]}, \zeta_{4[1]}]$	$\vec{\tilde{p}}_{II[1]}$
1	[25, 35, 8, 49]	[0.0005, 0.0005, 0.0002, 0.0002]	[0.2222, 0.2904, 0.0596, 0.4273]	[0.97, 0.009, 0.009, 0.009]	[0.21, 0.28, 0.05, 0.41]
2	[24, 36, 9, 48]	[0.002, 0.002, 0.0008, 0.0008]	[0.2221, 0.2899, 0.0591, 0.4273]	[0.002, 0.95, 0.002, 0.002]	[0.20, 0.26, 0.04, 0.40]
3	[23, 37, 10, 47]	[0.005, 0.005, 0.002, 0.002]	[0.2220, 0.2890, 0.0582, 0.4371]	[0.03, 0.03, 0.92, 0.03]	[0.19, 0.25, 0.03, 0.38]
4	[22, 38, 11, 46]	[0.008, 0.009, 0.003, 0.003]	[0.2219, 0.2878, 0.0546, 0.4270]	[0.03, 0.03, 0.03, 0.90]	[0.17, 0.24, 0.02, 0.36]
5	[21, 39, 12, 45]	[0.01, 0.01, 0.005, 0.005]	[0.2217, 0.2862, 0.0551, 0.4268]	[0.87, 0.04, 0.04, 0.04]	[0.16, 0.22, 0.01, 0.35]

Table 7.19 The odds ratio for five CF true frequency models under two scenarios for controls

CF true model	$[n_{011}, n_{010}, n_{001}, n_{000}]$	Scenario I $[\gamma_{E[0]}, \eta_{E[0]}, \gamma_{C[0]}, \eta_{C[0]}]$	$\vec{\tilde{p}}_{I[0]}$	Scenario II $[\zeta_{1[0]}, \zeta_{2[0]}, \zeta_{3[0]}, \zeta_{4[0]}]$	$\vec{\tilde{p}}_{II[0]}$
1	[37, 152, 67, 212]	$[5.1 \cdot 10^{-5}, 3.4 \cdot 10^{-5}, 1.5 \cdot 10^{-5}, 9.8 \cdot 10^{-6}]$	[0.2222, 0.2906, 0.0598, 0.4274]	[0.9936, 0.0021, 0.0021, 0.0021]	[0.2191, 0.2872, 0.0574, 0.4234]
2	[36, 153, 68, 211]	$[0.0002, 0.0001, 5.8 \cdot 10^{-5}, 3.9 \cdot 10^{-5}]$	[0.2223, 0.2907, 0.0598, 0.4276]	[0.0043, 0.9872, 0.0043, 0.0043]	[0.2160, 0.2838, 0.0550, 0.4174]
3	[35, 154, 69, 210]	$[0.0005, 0.0003, 0.0001, 8.9 \cdot 10^{-5}]$	[0.2225, 0.2908, 0.0598, 0.4278]	[0.0064, 0.0064, 0.9808, 0.0064]	[0.2130, 0.2805, 0.0527, 0.4155]
4	[34, 155, 70, 209]	[0.0008, 0.0006, 0.0002, 0.0002]	[0.2227, 0.2910, 0.0598, 0.4282]	[0.0085, 0.0085, 0.0085, 0.9744]	[0.2099, 0.2771, 0.0503, 0.4115]
5	[33, 156, 71, 208]	[0.0013, 0.0009, 0.0004, 0.0002]	[0.2230, 0.2912, 0.0597, 0.4287]	[0.9679, 0.0107, 0.0107, 0.0107]	[0.2068, 0.2737, 0.0474, 0.4075]

variable (the use of prescribed fenoterol) [24]. Furthemore, it was shown to be an effect modifier by the value of $\widehat{\psi}_{homo}$ or $\widehat{R}_{mult\,|\,DEC}$. Once an effect modifier is present, whether C is a confounder becomes not a concern. Rather, stratum-specific odds ratio estimates ($\widehat{R}_{E\,|\,C=i}$) should be reported because summary estimates do not convey information on the pattern of variation about stratum-specific estimates.

Table 7.20 Bias-adjusted estimator with 95% confidence interval under scenario I

BA estimator/ 95%CI	CF true model (case, control)				
	(1)	(2)	(3)	(4)	(5)
$\tilde{R}_E$	1.55 [1.50, 1.62]	1.55 [1.50, 1.61]	1.55 [1.5538, 1.5540]	1.55 [1.5538, 1.5540]	1.55 [1.5538, 1.5540]
$\tilde{R}_{E\mid C=1}$	5.66 [5.23, 6.13]	5.04 [4.62, 5.49]	4.53 [4.18, 4.91]	4.12 [3.77, 4.50]	3.77 [3.47, 4.09]
$\tilde{R}_{E\mid C=0}$	0.996 [0.97, 1.02]	1.03 [1.01, 1.06]	1.07 [1.03, 1.12]	1.11 [1.09, 1.14]	1.15 [1.13, 1.18]
$\tilde{R}_{E\mid MH}$	1.53 [1.49, 1.57]	1.54 [1.43, 1.66]	1.55 [1.44, 1.66]	1.55 [1.4, 1.68]	1.56 [1.44, 1.69]
$\tilde{\psi}_{E\mid C}$	0.99 [0.94, 1.03]	0.99 [0.91, 1.07]	0.99 [0.93, 1.07]	1.00 [0.93, 1.08]	1.01 [0.93, 1.09]
$\tilde{\psi}_{homo}$	5.68 [5.23, 6.17]	4.87 [4.45, 5.33]	4.22 [3.87, 4.61]	3.70 [3.37, 4.05]	3.26 [2.99, 3.55]
$\tilde{R}_{[1]mult\mid EC}$	4.38 [4.36, 4.39]	3.56 [3.54, 3.57]	2.92 [2.91, 2.93]	2.42 [2.418, 2.424]	2.02 2.01, 2.03]
$\tilde{R}_{[0]mult\mid EC}$	0.77 [0.77, 0.77]	0.73 [0.73, 0.73]	0.69 [0.69, 0.69]	0.65 [0.65, 0.65]	0.62 [0.62, 0.62]
$\tilde{R}_{mult\mid DEC}$	5.68 [5.19, 6.21]	4.87 [4.45, 5.33]	4.22 [3.86, 4.63]	3.70 [3.52, 3.88]	3.26 [2.97, 3.57]
$\tilde{R}_C$	0.22 [0.211, 0.226]	0.23 [0.221, 0.235]	0.24 [0.230, 0.245]	0.25 [0.244, 0.253]	0.26 [0.251, 0.267]

For other references on the confounder, see Wickramaratne-Holford [27]; Weinberg [26]; or Yiostalo-Knuuttila [28].

Remarks

1. The calculation of the misclassification error probabilities is inaccurate in Lee [20].
2. Advantages in using counterfactual true models to conduct a sensitivity analysis are multifold. First, it solves the problem that we need to find a gold standard in order to calculate the misclassification error probability. Second, an assumption of nondifferential misclassification is not needed on any factor under study. Third, all results are strictly restricted to the observed data. Hence, the final conclusion is drawn from real data-based rather than hypothetical data used by Greenland [16] or Greenland-Robins [17].

Appendix 7.3A

By adapting the variance formula in Lee [14, 20], the variance formula is readily given for the crude and bias-adjusted estimators for the 2-way multiplicative interaction by

Table 7.21 Bias-adjusted estimator with 95% confidence interval under scenario II

BA estimator/95% CI	CF true model (case, control)				
	(1)	(2)	(3)	(4)	(5)
$\tilde{R}_E$	1.55 [1.50, 1.61]	1.55 [1.50, 1.61]	1.55 [1.50, 1.61]	1.55 [1.50, 1.61]	1.55 [1.49, 1.62]
$\tilde{R}_{E\mid C=1}$	5.66 [5.17, 6.18]	5.04 [4.54, 5.59]	4.53 [3.99, 5.15]	4.11 [3.46, 4.89]	3.77 [2.83, 107.9]
$\tilde{R}_{E\mid C=0}$	0.996 [0.47, 2.12]	1.03 [1.01, 1.06]	1.07 [1.05, 1.10]	1.11 [1.09, 1.14]	1.16 [1.13, 1.19]
$\tilde{R}_{E\mid MH}$	1.53 [1.49, 1.58]	1.54 [1.48, 1.60]	1.55 [1.50, 1.60]	1.55 [1.52, 1.59]	1.56 [1.51, 1.62]
$\tilde{\psi}_{E\mid C}$	0.99 [0.94, 1.03]	0.99 [0.989, 0.991]	0.99 [0.95, 1.05]	1.00 [0.96, 1.05]	1.01 [0.95, 1.06]
$\tilde{\psi}_{homo}$	5.68 [2.66, 12.2]	4.87 [4.38, 5.42]	4.22 [3.71, 4.81]	3.70 [3.10, 4.40]	3.26 [2.44, 4.34]
$\tilde{R}_{[1]mult\mid EC}$	4.38 [4.35, 4.40]	3.56 [3.54, 3.57]	2.92 [2.91, 2.93]	2.42 [2.41, 2.44]	2.02 [1.93, 2.11]
$\tilde{R}_{[0]mult\mid EC}$	0.77 [0.77, 0.77]	0.73 [0.73, 0.73]	0.69 [0.69, 0.69]	0.65 [0.65, 0.66]	0.62 [0.62, 0.62]
$\tilde{R}_{mult\mid DEC}$	5.68 [5.65, 5.71]	4.87 [4.85, 4.89]	4.22 [4.21, 4.24]	3.70 [3.68, 3.71]	3.26 [3.12, 3.41]
$\tilde{R}_C$	0.22 [0.21, 0.23]	0.23 [0.22, 0.23]	0.24 [0.23, 0.24]	0.25 [0.24, 0.25]	0.26 [0.25, 0.27]

$$\sigma^2\left(\ln\left(\widehat{R}_{[i]mult\mid EC}\right)\right) = n_{[i]}^{-1}\widehat{\vec{a}}_{[i]}^{T}\Sigma_{[i]}\widehat{\vec{a}}_{[i]}, \tag{7.114}$$

where $\widehat{\vec{a}}_{[i]} = \left[\widehat{p}_{i11}^{-1}, \widehat{p}_{i10}^{-1}, \widehat{p}_{i01}^{-1}, \widehat{p}_{i00}^{-1}\right]^T$.

$$\sigma^2\left(\ln\left(\tilde{R}_{[i]mult\mid EC}\right)\right) = n_{[i]}^{-1}\tilde{\vec{a}}_{[i]}^{T}\Sigma_{[i]}\tilde{\vec{a}}_{[i]}, \tag{7.115}$$

where $\tilde{\vec{a}}_{[i]} = \left[v_{11[.;i]}\tilde{p}_{i11}^{-1}, -v_{22[.;i]}\tilde{p}_{i10}^{-1}, -v_{33[.;i]}\tilde{p}_{i01}^{-1}, v_{44[.;i]}\tilde{p}_{i00}^{-1}\right]^T$, $\left\{v_{jj[.;i]}\right\}$ are the jth diagonal entry of the inverse matrix $\mathcal{V}_{.[i]} = \mathcal{W}_{.[i]}^{-1}$, $\mathcal{W}_{.[i]} = \mathcal{W}_{I[i]}$ or $\mathcal{W}_{II[i]}$, $\tilde{\vec{p}}_{[i]} = \mathcal{V}_{.[i]}\widehat{\vec{p}}_{[i]}$, and $\Sigma_{[i]}$ is given by Eq. (7.89). The variance formula for the crude and bias-adjusted estimators for the 3-way multiplicative interaction are given by

$$\sigma^2\left(\ln\left(\widehat{R}_{mult\mid DEC}\right)\right) = \sum\nolimits_{i=0}^{1}\sigma^2\left(\ln\left(\widehat{R}_{[i]mult\mid EC}\right)\right), \tag{7.116}$$

and

$$\sigma^2\left(\ln\left(\tilde{R}_{mult\,|\,DEC}\right)\right)=\sum\nolimits_{i=0}^{1}\sigma^2\left(\ln\left(\tilde{R}_{[i]mult\,|\,EC}\right)\right). \tag{7.117}$$

Similarly, we have the variance for the crude and bias-adjusted odds ratio ignoring the confounding factor C are given, respectively, by applying the delta method [2]

$$\sigma^2\left(\ln\left(\widehat{R}_E\right)\right)=\sum\nolimits_{i=0}^{1}n_{[i]}^{-1}\widehat{\vec{b}}_{[i]}^{T}\Sigma_{[i]}\widehat{\vec{b}}_{[i]}, \tag{7.118}$$

where $\widehat{\vec{b}}_{[1]}=\left[\widehat{p}_{11+}^{-1},\widehat{p}_{11+}^{-1},-\widehat{p}_{10+}^{-1},-\widehat{p}_{10+}^{-1}\right]^T$, and $\widehat{\vec{b}}_{[0]}=\left[-\widehat{p}_{01+}^{-1},-\widehat{p}_{01+}^{-1},\widehat{p}_{00+}^{-1},\widehat{p}_{00+}^{-1}\right]^T$, and

$$\sigma^2\left(\ln\left(\tilde{R}_E\right)\right)=\sum\nolimits_{i=0}^{1}n_{[i]}^{-1}\tilde{\vec{b}}_{[i]}^{T}\Sigma_{[i]}\tilde{\vec{b}}_{[i]}, \tag{7.119}$$

where $\tilde{\vec{b}}_{[1]}=\left[v_{11[.;1]}\tilde{p}_{11+}^{-1},v_{22[.;1]}\tilde{p}_{11+}^{-1},-v_{33[.;1]}\tilde{p}_{10+}^{-1},-v_{44[.;1]}\tilde{p}_{10+}^{-1}\right]^T$, and $\vec{b}_{[0]}=\left[-v_{11[.;0]}\tilde{p}_{01+}^{-1},-v_{22[.;0]}\tilde{p}_{01+}^{-1},v_{33[.;0]}\tilde{p}_{00+}^{-1},v_{44[.;0]}\tilde{p}_{00+}^{-1}\right]^T$, $\tilde{\vec{p}}_{[i]}$ is defined by Eq. (7.115).

The variance of the crude and bias-adjusted odds ratio stratified by the confounder C are given by

$$\sigma^2\left(\ln\left(\widehat{R}_{E\,|\,C=1}\right)\right)=\sum\nolimits_{i=0}^{1}n_{[i]}^{-1}\widehat{\vec{c}}_{[i]\,|\,C=1}\Sigma_{[i]}\widehat{\vec{c}}_{[i]\,|\,C=1}, \tag{7.120}$$

where $\widehat{\vec{c}}_{[i]\,|\,C=1}=\left[\widehat{p}_{i11}^{-1},0,-\widehat{p}_{i01}^{-1},0\right]^T$, and $\widehat{\vec{c}}_{[i]\,|\,C=0}=\left[0,-\widehat{p}_{i10}^{-1},0,-\widehat{p}_{i00}^{-1}\right]^T$, and

$$\sigma^2\left(\ln\left(\tilde{R}_{E\,|\,C=1}\right)\right)=\sum\nolimits_{i=0}^{1}n_{[i]}^{-1}\tilde{\vec{c}}_{[i]\,|\,C=1}\Sigma_{[i]}\tilde{\vec{c}}_{[i]\,|\,C=1}, \tag{7.121}$$

where $\tilde{\vec{c}}_{[i]\,|\,C=1}=\left[v_{11[.;i]}\tilde{p}_{i11}^{-1},0,-v_{33[.;i]}\tilde{p}_{i01}^{-1},0\right]^T$ and $\vec{c}_{[i]\,|\,C=0}=\left[0,-v_{22[.;i]}\tilde{p}_{i10}^{-1},0,-v_{44[.;i]}\tilde{p}_{i00}^{-1}\right]^T$.

The variance of the crude Mantel-Haenszel summary odds ratio is given by

$$\sigma^2\left(\ln\left(\widehat{R}_{E\,|\,MH}\right)\right)=\sum\nolimits_{i=0}^{1}n_{[i]}^{-1}\widehat{\vec{d}}_{[i]}^{T}\Sigma_{[i]}\widehat{\vec{d}}_{[i]}, \tag{7.122}$$

where $\widehat{\vec{d}}_{[i]}=\left[\widehat{d}_{1[i]},\widehat{d}_{2[i]},\widehat{d}_{3[i]},\widehat{d}_{4[i]}\right]^T$ and each component in $\widehat{\vec{d}}_{[i]}$ is given by

$$\widehat{d}_{1[1]} = \frac{\widehat{p}_{++0}}{\widehat{p}_{++1}} [\widehat{\rho}_1 \widehat{p}_{001} (\widehat{p}_{101} + \widehat{p}_{011} + \widehat{p}_{001}) + \widehat{\rho}_0 \widehat{p}_{101} \widehat{p}_{011}],$$

$$\widehat{d}_{2[1]} = \frac{\widehat{p}_{++1}}{\widehat{p}_{++0}} [\widehat{\rho}_1 \widehat{p}_{000} (\widehat{p}_{100} + \widehat{p}_{010} + \widehat{p}_{000}) + \widehat{\rho}_0 \widehat{p}_{100} \widehat{p}_{010}],$$

$$\widehat{d}_{3[1]} = -\frac{\widehat{p}_{++0}}{\widehat{p}_{++1}} [\widehat{\rho}_1 \widehat{p}_{111} \widehat{p}_{001} + \widehat{\rho}_0 \widehat{p}_{011} (\widehat{p}_{111} + \widehat{p}_{011} + \widehat{p}_{001})],$$

$$\widehat{d}_{4[1]} = -\frac{\widehat{p}_{++1}}{\widehat{p}_{++0}} [\widehat{\rho}_1 \widehat{p}_{110} \widehat{p}_{000} + \widehat{\rho}_0 \widehat{p}_{010} (\widehat{p}_{110} + \widehat{p}_{010} + \widehat{p}_{000})],$$

$$\widehat{d}_{1[0]} = -\frac{\widehat{p}_{++0}}{\widehat{p}_{++1}} [\widehat{\rho}_1 \widehat{p}_{111} \widehat{p}_{001} + \widehat{\rho}_0 \widehat{p}_{101} (\widehat{p}_{111} + \widehat{p}_{101} + \widehat{p}_{001})],$$

$$\widehat{d}_{2[0]} = -\frac{\widehat{p}_{++1}}{\widehat{p}_{++0}} [\widehat{\rho}_1 \widehat{p}_{110} \widehat{p}_{000} + \widehat{\rho}_0 \widehat{p}_{100} (\widehat{p}_{110} + \widehat{p}_{100} + \widehat{p}_{000})],$$

$$\widehat{d}_{3[0]} = \frac{\widehat{p}_{++0}}{\widehat{p}_{++1}} [\widehat{\rho}_1 \widehat{p}_{111} (\widehat{p}_{111} + \widehat{p}_{101} + \widehat{p}_{001}) + \widehat{\rho}_0 \widehat{p}_{101} \widehat{p}_{011}],$$

$$\widehat{d}_{4[0]} = \frac{\widehat{p}_{++1}}{\widehat{p}_{++0}} [\widehat{\rho}_1 \widehat{p}_{110} (\widehat{p}_{110} + \widehat{p}_{100} + \widehat{p}_{010}) + \widehat{\rho}_0 \widehat{p}_{100} \widehat{p}_{010}],$$

$$\widehat{\rho}_1 \equiv \left(\widehat{p}_{++0} \widehat{p}_{111} \widehat{p}_{001} + \widehat{p}_{++1} \widehat{p}_{110} \widehat{p}_{000}\right)^{-1},$$

$$\widehat{\rho}_0 = \left(\widehat{p}_{++0} \widehat{p}_{101} \widehat{p}_{011} + \widehat{p}_{++1} \widehat{p}_{100} \widehat{p}_{000}\right)^{-1}.$$

The variance for the BACP of the Mantel-Haenszel summary odds ratio is given by

$$\sigma^2\left(\ln\left(\tilde{R}_{E\,|\,MH}\right)\right) = \sum\nolimits_{i=0}^{1} n_{[i]}^{-1} \vec{\tilde{d}}_{[i]}^{T} \Sigma_{[i]} \vec{\tilde{d}}_{[i]}, \tag{7.123}$$

where $\vec{\tilde{d}}_{[i]} = \left[\tilde{d}_{1[i]}, \tilde{d}_{2[i]}, \tilde{d}_{3[i]}, \tilde{d}_{4[i]}\right]^T$ and each component in $\vec{\tilde{d}}_{[i]}$ is given by

$$\tilde{d}_{1[1]} = v_{11[.;1]} \cdot \frac{\tilde{p}_{++0}}{\tilde{p}_{++1}} [\tilde{\rho}_1 \tilde{p}_{001} (\tilde{p}_{101} + \tilde{p}_{011} + \tilde{p}_{001}) + \tilde{\rho}_0 \tilde{p}_{101} \tilde{p}_{011}],$$

$$\tilde{d}_{2[1]} = v_{22[.;1]} \cdot \frac{\tilde{p}_{++1}}{\tilde{p}_{++0}} [\tilde{\rho}_1 \tilde{p}_{000} (\tilde{p}_{100} + \tilde{p}_{010} + \tilde{p}_{000}) + \tilde{\rho}_0 \tilde{p}_{100} \tilde{p}_{010}],$$

$$\tilde{d}_{3[1]} = -v_{33[.;1]} \cdot \frac{\tilde{p}_{++0}}{\tilde{p}_{++1}} [\tilde{\rho}_1 \tilde{p}_{111} \tilde{p}_{001} + \tilde{\rho}_0 \tilde{p}_{011} (\tilde{p}_{111} + \tilde{p}_{011} + \tilde{p}_{001})],$$

$$\tilde{d}_{4[1]} = -v_{44[\cdot;1]} \cdot \frac{\tilde{p}_{++1}}{\tilde{p}_{++0}} [\tilde{\rho}_1 \tilde{p}_{110} \tilde{p}_{000} + \tilde{\rho}_0 \tilde{p}_{010} (\tilde{p}_{110} + \tilde{p}_{010} + \tilde{p}_{000})],$$

$$\tilde{d}_{1[0]} = -v_{11[\cdot;0]} \cdot \frac{\tilde{p}_{++0}}{\tilde{p}_{++1}} [\tilde{\rho}_1 \tilde{p}_{111} \tilde{p}_{001} + \tilde{\rho}_0 \tilde{p}_{101} (\tilde{p}_{111} + \tilde{p}_{101} + \tilde{p}_{001})],$$

$$\tilde{d}_{2[0]} = -v_{22[\cdot;0]} \cdot \frac{\tilde{p}_{++1}}{\tilde{p}_{++0}} [\tilde{\rho}_1 \tilde{p}_{110} \tilde{p}_{000} + \tilde{\rho}_0 \tilde{p}_{100} (\tilde{p}_{110} + \tilde{p}_{100} + \tilde{p}_{000})],$$

$$\tilde{d}_{3[0]} = v_{33[\cdot;0]} \cdot \frac{\tilde{p}_{++0}}{\tilde{p}_{++1}} [\tilde{\rho}_1 \tilde{p}_{111} (\tilde{p}_{111} + \tilde{p}_{101} + \tilde{p}_{001}) + \tilde{\rho}_0 \tilde{p}_{101} \tilde{p}_{011}],$$

$$\tilde{d}_{4[0]} = v_{44[\cdot;0]} \cdot \frac{\tilde{p}_{++1}}{\tilde{p}_{++0}} [\tilde{\rho}_1 \tilde{p}_{110} (\tilde{p}_{110} + \tilde{p}_{100} + \tilde{p}_{010}) + \tilde{\rho}_0 \tilde{p}_{100} \tilde{p}_{010}],$$

$$\tilde{\rho}_1 \equiv \left(\tilde{p}_{++0} \tilde{p}_{111} \tilde{p}_{001} + \tilde{p}_{++1} \tilde{p}_{110} \tilde{p}_{000}\right)^{-1},$$

$$\tilde{\rho}_0 = \left(\tilde{p}_{++0} \tilde{p}_{101} \tilde{p}_{011} + \tilde{p}_{++1} \tilde{p}_{100} \tilde{p}_{000}\right)^{-1}.$$

The variance of $\ln\left(\widehat{R}_C\right)$ is given by

$$\sigma^2\left(\ln\left(\widehat{R}_C\right)\right) = \sum\nolimits_{i=0}^{1} n_{[i]}^{-1} \widehat{\vec{e}}_{[i]}^{\,T} \Sigma_{[i]} \widehat{\vec{e}}_{[i]}, \tag{7.124}$$

where each component of the vector $\widehat{\vec{e}}_{[i]} = \left[\widehat{e}_{1[i]}, \widehat{e}_{2[i]}, \widehat{e}_{3[i]}, \widehat{e}_{4[i]}\right]^T$ is given by

$$\widehat{e}_{1[1]} = 0,$$

$$\widehat{e}_{2[1]} = \widehat{\rho}_0 \widehat{p}_{101} \widehat{p}_{000},$$

$$\widehat{e}_{3[1]} = \widehat{\rho}_0 \widehat{p}_{10+}^{-1} \widehat{p}_{100} (\widehat{p}_{110} \widehat{p}_{000} - \widehat{p}_{010} \widehat{p}_{001}),$$

$$\widehat{e}_{4[1]} = \widehat{\rho}_0 \widehat{p}_{10+}^{-1} \widehat{p}_{100}^{-1} \left(\widehat{p}_{110} \widehat{p}_{000} \widehat{p}_{101}^2 - \widehat{p}_{010} \widehat{p}_{001} \widehat{p}_{100}^2\right),$$

$$\widehat{e}_{1[0]} = -\widehat{p}_{01+}^{-1},$$

$$\widehat{e}_{2[0]} = \widehat{\rho}_0 \widehat{p}_{01+}^{-1} (\widehat{p}_{100} \widehat{p}_{001} \widehat{p}_{011} - \widehat{p}_{000} \widehat{p}_{110} \widehat{p}_{101}),$$

$$\widehat{e}_{3[0]} = \widehat{\rho}_0 [\widehat{p}_{000} (\widehat{p}_{110} \widehat{p}_{101} + \widehat{p}_{100} \widehat{p}_{010}) + 2 \widehat{p}_{100} \widehat{p}_{010} \widehat{p}_{001}],$$

$$\widehat{e}_{4[0]} = \widehat{\rho}_0 \widehat{p}_{00+}^{-1} \widehat{p}_{000} \widehat{p}_{001} \left(\widehat{p}_{110} \widehat{p}_{000}^2 - \widehat{p}_{100} \widehat{p}_{010} \widehat{p}_{001}\right),$$

$$\widehat{\rho}_0 = (\widehat{p}_{000} \widehat{p}_{110} \widehat{p}_{101} + \widehat{p}_{100} \widehat{p}_{010} \widehat{p}_{001})^{-1}.$$

The variance of $\ln(\tilde{R}_C)$ is given by

$$\sigma^2\left(\ln\left(\tilde{R}_C\right)\right)=\sum\nolimits_{i=0}^{1} n_{[i]}^{-1}\vec{\tilde{e}}_{[i]}^{\,T}\Sigma_{[i]}\vec{\tilde{e}}_{[i]}, \tag{7.125}$$

where each component of the vector $\vec{\tilde{e}}_{[i]}=\left[\tilde{e}_{1[i]},\tilde{e}_{2[i]},\tilde{e}_{3[i]},\tilde{e}_{4[i]}\right]^T$ is given by

$$\begin{aligned}
\tilde{e}_{1[1]}&=0,\\
\tilde{e}_{2[1]}&=\tilde{\rho}_0 v_{22[.;1]}\tilde{p}_{101}\tilde{p}_{000},\\
\tilde{e}_{3[1]}&=\tilde{\rho}_0 v_{33[.;1]}\tilde{p}_{10+}^{-1}\tilde{p}_{100}\left(\tilde{p}_{110}\tilde{p}_{000}-\tilde{p}_{010}\tilde{p}_{001}\right),\\
\tilde{e}_{4[1]}&=\tilde{\rho}_0 v_{44[.;1]}\tilde{p}_{10+}^{-1}\tilde{p}_{100}^{-1}\left(\tilde{p}_{110}\tilde{p}_{000}\tilde{p}_{101}^2-\tilde{p}_{010}\tilde{p}_{001}\tilde{p}_{100}^2\right),\\
\tilde{e}_{1[0]}&=-v_{11[.;0]}\tilde{p}_{01+}^{-1},\\
\tilde{e}_{2[0]}&=\tilde{\rho}_0 v_{22[.;0]}\tilde{p}_{01+}^{-1}\left(\tilde{p}_{100}\tilde{p}_{001}\tilde{p}_{011}-\tilde{p}_{000}\tilde{p}_{110}\tilde{p}_{101}\right),\\
\tilde{e}_{3[0]}&=\tilde{\rho}_0 v_{33[.;0]}\left[\tilde{p}_{000}\left(\tilde{p}_{110}\tilde{p}_{101}+\tilde{p}_{100}\tilde{p}_{010}\right)+2\tilde{p}_{100}\tilde{p}_{010}\tilde{p}_{001}\right],\\
\tilde{e}_{4[0]}&=\tilde{\rho}_0 v_{44[.;0]}\tilde{p}_{00+}^{-1}\tilde{p}_{000}\tilde{p}_{001}\left(\tilde{p}_{110}\tilde{p}_{000}^2-\tilde{p}_{100}\tilde{p}_{010}\tilde{p}_{001}\right),\\
\tilde{\rho}_0&=\left(\tilde{p}_{000}\tilde{p}_{110}\tilde{p}_{101}+\tilde{p}_{100}\tilde{p}_{010}\tilde{p}_{001}\right)^{-1}.
\end{aligned}$$

Lastly, the variances of the crude and bias-adjusted estimators for Eqs. (7.94) and (7.95) are given, respectively, by

$$\begin{aligned}
\sigma^2\left(\ln\left(\widehat{\psi}_{E|C}\right)\right)&=\sigma^2\left(\ln\left(\widehat{R}_{E|MH}\right)\right)+\sigma^2\left(\ln\left(\widehat{R}_E\right)\right),\\
\sigma^2\left(\ln\left(\tilde{\psi}_{E|C}\right)\right)&=\sigma^2\left(\ln\left(\tilde{R}_{E|MH}\right)\right)+\sigma^2\left(\ln\left(\tilde{R}_E\right)\right),\\
\sigma^2\left(\ln\left(\widehat{\psi}_{homo}\right)\right)&=\sigma^2\left(\ln\left(\widehat{R}_{E|C=1}\right)\right)+\sigma^2\left(\ln\left(\widehat{R}_{E|C=0}\right)\right),\\
\sigma^2\left(\ln\left(\tilde{\psi}_{homo}\right)\right)&=\sigma^2\left(\ln\left(\tilde{R}_{E|C=1}\right)\right)+\sigma^2\left(\ln\left(\tilde{R}_{E|C=0}\right)\right).
\end{aligned} \tag{7.126}$$

7.4 Misclassified Fisher-Irwin's Exact Test

Let X and Y be two independent binomial random variables with parameters (n_{+X}, p_X) and (n_{+Y}, p_Y), respectively. Suppose that the observed cell absolute frequencies be wrongly classified in Table 7.22. The question now is that how do we adjust the Fisher-Irwin's test with the misclassified data in Table 7.22.

If we wish to find an exact test for the null hypotheses $H_0: p_X = p_Y$ versus the one-sided alternative hypothesis $H_1: p_X > p_Y$, or equivalently, $H_0: \gamma = 1$ versus $H_1: \gamma > 1$, where γ is the odds ratio defined by [14]

Table 7.22 The observations of two binomial random variables

	X	Y
Success	n_{1X}	n_{1Y}
Failure	n_{2X}	n_{2Y}
Column total	n_{+X}	n_{+Y}

Where $n_{+X} = \sum_{i=1}^{2} n_{iX}$, $n_{+Y} = \sum_{i=1}^{2} n_{iY}$, $n_{ij} \geq 0$ for i = 1, 2, j = X, Y

$$\gamma = \frac{p_X q_Y}{p_Y q_X}. \tag{7.127}$$

Let the observed number of successes be x and y among n_X and n_Y subjects. By conditioning on that $x + y = z$ is fixed, the conditional distribution of $X = x$ is given by noncentral hypergeometric distribution under the alternative hypothesis [9, 10]

$$\Pr(X = x|z;\gamma) = \frac{\binom{n_X}{x}\binom{n_Y}{z-x}\gamma^x}{\sum_{j=0}^{z}\binom{n_X}{j}\binom{n_Y}{z-j}\gamma^j}, \tag{7.128}$$

where $x = \max(0, z - n_Y), \ldots, \min(z, n_X)$, or the conditional distribution of Y = y is given by

$$\Pr(Y = y|z;\gamma) = \frac{\binom{n_X}{z-y}\binom{n_Y}{y}\gamma^{-y}}{\sum_{j=0}^{z}\binom{n_X}{z-j}\binom{n_Y}{j}\gamma^{-j}}, \tag{7.129}$$

where $y = \max(0, z - n_X), \ldots, \min(z, n_Y)$. In practical applications, Eq. (7.128) is used if x < y; otherwise, Eq. (7.129) is used. By the way, Eqs. (7.128) and (7.129) were first introduced by Fisher [5].

If x > y, the p-value of Fisher-Irwin's test is given by

$$p - value = \sum_{k=y}^{z} \Pr(Y = k|z;\gamma = 1), \tag{7.130}$$

where $\Pr(Y = k|z;\gamma = 1)$ is given by Eq. (7.129) that yields an ordinary hypergeometric distribution as follows:

$$\Pr(Y = y|z;\gamma = 1) = \frac{\binom{n_X}{z-y}\binom{n_Y}{y}}{\binom{n_X+n_Y}{z}}, \mathrm{y} = 0, 1, \ldots, \mathrm{z} \tag{7.131}$$

On which the Fisher-Irwin's test is based.

For small frequencies, the critical value of Y has been provided by choosing y_c for the right-sided alternative ($p_X > p_Y$) such that

$$\begin{aligned} &\Pr(Y \le y_c|z) = \sum\nolimits_{y=0}^{y_c} \Pr(Y = y|z; \gamma = 1) \le \alpha, \text{ and} \\ &\Pr(Y \le y_c + 1|z) > \alpha. \end{aligned} \tag{7.132}$$

For nominal levels of significance $\alpha = 0.05, 0.025, 0.01, 0.005$, x_c is tabulated for $n_Y \le n_X \le 25$ (Bennet-Hsu [1]). For the two-sided alternative ($p_X \ne p_Y$), the tabular exact probabilities are doubled accordingly.

If x > y, the (conditional) power function of the Fisher-Irwin's test is then given by

$$\beta(\gamma|z) = \Pr(y \le y_c|H_1) = \sum\nolimits_{y=0}^{y_c} \Pr(Y = y|\gamma) = \frac{\sum\nolimits_{y=0}^{y_c} \binom{n_X}{z-y}\binom{n_Y}{y}\gamma^{-y}}{\sum\nolimits_{j=z_1}^{z_2} \binom{n_X}{z-j}\binom{n_Y}{j}\gamma^{-j}}, \tag{7.133}$$

where $z_1 = \max(0, z - n_X)$ and $z_2 = \max(z, n_Y)$. The expected power of the Fisher-Irwin's test is

$$\begin{aligned} \beta(\gamma) &= \sum_z \beta(\gamma|z)\Pr(Z = z) \\ &= q_X^{n_X} q_Y^{n_Y} \left\{ \sum_z \left(\frac{p_X}{q_X}\right)^z \left[\sum\nolimits_{y=z_1}^{y_c} \binom{n_X}{z-y}\binom{n_Y}{y}\gamma^{-y}\right]\right\}, \end{aligned} \tag{7.134}$$

where Pr(Z = z) is given by

$$\Pr(Z = z) = \sum\nolimits_{i=L}^{U} \binom{n_X}{z-i} p_X^{z-i} q_X^{n_X - z + i} \binom{n_Y}{i} p_Y^i q_Y^{n_Y - i}, \tag{7.135}$$

where $L = \max(0, z - n_X)$, $U = \min(z, n_Y)$,and the summation in z is over all significance pairs of points on the diagonal, $z = x + y$, in the (x, y) sample space at the level of significance equals to α at most [9, 10].

Now when both the number of successes for X and Y is misclassified with errors, how do we adjust Eq. (7.127) to account for the misclassification error? Let Z^* denote the surrogate classified variable for Z and let φ_Z and ψ_Z, where Z = X, Y, be the misclassification (false negative and false positive) probabilities of Z with respect to the number of success and failure respectively, that is,

$$\begin{aligned} \varphi_Z &= \Pr(Z^* = 0|Z = 1), \text{ and} \\ \psi_Z &= \Pr(Z^* = 1|Z = 0). \end{aligned} \tag{7.136}$$

From Table 7.22, the maximum likelihood estimators for the unknown p_X and p_Y are given, respectively, by

$$\widehat{p}_X = \frac{n_{1X}}{n_{+X}}, \tag{7.137}$$

and

$$\widehat{p}_Y = \frac{n_{1Y}}{n_{+Y}}. \tag{7.138}$$

It is well known that Eqs. (7.137) and (7.138) are no longer unbiased estimators for the true unknown prevalence rates p_X and p_Y. As a result, the classical crude odds ratio defined by [14]

$$\widehat{\gamma} = \frac{\widehat{p}_X \widehat{q}_Y}{\widehat{p}_Y \widehat{q}_X}, \tag{7.139}$$

as a point estimator for the true unknown odds ratio γ of Eq. (7.127) could have a substantial bias [8].

To account for the misclassification bias, the bias-adjusted estimator for the true unknown p_Z and q_Z can be obtained from Eq. (6.9)

$$\tilde{p}_Z = \frac{\widehat{p}_Z - \psi_Z}{\Delta_Z}, \tag{7.140}$$

and

$$\tilde{q}_Z = \frac{\widehat{q}_Z - \varphi_Z}{\Delta_Z}, \tag{7.141}$$

where $\widehat{q}_Z = 1 - \widehat{p}_Z$, Δ_Z is given by

$$\Delta_Z = 1 - \varphi_Z - \psi_Z. \tag{7.142}$$

Conditioning on that φ_Z and ψ_Z are given, it is easily shown that Eqs. (7.140) and (7.141) are unbiased estimators for the true unknown p_Z and q_Z, respectively. The bias-adjusted estimators of Eqs. (7.140) and (7.141) are said to be plausible if they satisfy the following constraints:

$$\psi_Z < \widehat{p}_Z, \varphi_Z < \widehat{q}_Z, \text{and } \Delta_Z > 0. \tag{7.143}$$

Note that the third constraint in Eq. (7.143) is a redundant one once the first two constraints are satisfied. A set of φ_Z and ψ_Z is said to be admissible if Eq. (7.143) holds and $\tilde{p}_Z$ and $\tilde{q}_Z$ lie between 0 and 1. To calculate the misclassification probabilities φ_Z and ψ_Z, we utilize the creation of the counterfactual true models for the observations of Z just like what we did in Examples 6.3 and 6.7. Let $\{N_{ij(k)}\}$ be the kth counterfactual true frequencies, where $N_{+1(k)} = n_{+X}$ and $N_{+2(k)} = n_{+Y}$. Then, compute

$$\varphi_{X(k)} = \frac{|N_{11(k)} - n_{11}|}{n_{+X}}, \text{ and}$$
$$\psi_{X(k)} = \frac{|N_{01(k)} - n_{01}|}{n_{+X}}. \tag{7.144}$$

Similarly, compute $\varphi_{Y(k)}$ and $\psi_{Y(k)}$ accordingly.

The bias-adjusted odds ratio (BAOR) estimator for the true unknown γ is then given by

$$\tilde{\gamma} = \frac{\tilde{p}_X \tilde{q}_Y}{\tilde{p}_Y \tilde{q}_X} = \frac{(\widehat{p}_X - \psi_X)(\widehat{q}_Y - \varphi_Y)}{(\widehat{p}_Y - \psi_Y)(\widehat{q}_X - \varphi_X)}, \tag{7.145}$$

and its asymptotic variance is given by

$$\sigma^2_{ln\,\tilde{\gamma}} = \sigma^2_{\ln(\widehat{p}_X - \psi_X)} + \sigma^2_{\ln(\widehat{q}_X - \varphi_X)} + \sigma^2_{\ln(\widehat{p}_Y - \psi_Y)} + \sigma^2_{\ln(\widehat{q}_Y - \varphi_Y)} = \frac{\sigma^2_{\widehat{p}_X}}{\mu^2_{\widehat{p}_X - \psi_X}}$$
$$+ \frac{\sigma^2_{\widehat{q}_X}}{\mu^2_{\widehat{q}_X - \varphi_X}} + \frac{\sigma^2_{\widehat{p}_Y}}{\mu^2_{\widehat{p}_Y - \psi_Y}} + \frac{\sigma^2_{\widehat{q}_Y}}{\mu^2_{\widehat{q}_Y - \varphi_Y}} = \frac{\sigma^2_{\widehat{p}_X}}{(p_X - \psi_X)^2} + \frac{\sigma^2_{\widehat{p}_X}}{(q_X - \varphi_X)^2}$$
$$+ \frac{\sigma^2_{\widehat{p}_Y}}{(p_Y - \psi_Y)^2} + \frac{\sigma^2_{\widehat{p}_Y}}{(q_Y - \varphi_Y)^2}, \tag{7.146}$$

where $\sigma^2_{\widehat{p}_z}$ is given by

$$\sigma^2_{\widehat{p}_z} = \frac{(p_Z \Delta_Z + \psi_Z)(q_Z \Delta_Z + \varphi_Z)}{n_Z}. \tag{7.147}$$

Using Eqs. (7.144) to (7.146), the 100%·(1 − α) confidence interval (LCL, UCL) for the true γ is given as follows: (0 < α < 1)

$$(\text{LCL}, \text{UCL}) = \exp\left\{\ln(\tilde{\gamma}) \pm z_{1-\alpha} \cdot \sqrt{\sigma_{ln\,\tilde{\gamma}}}\right\}. \tag{7.148}$$

Example 7.4

The Lange's data [13] on criminality among twin brothers/sisters of criminals is used to illustrate the Fisher-Irwin's test with the misclassified data. Table 7.23 provides the number of twin brothers/sisters who had been convicted, separately for dizygotic

Table 7.23 The criminal data of monozygotic and dizygotic twins

	Dizygotic (= X)	Monozygotic (= Y)	Row total
Not convicted (success)	13	3	16
Convicted (failure)	2	10	12
Column total	15	13	28

but like-sexed (= X) and monozygotic twins (= Y). By using Eqs. (7.137) and (7.138), $\widehat{p}_X = \frac{13}{15} > \widehat{p}_Y = \frac{3}{13}$, the phrase of not convicted is taken as a success. From Table 7.23, the COR of Eq. (7.139) is obtained as $\widehat{\gamma} = 21.7$ with p = 0.001. As a result, the null hypothesis is rejected. It thus indicates that criminality is more frequent among monozygotic twins than dizygotic twins [13].

Suppose that the classification error exists in Table 7.23. Since validation data are not available, we take a counterfactual approach to estimate the true misclassification probabilities.

From Table 7.23, $\widehat{p}_X = 0.87$ and $\widehat{q}_X = 0.13$. Also, $\widehat{p}_Y = 0.23$ and $\widehat{q}_Y = 0.77$. The values of Δ_Z for model 8 to 12 for X and model 7 to 9 for Y violate the constraints that must be positive in Eq. (7.143). As a result, those counterfactual true models are not feasible. Furthermore, the values of φ_X or ψ_Y for model 2 to 7 for X and model 3 to 6 for Y violate the constraints that they must be less than that of $\widehat{q}_X$ and $\widehat{p}_Y$ in Eq. (7.143). Hence, those counterfactual true models are not feasible either. They are boldface in Tables 7.24 and 7.25.

In Table 7.24, only model 1 is feasible and an admissible pairs of misclassification probabilities calculated from using Eq. (7.144) is $\varphi_{X(1)} = \psi_{x(1)}$- $= 0.07$, while in Table 7.25 models 1 and 2 are feasible and two amissible pairs of misclassification probabilities are $\psi_{Y(1)} = \varphi_{Y(1)} = 0.08$ and $\psi_{Y(2)} = \varphi_{Y(2)} = 0.15$. By using Eqs. (7.140) and (7.141),

$$\begin{aligned} \tilde{p}_{X(1)} &= \frac{0.87 - 0.07}{1 - 0.07 - 0.07} = 0.930232 \approx 0.93, \text{and} \\ \tilde{q}_{X(1)} &= \frac{0.13 - 0.07}{1 - 0.07 - 0.07} = 0.06976 \approx 0.07. \end{aligned} \tag{7.149}$$

Similarly, two bias-adjusted prevalence rates for Y are

$$\begin{aligned} &\tilde{p}_{Y(1)} = 0.18 \text{ and } \tilde{q}_{Y(1)} = 0.82, \text{and} \\ &\tilde{p}_{Y(2)} = 0.11 \text{ and } \tilde{q}_{Y(2)} = 0.89. \end{aligned} \tag{7.150}$$

By substituting Eqs. (7.149) and (7.150) into Eq. (7.145), two adjusted odds ratio values are given by

Table 7.24 Pairs of admissible misclassification probabilities for X

Model k	$N_{01(k)}$	$N_{11(k)}$	$\varphi_{X(k)}$	$\psi_{X(k)}$	$\Delta_{X(k)}$
1	3	12	0.07	0.07	0.86
2	4	11	**0.13**	0.13	0.74
3	5	10	**0.2**	0.2	0.6
4	6	9	**0.27**	0.27	0.46
5	7	8	**0.33**	0.33	0.34
6	8	7	**0.4**	0.4	0.2
7	9	6	**0.47**	0.47	0.06
8	10	5	**0.53**	**0.53**	–
9	11	4	**0.6**	**0.6**	–
10	12	3	**0.67**	**0.67**	–
11	13	2	**0.73**	**0.73**	–
12	14	1	**0.8**	**0.8**	–

Table 7.25 Pairs of admissible misclassification probabilities for Y

Model k	$N_{10(k)}$	$N_{00(k)}$	$\varphi_{Y(k)}$	$\psi_{Y(k)}$	$\Delta_{Y(k)}$
1	4	9	0.08	0.08	0.84
2	5	8	0.15	0.15	0.7
3	6	7	0.23	**0.23**	0.54
4	7	6	0.31	**0.31**	0.38
5	8	5	0.38	**0.38**	0.24
6	9	4	0.46	**0.46**	0.08
7	10	3	**0.54**	**0.54**	–
8	11	2	**0.62**	**0.62**	–
9	12	1	**0.69**	**0.69**	–

$$\tilde{\gamma}_{(1)} = \frac{0.93 \cdot 0.82}{0.18 \cdot 0.07} = 60.5238 \approx 60.5, \text{ and}$$
$$\tilde{\gamma}_{(2)} = \frac{0.93 \cdot 0.89}{0.11 \cdot 0.07} = 107.4935 \approx 107.5. \tag{7.151}$$

By substituting Eqs (7.149). and (7.150) into Eq. (7.147),

$$\tilde{\sigma}^2_{\widehat{p_{X(1)}}} = \frac{\left(\tilde{p}_{X(1)}\Delta_{X(1)} + \psi_{X(1)}\right)\left(\tilde{q}_{X(1)}\Delta_{X(1)} + \varphi_{X(1)}\right)}{n_X} = \frac{(0.93 \cdot 0.86 + 0.07)(0.07 \cdot 0.86 + 0.07)}{15} \approx 0.0077$$
$$\tilde{\sigma}^2_{\widehat{p_{Y(1)}}} = \frac{(0.18 \cdot 0.84 + 0.08)(0.82 \cdot 0.84 + 0.08)}{13} \approx 0.0134 \text{ and}$$
$$\tilde{\sigma}^2_{\widehat{p_{Y(2)}}} = \frac{(0.11 \cdot 0.7 + 0.15)(0.89 \cdot 0.7 + 0.15)}{13} \approx 0.0134. \tag{7.152}$$

By substituting Eq. (7.152) into Eq. (7.146),

$$\sigma^2_{ln\,\tilde{\gamma}_{(1)}} = \tilde{\sigma}^2_{\widehat{p_{X(1)}}}\left(\frac{1}{\left(\tilde{p}_{X(1)} - \psi_{X(1)}\right)^2} + \frac{1}{\left(\tilde{q}_{X(1)} - \varphi_{X(1)}\right)^2}\right)$$

$$+ \tilde{\sigma}^2_{\widehat{p_{Y(1)}}}\left(\frac{1}{\left(\tilde{p}_{Y(1)} - \psi_{Y(1)}\right)^2} + \frac{1}{\left(\tilde{q}_{Y(1)} - \varphi_{Y(1)}\right)^2}\right)$$

$$= 0.0077 \cdot \left(\frac{1}{(0.93 - 0.07)^2} + \frac{1}{(0.17 - 0.07)^2}\right)$$

$$+ 0.0134 \cdot \left(\frac{1}{(0.18 - 0.08)^2} + \frac{1}{(0.82 - 0.08)^2}\right) = 73.2993,$$

$$\sigma^2_{ln\,\tilde{\gamma}_{(2)}} = 0.0077 \cdot \left(\frac{1}{(0.93 - 0.07)^2} + \frac{1}{(0.17 - 0.07)^2}\right)$$

$$+ 0.0134 \cdot \left(\frac{1}{(0.11 - 0.08)^2} + \frac{1}{(0.89 - 0.08)^2}\right) = 74.5907.$$

As a result,

$$\begin{aligned}\sigma_{ln\,\tilde{\gamma}_{(1)}} &= \sqrt{73.2993} \approx 8.56, \text{ and} \\ \sigma_{ln\,\tilde{\gamma}_{(2)}} &= \sqrt{74.5907} \approx 8.64.\end{aligned} \tag{7.153}$$

By substituting Eq. (7.153) into Eq. (7.148), the 95% confidence interval for the odds ratio γ is given by

$$\begin{aligned}2.8 \cdot 10^{-6} \le \gamma_{(1)} \le 1.04 \cdot 10^9, \text{ and} \\ 4.3 \cdot 10^{-6} \le \gamma_{(2)} \le 2.15 \cdot 10^9.\end{aligned} \tag{7.154}$$

Equation (7.154) indicates that the convicted criminality between dizygotic and monozygotic twins is the same. Since this contradicts to the classical conclusion obtained by assuming the data is without misclassification. Our assumption that the data supposed to be misclassified is invalid.

Remark
The calculation of the misclassification probability is inaccurate in Lee [19].

7.5 Exercise

1. Show that Eqs. (7.95) and (7.97) equal one another.
2. Verify the computation of misclassification error probabilities for cases and controls in Tables 7.18 and 7.19 by applying the CF true tables to the observed table.

References

1. Acheson, E. D., & Gardner, M. J. (1979). Mesothelioma and exposure to mixtures of chrysotile and amphibole. *Archives of Environmental Health, 34*, 240–242.
2. Agresti, A. (2002). *Categorical data analysis* (2nd ed.). Wiley.
3. Anderson, T. W. (2003). *An introduction to multivariate statistical analysis* (3rd ed.). Wiley.
4. Barlett, M. S. (1935). Contingency table interaction. *Supplement to the Journal of the Royal Statistical Society, 2*, 248–252.
5. Barron, B. A. (1977). The effects of misclassification on the estimation of relative risk. *Biometrics, 33*, 414–418.
6. Bennet, B. M., & Hsu, P. (1960). On the power function of the exact test for the 2 × 2 contingency table. *Biometrika, 47*, 393–398.
7. Bhapkar, V. P., & Koch, G. G. (1968). On the hypothesis of 'no interaction' in contingency tables. *Biometrics, 24*, 567–594.
8. Birch, M. W. (1964). The detection of partial association, I: The 2 × 2 case. *Journal of the Royal Statistical Society Series B, 26*, 313–324.
9. Casagrande, J. T., Pike, M. C., & Smith, P. G. (1978a). The power function of the exact test for comparing two binomial distributions. *Applied Statistics, 27*, 176–180.
10. Casagrande, J. T., Pike, M. C., & Smith, P. G. (1978b). Algorithm AS 129: The power function of the exact test for comparing two binomial distributions. *Applied Statistics, 27*, 212–219.
11. Crane, J., Pearce, N., Flatt, A., et al. (1989). Prescribed fenoterol and death from asthma in New Zealand, 1981–1983: Case-control study. *Lancet, 1*, 917–922.
12. Darroch, J. N., & Borkent, M. (1994). Synergism, attributable risk and interaction for two binary factors. *Biometrika, 81*, 259–270.
13. Fisher, A. L. (1946). *Statistcal methods for research workers* (10th ed.). Oliver and Boyd.
14. Fleiss, J. L., Levin, B., & Paik, M. C. (2003). *Statistical methods for rates and proportions*. Wiley & Sons, Inc..
15. Gardner, M. J., & Munford, A. G. (1980). The combined effect of two factors on disease in a case-control study. *Applied Statistics, 29*, 276–281.
16. Greenland, S. (1980). The effect of misclassification in the presence of covariates. *American Journal of Epidemiology, 112*, 564–569.
17. Greenland, S., & Robins, J. M. (1985). Confounding and misclassification. *American Journal of Epidemiology, 122*, 495–506.
18. Kleinbaum, D. G., Kupper, L. L., & Morgenstern, H. (1982). *Epidemiologic research: Principles and quantitative methods*. Wiley.
19. Lee, T.-S. (2011). Fisher's exact test for misclassified data. *Journal of Modern Applied Statistical Methods, 10*, 1–7.
20. Lee, T.-S. (2013). Case-control studies with jointly misclassified exposure and confounding variables. *Journal of Modern Applied Statistical Methods, 12*, 191–210.
21. Lee, T.-S. (2020). *Medical statistics: A practical approach*. World Scientific Publishing Company.

22. Mantel, N., & Haenszel, W. (1959). Statistical aspects of the analysis of data from retrospective studies of disease. *Journal of the National Cancer Institute, 22*, 719–748.
23. Miettinen, O. S. (1974). Confounding and effect modification. *American Journal of Epidemiology, 100*, 350–353.
24. O'Donnel, T. V., Rea, H. H., Holst, & Sears, M. R. (1989). Fenoterol and fatal asthma. *The Lancet, 1*, 1070–1071.
25. Psaty, B. M., Koepsell, T. D., Lin, T. D., et al. (1999). Assessment and control for confounding by indication in observational studies. *Journal of the American Geriatrics Society, 47*, 749–754.
26. Weinberg, C. R. (1993). Toward a clearer definition of cofounding. *American Journal of Epidemiology, 137*, 1–8.
27. Wickramarantne, P. J., & Holford, T. R. (1987). Confounding in epidemiologic studies: The adequacy of control group as a measure of confounding. *Biometrics, 43*, 751–765.
28. Yiostalo, P. V., & Knuuttila, M. L. (2006). Confounding and effect modification: Possible explanation for variation in the results on the association between oral and systemic diseases. *Journal of Clinical Periodontology, 33*, 104–108.

Part IV
Hypothesis Testing on the Data

Chapter 8
No Misclassification

8.1 Bayes Factor

In inferential statistics, it is a headache problem how to measure the evidential strength of the collected data. The p-value proposed by R. A. Fisher [8] in the 1920 as an informal index to be used as a measure of discrepancy between the data and the null hypothesis. It was not part of a formal inferential method. Fisher suggested that it be used as part of the fluid, non-quantifiable process of drawing conclusions from the data, a process that included combining the p-value in some unspecified way with background information. However, most researchers and readers have an unfortunate misinterpretation and think that a p-value of 0.05 means that the null hypothesis has a probability to be true of only 5%. This is an understandable but categorically wrong interpretation because the p-value is calculated on the assumption that the null hypothesis is true. Hence, it cannot be a direct measure of the probability that the null hypothesis is false. This logical error reinforces the mistaken notion that the data alone can tell us that the probability that a hypothesis is true [3].

Determining which underlying truth is most likely on the basis of the data is a problem in inverse probability or inductive inference. It was solved quantitatively more than 200 years ago by the Reverend Thomas Bayes in his famous Bayes theorem. Figure 8.1 shows that Bayes theorem in words.

As a mathematical equation, Bayes theorem is not controversial. However, as a model, it is criticized because it requires assigning a prior probability to the truth of an idea, a number whose objective scientific meaning is unclear.

Let D denote the data, while H_0 and H_1 be the null and alternative hypotheses, respectively. In fact, the Bayes factor is embedded in the Bayes theorem (Fig. 8.1).

T.-S. Lee, *Misclassification in Epidemiology*, Emerging Topics in Statistics and Biostatistics, https://doi.org/10.1007/978-3-032-12563-7_8

Prior odds of null hypothesis being true (before seeing data)	Subjective component
×	
Bayes factor	Data component
⇓	
Posterior odds of null hypothesis being true	Probability of truth

Fig. 8.1 Bayes theorem in words

Definition 8.1
The Bayes factor BF(D) is given by

$$BF(D) = \frac{\Pr(D|H_0)}{\Pr(D|H_1)}, \tag{8.1}$$

where Pr(.|.) denotes the conditional probability [17].

Remarks
1. When both H_0 and H_1 are simple hypotheses, Eq. (8.1) is nothing but the likelihood ratio.
2. The Bayes factor differs in many ways from the p-value. First, the Bayes factor is not a probability itself but a ratio of probabilities, and it can vary from zero to infinity. It requires two hypotheses, making it clear that for evidence to be against the null hypothesis, it must be for some alternative. Second, the Bayes factor depends on the probability of the observed data alone, not including unobserved "long run" results that are part of the p-value calculation. Thus, factors unrelated to the data that affect the p-value, such as the stopping rule in a sequential medical trial, do not affect the Bayes factor.

Example 8.1
In this example, we are going to show how far Bayes factors (BF) move prior probabilities, on the null hypothesis (H_0), of 90%, 50%, and 25%. These correspond, respectively, to high initial confidence in H_0 equivocal confidence, and moderate suspicion that H_0 is not true. The final posterior probability of the null hypothesis after observing various Bayes factors as a function of the prior probability of the null hypothesis is given Table 8.1.

The values in the fourth column of Table 8.1 are calculated as follows. The prior probability of 90% is equivalent to the prior odds of $\frac{90\%}{1-90\%} = 9$. Then the posterior odds is given by

$$\text{Posterior odds} = \text{BF} \cdot (\text{Prior odds}) = \frac{1}{5} \cdot 9 = 1.8.$$

Thus,

$$\text{Posterior probability} = \frac{\text{posterior odds}}{1 + \text{posterior odds}} = \frac{1.8}{2.8} = 0.642857 \approx 0.64,$$

Table 8.1 Bayes factor as a function of the prior probability of the null hypothesis

		Decrease in probability of H_0	
		From	To no less than
Strength of evidence	BF	%	
Weak	$\frac{1}{5}$	90	64
		50	17
		25	7
Moderate	$\frac{1}{10}$	90	47
		50	9
		25	3
Moderate to strong	$\frac{1}{20}$	90	31
		50	5
		25	2
Strong to very strong	$\frac{1}{100}$	90	8
		50	1
		25	0.3

which is the first entry of the fourth column. The rest of the entries are calculated accordingly.

If one is highly convinced of no effect (90% prior probability of H_0) before starting the experiment, a Bayes factor of $\frac{1}{10}$ will move one to equivocal (47% posterior probability of H_0), but if one is equivocal at the start (50% prior probability of H_0), that same amount of evidence will be moderately convincing that H_0 is not true (9% posterior probability). A Bayes factor of $\frac{1}{100}$ is strong enough to move one from 90% sure of H_0 to being only 8% sure.

As the strength of the evidence increases, the data are more able to convert a skeptic into a believer or a tentative suggestion into an accepted truth. This implies that as the experimental evidence gets stronger, the amount of external evidence needed to support a scientific claim decreases. This phenomenon was observed empirically in the medical community's reluctance to accept the results of clinical trials that were counter to strong prior beliefs.

The simplest relation between p-values and Bayes factors exists when statistical tests are based on a normal approximation. The minimum Bayes factor is calculated with the same numbers used to calculate a p-value. For a random variable X with a normal distribution, that is, $X \sim N(\mu_X, \sigma_X^2)$, the hypothesis test typically concerns μ_X. The probability of the observed data x is given by

$$\Pr(x) = \frac{1}{\sigma_X\sqrt{2\pi}} \cdot \exp\left(-\frac{1}{2}\left(\frac{x-\mu_X}{\sigma_X}\right)^2\right). \tag{8.2}$$

Table 8.2 Minimum Bayes factor as a function of p-value

p-value (Z-score)	Minimum BF(x)	Decrease in probability of H_0 From (%)	To no less than	Strength of evidence
0.10 ($\pm$1.64)	3.8374^{-1} $\approx 0.2606 \approx 0.26$	75	$0.4382 \approx 0.44$	Weak
		50	$0.2063 \approx 0.21$	
		25	$0.0796 \approx 0.08$	
0.05 ($\pm$1.96)	6.8264^{-1} $\approx 0.1465 \approx 0.15$	75	$0.3103 \approx 0.31$	Moderate
		50	$0.1304 \approx 0.13$	
		25	$0.0476 \approx 0.05$	
0.01 ($\pm$2.58)	27.888^{-1} $\approx 0.0359 \approx 0.036$	75	$0.0975 \approx 0.1$	Moderate to strong
		50	$0.0347 \approx 0.03$	
		25	$0.0119 \approx 0.01$	
0.001 ($\pm$3.28)	216.848^{-1} $\approx 0.0046 \approx 0.005$	75	$0.0148 \approx 0.01$	Strong to very strong
		50	0.005	
		25	$0.0017 \approx 0.002$	

Equation (8.2) is maximized when the exponent is zero. As a result, $\mu_X = x$. The likelihood ratio for $H_0 : \mu_X = 0$ versus the maximally supported alternative hypothesis $H_1 : \mu_X = x$ is the minimum Bayes factor given by using Eq. (8.2):

$$\frac{\Pr(x|H_0)}{\Pr(x|H_1)} = \exp\left(-\frac{1}{2}\left(\frac{x}{\sigma_X}\right)^2\right). \tag{8.3}$$

Because the value of $\frac{x}{\sigma_X}$ is the so-called Z-score z, Eq. (8.3) reduces to

$$\text{Minimum BF}(x) = \left(\exp\left(\frac{z^2}{2}\right)\right)^{-1}. \tag{8.4}$$

Example 8.2
Let us use Eq. (8.4) to find the relation between the fixed sample size p-values and the minimum Bayes factors with their effect of such evidence on the probability of $H_0 : \mu_X = 0$ for the observation of x from Eq. (8.2). The result is given by Table 8.2.

Table 8.2 provides the minimum Bayes factor and the two-sided p-value for any given Z-score. For instance, when a result is ± 1.96 from its null value (p-value = 0.05), the minimum Bayes factor is 0.15, meaning that H_0 gets 15% as much support as the best-supported hypothesis. This is threefold higher than the p-value = 0.05, implying that the evidence against H_0 is not nearly as strong as p-value = 0.05 suggests. These calculations show that p-values of 0.05 represent at best moderate evidence against H_0; those between 0.01 and 0.001 represent moderate to strong evidence; and those less than 0.001 represent strong to very strong evidence.

These tables show us what many researchers learn from experience that the weight of evidence against $H_0$is not nearly as strong as the magnitude of p-value suggests. They conclude this not always because contradictory prior evidence outweighed the trial evidence but because the trial evidence was not very strong in the first place. It also provides justification for the judgment of many experienced meta-analysts who have suggested that the threshold for significance in a meta-analysis should be more than two standard errors away from the null effect rather than just two.

Remarks

1. When the alternative hypothesis H_1 is a composite hypothesis, the Bayes factors differ from likelihood ratios. But the machinery of Bayes theorem allows measurement of the evidence for composite hypotheses [11].
2. Many scientists have noted that testing a hypothesis of exact null effect is artificial because it is unlikely to be exactly true and because other scientific questions may be of more interest. For example, "What is the evidence that the treatment is harmful?" instead of "What is the evidence that the treatment has no effect?" These questions have different answers because the question about harmful includes all treatment differences that are not beneficial. This changes the null hypothesis from a simple hypothesis into a composite hypothesis. When this is done, under certain conditions, the one-sided p-value can be reasonable approximate the Bayes factor [4].

8.2 Bayes Factor for No Misclassification Errors in a Case-Control Study

Misclassification is a ubiquitous problem in epidemiologic case-control studies. It often occurs if the data are collected from the proxy or surrogate. Almost all studies make an assumption in the beginning that the collected data are not misclassified. Yet the validity of this assumption has not been addressed except Lee [14]. In this section, I will address this problem specifically.

First, I include the misclassification error probability into both the null and alternative hypotheses. Second, bias-adjusted estimators for the prevalence of exposure in cases or controls are presented. Third, the uniform and Beta distribution are adopted respectively as the prior distribution for the misclassification error probability and the prevalence in cases or controls. Finally, the minimum Bayes factor is calculated. A real-world data set is used as an example to illustrate the proposed method. A comparison between the Bayes factor and the p-value is also made.

Consider the data for case-control studies given in Table 8.3. Let E^* be the surrogate for the true exposure variable E, while D indicates the disease status of the subjects with D $= 1$ and D $= 0$ representing cases and controls respectively. Suppose that E^* is misclassified, but D is not.

Let p_i, i $= 1, 0$ be the true unknown prevalence for the exposed group of cases and controls, respectively. It is well known that the classical prevalence estimators for cases and controls are given by

Table 8.3 The observed data of cases and controls

	Group of subjects	
Classified exposure status	D = 1 (cases)	D = 0 (controls)
$E^* = 1$ (exposed)	n_{11}	n_{10}
$E^* = 0$ (unexposed)	n_{01}	n_{00}
Sample size	n_{+1}	n_{+0}

$$\hat{p}_i = \frac{n_{1i}}{n_{+i}}, \tag{8.5}$$

where $\hat{q}_i = 1 - \hat{p}_i$.

Let the misclassification error (false negative and false positive) probability φ_i and ψ_i be defined, respectively, by

$$\varphi_i = \Pr(E^* = 0|E = 1, D = i), \tag{8.6}$$

and

$$\psi_i = \Pr(E^* = 1|E = 0, D = i). \tag{8.7}$$

In term of the misclassification error probabilities of Eqs. (8.6) and (8.7), it is easily shown that

$$E(\hat{p}_i) = p_i\Delta_i + \psi_i. \tag{8.8}$$

where Δ_i is defined by

$$\Delta_i = 1 - \varphi_i - \psi_i. \tag{8.9}$$

Remarks

1. From Eq. (8.8), $\hat{p}_i$ is not an unbiased estimator of p_i unless the method of surrogate classification is perfect, namely, $\varphi_i = \psi_i = 0$, $i = 0, 1$.
2. Assume that $n_{+i}\hat{p}_i$ follows a binomial distribution with mean $n_{+i}[p_i\Delta_i + \psi_i]$, the variance of $\hat{p}_i$, $i = 0, 1$ is similar to Eq. (6.6) that is given by

$$\sigma^2(\hat{p}_i) = \frac{[p_i\Delta_i + \psi_i][q_i\Delta_i + \varphi_i]}{n_{+i}}. \tag{8.10}$$

3. A bias-adjusted prevalence (BAP) estimates are given by

$$\tilde{p}_i = \frac{\widehat{p}_i - \psi_i}{\Delta_i}, \tag{8.11}$$

and

$$\tilde{q}_i = \frac{\widehat{q}_i - \varphi_i}{\Delta_i}, \tag{8.12}$$

where $\widehat{p}_i$, ψ_i, and Δ_i are given, respectively, by Eqs. (8.5), (8.7), and (8.9). It can be shown that Eq. (8.11) is an unbiased estimator of p_i, provided that φ_i and ψ_i are given.

Now, let us return to what concerns us, namely, whether the given data in Table 8.3 are misclassified. Ordinarily, we're concerned with the issue if the exposure prevalence for cases and controls are not different. This issue can be tested through the hypothesis testing as follows:

$$H_0 : \varepsilon_{RD} = 0 \text{ versus } H_1 : \varepsilon_{RD} \neq 0, \tag{8.13}$$

where $\varepsilon_{RD} = p_1 - p_0$, the subscript "RD" means that the prevalence difference between "cases" and "controls." Eq. (8.13) cannot be used to test if the observed data in Table 8.3 are classified. In order to test the assumption if the data are misclassified, Eq. (8.13) has to be expanded as for i = 0, 1

$$H_0 : \varepsilon_{RD} = 0, \varphi_i = \psi_i = 0 \text{ versus } H_1 : \varepsilon_{RD} \neq 0, \varphi_i \neq 0, \psi_i \neq 0. \tag{8.14}$$

To test Eq. (8.14), we will take a mixed Bayesian approach to solve this problem [12]. Define

$$\tilde{\varepsilon}_{RD} = \tilde{p}_1 - \tilde{p}_0 - \varepsilon_{RD}, \tag{8.15}$$

where ε_{RD} is given by Eq. (8.13). It can be shown that

$$E(\tilde{\varepsilon}_{RD}) = 0, \tag{8.16}$$

and

$$\sigma^2_{\tilde{\varepsilon}_{RD}} = \sum\nolimits_{i=0}^{1} \frac{(p_i\Delta_i + \psi_i)(q_i\Delta_i + \varphi_i)}{n_{+i}}. \tag{8.17}$$

Define

$$\tilde{\mathfrak{X}}_{RD} = \frac{\tilde{\varepsilon}^2_{RD}}{\sigma^2_{\tilde{\varepsilon}_{RD}}}. \tag{8.18}$$

To assess the evidence in favor of H_0 against H_1 in Eq. (8.14), the Bayes factor for favoring H_0 against H_1 from using Eq. (8.18) is calculated as follows:

$$B_g(\tilde{\mathfrak{X}}_{RD}) = \frac{f(\tilde{\mathfrak{X}}_{RD}|H_0)}{m_g(\tilde{\mathfrak{X}}_{RD})}, \tag{8.19}$$

where

$$m_g(\tilde{\mathfrak{X}}_{RD}) = \iint_{R\times\Omega} f(\tilde{\mathfrak{X}}_{RD}|H_1)\prod_{i=0}^{1} h_0(\varphi_i,\psi_i)g(p_i,q_i)d\varphi_i d\psi_i dp_i dq_i, \tag{8.20}$$

$f(\tilde{\mathfrak{X}}_{RD}|H_1)$ is the central chi-square distribution with one degree of freedom, $g(p_i,q_i) = \Gamma(\eta+\tau)p_i^{\eta-1}q_i^{\tau-1}/[\Gamma(\eta)\Gamma(\tau)]$ is the beta distribution with the parameters η and τ over [0, 1], and $h_0(\varphi_i,\psi_i) = [\varphi_i\psi_i]^{-1}$ is the uniform distribution over $\Omega_i = [0, a_i] \times [0, b_i]$, a_i and b_i are specified in the appendix.

Although the posterior marginal probability density function of m_g depends on two hyper-parameters η and τ, we adopt a Bayes/non-Bayes compromise rather than a type III hyper-distribution for η and τ [9]. As a result, the parameters η and τ are estimated by applying the likelihood method. The maximum likelihood estimators for η and τ and the relative maximum value of m_g are denoted respectively by $\widehat{\eta}$, $\widehat{\tau}$, and $m_g^{max} = m_g(\widehat{\eta},\widehat{\tau})$. Thus, define the minimum Bayes factor as follows:

$$B_g^{min} = \frac{f(\tilde{\mathfrak{X}}_{RD}|H_0)}{m_g^{max}}. \tag{8.21}$$

The details of calculating Eq. (8.21) are given in the appendix.

Example 8.3
The data in Table 8.4 is taken from Cornfield [5] which is adapted from a study of the lung cancer in physicians related to their smoking status. We are interested in testing if the data concerning the smoking status in Table 8.4 for both cases and controls are misclassified. If the smoking status in Table 8.4 is misclassified, the true (not misclassified) table is the counterfactual (CF) one. Undoubtedly, there exist many possible CF models that could be the true table. Of course, not all CF models are admissible. A CF model is said to be admissible if the corresponding BAP estimators of Eqs. (8.11) and (8.12) are admissible.

In order to construct CF models, we first let the number of nonsmokers in Table 8.4 varying in increasing or decreasing direction and the number of smokers is obtained afterwards by subtracting respectively the number of nonsmokers from the column marginal total number of subjects for cases and controls.

By applying the technique used in Sect. 8.2, we then calculate the misclassification error probabilities φ_i and ψ_i from treating the CF model as the true table and the Table 8.4 as the factual misclassified table. By using Eqs. (8.11)

Table 8.4 The lung cancer data of physicians whether he/she is a smoker

Exposure status	Cases (lung cancer patients)	Controls
Smoker	60	32
Non-smoker	3	11
Total	63	43

Table 8.5 The admissible CF models for cases

CF model	(n_{11}, n_{01})	(φ_1, ψ_1)	Δ_1	$(\tilde{p}_1, \tilde{q}_1)$
1	(62, 1)	(0.016, 0.016)	0.9683	(0.97, 0.03)
2	(61, 2))	(0.032, 0.032)	0.9365	(0.98, 0.02)

Table 8.6 The admissible CF models for controls

CF model	(n_{10}, n_{00})	(φ_0, ψ_0)	Δ_0	$(\tilde{p}_0, \tilde{q}_0)$
1	(33, 10)	(0.023, 0.023)	0.9535	(0.76, 0.24)
2	(34, 9)	(0.047, 0.047)	0.9070	(0.77, 0.23)
3	(35, 8)	(0.070, 0.070)	0.8605	(0.78, 0.22)
4	(36, 7)	(0.093, 0.093)	0.8140	(0.8, 0.2)
5	(37, 6)	(0.116, 0.116)	0.7674	(0.82, 0.18)
6	(38, 5)	(0.140, 0.140)	0.7209	(0.84, 0.16)
7	(39, 4)	(0.163, 0.163)	0.6744	(0.86, 0.14)
8	(40, 3)	(0.186, 0.186)	0.6279	(0.89, 0.11)
9	(41, 2)	(0.209, 0.209)	0.5814	(0.92, 0.08)
10	(42, 1)	(0.233, 0.233)	0.5349	(0.96, 0.04)

and (8.12), the BA estimators $\tilde{p}_i$ and $\tilde{q}_i$ are obtained and given in fifth column of Tables 8.5 and 8.6.

Admissible CF models for cases and controls are given in the second column of Tables 8.5 and 8.6. There are two and ten admissible CF models for cases and controls, respectively.

After checking the validity of (φ_i, ψ_i), all CF models are feasible for cases and controls. Altogether there are 20 combined models for cases and controls.

Before calculating the Bayes factor, we substitute $n_{+1} = 63$, $n_{+0} = 43$, $\widehat{p}_1 = 0.952$, $\widehat{q}_1 = 0.048$, $\widehat{p}_0 = 0.744$, and $\widehat{q}_0 = 0.256$, into Eqs. (8.41) and (8.42), we have from Eq. (8.43)

$$m_g(\tilde{\mathfrak{X}}_{RD}) = \frac{1}{\sqrt{2\pi}}\left[m_g^{(1)}(\eta,\tau) - \frac{1}{2}m_g^{(2)}(\eta,\tau)\right]$$
$$= \frac{\eta[0.04\eta^3 + \eta\tau(0.001\eta^2 - 0.001\eta\tau) - 0.018\eta - 0.062\tau - 0.0095) + 0.0026\tau^3 + 0.0045\tau^2 + 0.005\eta^2 - 0.0025\tau] - 0.00005\tau^4}{\eta^2\sqrt{2\pi\eta\tau}}, \tag{8.22}$$

where

Table 8.7 The computed values of Eqs. (8.18) and (8.19) for 20 combined CF models

CF model	$(n_{11}, n_{01}, n_{10}, n_{00})$	$\widehat{\mathfrak{X}}_{RD}$/p-value	$f\left(\widehat{\mathfrak{X}}_{RD}\right)$	$B_g^{min}\left(\tilde{\mathfrak{X}}_{RD}\right)$
1	(61, 2, 33, 10)	8.69/0.003	0.002	0.11
2	(61, 2, 34, 9)	7.27/0.007	0.004	0.24
3	(61, 2, 35, 8)	5.94/0.015	0.008	0.52
4	(61, 2, 36, 7)	4.70/0.03	0.018	1.08
5	(61, 2, 37, 6)	3.54/0.06	0.036	2.21
6	(61, 2, 38, 5)	2.48/0.12	0.073	4.49
7	(61, 2, 39, 4)	1.53/0.22	0.15	9.19
8	(61, 2, 40, 3)	0.72/0.39	0.33	20.03
9	(61, 2, 41, 2)	0.14/0.70	0.98	60.13
10	(61, 2, 42, 1)	0.07/0.79	1.45	88.69
11	(62, 1, 33, 10)	10.67/0.001	0.0006	0.04
12	(62, 1, 34, 9)	9.13/0.003	0.001	0.08
13	(62, 1, 35, 8)	7.68/0.006	0.003	0.19
14	(62, 1, 36, 7)	6.32/0.012	0.007	0.41
15	(62, 1, 37, 6)	5.30/0.025	0.014	0.88
16	(62, 1, 38, 5)	3.82/0.051	0.030	1.85
17	(62, 1, 39, 4)	2.69/0.10	0.063	3.88
18	(62, 1, 40, 3)	1.65/0.20	0.136	8.33
19	(62, 1, 41, 2)	0.73/0.39	0.323	19.80
20	(62, 1, 42, 1)	0.07/0.79	1.454	89.17
Observed table	(60, 3, 32, 11)	8.42/0.004	0.002	0.13

$$m_g^{(1)}(\eta,\tau) \equiv \frac{\left\{0.05\eta^3+\eta\tau[0.001\eta(\eta-\tau)-0.1\eta-0.15\tau]+0.005(\eta+\tau)^2\right.}{\eta\sqrt{\eta\tau}},$$

$$m_g^{(2)}(\eta,\tau) \equiv \frac{\eta\left[0.02\eta^3-\eta\tau(0.1639\eta+0.1818\tau-0.0001)+\tau\left(0.0052\tau^2+0.001\tau+0.005\right)\right]+0.0001\tau^4}{\eta^2\sqrt{\eta\tau}}.$$

To find the relative maximum/minimum of Eq. (8.22), we partition the unit square [0, 1] × [0, 1] into 100 lattice points (0.1, 0.1), (0.1, 0.2), …, (0.9, 0.8), (0.9, 0.9) and then evaluated the function value of Eq. (8.20) at these lattice points. After identifying the proximity of the relative maximum, we then search in a finer neighborhood to locate them. Eq. (8.20) has a relative maximum: $m_g^{\max}(0.705, 0.105) = 0.0163$. After substituting the relative maximum of m_g into Eq. (8.20), the minimum Bayes factor was obtained by dividing the value of $f(\tilde{x}_{RD}|H_0)$ by $m_g^{max} = 0.0163$ that are given in column 5 of Table 8.7.

Note that the value of $\tilde{\mathfrak{X}}_{RD} \,|\, H_0$ is reduced to that of $\widehat{\mathfrak{X}}_{RD} = \widehat{\varepsilon}_{RD}^2 \cdot \widehat{\sigma}_{\widehat{\varepsilon}_{RD}}^{-2}$, where $\widehat{\varepsilon}_{RD} = \widehat{p}_1 - \widehat{p}_0$, and their p-values were computed from the central chi-square distribution with one degree of freedom (column 3 in Table 8.7). The value of $f\left(\tilde{\mathfrak{X}}_{RD}|H_0\right)$ was evaluated directly from the probability density function of the central chi-square distribution with one degree of freedom (column 4 in Table 8.7).

In general, all the minimum Bayes factors $\left(B_g^{min}(\tilde{x}_{RD})\right)$ confirms by theory that their values are much greater than the corresponding p-values. CF models 1–10 behave very similar to models 11–20. Although H_0 are rejected for models 1–4 and 11–15, yet its minimum Bayes factor values do not provide strong evidence in supporting a favor for the alternative hypothesis H_1. By taking the reciprocal of the calculated values of minimum Bayes factor given in the last row of Table 8.7, the evidence for supporting H_1 against H_0 in Eq. (8.14) is at most the odds of 10 to 1 or 25 to 1 which are not very strong to support a favor for the alternative hypothesis. Therefore, the evidence provided by Table 8.4 merely support that the observed data are possibly not misclassified.

Remark
The calculation of the misclassification error is inaccurate in Lee [14].

Appendix 8.2A
By applying the linear approximation to the probability density function of the central chi-square distribution with one degree of freedom in Eq. (8.20), we have

$$f\left(\tilde{\mathfrak{X}}_{RD}|\varepsilon_{RD},\varphi_0,\psi_0,\varphi_1,\psi_1\right)=\frac{1}{\sqrt{2\pi}}\tilde{\mathfrak{X}}_{RD}^{-\frac{1}{2}}e^{-\frac{1}{2}\tilde{\mathfrak{X}}_{RD}}\approx\frac{1}{\sqrt{2\pi\tilde{\mathfrak{X}}_{RD}}}$$
$$\cdot\left(1-\frac{1}{2}\cdot\tilde{\mathfrak{X}}_{RD}\right)=\frac{1}{\sqrt{2\pi}}\left[\frac{\sigma_{\tilde{\varepsilon}_{RD}}}{\tilde{\varepsilon}_{RD}}-\frac{1}{2}\cdot\frac{\tilde{\varepsilon}_{RD}}{\sigma_{\tilde{\varepsilon}_{RD}}}\right], \tag{8.23}$$

where $\tilde{\varepsilon}_{RD}$ and $\sigma^2_{\tilde{\varepsilon}_{RD}}$ are given, respectively, by Eqs. (8.15) and (8.17).

By using the linear approximation: $\left[1-\varepsilon_{RD}^{-1}(\tilde{p}_1-\tilde{p}_0)\right]^{-1}\approx 1+\varepsilon_{RD}^{-1}(\tilde{p}_1-\tilde{p}_0)$, we have

$$\begin{aligned}
\frac{\sigma_{\tilde{\varepsilon}_{RD}}}{\tilde{\varepsilon}_{RD}}&=\frac{\sqrt{\sum_{i=0}^{1}\Delta_i^{-2}n_{+i}^{-1}(p_i\Delta_i+\psi_i)(q_i\Delta_i+\varphi_i)}}{\tilde{p}_1}-\tilde{p}_0-\varepsilon_{RD}=-\frac{\sqrt{n_{+1}^{-1}p_1q_1}}{\varepsilon_{RD}(1-\varepsilon_{RD}^{-1}\tilde{\varepsilon}_{RD})}\\
&\cdot\sqrt{1+\frac{p_1\varphi_1+q_1\psi_1}{n_{+1}^{-1}p_1q_1\Delta_1}+\frac{\varphi_1\psi_1}{n_{+1}^{-1}p_1q_1\Delta_1^2}+\frac{n_{+0}^{-1}p_0q_0}{n_{+1}^{-1}p_1q_1}\left(1+\frac{p_0\varphi_0+q_0\psi_0}{p_0q_0\Delta_0}+\frac{\varphi_0\psi_0}{p_0q_0\Delta_0^2}\right)}\}\approx\\
&-\frac{\sqrt{n_{+1}^{-1}p_1q_1}}{\varepsilon_{RD}}\left[1+\varepsilon_{RD}^{-1}\left(\frac{p_1-\psi_1}{\Delta_1}-\frac{p_0-\psi_0}{\Delta_0}\right)\right]\left\{1+\frac{n_{+1}}{2p_1q_1}\left(\frac{p_1\varphi_1+q_1\psi_1}{\Delta_1}+\frac{\varphi_1\psi_1}{\Delta_1^2}\right)+\frac{n_{+1}p_0q_0}{n_{+0}p_1q_1}\left[1+\frac{1}{p_0q_0}\left(\frac{p_0\varphi_0+q_0\psi_0}{\Delta_0}+\frac{\varphi_0\psi_0}{\Delta_0^2}\right)\right]\right\}\\
&=-\frac{\sqrt{n_{+1}^{-1}p_1q_1}}{\varepsilon_{RD}}\{[1+\frac{n_{+1}}{2p_1q_1}\left[\frac{p_1\varphi_1+q_1\psi_1}{\Delta_1}+\frac{\varphi_1\psi_1}{\Delta_1^2}+\frac{n_{+1}}{n_{+0}p_1q_1}\left(p_0q_0+\frac{p_0\varphi_0+q_0\psi_0}{\Delta_0}+\frac{\varphi_0\psi_0}{\Delta_0^2}\right)\right]\\
&+\varepsilon_{RD}^{-1}\left(\frac{p_1-\psi_1}{\Delta_1}-\frac{p_0-\psi_0}{\Delta_0}\right)\left[1+\frac{1}{2p_1q_1}\left[\frac{p_1\varphi_1+q_1\psi_1}{\Delta_1}+\frac{\varphi_1\psi_1}{\Delta_1^2}+\frac{n_{+1}}{n_{+0}p_1q_1}\left(p_0q_0+\frac{p_0\varphi_0+q_0\psi_0}{\Delta_0}+\frac{\varphi_0\psi_0}{\Delta_0^2}\right)\right]\right]\}.
\end{aligned} \tag{8.24}$$

By calculating the terms over the misclassification error probabilities inside the bracket of Eq. (8.24) one by one, we have

$$\int_0^{\widehat{q}_0-0.005}\int_0^{\widehat{p}_0}\int_0^{\widehat{q}_1-0.005}\int_0^{\widehat{p}_1}\left(\frac{p_1\varphi_1+q_1\psi_1}{\Delta_1}+\frac{\varphi_1\psi_1}{\Delta_1^2}\right)d\psi_1 d\varphi_1 d\psi_0 d\varphi_0$$
$$\approx\widehat{p}_0\widehat{q}_0[\mathcal{A}(p_1,q_1;\widehat{p}_1,\widehat{q}_1)+\mathcal{B}(\widehat{p}_1,\widehat{q}_1)], \tag{8.25}$$

where $\mathcal{A}$ and $\mathcal{B}$ are given, respectively, by

$$\begin{aligned}
&\mathcal{A}(p_1,q_1;\widehat{p}_1,\widehat{q}_1)=a(\widehat{p}_1,\widehat{q}_1)p_1+b(\widehat{p}_1,\widehat{q}_1)q_1,\\
&a(\widehat{p}_1,\widehat{q}_1)=0.5\left[(\widehat{p}_1-2)\widehat{p}_1\ln\widehat{p}_1-\widehat{q}_1^2\ln\widehat{q}_1-0.5\widehat{p}_1^2+1.5\widehat{q}_1^2\right],\\
&b(\widehat{p}_1,\widehat{q}_1)=0.5\left[\widehat{p}_1^2\ln\widehat{p}_1+\left(\widehat{q}_1^2+2\widehat{p}_1\right)\ln\widehat{q}_1-0.5(2+\widehat{p}_1)\widehat{p}_1-0.5\widehat{q}_1^2\right],
\end{aligned} \tag{8.26}$$

and

$$\begin{aligned}
\mathcal{B}(\widehat{p}_1,\widehat{q}_1)=&\,\widehat{p}_1\widehat{q}_1(6.3+\ln\widehat{q}_1)-0.25\widehat{p}_1^2-0.5\widehat{q}_1^2\\
&+\widehat{p}_1[2-(1+0.5\widehat{p}_1)\ln\widehat{p}_1]-1.25.
\end{aligned} \tag{8.27}$$

Similarly, we have by using Eq. (8.25)

$$\int_0^{\widehat{q}_1-0.005}\int_0^{\widehat{p}_1}\int_0^{\widehat{q}_0-0.005}\int_0^{\widehat{p}_0}\left(\frac{p_0\varphi_0+q_0\psi_0}{\Delta_0}+\frac{\varphi_0\psi_0}{\Delta_0^2}\right)d\psi_0 d\varphi_0 d\psi_1 d\varphi_1$$
$$\approx\widehat{p}_1\widehat{q}_1[\mathcal{A}(p_0,q_0;\widehat{p}_0,\widehat{q}_0)+\mathcal{B}(\widehat{p}_0,\widehat{q}_0)], \tag{8.28}$$

where $\mathcal{A}(p_0,q_0;\widehat{p}_0,\widehat{q}_0)$ is given by Eq. (8.26) with the argument $(p_1,q_1;\widehat{p}_1,\widehat{q}_1)$ being replaced by $(p_0,q_0;\widehat{p}_0,\widehat{q}_0)$, $\mathcal{B}(\widehat{p}_0,\widehat{q}_0)$is given by Eq. (8.27) with the argument $(\widehat{p}_1,\widehat{q}_1$) being replaced by $(\widehat{p}_0,\widehat{q}_0)$ accordingly.

Further,

$$\int_0^{\widehat{q}_0-0.005}\int_0^{\widehat{p}_0}\int_0^{\widehat{q}_1-0.005}\int_0^{\widehat{p}_1}\frac{(\widehat{p}_1-\psi_1)(p_1\varphi_1+q_1\psi_1)}{\Delta_1^2}d\psi_1 d\varphi_1 d\psi_0 d\varphi_0$$
$$\approx\widehat{p}_0\widehat{q}_0 C(p_1,q_1;\widehat{p}_1,\widehat{q}_1), \tag{8.29}$$

where C is given by

$$\begin{aligned}
&C(p_1,q_1;\widehat{p}_1,\widehat{q}_1)=c(\widehat{p}_1,\widehat{q}_1)p_1+d(\widehat{p}_1,\widehat{q}_1)q_1+e(\widehat{p}_1),\\
&c(\widehat{p}_1,\widehat{q}_1)=\widehat{p}_1(\widehat{p}_1+2)+\widehat{q}_1^2-3+\widehat{q}_1(1-0.5\widehat{q}_1)\ln\widehat{q}_1,\\
&d(\widehat{p}_1,\widehat{q}_1)=\widehat{p}_1[\ln\widehat{q}_1-\widehat{q}_1(\ln\widehat{p}_1+2)]-\widehat{q}_1^2(\ln\widehat{q}_1-2),\\
&e(\widehat{p}_1)=-\widehat{p}_1\ln\widehat{p}_1.
\end{aligned} \tag{8.30}$$

$$\int_0^{\widehat{q}_0-0.005}\int_0^{\widehat{p}_0}\int_0^{\widehat{q}_1-0.005}\int_0^{\widehat{p}_1}\frac{(\widehat{p}_1-\psi_1)\varphi_1\psi_1}{\Delta_1^3}d\psi_1 d\varphi_1 d\psi_0 d\varphi_0$$
$$\approx\widehat{p}_0\widehat{q}_0\mathcal{D}(p_1,q_1;\widehat{p}_1,\widehat{q}_1) \tag{8.31}$$

where $\mathcal{D}$ is given by

$$\mathcal{D}(\widehat{p}_1,\widehat{q}_1)=\widehat{q}_1\Big\{4.675+3.3\widehat{p}_1+0.25\widehat{q}_1+0.125\widehat{p}_1^2-0.5[\widehat{q}_1(\widehat{q}_1-\widehat{p}_1)\,ln\,\widehat{q}_1$$
$$+\left(1+2\widehat{p}_1-2\widehat{q}_1-0.5\widehat{p}_1^2\right)ln\,\widehat{p}_1]\Big\}. \tag{8.32}$$

Similarly, by using Eqs. (8.29) and (8.31) we have

$$\int_0^{\widehat{q}_1-0.005}\int_0^{\widehat{p}_1}\int_0^{\widehat{q}_0-0.005}\int_0^{\widehat{p}_0}\frac{(\widehat{p}_0-\psi_0)(p_0\varphi_0+q_0\psi_0)}{\Delta_0^2}d\psi_0 d\varphi_0 d\psi_1 d\varphi_1$$
$$\approx\widehat{p}_1\widehat{q}_1\mathcal{C}(p_0,q_0;\widehat{p}_0,\widehat{q}_0), \tag{8.33}$$

and

$$\int_0^{\widehat{q}_1-0.005}\int_0^{\widehat{p}_1}\int_0^{\widehat{q}_0-0.005}\int_0^{\widehat{p}_0}\frac{(\widehat{p}_0-\psi_0)\varphi_0\psi_0}{\Delta_0^3}d\psi_0 d\varphi_0 d\psi_1 d\varphi_1$$
$$\approx\widehat{p}_1\widehat{q}_1\mathcal{D}(\widehat{p}_0,\widehat{q}_0) \tag{8.34}$$

where $\mathcal{C}$ and $\mathcal{D}$ are given by Eqs. (8.30) and (8.32) with their arguments being replaced accordingly.

$$\int_0^{\widehat{q}_0-0.005}\int_0^{\widehat{p}_0}\int_0^{\widehat{q}_1-0.005}\int_0^{\widehat{p}_1}\frac{(\widehat{p}_0-\psi_0)}{\Delta_0}$$
$$\times\left(\frac{p_1\varphi_1+q_1\psi_1}{\Delta_1}+\frac{\varphi_1\psi_1}{\Delta_1^2}\right)d\psi_1 d\varphi_1 d\psi_0 d\varphi_0$$
$$=\int_0^{\widehat{q}_0-0.005}\int_0^{\widehat{p}_0}\frac{\widehat{p}_0-\psi_0}{\Delta_0}d\psi_0 d\varphi_0$$
$$\cdot\int_0^{\widehat{q}_1-0.005}\int_0^{\widehat{p}_1}\left(\frac{p_1\varphi_1+q_1\psi_1}{\Delta_1}+\frac{\varphi_1\psi_1}{\Delta_1^2}\right)d\psi_1 d\varphi_1\approx\mathcal{E}(\widehat{p}_0,\widehat{q}_0)$$
$$\times[\mathcal{A}(p_1,q_1;\widehat{p}_1,\widehat{q}_1)+\mathcal{B}(\widehat{p}_1,\widehat{q}_1)], \tag{8.35}$$

where $\mathcal{A}$ and $\mathcal{B}$ are given, respectively, by Eqs. (8.26) and (8.27), $\mathcal{E}$ is given by

$$\mathcal{E}(\widehat{p}_0, \widehat{q}_0) \approx 0.5\widehat{q}_0^3(\ln \widehat{q}_0 - 0.5) + (\widehat{p}_0 - \widehat{q}_0)\widehat{p}_0 \ln \widehat{p}_0 - 0.5\widehat{p}_0^2 - 1.5\widehat{q}_0^2 + \widehat{p}_0\widehat{q}_0 + 0.5. \tag{8.36}$$

Similarly, we have by using Eq. (8.35)

$$\int_0^{\widehat{q}_0 - 0.005} \int_0^{\widehat{p}_0} \int_0^{\widehat{q}_1 - 0.005} \int_0^{\widehat{p}_1} \frac{(\widehat{p}_1 - \psi_1)}{\Delta_1} \times \left[\frac{(p_0\varphi_0 + q_0\psi_0)}{\Delta_0} + \frac{\varphi_0\psi_0}{\Delta_0^2} \right] d\psi_0 d\varphi_0 d\psi_1 d\varphi_1 \approx \mathcal{E}(\widehat{p}_1, \widehat{q}_1) \times [\mathcal{A}(p_0, q_0; \widehat{p}_0, \widehat{q}_0) + \mathcal{B}(\widehat{p}_0, \widehat{q}_0)], \tag{8.37}$$

where $\mathcal{E}$ is given by Eq. (8.36) with the argument $(\widehat{p}_0, \widehat{q}_0)$ being replaced by $(\widehat{p}_1, \widehat{q}_1)$ accordingly.

In addition, by using Eqs. (8.36) and (8.27), we have

$$\int_0^{\widehat{q}_1 - 0.005} \int_0^{\widehat{p}_1} \int_0^{\widehat{q}_0 - 0.005} \int_0^{\widehat{p}_0} \frac{(\widehat{p}_0 - \psi_0)\varphi_1\psi_1}{\Delta_0\Delta_1^2} d\psi_0 d\varphi_0 d\psi_1 d\varphi_1 \approx \mathcal{E}(\widehat{p}_0, \widehat{q}_0)\mathcal{B}(\widehat{p}_1, \widehat{q}_1), \tag{8.38}$$

where $\mathcal{E}$ is given by Eq. (8.36) and $\mathcal{B}$ by Eq. (8.27).

Similarly, by using Eq. (8.38) we have

$$\int_0^{\widehat{q}_0 - 0.005} \int_0^{\widehat{p}_0} \int_0^{\widehat{q}_1 - 0.005} \int_0^{\widehat{p}_1} \frac{(\widehat{p}_1 - \psi_1)\varphi_0\psi_0}{\Delta_1\Delta_0^2} d\psi_1 d\varphi_1 d\psi_0 d\varphi_0 \approx \mathcal{E}(\widehat{p}_1, \widehat{q}_1)\mathcal{B}(\widehat{p}_0, \widehat{q}_0), \tag{8.39}$$

where $\mathcal{E}$ is given by Eq. (8.36) with the argument $(\widehat{p}_0, \widehat{q}_0)$ being replaced by $(\widehat{p}_1, \widehat{q}_1)$ and $\mathcal{B}$ by Eq. (8.27) with the argument $(\widehat{p}_1, \widehat{q}_1)$ being replaced by $(\widehat{p}_0, \widehat{q}_0)$ accordingly.

By using the quadratic approximation to ε_{RD}^{-1} and ε_{RD}^{-2} with an assumption that $p_1 > p_0$, we have

$$\varepsilon_{RD}^{-1} = p_1^{-1} + p_0 p_1^{-2} + p_0^2 p_1^{-3}, \tag{8.40}$$

and

$$\varepsilon_{RD}^{-2} = p_1^{-2} - 2p_0^{-1} p_1^{-1} + 3p_0^{-2}. \tag{8.41}$$

By using Eq. (8.24) and integrating over the prior Beta distribution after applying the integration on the misclassification error probabilities on φ_i and ψ_i, we have

$$
\begin{aligned}
m_g^{(1)}(\eta,\tau) \equiv & \int_0^1 \int_0^1 \int_0^{\hat{q}_0-0.005} \int_0^{\hat{p}_0} \int_0^{\hat{q}_1-0.005} \int_0^{\hat{p}_1} \frac{\sigma_{\tilde{\varepsilon}_{RD}}}{\tilde{\varepsilon}_{RD}} \prod\nolimits_{i=1}^{0} d\psi_i d\varphi_i \prod\nolimits_{i=0}^{1} p_i^{\eta-1} q_i^{\tau-1} dp_i \\
= & -\sqrt{n_{+1}^{-1}} \Big\{ \frac{\mathcal{K}\tau}{\sqrt{\eta\tau}} \Big(2+\eta+\tau+\frac{3n_{+1}}{2n_{+0}} \Big) + \Big[\frac{3(\eta+\tau)}{2\eta\sqrt{\eta\tau}} \Big(\hat{p}_0\hat{q}_0 + \frac{n_{+1}}{n_{+0}} \hat{p}_1\hat{q}_1 \Big) \\
& \big(a(\hat{p}_1,\hat{q}_1)\eta + b(\hat{p}_1,\hat{q}_1)\tau + (\eta+\tau)\mathcal{B}(\hat{p}_1,\hat{q}_1) \big) + \frac{\mathcal{K}(\eta+\tau)^2}{\eta^2\sqrt{\eta\tau}} \Big(\hat{p}_0\hat{q}_0 - \frac{n_{+1}}{n_{+0}} \hat{p}_1\hat{q}_1 \Big) \\
& \big(c(\hat{p}_1,\hat{q}_1)\eta + d(\hat{p}_1,\hat{q}_1)\tau + (\eta+\tau)\big(e(\hat{p}_1,\hat{q}_1) + \mathcal{D}(\hat{p}_1,\hat{q}_1) \big) \big) \Big] \\
& + \frac{\mathcal{K}(\eta+\tau)^2}{\eta^2\sqrt{\eta\tau}} \cdot \Big[\frac{n_{+1}}{n_{+0}} \mathcal{E}(\hat{p}_1,\hat{q}_1) \big(a(\hat{p}_0,\hat{q}_0)\eta + b(\hat{p}_0,\hat{q}_0)\tau + (\eta+\tau)\mathcal{B}(\hat{p}_0,\hat{q}_0) \big) \\
& - \mathcal{E}(\hat{p}_0,\hat{q}_0) \big(a(\hat{p}_1,\hat{q}_1)\eta + b(\hat{p}_1,\hat{q}_1)\tau + (\eta+\tau)\mathcal{B}(\hat{p}_1,\hat{q}_1) \big) \Big] \\
& + \frac{2(\eta+\tau)\tau}{\eta\sqrt{\eta\tau}} \Big(\frac{n_{+1}}{n_{+0}} + 1 \Big) \big[\hat{p}_0\hat{q}_0 \mathcal{E}(\hat{p}_1,\hat{q}_1) - \hat{p}_1\hat{q}_1 \mathcal{E}(\hat{p}_0,\hat{q}_0) \big] \Big\},
\end{aligned}
\tag{8.42}
$$

where $\mathcal{K} = \widehat{p}_0\widehat{q}_0\widehat{p}_1\widehat{q}_1$, $\mathcal{B}$, $\mathcal{D}$, and $\mathcal{E}$ are given, respectively, by Eqs. (8.27), (8.30), (8.32), and (8.36), a, b, c, d, and e are given, respectively, by Eqs. (8.26) and (8.30). Note that in Eq. (8.42) the approximation of $\Gamma(x+a) = x^a\Gamma(x)$ [2] was used to get the last line [1].

On the other hand, if we integrate the second term inside the bracket of Eq. (8.23) over (p_i, q_i) with the prior Beta distribution and misclassification error probabilities (φ_i, ψ_i), we get

$$
\begin{aligned}
m_g^{(2)}(\eta,\tau) \equiv & \int_0^1 \int_0^1 \int_0^{\hat{q}_0-0.005} \int_0^{\hat{p}_0} \int_0^{\hat{q}_1-0.005} \int_0^{\hat{p}_1} \frac{\tilde{\varepsilon}_{RD}}{\sigma_{\tilde{\varepsilon}_{RD}}} p_i^{\eta-1} q_i^{\tau-1} \prod\nolimits_{i=0}^{1} p_i \prod\nolimits_{i=0}^{1} d\psi_i d\varphi_i \\
= & \sqrt{n_{+1}^{-1}} \Big\{ \frac{\sqrt{\eta\tau}}{\eta+\tau} \big[\hat{p}_1\hat{q}_1 \mathcal{E}(\hat{p}_0,\hat{q}_0) - \hat{p}_0\hat{q}_0 \mathcal{E}(\hat{p}_1,\hat{q}_1) \big] + \frac{1}{\sqrt{\eta\tau}} \Big[\frac{n_{+1}}{n_{+0}} \mathcal{K}\mathcal{E}(\hat{p}_1,\hat{q}_1) \big(a(\hat{p}_0,\hat{q}_0)\eta \\
& + b(\hat{p}_0,\hat{q}_0)\tau + \mathcal{B}(\hat{p}_0,\hat{q}_0)(\eta+\tau) \big) - 0.5\mathcal{K}\mathcal{E}(\hat{p}_0,\hat{q}_0) \big(a(\hat{p}_1,\hat{q}_1)\eta \\
& + b(\hat{p}_1,\hat{q}_1)\tau + \mathcal{B}(\hat{p}_1,\hat{q}_1)(\eta+\tau) \big) \Big] + \frac{1}{\sqrt{\eta\tau}} \Big[0.5\hat{p}_0\hat{q}_0 \big(c(\hat{p}_1,\hat{q}_1)\eta + d(\hat{p}_1,\hat{q}_1)\tau \\
& + \big(e(\hat{p}_1,\hat{q}_1) + \mathcal{D}(\hat{p}_1,\hat{q}_1) \big)(\eta+\tau) \big) - \frac{n_{+1}}{n_{+0}} \hat{p}_1\hat{q}_1 \big(c(\hat{p}_0,\hat{q}_0)\eta + d(\hat{p}_0,\hat{q}_0)\tau \\
& + \big(e(\hat{p}_0,\hat{q}_0) + \mathcal{D}(\hat{p}_0,\hat{q}_0) \big)(\eta+\tau) \big) \Big] \Big\},
\end{aligned}
\tag{8.43}
$$

where $\mathcal{K} = \widehat{p}_0\widehat{q}_0\widehat{p}_1\widehat{q}_1$, $\mathcal{B}$ $\mathcal{D}$, and $\mathcal{E}$ are given, respectively, by Eqs. (8.27), (8.32), and (8.36).

Finally, Eq. (8.20) is given by

$$
m_g(\eta,\tau) = \left(\sqrt{2\pi}\right)^{-1} \left[m_g^{(1)}(\eta,\tau) - 0.5 m_g^{(2)}(\eta,\tau) \right], \tag{8.44}
$$

where $m_g^{(1)}$ and $m_g^{(2)}$are given, respectively, by Eqs. (8.42) and (8.43). Incidentally, the derivation of Eqs. (8.42) and (8.43) has made an error in Good [9].

8.3 Bayes Factor for *No Misclassification Errors in* Categorical Data

In this section, we are going to calculate the Bayes factor to test the hypothesis of no misclassification error in the data of a categorical variable.

Given that X is a categorical variable with K (K ≥ 3) categories and the data are collected by a simple random sampling of size N, where $N = \sum_{i=1}^{K} n_i$ (Table 8.8). The crude estimator $\widehat{p}_j$ for the population cell proportion p_j in the jth category is given by

$$\widehat{p}_j = \frac{n_j}{N}. \tag{8.45}$$

Assume that $\widehat{p}_j$ is distributed as a multinomial distribution with the population size N and the cell proportion of the jth category p_j. It is well known that Eq. (8.45) is an unbiased estimator for p_j, provided that the observed data are not misclassified [1]. However, it is easily shown that Eq. (8.45) is no longer unbiased, once the observed data are misclassified.

Suppose that the observed data are misclassified. Let w_{jk} (j $\neq k$) be the misclassification error probability of an observation belonging to the jth category being incorrectly classified into the kth category and w_{jj} the correct classification probability that an observation belonging to the jth category being correctly classified into the jth category. Thus, it is easily shown that the expected value of $\widehat{p}_j$ is

$$E\left(\widehat{\vec{p}}\right) = \mathcal{W}\vec{p}, \tag{8.46}$$

where $\vec{p} = (p_1, p_2, \ldots, p_K)^T$, $\widehat{\vec{p}} = (\widehat{p}_1, \widehat{p}_2, \ldots, \widehat{p}_K)^T$, and $\mathcal{W} = \left[w_{jk}\right], j, k = 1, 2, \ldots, K$ is the misclassification error matrix, in which $\sum_{k=1}^{K} w_{jk} = 1$ for j = 1, 2, …, K. Eq. (8.46) shows that the crude estimator $\widehat{p}_k$ is no longer unbiased for the true population parameter p_k, provided that $\mathcal{W} \neq$ I, where I is the K × K identity matrix. A set of misclassification error probability $\left\{w_{jk}\right\}$ is said to be feasible if the misclassification error matrix in Eq. (8.46) is invertible (or nonsingular) for $0 < w_{jk} < 1$.

Assume that $\mathcal{W}$ is invertible. Then the bias-adjusted cell proportion (BACP) estimators $(\tilde{p}_k)$ are defined by

Table 8.8 The data of categorical variable X

Variable	Categories				
X	1	2	…	…	K
Observation	n_1	n_2	…	…	n_K

$$\tilde{\vec{p}} = \mathcal{W}^{-1}\widehat{\vec{p}} = \mathcal{V}\widehat{\vec{p}}\,, \tag{8.47}$$

where $\tilde{\vec{p}} = (\tilde{p}_1, \tilde{p}_2, \ldots, \tilde{p}_K)^T$, $\mathcal{V} = [v_{jk}]$, j, k = 1, 2, …, K, denotes the inverse matrix of $\mathcal{W}$, and $\tilde{\vec{n}} = \mathcal{V}\vec{n}$, $\tilde{\vec{n}} = (\tilde{n}_1, \tilde{n}_2, \ldots, \tilde{n}_K)^T$, and $\vec{n} = (n_1, n_2, \ldots, n_K)^T$. Note that from Eqs. (8.46) and (8.47) it is easily shown that $E\left(\tilde{\vec{p}}\right) = \vec{p}$, that is, $\tilde{\vec{p}}$ is an unbiased estimator for $\vec{p}$, provided that $\mathcal{W}$ is known. The BACP estimator $\{\tilde{p}_k\}$ is said to be admissible if for feasible w_{jk} we have $\tilde{p}_k$ lying between zero and one such that $\sum_{k=1}^{K}\tilde{p}_k = 1$. Furthermore, a set of misclassification error probability $\{w_{jk}\}$ is said to be admissible if the corresponding BACP estimators $\{\tilde{p}_k\}$ are admissible.

The misclassification error matrix $\mathcal{W}$ has two possible forms depending on how the categorical variable X is misclassified. These two possible scenarios are given as follows:

Scenario I The misclassification occurs after classifying one category incorrectly into all other categories. Because a misclassification can occur equally likely from any true jth category into the wrong kth observed category, we thus have for fixed j

$$w_{jk} \equiv s_j > 0, \mathrm{k} \neq \mathrm{j}, \text{and } w_{jj} = 1 - \sum\nolimits_{k \neq j, k=1}^{K} w_{jk}, \mathrm{j} = 1, \ldots, \mathrm{K}; \tag{8.48}$$

Scenario II The misclassification occurs after classifying one category incorrectly only into its neighboring categories. Thus, we have for fixed j

$$w_{jk} = 0 \text{ for } |\mathrm{k} - \mathrm{j}| > 1, \text{and } w_{jj} = 1 - \sum\nolimits_{k \neq j, k=1}^{K} w_{jk}, \mathrm{j} = 1, \ldots, \mathrm{K}. \tag{8.49}$$

When K = 3, the associated misclassification error matrix with its determinant and inverse matrix for scenarios I and II are obtained respectively. An explicit form of the misclassification error matrix $\mathcal{W}_I$ and its inverse $\mathcal{V}_I$ for scenario I are given respectively by

$$\mathcal{W}_I = \begin{bmatrix} 1 - s_2 - s_3 & s_2 & s_3 \\ s_1 & 1 - s_1 - s_3 & s_3 \\ s_1 & s_2 & 1 - s_1 - s_2 \end{bmatrix}, \tag{8.50}$$

$$d_I \equiv \det(\mathcal{W}_I) = (1 - s_1 - s_2 - s_3)^2 \neq 0, \tag{8.51}$$

and

$$\mathcal{V}_I \equiv \left[v_{jk(I)}\right] = d_I^{-1} \cdot \begin{bmatrix} 1 - s_1 & -s_1 & -s_1 \\ -s_2 & 1 - s_2 & -s_2 \\ -s_3 & -s_3 & 1 - s_3 \end{bmatrix}, \tag{8.52}$$

where $s_1 \equiv w_{12} = w_{13}$, $s_2 \equiv w_{21} = w_{23}$, and $s_3 \equiv w_{31} = w_{32}$.

The BACP estimators for scenario I are given by

$$\tilde{p}_{k(I)} = \sum\nolimits_{j=1}^{K} v_{jk(I)}\widehat{p}_j, \mathrm{k} = 1, 2, \ldots, \mathrm{K} \tag{8.53}$$

By using Eqs. (8.51) and (8.53), the feasibility and admissibility constraints for the misclassification error probability and BACP estimator are given by

$$s_1 + s_2 + s_3 < 1, \tag{8.54}$$

and

$$s_1 < 1, s_2 < 1, \text{and } s_3 < 1. \tag{8.55}$$

For scenario II, an explicit form for the misclassification error matrix $\mathcal{W}_{II}$ and its inverse $\mathcal{V}_{II}$ are given, respectively, by

$$\mathcal{W}_{II} = \begin{bmatrix} 1-t_2 & t_2 & 0 \\ t_1 & 1-t_1-t_3 & t_3 \\ 0 & t_2 & 1-t_2 \end{bmatrix}, \tag{8.56}$$

$$d_{II} \equiv \det(\mathcal{W}_{II}) = (1-t_2)(1-t_1-t_2-t_3) \neq 0, \tag{8.57}$$

and

$$\mathcal{V}_{II} \equiv \left[v_{jk(II)}\right] = d_{II}^{-1} \cdot \begin{bmatrix} (1-t_1)(1-t_2) & -t_1(1-t_2) & t_1 t_2 \\ -t_2(1-t_2) & (1-t_2)^2 & -t_2(1-t_2) \\ t_2 t_3 & -t_3(1-t_2) & (1-t_2)(1-t_3)-t_1 \end{bmatrix}, \tag{8.58}$$

where $t_1 \equiv w_{12}$, $t_2 \equiv w_{21} = w_{23}$, $t_3 \equiv w_{32}$, and $w_{13} = w_{31} \equiv 0$.

The BACP estimator for scenario II is given by

$$\tilde{p}_{j(II)} = \sum\nolimits_{k=1}^{K} v_{jk(II)}\widehat{p}_k, \mathrm{j} = 1, 2, \ldots, \mathrm{K}. \tag{8.59}$$

From Eqs. (8.57) and (8.59), the feasibility and admissibility constraints for the misclassification error probability and BACP are given, respectively, as

$$t_1 + t_2 + t_3 < 1, \tag{8.60}$$

and

$$t_2 < \widehat{p}_2. \tag{8.61}$$

To test if the data in Table 8.8 are misclassified, we need to test the null hypothesis that the data has no misclassification at $\vec{p} = \vec{p}^{(0)}$ versus the alternative hypothesis that the data are misclassified [3]

$$H_0 : \vec{p} = \vec{p}^{(0)}, \vec{w} = \vec{0} \text{ versus } H_1 : \vec{p} \neq \vec{p}^{(0)}, \vec{w} > \vec{0}, \tag{8.62}$$

where $\vec{w} = (w_{11}, \ldots, w_{1K}, w_{21}, \ldots, w_{2K}, \ldots, w_{K1}, \ldots, w_{KK})^T$, $\{w_{jk}\}$ are the entries of W given in Eq. (8.46), $\vec{p} = (p_1, p_2, \ldots, p_K)^T$, and $\vec{p}^{(0)} = \left(p_1^{(0)}, p_2^{(0)}, \ldots, p_K^{(0)}\right)^T$.

To test Eq. (8.62), the bias-adjusted chi-square test (BACPT) is given by

$$\tilde{X}_K = \sum_{k=1}^{K} N\left[\left(\tilde{p}_k - p_k^{(0)}\right)^2 / p_k^{(0)}\right] = \sum_{k=1}^{K} \left(\tilde{n}_k^2 / n_k^{(0)}\right) - N, \tag{8.63}$$

where $\tilde{n}_k = \sum_{j=1}^{K} v_{jk} n_j$, $\{v_{jk}\}$ denotes the entry of the jth row and the kth column of the inverse matrix $\mathcal{V}$ Of the the misclassification error matrix $\mathcal{W}$ in Eq. (8.46) and $n_k^{(0)} = N p_k^{(0)}$, k = 1, 2, …, K.

For large samples, Eq. (8.63) is distributed asymptotically under H_0 as the central chi-square distribution with K – 1 degrees of freedom (df). However, Eq. (8.63) is distributed asymptotically under H_1 as the noncentral chi-square distribution with K – 1 degree of freedom and the non-centrality parameter given by [13]

$$\tilde{r}_k = \sum_{j=1}^{K} \left(p_j - p_j^{(0)}\right)^2 = \sum_{j=1}^{K} \left(p_j^2 - 2p_j^{(0)} p_j + p_j^{(0)2}\right), \tag{8.64}$$

When $w_{jk} = 0$ for all j and k, Eq. (8.63) is reduced to

$$\widehat{X}_K = \sum_{j=1}^{K} \left(\frac{n_j^2}{n_j^{(0)}}\right) - N. \tag{8.65}$$

Reject H_0 if $\widehat{X}_K > c_0$, where $\widehat{X}_K$ is given by Eq. (8.65) and c_0 is the critical value of the central chi-square distribution with K – 1 degree of freedom at the significance level α.

As is well known from the Bayesian viewpoint, the p-value is not an adequate measure of the evidence to support H_0 [10, 11]. Hence the Bayes factor is calculated instead as a measure of the evidence for the observed data. To formulate the hypothesis testing problem in a Bayesian setting, we assume that the probability distribution of the observed data follows a family of distributions which are parametrized by $\left(\vec{p}, \vec{w}\right) \in \Sigma \times \Omega$, where $\Sigma = \left\{\vec{p} \mid \sum_{k=1}^{K} p_k = 1, p_k > 0\right\}$ is the K-dimensional simplex.

To test Eq. (8.62), we assume that there exists a prior probability density function (pdf) $h_0\left(\vec{w}\right)$ and another joint density $h\left(\vec{p}, \vec{w}\right)$ under H_1. Since $\vec{p}$ and $\vec{w}$ are a priori independent under H_1, we have

$$h\left(\vec{p}, \vec{w}\right) = h_0\left(\vec{w}\right)g\left(\vec{p}\right), \tag{8.66}$$

where g is a priori pdf for $\vec{p} \in \Sigma$ which assigns a mass π_0 to $\left\{\vec{p} = \vec{p}^{(0)}\right\}$ and 1 - π_0 to $\left\{\vec{p} \neq \vec{p}^{(0)}\right\}$. Define $g\left(\vec{p}^{(0)}\right) = 0$ and writing the pdf of $\tilde{X}_K$ given $\vec{p}$ and $\vec{w}$ as $f\left(\tilde{X}_K|\vec{p}, \vec{w}\right)$, the Bayes factor is given by [12]

$$\mathcal{B}_g(\tilde{X}_K) = \frac{f\left(\tilde{X}_K|\vec{p}^{(0)}, \vec{w} = \vec{0}\right)}{m_g(\tilde{X}_K)}, \tag{8.67}$$

where m_g is given by

$$m_g(\tilde{X}_K) = \iint_{\Sigma \times \Omega} f\left(\tilde{X}_K|\vec{p}, \vec{w}\right)h_0\left(\vec{w}\right)g\left(\vec{p}\right)d\vec{w}d\vec{p} \tag{8.68}$$

Note that in Eq. (8.67), $f\left(\tilde{X}_K|\vec{p}^{(0)}, \vec{w} = \vec{0}\right)$ is the pdf of the central chi-square distribution with K − 1 df, while $f\left(\tilde{X}_K|\vec{p}, \vec{w}\right)$ in Eq. (8.68) is the pdf of the noncentral chi-square distribution with K − 1 df and the non-centrality parameter $\tilde{r}_K$ given by Eq. (8.64).

When K = 3, $m_g\left(\tilde{X}_{3(I)}\right)$ of Eq. (8.68) is calculated for scenario I with the assumption of $s_1 = s_2 = s_3 \equiv s$ and $h_0(s) = a^{-1}$, the pdf of the uniform distribution on $[0, a]$, where a is the upper bound on the admissible BACP for scenario I, we have

$$m_g\left(\tilde{X}_{3(I)}\right) = \int_{\Sigma}\int_0^a \frac{1}{a} \cdot \frac{1}{2 + \tilde{r}_3} \cdot \exp\left(-\frac{s}{2 + \tilde{r}_3}\right)ds \cdot g\left(\vec{p}\right)d\vec{p}, \tag{8.69}$$

where an approximation to the noncentral chi-square distribution is applied by using the central chi-square distribution [6]. The lower bound for the Bayes factor after applying a symmetric Dirichlet's prior for $g\left(\vec{p}\right)$ are obtained under scenarios I and II as

$$B_g^{(i)} = \frac{\frac{1}{2}\exp\left\{-\frac{1}{2}\left[\sum_{j=1}^{3}\left(\frac{n_j^2}{n_j^{(0)}}\right)-N\right]\right\}}{m_g\left(\tau_{\max(i)}|\widetilde{X}_{3(i)}\right)}, \mathrm{i}=\mathrm{I} \text{ or II}. \tag{8.70}$$

The details for obtaining the value of $\tau_{\max(i)}$, i = I or II, are given in the appendix [15].

Example 8.4
The data in Table 8.9 are taken from Table C.1 in Woodward [18]. It represents the lung cancer data collected by the Bombay Cancer Registry from all cancer patients registered in the 168 government and private hospitals and nursing homes in Bombay, Australia, and from death records maintained by the Bombay Municipal Corporation. The survival times of each subject with lung cancer from time of first diagnosis to death (or censoring) were recorded over the period from first January 1989 to 31st December 1991. Here we are only concerned with type of tumor of 682 subjects grouped by gender:

The issue of concern is whether the data are misclassified separately for males and females. Because we do not have any prior belief on the value of $\vec{p}^{(0)}$ in Eq. (8.62), they are thereby determined empirically from the observed data. As a result, the values of $\vec{p}^{(0)}$ are chosen differently for males and females. For females the value of $\vec{p}^{(0)}$ are chosen to be that of equiprobability, that is $\vec{p}_F^{(0)} = \left(\frac{1}{3}, \frac{1}{3}, \frac{1}{3}\right)^T$, while for males it is chosen as $\vec{p}_M^{(0)} = (0.3, 0.3, 0.4)^T$. The null and alternative hypotheses for males and females are set up respectively as follows:

$$H_{0(M)} : \vec{p} = \vec{p}_M^{(0)}, \vec{w} = \vec{0} \text{ versus } H_{1(M)} : \vec{p} \neq \vec{p}_M^{(0)}, \vec{w} > \vec{0}; \tag{8.71}$$

and

$$H_{0(F)} : \vec{p} = \vec{p}_F^{(0)}, \vec{w} = \vec{0} \text{ versus } H_{1(F)} : \vec{p} \neq \vec{p}_F^{(0)}, \vec{w} > \vec{0}. \tag{8.72}$$

Because the misclassification error probabilities are zero under $H_{0(M)}$ in Eq. (8.71) or $H_{0(F)}$, the BACST values of Eq. (8.65) are given respectively by $\widehat{X}_{3(M)} = 0.15$ (p-value = 0.93) and $\widehat{X}_{3(F)} = 0.47$ (p-value = 0.79) for males and females. Therefore, $H_{0(M)}$ or $H_{0(F)}$ are not rejected at the significance level of 0.05. Yet, we would like to calculate the Bayes factor as a comparison with the p-value.

Table 8.9 Cancer data collected from 168 hospitals and nursing homes in Bombay, Australia

	Type of tumor			
Gender	Local	Regional	Advanced	Total
Male	165	169	229	563
Female	37	39	43	119

Table 8.10 The calculated result of τ_{max}, m_g, and $\mathcal{B}_g$

Scenario II					
Males	a_2	$\tau_{\max(II)}$	$m_g(\tau_{\max(II)})$	$\mathcal{B}_{g(II)}$	p-value
	0.2931	0.0553	61	0.053	0.93
Scenario I					
Females	a_1	$\tau_{\max(I)}$	$m_g(\tau_{\max(I)})$	$\mathcal{B}_{g(I)}$	p-value
	0.309	0.0540	1.8	0.22	0.79

For both males and females under scenarios I or II, Eq. (8.82) in the appendix has three negative and one positive, and a pair of complex roots. Due to the constraint that $\tau > 0$, only the positive root is a stationary point for Eq. (8.81). For males Eq. (8.81) has only a unique positive local maximum under scenario II, while it has a unique positive local maximum under scenario I for females.

By taking the reciprocal of the lower bound of the Bayes factor (column 4 in Table 8.10), we are able to assess the evidence provided by Table 8.9. The collected data for males are in favor of supporting $H_{1(M)}$ against $H_{0(M)}$ in Eq. (8.71) by at most the odds of 19 to 1, whereas for females by at most the odds of 5 to 1 of supporting $H_{1(F)}$ against $H_{0(F)}$ in Eq. (8.72). Both of their odds ratios are not strong enough to support the favor of the alternative hypothesis.

Remarks

1. So far, we are not aware of any guideline available in the literature on judging how large the lower bound for the Bayes factor should be so that we are confident the evidence provided by the data surely supporting a favor of H_1 against H_0. All we can say is that the larger the odds are, the stronger the support is. From the magnitude of the odds, the data for males under scenario II are possibly misclassified, but possibly not misclassified under scenario I for females.
2. From this example, the existence of Bayes factor seems to depend not only on the scenario (I or II), but also on the value of $\vec{p}^{(0)}$. To clarify this issue, another data set involves the degree of severity of myocardial infarction [16] is studied, where $\vec{p}^{(0)}$ is chosen as $\vec{p}_T^{(0)} = (0.4, 0.4, 0.2)^T$ or $\vec{p}_C^{(0)} = (0.3, 0.4, 0.3)^T$ respectively for the treated or control groups. It was found that the Bayes factor exists for the treated group under scenario I, but not under scenario II, whereas it exists under both scenarios for the control group [15].

Appendix 7.3A

With an assumption $s_1 = s_2 = s_3 \equiv s$ and $\tilde{\vec{n}} = N\tilde{\vec{p}}$, we have under scenario I

$$\tilde{\vec{n}}_{(I)} \equiv \begin{bmatrix} \tilde{n}_{1(I)} \\ \tilde{n}_{2(I)} \\ \tilde{n}_{3(I)} \end{bmatrix} = (1-3s)^{-1} \begin{bmatrix} (1-s)n_1 - sn_2 - sn_3 \\ -sn_1 + (1-s)n_2 - sn_3 \\ -sn_1 - sn_2 + (1-s)n_3 \end{bmatrix}, \quad 0 < s < a_1, \tag{8.73}$$

where $a_1 = \min_{j=1,2,3} \left\{ \frac{1}{3}, \widehat{p}_j \right\}$.

By substituting Eq. (8.73) into Eq. (8.63),

$$\tilde{X}_{3(I)} = \sum_{j=1}^{3} \mathit{b}_{j(I)} n_j^2 - 2\sum_{j\neq k} \mathit{b}_{jk(I)} n_j n_k - N, \tag{8.74}$$

where

$$\mathit{b}_{1(I)} = \frac{1}{(1-3s)^2}\left[\frac{(1-s)^2}{n_1^{(0)}} + s^2\left(\frac{1}{n_2^{(0)}} + \frac{1}{n_3^{(0)}}\right)\right],$$

$$\mathit{b}_{2(I)} = \frac{1}{(1-3s)^2}\left[\frac{(1-s)^2}{n_2^{(0)}} + s^2\left(\frac{1}{n_1^{(0)}} + \frac{1}{n_3^{(0)}}\right)\right],$$

$$\mathit{b}_{3(I)} = \frac{1}{(1-3s)^2}\left[\frac{(1-s)^2}{n_3^{(0)}} + s^2\left(\frac{1}{n_1^{(0)}} + \frac{1}{n_2^{(0)}}\right)\right],$$

$$\mathit{b}_{12(I)} = \frac{1}{(1-3s)^2}\left[s(1-s)\left(\frac{1}{n_1^{(0)}} + \frac{1}{n_2^{(0)}}\right) - \frac{s^2}{n_3^{(0)}}\right],$$

$$\mathit{b}_{13(I)} = \frac{1}{(1-3s)^2}\left[s(1-s)\left(\frac{1}{n_1^{(0)}} + \frac{1}{n_3^{(0)}}\right) - \frac{s^2}{n_2^{(0)}}\right],$$

$$\mathit{b}_{23(I)} = \frac{1}{(1-3s)^2}\left[s(1-s)\left(\frac{1}{n_2^{(0)}} + \frac{1}{n_3^{(0)}}\right) - \frac{s^2}{n_1^{(0)}}\right].$$

By using Eq. (8.64), we have

$$\tilde{r}_3 = \sum_{j=1}^{3} \left(p_j^2 - 2p_j^{(0)} p_j + p_j^{(0)2}\right). \tag{8.75}$$

Note that $m_g(\tilde{X}_K)$ of Eq. (8.69) with a choice of $h_0(s)$ that equals the pdf of a uniform distribution over $[0, a_1]$ is reduced to

$$m_g(\tilde{X}_3) = \int_{\Sigma}\int_0^{a_1} \frac{1}{a_1(2+\tilde{r}_3)} \cdot \exp\left(-\frac{\tilde{X}_3}{2+\tilde{r}_3}\right) ds \cdot g\left(\vec{p}\right) d\vec{p}, \tag{8.76}$$

where $\tilde{X}_{3(I)}$ and $\tilde{r}_3$ are given by Eqs. (8.74) and (8.75). By applying a linear approximation from the Taylor series expansion of $\exp\left(-\frac{\tilde{X}_3}{2+\tilde{r}_3}\right)$ and another linear approximation to $\frac{1}{2+\tilde{r}_3}$, Eq. (8.76) simplifies under scenario I to

$$m_g\left(\tilde{x}_{3(I)}\right) \approx \int_\Sigma \int_0^{a_1} \left[\frac{1}{4}\tilde{r}_3^3 - \frac{1}{4}\left(2+\tilde{x}_{3(I)}\right)\tilde{r}_3^2 + \left(\tilde{x}_{3(I)}-1\right)\tilde{r}_3 + 2 - \tilde{x}_{3(I)}\right] a_1^{-1} ds$$
$$\cdot g\left(\vec{p}\right) d\vec{p}\,.$$

By substituting Eqs. (8.74) and (8.75) into the above equation and integrating $\tilde{x}_{3(I)}$ with respect to s, we have after algebraic simplification

$$m_g(\dot{\mathcal{X}}_{3(I)}) = \frac{1}{\dashv_1}\int_\Sigma g(\vec{p})\{\frac{1}{4}[\sum_{j=1}^3 p_j^6 + 3\sum_{j\neq k\neq \ell} p_j^4(p_k^2+p_\ell^2) + 6\prod_{j=1}^3 p_j^2$$
$$-6\left(\sum_{j=1}^3 p_j^{(0)} p_j^5 + \sum_{j\neq k\neq \ell} p_j^4\left(p_k^{(0)}p_k + p_\ell^{(0)}p_\ell\right)\right)$$
$$-12\left(\sum_{j\neq k\neq \ell} p_j^{(0)} p_j^3(p_k^2+p_\ell^2) + \sum_{j\neq k\neq \ell} p_j^{(0)} p_j p_k^2 p_\ell^2\right)$$
$$+12\left[\sum_{j=1}^3 p_j^{(0)2} p_j^4 + \sum_{j\neq k}\left(p_j^{(0)2} + p_k^{(0)2}\right)p_j^2 p_k^2\right.$$
$$\left.+2\left(\sum_{j\neq k} p_j^{(0)} p_k^{(0)}\left(p_j^3 p_k + p_j p_k^3\right) + \sum_{j\neq k\neq \ell} p_j^{(0)} p_k^{(0)} p_j p_k p_\ell^2\right)\right]$$
$$+\frac{1}{4}(3\rho_0 - 2 - \dot{\mathcal{X}}_{3(I)})\sum_{j=1}^3 p_j^4 + \frac{1}{2}(3\rho_0 - 2 - \dot{\mathcal{X}}_{3(I)})\sum_{j\neq k} p_j^2 p_k^2$$
$$-2\left[\sum_{j=1}^3 p_j^{(0)3} p_j^3 + 3\sum_{j\neq k\neq \ell} p_j^{(0)2} p_j^2\left(p_k^{(0)}p_k + p_\ell^{(0)}p_\ell\right) + 6\prod_{j=1}^3 p_j^{(0)}p_j\right]\}d\vec{p}$$
$$+\frac{1}{\dashv_1}\int_\Sigma g(\vec{p})\{-(3\rho_0 - 2 - \dot{\mathcal{X}}_{3(I)})\left[\sum_{j=1}^3 p_j^{(0)} p_j^3 + \sum_{j\neq k\neq \ell} p_j^{(0)} p_j(p_k^2+p_\ell^2)\right] + 3\rho_0\sum_{j=1}^3 p_j^{(0)2}$$
$$-(2+\dot{x}_{3(I)})\sum_{j=1}^3 p_j^{(0)} p_j^2 + \frac{1}{4}\left[3\rho_0^2 - 4\rho_0 - 4 + 2(2-\rho_0)\dot{x}_{3(I)}\right]\sum_{j=1}^3 p_j^2$$
$$+\left[6\rho_0 - 2(2+\dot{x}_{3(I)})\right]\sum_{j\neq k} p_j^{(0)} p_k^{(0)} p_j p_k$$
$$+\left[2(\rho_0+1) + (\rho_0-2)\dot{x}_{3(I)}\right]\sum_{j=1}^3 p_j^{(0)} p_j$$
$$+\frac{1}{4}\rho_0\left[\rho_0^2 - 2\rho_0 - 4 + (4-\rho_0)\dot{x}_{3(I)}\right]\}d\vec{p}\,, \tag{8.77}$$

where

$$\dot{x}_{3(I)} = \int_0^{a_1} \tilde{x}_{3(I)} ds = \sum_{j=1}^{3} \dot{b}_{j(I)} n_j^2 - 2\sum_{j \neq k} \dot{b}_{jk(I)} n_j n_k - N a_1,$$

$$\dot{b}_{1(I)} = \frac{c_{1(I)}}{n_1^{(0)}} + c_{2(I)} \left(\frac{1}{n_2^{(0)}} + \frac{1}{n_3^{(0)}} \right),$$

$$\dot{b}_{2(I)} = \frac{c_{1(I)}}{n_2^{(0)}} + c_{2(I)} \left(\frac{1}{n_1^{(0)}} + \frac{1}{n_3^{(0)}} \right),$$

$$\dot{b}_{3(I)} = \frac{c_{1(I)}}{n_3^{(0)}} + c_{2(I)} \left(\frac{1}{n_1^{(0)}} + \frac{1}{n_2^{(0)}} \right),$$

$$\dot{b}_{12(I)} = c_{3(I)} \left(\frac{1}{n_1^{(0)}} + \frac{1}{n_2^{(0)}} \right) - \frac{c_{2(I)}}{n_3^{(0)}},$$

$$\dot{b}_{13(I)} = c_{3(I)} \left(\frac{1}{n_1^{(0)}} + \frac{1}{n_3^{(0)}} \right) - \frac{c_{2(I)}}{n_2^{(0)}},$$

$$\dot{b}_{23(I)} = c_{3(I)} \left(\frac{1}{n_2^{(0)}} + \frac{1}{n_3^{(0)}} \right) - \frac{c_{2(I)}}{n_1^{(0)}},$$

$$c_{1(I)} = \frac{1}{9}\left[a_1(5-3a_1)(1-3a_1)^{-1} - \frac{4}{3}\ln(1-3a_1) \right],$$

$$c_{2(I)} = \frac{1}{9}\left[\frac{2}{3}\ln(1-3a_1) + a_1(2-3a_1)(1-3a_1)^{-1} \right],$$

$$c_{3(I)} = \frac{1}{9}\left[\frac{2}{3}\ln(1-3a_1) + a_1(1+3a_1)(1-3a_1)^{-1} \right],$$

$$\rho_0 = \sum_{j=1}^{3} p_j^{(0)2}.$$

With an assumption of $t_1 = t_2 = t_3 \equiv t$, we have under scenario II

$$\vec{\tilde{n}}_{(II)} \equiv \begin{bmatrix} \tilde{n}_{1(II)} \\ \tilde{n}_{2(II)} \\ \tilde{n}_{3(II)} \end{bmatrix} = \frac{1-t}{1-3t} \begin{bmatrix} (1-t)^2 n_1 - t(1-t)n_2 + t^2 n_3 \\ -t(1-t)n_1 + (1-t)^2 n_2 - t(1-t)n_3 \\ t^2 n_1 - t(1-t)n_2 + \left(1-3t+t^2\right)n_3 \end{bmatrix}, \quad 0 < t < a_2, \tag{8.78}$$

where $a_2 \equiv a_1 = \min_{j=1,2,3} \left\{ \frac{1}{3}, \widehat{p}_j \right\}$.
By using Eq. (8.78), we have

$$\sum_{j=1}^{3} \tilde{n}_{j(II)}^2 = \sum_{j=1}^{3} b_{j(II)} n_j^2 - 2\left[b_{12(II)} n_1 n_2 + b_{23(II)} n_2 n_3 - b_{13(II)} n_1 n_3 \right], \tag{8.79}$$

where

$$\tilde{b}_{1(II)} = \frac{1}{[(1-t)(1-3t)]^2}\left[\frac{(1-t)^4}{n_1^{(0)}} + \frac{t^2(1-t)^2}{n_2^{(0)}} + \frac{t^4}{n_3^{(0)}}\right],$$

$$\tilde{b}_{2(II)} = \frac{1}{[(1-t)(1-3t)]^2}\left[t^2(1-t)^2\left(\frac{1}{n_1^{(0)}} + \frac{1}{n_3^{(0)}}\right) + \frac{(1-t)^4}{n_2^{(0)}}\right],$$

$$\tilde{b}_{3(II)} = \frac{1}{[(1-t)(1-3t)]^2}\left[\frac{t^4}{n_1^{(0)}} + \frac{t^2(1-t)^2}{n_2^{(0)}} + \frac{(t^2-3t+1)^2}{n_3^{(0)}}\right],$$

$$\tilde{b}_{12(II)} = \frac{1}{[(1-t)(1-3t)]^2}\left[t(1-t)^3\left(\frac{1}{n_1^{(0)}} + \frac{1}{n_2^{(0)}}\right) + \frac{t^3(1-t)}{n_3^{(0)}}\right],$$

$$\tilde{b}_{23(II)} = \frac{1}{[(1-t)(1-3t)]^2}\left[\frac{t^3(1-t)}{n_1^{(0)}} + \frac{t(1-t)^3}{n_2^{(0)}} + \frac{t(1-t)(t^2-3t+1)}{n_3^{(0)}}\right],$$

$$\tilde{b}_{13(II)} = \frac{1}{[(1-t)(1-3t)]^2}\left[t^2(1-t)^2\left(\frac{1}{n_1^{(0)}} + \frac{1}{n_2^{(0)}}\right) + \frac{t^2(t^2-3t+1)}{n_3^{(0)}}\right].$$

By substituting Eq. (8.79) into Eq. (8.63) and integrating $\tilde{X}_{3(II)}$ with respect to t over $[0, a_2]$, we have

$$\dot{X}_{3(II)} = \int_0^{a_2} \tilde{X}_{3(II)}dt = \sum\nolimits_{j=1}^{3} \dot{b}_{j(II)}n_j^2 - 2\left[\dot{b}_{12(II)}n_1n_2 + \dot{b}_{23(II)}n_2n_3 - \dot{b}_{13(II)}n_1n_3\right] - Na_2, \tag{8.80}$$

where

$$\dot{b}_{1(II)} = \frac{c_{1(II)}}{n_1^{(0)}} + \frac{c_{2(II)}}{n_2^{(0)}} + \frac{c_{3(II)}}{n_3^{(0)}},$$

$$\dot{b}_{2(II)} = \frac{c_{1(II)}}{n_2^{(0)}} + c_{2(II)}\left(\frac{1}{n_1^{(0)}} + \frac{1}{n_3^{(0)}}\right),$$

$$\dot{b}_{3(II)} = \frac{c_{3(II)}}{n_1^{(0)}} + \frac{c_{2(II)}}{n_2^{(0)}} + \frac{c_{4(II)}}{n_3^{(0)}},$$

$$\dot{b}_{12(II)} = c_{5(II)}\left(\frac{1}{n_1^{(0)}} + \frac{1}{n_2^{(0)}}\right) + \frac{c_{6(II)}}{n_3^{(0)}},$$

$$\dot{b}_{23(II)} = \frac{c_{6(II)}}{n_1^{(0)}} + \frac{c_{5(II)}}{n_2^{(0)}} + \frac{c_{7(II)}}{n_3^{(0)}},$$

$$\dot{b}_{13(II)} = c_{2(II)}\left(\frac{1}{n_1^{(0)}} + \frac{1}{n_2^{(0)}}\right) + \frac{c_{8(II)}}{n_3^{(0)}},$$

$$c_{1(II)} = \int_0^{a_2} \frac{(1-t)^2}{(1-3t)^2}dt = \frac{1}{27}\left[\frac{3a_2(5-3a_2)}{1-3a_2} - 4\ln(1-3a_2),\right.$$

$$c_{2(II)} = \int_0^{a_2} \frac{t^2}{(1-3t)^2}dt = \frac{1}{27}\left[\frac{3a_2(2-3a_2)}{1-3a_2} + 2\ln(1-3a_2),\right.$$

$$c_{3(II)} = \int_0^{a_2} \frac{t^4}{[(1-t)(1-3t)]^2}dt = \frac{1}{108}$$
$$\times\left[\frac{3a_2\left(12a_2^2 - 44a_2 + 14\right)}{(1-a_2)(1-3a_2)} + 27\ln(1-a_2) + 5\ln(1-3a_2)\right],$$

$$c_{4(II)} = \int_0^{a_2} \frac{\left(t^2 - 3t + 1\right)^2}{[(1-t)(1-3t)]^2}dt = \frac{1}{108}$$
$$\times\left[\frac{3a_2\left(12a_2^2 - 44a_2 + 14\right)}{(1-a_2)(1-3a_2)} - 27\ln(1-a_2) - 23\ln(1-3a_2)\right],$$

$$c_{5(II)} = \int_0^{a_2} \frac{t(1-t)}{(1-3t)^2}dt = \frac{1}{27}\left[\frac{3a_2(1+3a_2)}{1-3a_2} + \ln(1-3a_2),\right.$$

$$c_{6(II)} = \int_0^{a_2} \frac{t^3}{(1-t)(1-3t)^2}dt = \frac{1}{108}$$
$$\times\left[\frac{3a_2(6a_2+1)}{1-3a_2} - 27\ln(1-a_2) + 7\ln(1-3a_2)\right],$$

$$c_{7(II)} = \int_0^{a_2} \frac{t\left(t^2-3t+1\right)}{(1-t)(1-3t)^2}dt = \frac{1}{108}$$
$$\times\left[\frac{6a_2(3a_2-2)}{1-3a_2} + 63\ln(1-a_2) - 31\ln(1-3a_2)\right],$$

$$c_{8(II)} = \int_0^{a_2} \frac{t^2\left(t^2-3t+1\right)}{[(1-t)(1-3t)]^2}dt = \frac{1}{54}\left[\frac{3a_2\left(6a_2^2+5a_2-2\right)}{(1-a_2)(1-3a_2)} - 2\ln(1-3a_2)\right].$$

If the prior distribution for $g\left(\vec{p}\right)$ is taken to be a symmetric Dirichlet's distribution with the flattening constant (or hyper-parameter) τ ($\tau > 0$) [8], Eq. (8.77) is reduced to

$$m_g\left(\tau|\dot{X}_{3(I)}\right) = \frac{1}{a_1} \cdot \frac{d_4\tau^4 + d_3\tau^3 + d_2\tau^2 + d_1\tau + d_0}{12(3\tau+1)(3\tau+2)(3\tau+4)(3\tau+5)}, \tag{8.81}$$

where

$$d_0 = 40\left[3\rho_0^3 - 15\rho_0^2 + 48\rho_0 - 24\rho_3 - \left(3\rho_0^2 - 18\rho_0 - 14\right)\dot{X}_{3(I)} + 3\right],$$

$$d_1 = 702\rho_0^3 + 2450\rho_0^2 + 138\rho_0 + (960\rho_0 + 1920)\rho_1 - 1440\rho_2 - 2736\rho_3 - \left(702\rho_0^2 - 4692\rho_0 + 320\rho_1 - 5274\right)\dot{X}_{3(I)} + 2722,$$

$$d_2 = 1323\rho_0^3 - 6101\rho_0^2 + 5307\rho_0 + (2736\rho_0 + 1728)\rho_1 - 1128\rho_2 - 1240\rho_3 - \left(1323\rho_0^2 - 9306\rho_0 + 912\rho_1 + 8425\right)\dot{X}_{3(I)} + 5943,$$

$$d_3 = 972\rho_0^3 - 5130\rho_0^2 + 2568\rho_0 + (1176\rho_0 + 464)\rho_1 - 864\rho_2 - 432\rho_3 - \left(972\rho_0^2 - 7020\rho_0 + 392\rho_1 + 6470\right)\dot{X}_{3(I)} + 4382,$$

$$d_4 = 243\rho_0^3 - 1377\rho_0^2 + 891\rho_0 + (648\rho_0 - 432)\rho_1 - 216\rho_2 - 72\rho_3 - \left(243\rho_0^2 - 1782\rho_0 + 432\rho_1 + 1647\right)\dot{X}_{3(I)} + 1059,$$

$$\rho_1 = \sum_{j \neq k} p_j^{(0)} p_k^{(0)},$$

$$\rho_2 = \sum_{j \neq k \neq \ell} \left(p_j^{(0)} + p_k^{(0)}\right) p_\ell^{(0)2},$$

$$\rho_3 = \sum\nolimits_{j=1}^{3} p_j^{(0)3}.$$

Similarly, $m_g\left(\tau|\dot{X}_{3(II)}\right)$ has exactly the same expression like Eq. (8.81) except that $\dot{X}_{3(I)}$ and a_1 are replaced by $\dot{X}_{3(II)}$ and a_2 accordingly.

To avoid the use of hyper-prior distribution on τ [9], the non-Bayesian approach is used to find the stationary point $\tau_{\max(.)}$ for $m_g\left(\tau|\dot{X}_{3(.)}\right)$. By using elementary technique in calculus to find the first derivative of $m_g\left(\tau|\dot{X}_{3(I)}\right)$ and set it equal zero, we have after simplification

$$\begin{aligned}&(324d_4 - 81d_3)\tau^6 + (882d_4 - 162d_2)\tau^5 \\ &+ (702d_4 + 441d_3 - 324d_2 - 243d_1)\tau^4 \\ &+ (160d_4 + 468d_3 - 648d_1 - 324d_0)\tau^3 \\ &+ (120d_3 + 234d_2 - 441d_1 - 972d_0)\tau^2 + (80d_2 - 882d_0)\tau + 40d_1 \\ &- 234d_0 = 0.\end{aligned} \tag{8.82}$$

The subroutine "ROOTS" in the MATLAB was used to solve Eq. (8.82) [16].

According to the terms of Good [7], the way to estimate τ_{max} is called as the type II maximum likelihood or the maximum -hyper-prior likelihood method.

8.4 Exercises

1. Show that Eqs. (8.26), (8.27), (8.30), (8.31), (8.36), (8.42), and (8.43) hold.
2. Show that Eq. (8.22) in Example 8.3 hold.

References

1. Agresti, A. (2002) Categorical data analysis, 2, Wiley, New York.
2. Askey, R. A., & Roy, R. (2010). Chapter 5: Gamma function. In F. W. Olver et al. (Eds.), *NIST handbook of mathematical functions*. National Institute of Standards and Technology, Cambridge University Press.
3. Berger, J. O., & Sellcke, T. (1987). Testing a point null hypothesis: The irreconcilability of p values and evidence. *Journal of the American Statistical Association, 82*, 112–122.
4. Casella, G., & Berger, R. (1987). Reconciling Bayesian and frequentist evidence in the one-sided testing problem. *Journal of the American Statistical Association, 82*, 106–111.
5. Cornfield, J. (1956). A statistical problem arising from retrospective studies. In *The third Berkeley symposium* (pp. 135–148). University of California Press.
6. Cox, D. R., & Reid, N. (1987). Approximations to noncentral distributions. *Canadian Journal of Statistics, 15*, 105–114.
7. Fisher, R. A. (1922). On the interpretation of the chi-square from contingency tables, and the calculation of p. *Journal of the Royal Statistical Society, 85*, 87–94.
8. Good, I. J. (1975). The Bayes factor against equiprobability of a multinomial population assuming a symmetric Dirichlet prior. *The Annals of Statistics, 3*, 246–250.
9. Good, I. J., & Crook, J. F. (1974). The Bayes/Non-Bayes compromise and the multinomial distribution. *Journal of the American Statistical Association, 69*, 711–720.
10. Goodman, S. (1999a). Toward evidence-based medical statistics. 1: The p value fallacy. *Annals of Internal Medicine, 130*, 995–1004.
11. Goodman, S. (1999b). Toward evidence-based medical statistics. 2: The Bayes factor. *Annals of Internal Medicine, 130*, 1005–1013.
12. Kass, R. E., & Raftery, A. E. (1995). Bayes factor. *Journal of the American Statistical Association, 90*, 773–795.
13. Lancaster, H. O. (1969). *The chi-squared distribution*. Wiley.
14. Lee, T.-S. (2015). The Bayes factor for case-control studies with misclassified data. *Journal of Modern Applied Statistical Methods, 14*, 201–218.
15. Lee, T.-S. (2018). The Bayes factor for the misclassified categorical data. *International Journal of Statistics and Probability (IJSP), 7*(4), 91–98.
16. Lee, T.-S. (2020). *Medical statistics: A practical approach*. World Scientific Publishing Company.
17. Redfern, D., & Campbell, C. (1998). *The MATLAB 5 handbook*. Springer.
18. Woodward, M. (2005). *Epidemiology: Study design and data analysis* (2nd ed.). Chapman & Hall/CRC Press.

Part V
Contingency Tables

Chapter 9
Misclassification in Two-Way Tables

9.1 The Double Sampling Scheme

The double sampling scheme [6] is described as follows:

Step 1 A random sample of N units is drawn from the population of interest.
Step 2 A subsample of n units is drawn from the main sample and each of these n units is measured by both diagnostic methods. Let n_{ij} denote the number of measured units, i, j = 1, 0.
Step 3 The remaining N—n units are measured only by the fallible diagnostic method. Let X denotes the number of units whose true measurements is "1" and let Y denote the number of units whose fallible measurements is "0."

The resulting data is represented in Fig. 9.1

For each unit in the sample, we define the random variable F_i, $i = 1, 2, \ldots$ n, as follows:

$F_i = 1$ if the ith unit belongs to category 1; = 0 otherwise.

The random variables F_i, $i = 1, 2, \ldots$ N, are mutually independent. Let p = Pr (F_i = 1), where q = 1 − p. The random variable F_i^* are similarly defined as F_i. Misclassification occurs when $F_i \neq F_i^*$.

An assumption is assumed that the following conditions are satisfied:

1. The probability of misclassification is equal to φ_i for all sampling units having $F_i = 1$.
2. The probability of misclassification is equal to ψ_i for all sampling units having $F_i = 0$.
3. The misclassification errors are independent among all sampling units.

Since φ and ψ remain the same for all units, we drop the subscripts on F_i and F_i^*. Thus, p, φ, and ψ are represented by

T.-S. Lee, *Misclassification in Epidemiology*, Emerging Topics in Statistics and Biostatistics, https://doi.org/10.1007/978-3-032-12563-7_9

		F^* (Fallible diagnostic method)		Total
		1	0	
F (True diagnostic method)	1	n_{11}	n_{10}	n_{1+}
	0	n_{01}	n_{00}	n_{0+}
Total		n_{+1}	n_{+0}	n
		X	Y	N - n

Fig. 9.1 A graphic representation of the double sampling scheme

$$\mathrm{p} = \Pr(\mathrm{F} = 1) \tag{9.1}$$

$$\varphi = \Pr(F^* = 0 | \; F = 1) \tag{9.2}$$

$$\psi = \Pr(F^* = 1 | \; F = 0) \tag{9.3}$$

We also define

$$p^* = \Pr(F^* = 1). \tag{9.4}$$

Thus,

$$p^* = p \cdot (1 - \varphi) + q \cdot \psi = p \cdot \Delta + \psi, \tag{9.5}$$

where $\Delta = 1 - \varphi - \psi$.

To estimate the unknown parameters p, φ, and ψ, we apply the maximum likelihood estimation. The distribution of X is binomial with probability $p^*$and sample size N—n. Since the second sample of N—n units is independent of the first sample of n units, the joint distribution of n_{11}, n_{11}, n_{11}, n_{11}, X and Y is given by

$$\begin{aligned} \mathcal{L} &= C\left[\frac{p(1-\varphi)}{p^*}\right]^{n_{11}} \left(\frac{p\varphi}{1-p^*}\right)^{n_{10}} \left(\frac{q\psi}{p^*}\right)^{n_{01}} \left[\frac{q(1-\psi)}{1-p^*}\right]^{n_{00}} (p^*)^{X+n_{+1}} (1-p^*)^{Y+n_{+0}} \\ &= C v_1^{n_{11}} v_2^{n_{10}} (1-v_1)^{n_{01}} (1-v_2)^{n_{00}} (p^*)^{X+n_{+1}} (1-p^*)^{Y+n_{+0}}, \end{aligned} \tag{9.6}$$

where p^* is given by Eq. (9.5),

$$v_1 = \frac{p(1-\varphi)}{p^*}, \tag{9.7}$$

$$v_2 = \frac{p\varphi}{1-p^*}. \tag{9.8}$$

and C is a constant independent of p, φ, and ψ. By taking the partial differentiation of the logarithm of Eq. (9.6) with respect to p, φ, and ψ and set them equal to zero,

$$\frac{\partial \ln \mathcal{L}}{\partial p} = C\left\{ n_{11}\cdot\frac{\partial \ln v_1}{\partial p} + n_{10}\cdot\frac{\partial \ln v_2}{\partial p} + n_{01}\cdot\frac{\partial \ln(1-v_1)}{\partial p} + n_{00}\cdot\frac{\partial \ln(1-v_2)}{\partial p} + (X+n_{+1})\cdot\frac{\partial \ln p^*}{\partial p} + (Y+n_{+0})\cdot\frac{\partial \ln(1-p^*)}{\partial p} = 0. \right. \tag{9.9}$$

On the other hand,

$$\frac{\partial \ln v_1}{\partial p} = \frac{\partial \ln v_1}{\partial v_1}\cdot\frac{\partial v_1}{\partial p} = \frac{\psi}{p^* p}, \tag{9.10}$$

$$\frac{\partial \ln v_2}{\partial p} = \frac{\partial \ln v_2}{\partial v_2}\cdot\frac{\partial v_2}{\partial p} = \frac{1-\psi}{p(1-p^*)}, \tag{9.11}$$

$$\frac{\partial \ln(1-v_1)}{\partial p} = \frac{\partial \ln(1-v_1)}{\partial(1-v_1)}\cdot\frac{\partial(1-v_1)}{\partial p} = \frac{\varphi-1}{(1-p)p^*}, \tag{9.12}$$

$$\frac{\partial \ln(1-v_2)}{\partial p} = \frac{\partial \ln(1-v_2)}{\partial(1-v_2)}\cdot\frac{\partial(1-v_2)}{\partial p} = -\frac{\varphi}{(1-p)(1-p^*)}, \tag{9.13}$$

$$\frac{\partial \ln p^*}{\partial p} = \frac{\partial \ln p^*}{\partial p^*}\cdot\frac{\partial p^*}{\partial p} = \frac{1-\varphi-\psi}{p^*}, \tag{9.14}$$

$$\frac{\partial \ln(1-p^*)}{\partial p} = \frac{\partial \ln(1-p^*)}{\partial(1-p^*)}\cdot\frac{\partial(1-p^*)}{\partial p} = -\frac{1-\varphi-\psi}{1-p^*}. \tag{9.15}$$

By substituting Eqs. (9.10) to (9.15) into Eq. (9.9),

$$\begin{aligned}&(1-\psi)[n_{11}\psi(1-p) - n_{01}(1-\varphi)p] \\ &+ p^*\{(1-\psi)[(n_{10}-n_{11}\psi)(1-p) + p(1-\varphi)n_{01}] - n_{00}\varphi p\} = \\ &-p(1-p)(1-\psi)(1-\varphi-\psi)(X+n_{+1}-Np^*).\end{aligned} \tag{9.16}$$

Similarly, on one hand,

$$\frac{\partial \ln \mathcal{L}}{\partial \varphi} = C\left\{ n_{11}\cdot\frac{\partial \ln v_1}{\partial \varphi} + n_{10}\cdot\frac{\partial \ln v_2}{\partial \varphi} + n_{01}\cdot\frac{\partial \ln(1-v_1)}{\partial \varphi} + n_{00}\cdot\frac{\partial \ln(1-v_2)}{\partial \varphi} + (X+n_{+1})\cdot\frac{\partial \ln p^*}{\partial \varphi} + (Y+n_{+0})\cdot\frac{\partial \ln(1-p^*)}{\partial \varphi} = 0. \right. \tag{9.17}$$

On the other hand,

$$\frac{\partial \ln v_1}{\partial \varphi} = \frac{\partial \ln v_1}{\partial v_1}\cdot\frac{\partial v_1}{\partial \varphi} = \frac{-\psi(1-p)}{(1-\varphi)p^*}, \tag{9.18}$$

$$\frac{\partial\, ln\, v_2}{\partial \varphi} = \frac{\partial\, ln\, v_2}{\partial v_2} \cdot \frac{\partial v_2}{\partial \varphi} = \frac{(1-p)(1-\psi)}{\varphi(1-p^*)}, \tag{9.19}$$

$$\frac{\partial \ln(1-v_1)}{\partial \varphi} = \frac{\partial\, ln(1-v_1)}{\partial(1-v_1)} \cdot \frac{\partial(1-v_1)}{\partial \varphi} = \frac{p}{p^*}, \tag{9.20}$$

$$\frac{\partial \ln(1-v_2)}{\partial \varphi} = \frac{\partial\, ln(1-v_2)}{\partial(1-v_2)} \cdot \frac{\partial(1-v_2)}{\partial \varphi} = -\frac{p}{1-p^*}, \tag{9.21}$$

$$\frac{\partial \ln p^*}{\partial \varphi} = \frac{\partial\, ln p^*}{\partial p^*} \cdot \frac{\partial p^*}{\partial \varphi} = \frac{p}{p^*}, \tag{9.22}$$

$$\frac{\partial \ln(1-p^*)}{\partial \varphi} = \frac{\partial \ln(1-p^*)}{\partial(1-p^*)} \cdot \frac{\partial(1-p^*)}{\partial \varphi} = \frac{-p}{1-p^*}. \tag{9.23}$$

By substituting Eqs. (9.18) to (9.23) into Eq. (9.17),

$$(1-p) \times \{-\varphi\psi n_{11} + [\varphi\psi n_{1+} - (1-\varphi-\psi)\text{p}^*\} + p\varphi(1-\varphi)(n_{01} - n_{0+}p^*) = -\varphi(1-\varphi)p(X - n_{+1} - Np^*). \tag{9.24}$$

Again, on the one hand,

$$\frac{\partial\, ln\, L}{\partial \psi} = C\left\{ n_{11} \cdot \frac{\partial\, ln\, v_1}{\partial \psi} + n_{10} \cdot \frac{\partial\, ln\, v_2}{\partial \psi} + n_{01} \cdot \frac{\partial \ln(1-v_1)}{\partial \psi} + n_{00} \cdot \frac{\partial \ln(1-v_2)}{\partial \psi} + (X + n_{+1}) \cdot \frac{\partial\, lnp^*}{\partial \psi} + (Y + n_{+0}) \cdot \frac{\partial \ln(1-p^*)}{\partial \psi} \right. = 0. \tag{9.25}$$

On the other hand,

$$\frac{\partial\, ln\, v_1}{\partial \psi} = \frac{\partial\, ln\, v_1}{\partial v_1} \cdot \frac{\partial v_1}{\partial \psi} = \frac{-(1-p)}{p^*}, \tag{9.26}$$

$$\frac{\partial\, ln\, v_2}{\partial \psi} = \frac{\partial\, ln\, v_2}{\partial v_2} \cdot \frac{\partial v_2}{\partial \psi} = \frac{1-p}{1-p^*}, \tag{9.27}$$

$$\frac{\partial \ln(1-v_1)}{\partial \psi} = \frac{\partial\, ln(1-v_1)}{\partial(1-v_1)} \cdot \frac{\partial(1-v_1)}{\partial \psi} = -\frac{p(1-\varphi)}{\psi p^*}, \tag{9.28}$$

$$\frac{\partial \ln(1-v_2)}{\partial \psi} = \frac{\partial\, ln(1-v_2)}{\partial(1-v_2)} \cdot \frac{\partial(1-v_2)}{\partial \psi} = -\frac{\varphi p}{(1-\psi)(1-p^*)}, \tag{9.29}$$

$$\frac{\partial \ln p^*}{\partial \psi} = \frac{\partial\, ln p^*}{\partial p^*} \cdot \frac{\partial p^*}{\partial \psi} = \frac{1-p}{p^*}, \tag{9.30}$$

$$\frac{\partial \ln(1-p^*)}{\partial \psi} = \frac{\partial \ln(1-p^*)}{\partial (1-p^*)} \cdot \frac{\partial (1-p^*)}{\partial \psi} = -\frac{1-p}{1-p^*}. \tag{9.31}$$

By substituting Eqs. (9.26) to (9.31) into Eq. (9.25),

$$\begin{aligned}&\psi(1-\psi)(-n_{11}+n_{1+}p^*)\\&+p\{(1-\psi)[n_{11}\psi+n_{01}(1-\varphi)]-\{(1-\psi)[(n_{11}-n_{10})\psi+n_{01}(1-\varphi)]-n_{00}\varphi\psi\}p^*\}\}=-\psi(1-\psi)(1-p)(X+n_{+1}-Np^*).\end{aligned} \tag{9.32}$$

It is difficult to solve directly from Eqs. (9.16), (9.24), and (9.32) for the maximum likelihood estimators $\widehat{p}$, $\widehat{\varphi}$, and $\widehat{\psi}$. Instead, we can use the invariance property of the maximum likelihood estimation by noting that the maximum likelihood estimators of the N units which have been classified in category 1 and 0 by the fallible diagnostic instrument F^* are given respectively by $\widehat{p}_{F^*=1} = \frac{X+n_{+1}}{N}$ and $\widehat{p}_{F^*=0} = \frac{Y+n_{+0}}{N}$. Therefore, $\widehat{p}$ is the proportional addition of the above two maximum likelihood estimators, namely,

$$\widehat{p} = \frac{n_{11}}{n_{+1}}\widehat{p}_{F^*=1} + \frac{n_{10}}{n_{+0}}\widehat{p}_{F^*=0} = \frac{n_{11}(X+n_{+1})}{Nn_{+1}} + \frac{n_{10}(Y+n_{+0})}{Nn_{+0}}. \tag{9.33}$$

Again, from the relation $\varphi p = \frac{n_{10}}{n_{+0}} p_{F^*=0}$, we have

$$\begin{aligned}\widehat{\varphi p} &= \frac{n_{10}}{n_{+0}}\widehat{p}_{F^*=0}, \text{ or}\\ \widehat{\varphi} &= \frac{n_{10}(Y+n_{+0})}{n_{+0}\widehat{p}}.\end{aligned} \tag{9.34}$$

Similarly, from the relation $(1-p)\psi = \frac{n_{01}}{n_{+1}} p_{F^*=1}$,

$$\widehat{\psi} = \frac{n_{01}(X+n_{+1})}{n_{+1}(1-\widehat{p})}. \tag{9.35}$$

By applying the delta method [7], the asymptotic variance of $\widehat{p}$ is given by

$$\sigma^2_{\widehat{p}} = \frac{pq}{n}\left[1 - \frac{pq\Delta^2}{p^*(1-p^*)}\right] + \frac{(pq\Delta)^2}{Np^*(1-p^*)}. \tag{9.36}$$

where Δ is given by (Eq. 9.5).

Example 9.1

An arthritis study in the Arsenal Health District of Pittsburgh was conducted in July 1952 through a household morbidity survey by using a random sample of 3000 households. All the persons over 14 years of age in these households were classified based on the information regarding rheumatism and arthritis obtained by nonmedical

Table 9.1 The joint pain data were collected from nonmedical interview and the physician's examination

		Interview result			
		Yes	No	Total	
Physician's examination	Yes	247	77	324	First sample
	No	35	119	154	
	Total	282	196	478	
		272	206	478	Second sample
		X	Y		

interviews. This resulted in a total of 956 persons. Each person in the sample was visited in his/her home by a nonmedical interview equipped with a detailed arthritis questionnaire; the individuals who were interviewed were urged to have an examination by physicians in the arthritis clinic. Some persons refused or unavailable for an interview and some did not return to the clinic for examination. The final data included 478 persons who had had both the interview and the examination [3]. In this example, joint pain is an error-prone variable; the interview data is regarded as the fallible data, whereas the physician's examination information as the true data.

A second random sample of 478 persons was collected from the interview. The entire data are given in Table 9.1.

(a) Find the maximum likelihood estimators of the prevalence ($\widehat{p}$) of the joint pain variable, the false negative and false positive rates of the classification procedure.
(b) Find the 95% confidence interval of $\widehat{p}$.

Solution

(a) From Table 9.1, $n_{11} = 247$, $n_{10} = 77$, $n_{01} = 35$, $n_{00} = 119$, $n_{+1} = 282$, $n_{+01} = 196$, N = 956, X = 272, and Y = 206. By substituting the above information into Eqs. (9.33) to (9.35),

$$\widehat{p} = \frac{247(282+272)}{272 \cdot 956} + \frac{77(196+206)}{196 \cdot 956} = 0.672772 \approx 0.67, \tag{9.37}$$

$$\widehat{\varphi} = \frac{\left[\frac{(247*(282+272)}{282 \cdot 956}\right]}{0.67} = 0.245547 \approx 0.25, \tag{9.38}$$

$$\widehat{\psi} = \frac{\left[\frac{35(196+206)}{196 \cdot 956}\right]}{(1-0.67)} = 0.219796 \approx 0.22. \tag{9.39}$$

The maximum likelihood estimators are given, respectively, by Eqs. (9.37) to (9.39).

(b) By applying Eqs. (9.37) to (9.39) to Eq. (9.5),

$$\widehat{p}^* = 0.67(1 - 0.25 - 0.22) = 0.5751 \approx 0.58. \tag{9.40}$$

By substituting Eqs. (9.37) to (9.40) into Eq. (9.36),

$$\widehat{\sigma}^2_{\widehat{p}} = \frac{0.67 \cdot 0.33}{478}\left[1 - \frac{0.67 \cdot 0.33 \cdot 0.53^2}{0.58 \cdot 0.42}\right] + \frac{(0.67 \cdot 0.33 \cdot 0.53)^2}{956 \cdot 0.58 \cdot 0.42} = 0.000401, \text{ or}$$
$$\widehat{\sigma}_{\widehat{p}} = 0.02. \tag{9.41}$$

By using Eqs. (9.37) and (9.41), the 95% confidence interval for p is given by

$$0.63 < p < 0.71.$$

9.2 Two-Way Tables with Joint Misclassification and Double Sampling

There are two methods of data collection: one which is error-free but expensive and the second which is fallible but inexpensive. An obvious dilemma faced by the researcher is that funds are limited. Should they sacrifice quantity for accuracy or should they sacrifice accuracy for quantity [1]? In this section the double sampling scheme is presented that gives the researcher another alternative which incorporates a balance between both measurement methods and their respective costs.

Consider the following situation. There are two methods of classification on each of two dichotomous categorical factors, X and Y. For the purpose of this section, one classification procedure is assumed to be error free and the other fallible; but the theory does not limit the use of these procedures from being extended method to any relationship between a more reliable and a less reliable one.

The probabilities of X, Y, X^*, Y^* are denoted by

$$p_{ij} = \Pr(X = i, Y = j), \quad i,j = 1,0; \tag{9.42}$$

and

$$p^*_{ij} = \Pr(X^* = i, Y^* = j), \quad i,j = 1,0; \tag{9.43}$$

The misclassified probabilities are the conditional probabilities given by

$$\varphi^{(k\ell)}_{ij} = \Pr(X^* = i, Y^* = j | X = k, Y = \ell), \tag{9.44}$$

and

$$\psi_{k\ell}^{(ij)} = \Pr(X = k, Y = \ell | X^* = i, Y^* = j). \tag{9.45}$$

The values of $\varphi_{11}^{(11)}$ and $\varphi_{00}^{(00)}$ are, respectively, called the sensitivity and specificity of the error-free method of (X, Y), whereas that of $\psi_{11}^{(11)}$ and $\psi_{00}^{(00)}$ the positive and negative predictive value of (X, Y).

The joint probability of X* = *i*, Y* = *j*, X = *k*, and Y = ℓ can be written as

$$\Pr(X^* = i, Y^* = j, X = k, Y = \ell) = \psi_{k\ell}^{(ij)} p_{ij}^* = \varphi_{ij}^{(k\ell)} p_{k\ell} \tag{9.46}$$

For each set given by the error-free method, there are four possible classes into which the fallible method might place the experimental unit as given in Table 9.2.

Assume that a random sample of size n is taken from the population and classified using both methods of classification. A second random sample of size N—n is classified by the fallible method only. The resulting frequency table is given in Table 9.3.

Table 9.2 Misclassification and marginal probabilities

class	X = 1,Y = 1	X = 1,Y = 0	X = 0,Y = 1	X = 0,Y = 0	Marginal
$X^* = 1,Y^* = 1$	$\varphi_{11}^{(11)} p_{11}$	$\varphi_{10}^{(11)} p_{10}$	$\varphi_{01}^{(11)} p_{01}$	$\varphi_{00}^{(11)} p_{00}$	p_{11}^*
$X^* = 1,Y^* = 0$	$\varphi_{11}^{(10)} p_{11}$	$\varphi_{10}^{(10)} p_{10}$	$\varphi_{01}^{(10)} p_{01}$	$\varphi_{00}^{(10)} p_{00}$	p_{01}^*
$X^* = 0,Y^* = 1$	$\varphi_{11}^{(01)} p_{11}$	$\varphi_{10}^{(01)} p_{10}$	$\varphi_{01}^{(01)} p_{01}$	$\varphi_{00}^{(01)} p_{00}$	p_{01}^*
$X^* = 0,Y^* = 0$	$\varphi_{11}^{(00)} p_{11}$	$\varphi_{10}^{(00)} p_{10}$	$\varphi_{01}^{(00)} p_{01}$	$\varphi_{00}^{(00)} p_{00}$	p_{00}^*
Marginal	p_{11}	p_{10}	p_{01}	p_{00}	

Where X and Y are of the error-free method; X* and Y* are of the fallible method

Table 9.3 Frequency table for double sampling method

class	X = 1,Y = 1	X = 1,Y = 0	X = 0,Y = 1	X = 0,Y = 0	Total
	First sample				
$X^* = 1,Y^* = 1$	$n_{11}^{(11)}$	$n_{10}^{(11)}$	$n_{01}^{(11)}$	$n_{00}^{(11)}$	n_{11}^*
$X^* = 1,Y^* = 0$	$n_{11}^{(10)}$	$n_{10}^{(10)}$	$n_{01}^{(10)}$	$n_{00}^{(10)}$	n_{10}^*
$X^* = 0,Y^* = 1$	$n_{11}^{(01)}$	$n_{10}^{(01)}$	$n_{01}^{(01)}$	$n_{00}^{(01)}$	n_{01}^*
$X^* = 0,Y^* = 0$	$n_{11}^{(00)}$	$n_{10}^{(00)}$	$n_{01}^{(00)}$	$n_{00}^{(00)}$	n_{00}^*
Total	n_{11}	n_{10}	n_{01}	n_{00}	n
Second sample					
Grand total					
$X^* = 1,Y^* = 1$			m_{11}		$m_{11} + n_{11}^*$
$X^* = 1,Y^* = 0$			m_{10}		$m_{10} + n_{10}^*$
$X^* = 0,Y^* = 1$			m_{01}		$m_{01} + n_{01}^*$
$X^* = 0,Y^* = 0$			m_{00}		$m_{00} + n_{00}^*$
Total			N - n		N

From Table 9.2, the relation between $\{p_{ij}\}$ and $\{p^*_{ij}\}$ is given by

$$\vec{p}^{\,*} = \mathcal{W}\vec{p}, \tag{9.47}$$

where $\vec{p}^{\,*} = \left(p^*_{11}, p^*_{10}, p^*_{01}, p^*_{00}\right)^T$, $\vec{p} = \left(p_{11}, p_{10}, p_{01}, p_{00}\right)^T$, and the misclassification matrix is given by

$$\mathcal{W} = \left[\varphi_{ij}^{(k\ell)}\right]_{i,j,k,\ell=0}^{1}. \tag{9.48}$$

It is assumed that $\mathcal{W}$ is nonsingular. The joint likelihood function of $\{n_{ij}^{(k\ell)}\}$, $\{n_{k\ell} - n_{ij}^{(k\ell)}\}$ and $\{m_{k\ell}\}$ is given by

$$\mathcal{L}\left(\varphi_{ij}^{(k\ell)}, p_{ij}\right) = c\prod_{i=0}^{1}\prod_{j=0}^{1}\prod_{k=0}^{1}\prod\nolimits_{\ell=0}^{1}\left(\varphi_{ij}^{(k\ell)}p_{ij}\right)^{n_{ij}^{(k\ell)}}$$
$$\cdot\left(p^*_{k\ell} - \varphi_{ij}^{(k\ell)}p_{ij}\right)^{n^*_{k\ell} - n_{ij}^{(k\ell)}} \cdot \left(p^*_{k\ell}\right)^{m_{k\ell} + n^*_{k\ell}}, \tag{9.49}$$

where c is a constant factor for a given sample.

Let us re-express Eq. (9.48) in terms of the following variable

$$s_{ij}^{(k\ell)} = \frac{\varphi_{ij}^{(k\ell)}p_{ij}}{p^*_{k\ell}}, \tag{9.50}$$

and then taking the natural logarithm of the likelihood function

$$\mathcal{L}^* = \ln\left[\mathcal{L}\left(s_{ij}^{(k\ell)}, p^*_{k\ell}\right)\right] = \sum\nolimits_{i,j=0}^{1} n_{ij}^{(k\ell)}\ln\left(s_{ij}^{(k\ell)}\right)$$
$$+\sum\nolimits_{k,\ell=0}^{1}\left(n^*_{k\ell} - n_{ij}^{(k\ell)}\right)\ln\left(1 - s_{ij}^{(k\ell)}\right) + \sum\nolimits_{k,\ell=0}^{1}\left(m_{k\ell} + n^*_{k\ell}\right) ln\left(p^*_{kl}\right), \tag{9.51}$$

To find the maximum likelihood estimators of $\left\{s_{ij}^{(k\ell)}\right\}$ and $\{p^*_{k\ell}\}$, we need to maximize Eq. (9.50) subject to

$$\sum\nolimits_{k,\ell=0}^{1} p^*_{k\ell} = 1. \tag{9.52}$$

By solving Eq. (9.51) for p^*_{00} and then substituting it into Eq. (9.50), we set the partial derivative of Eq. (9.50) with respect to $s_{ij}^{(k\ell)}$ and $p^*_{k\ell}$ to equal zero:

$$\frac{\partial \mathcal{L}^*}{\partial p_{11}^*} = \frac{m_{11} + n_{11}^*}{p_{11}^*} + \frac{\left(m_{00} + n_{00}^*\right) \cdot (-1)}{1 - p_{11}^* - p_{10}^* - p_{01}^*} = 0, \tag{9.53}$$

$$\frac{\partial \mathcal{L}^*}{\partial p_{10}^*} = \frac{m_{10} + n_{10}^*}{p_{10}^*} + \frac{\left(m_{00} + n_{00}^*\right) \cdot (-1)}{1 - p_{11}^* - p_{10}^* - p_{01}^*} = 0, \tag{9.54}$$

$$\frac{\partial \mathcal{L}^*}{\partial p_{01}^*} = \frac{m_{01} + n_{01}^*}{p_{01}^*} + \frac{\left(m_{00} + n_{00}^*\right) \cdot (-1)}{1 - p_{11}^* - p_{10}^* - p_{01}^*} = 0, \tag{9.55}$$

$$\frac{\partial \mathcal{L}^*}{\partial s_{ij}^{(k\ell)}} = \frac{n_{ij}^{(k\ell)}}{s_{ij}^{(k\ell)}} + \frac{\left(n_{k\ell}^* - n_{ij}^{(k\ell)}\right)(-1)}{1 - s_{ij}^{(k\ell)}} = 0, \tag{9.56}$$

After solving Eq. (9.52) to (9.55), we have

$$\widehat{p}_{11}^* = \frac{m_{11} + n_{11}^*}{\sum_{k,\ell=0}^{1}\left(m_{k\ell} + n_{k\ell}^*\right)} = \frac{m_{11} + n_{11}^*}{N}, \tag{9.57}$$

$$\widehat{p}_{10}^* = \frac{m_{10} + n_{10}^*}{\sum_{k,\ell=0}^{1}\left(m_{k\ell} + n_{k\ell}^*\right)} = \frac{m_{10} + n_{10}^*}{N}, \tag{9.58}$$

$$\widehat{p}_{01}^* = \frac{m_{01} + n_{01}^*}{\sum_{k,\ell=0}^{1}\left(m_{k\ell} + n_{k\ell}^*\right)} = \frac{m_{01} + n_{01}^*}{N}, \tag{9.59}$$

$$\widehat{s}_{ij}^{(k\ell)} = \frac{n_{ij}^{(k\ell)}}{n_{k\ell}^*}. \tag{9.60}$$

After substituting Eqs. (9.56) to Eq. (9.58) into Eq. (9.51),

$$\widehat{p}_{00}^* = 1 - \widehat{p}_{11}^* - \widehat{p}_{10}^* - \widehat{p}_{01}^* = \frac{m_{00} + n_{00}^*}{N}. \tag{9.61}$$

After substituting Eq. (9.59) into Eq. (9.49),

$$\widehat{p}_{ij} = \sum_{k,\ell=0}^{1} \widehat{s}_{ij}^{(k\ell)} \widehat{p}_{k\ell}^* = N^{-1} \sum_{k,\ell=0}^{1} \frac{n_{ij}^{(k\ell)}\left(m_{k\ell} + n_{k\ell}^*\right)}{n_{k\ell}^*}. \tag{9.62}$$

The null hypothesis of independence in a 2 × 2 contingency table is given by

$$H_0 : p_{11}p_{00} = p_{10}p_{01}. \tag{9.63}$$

Under the assumption that $\mathcal{W}$ is nonsingular, the inverse of $\mathcal{W}$ is given by

$$\mathcal{V} = \mathcal{W}^{-1} = (\det(\mathcal{W}))^{-1}\left[w_{ij}^{(k\ell)}\right]^{T}, \tag{9.64}$$

where $w_{ij}^{(k\ell)}$ is the cofactor of $\varphi_{ij}^{(k\ell)}$ in $\mathcal{W}$ [5].

The logarithm of the likelihood function (Eq. (9.48)) can be written as

$$\ln(\mathcal{L}) = \ln(c) + \sum\nolimits_{i,j,k,\ell=0}^{1} n_{ij}^{(k\ell)} \ln\left(\varphi_{ij}^{(k\ell)}\right) + \sum\nolimits_{k,\ell=0}^{1}(m_{k\ell}+n_{k\ell}^{*}) \ln\left[\sum\nolimits_{r,s=0}^{1}(\det(\mathcal{W}))^{-1} w_{k\ell}^{(rs)} p_{rs}^{*}\right], \tag{9.65}$$

To obtain the maximum likelihood estimators of the parameters under H_0, we maximize Eq. (9.64) which is subject to the following constraints

$$\sum\nolimits_{k,\ell=0}^{1} p_{kl}^{*} = \sum\nolimits_{k,\ell=0}^{1} \varphi_{ij}^{(k\ell)} = 1, \tag{9.66}$$

and

$$p_{11}p_{00} - p_{10}p_{01} = 0. \tag{9.67}$$

Equation (9.66) can be re-expressed in terms of $p_{k\ell}^{*}$ by using Eq. (9.46) as follows:

$$\left(\sum\nolimits_{k,\ell=0}^{1} \frac{w_{k\ell}^{(11)}}{\det(\mathcal{W})} p_{k\ell}^{*11}\right)\cdot\left(\sum\nolimits_{k,\ell=0}^{1} \frac{w_{k\ell}^{(00)}}{\det(\mathcal{W})} p_{k\ell}^{*00}\right) - \left(\sum\nolimits_{k,\ell=0}^{1} \frac{w_{k\ell}^{(10)}}{\det(\mathcal{W})} p_{k\ell}^{*10}\right)\cdot\left(\sum\nolimits_{k,\ell=0}^{1} \frac{w_{k\ell}^{(01)}}{\det(\mathcal{W})} p_{k\ell}^{*01}\right) = 0, \text{or}$$
$$\left(\sum\nolimits_{k,\ell=0}^{1} w_{k\ell}^{(11)} p_{k\ell}^{*11}\right)\cdot\left(\sum\nolimits_{k,\ell=0}^{1} w_{k\ell}^{(00)} p_{k\ell}^{*00}\right) = \left(\sum\nolimits_{k,\ell=0}^{1} w_{k\ell}^{(10)} p_{k\ell}^{*10}\right)\cdot\left(\sum\nolimits_{k,\ell=0}^{1} w_{k\ell}^{(01)} p_{k*\ell}^{*01}\right). \tag{9.68}$$

From Eq. (9.65),

$$p_{00}^{*} = 1 - p_{11}^{*} - p_{10}^{*} - p_{01}^{*}, \tag{9.69}$$

and

$$\varphi_{ij}^{(00)} = 1 - \varphi_{ij}^{(11)} - \varphi_{ij}^{(10)} - \varphi_{ij}^{(01)}. \tag{9.70}$$

By substituting Eqs. (9.68) and (9.69) into Eq. (9.64) and then differentiating Eq. (9.64) with respect to its parameters $\{p_{11}^{*}, p_{10}^{*}, p_{01}^{*}\}$ and $\{\varphi_{ij}^{(11)}, \varphi_{ij}^{(10)}, \varphi_{ij}^{(01)}\}$, we have

$$\frac{\partial \ln(\mathcal{L})}{\partial p_{11}^{*}} = \sum\nolimits_{k,\ell=0}^{1}(m_{k\ell} + n_{k\ell}^{*})\left(w_{11}^{(k\ell)} - w_{00}^{(k\ell)}\right)\cdot\left[\sum\nolimits_{r,s=0}^{1} w_{rs}^{(k\ell)} p_{rs}^{*}\right]^{-1} = 0, \tag{9.71}$$

$$\frac{\partial \ln(\mathcal{L})}{\partial p_{10}^{*}} = \sum\nolimits_{k,\ell=0}^{1}(m_{k\ell} + n_{k\ell}^{*})\left(w_{k\ell}^{(10)} - w_{k\ell}^{(00)}\right)\cdot\left(\sum\nolimits_{r,s=0}^{1} w_{rs}^{(k\ell)} p_{rs}^{*}\right)^{-1} = 0, \tag{9.72}$$

$$\frac{\partial \ln(\mathcal{L})}{\partial p_{01}^*} = \sum\nolimits_{k,\ell=0}^{1} \left(m_{k\ell} + n_{k\ell}^*\right)\left(w_{k\ell}^{(01)} - w_{k\ell}^{(00)}\right) \cdot \left(\sum\nolimits_{r,s=0}^{1} w_{rs}^{(k\ell)}\right)^{-1} = 0, \quad (9.73)$$

$$\frac{\partial \ln(\mathcal{L})}{\partial \varphi_{11}^{(11)}} = \frac{n_{11}^{(11)}}{\varphi_{11}^{(11)}} - \frac{n_{11}^{(00)}}{\overline{\varphi}_{11}^{(00)}}$$

$$+\frac{\left(m_{10}+n_{10}^*\right)\Big[p_{10}^*\left(\varphi_{01}^{(01)}\varphi_{00}^{(00)}-\varphi_{01}^{(01)}\varphi_{01}^{(00)}\right)-p_{01}^*\left(\varphi_{10}^{(01)}\varphi_{00}^{(00)}-\varphi_{00}^{(01)}\varphi_{10}^{(00)}\right)+\overline{p}_{00}^*\left(\varphi_{10}^{(01)}\varphi_{01}^{(00)}-\varphi_{10}^{(00)}\varphi_{01}^{(01)}\right)}{\sum_{r,s=0}^{1} w_{11}^{(rs)} p_{rs}^*}$$

$$+\frac{\left(m_{01}+n_{01}^*\right)\Big[-p_{10}^*\left(\varphi_{01}^{(10)}\varphi_{00}^{(00)}-\varphi_{00}^{(10)}\varphi_{01}^{(00)}\right)+p_{01}^*\left(\varphi_{10}^{(10)}\varphi_{00}^{(00)}-\varphi_{00}^{(10)}\varphi_{10}^{(00)}\right)-\overline{p}_{00}^*\left(\varphi_{10}^{(10)}\varphi_{01}^{(00)}-\varphi_{01}^{(10)}\varphi_{11}^{(00)}\right)}{\sum_{r,s=0}^{1} w_{11}^{(rs)} p_{rs}^*}$$

$$+\frac{\left(m_{00}+n_{00}^*\right)\Big[-p_{10}^*\left(\varphi_{01}^{(10)}\varphi_{00}^{(01)}-\varphi_{00}^{(10)}\varphi_{01}^{(01)}\right)-p_{01}^*\left(\varphi_{10}^{(10)}\varphi_{00}^{(01)}-\varphi_{00}^{(10)}\varphi_{10}^{(01)}\right)+\overline{p}_{00}^*\left(\varphi_{10}^{(10)}\varphi_{01}^{(01)}-\varphi_{01}^{(10)}\varphi_{10}^{(01)}\right)}{\sum_{r,s=0}^{1} w_{11}^{(rs)} p_{rs}^*}=0, \quad (9.74)$$

$$\frac{\partial \ln(\mathcal{L})}{\partial \varphi_{11}^{(10)}} = \frac{n_{11}^{(10)}}{\varphi_{11}^{(10)}} - \frac{n_{11}^{(00)}}{\overline{\varphi}_{10}^{(00)}}$$

$$+\frac{\left(m_{10}+n_{10}^*\right)\Big[-p_{11}^*\left(\varphi_{01}^{(01)}\varphi_{00}^{(00)}-\varphi_{00}^{(01)}\varphi_{01}^{(00)}\right)+p_{01}^*\left(\varphi_{10}^{(11)}\varphi_{00}^{(00)}-\varphi_{00}^{(11)}\varphi_{01}^{(00)}\right)-\overline{p}_{00}^*\left(\varphi_{01}^{(11)}\varphi_{00}^{(01)}-\varphi_{00}^{(11)}\varphi_{01}^{(01)}\right)}{\sum_{r,s=0}^{1} w_{11}^{(rs)} p_{rs}^*}$$

$$+\frac{\left(m_{01}+n_{01}^*\right)\Big[p_{11}^*\left(\varphi_{10}^{(01)}\varphi_{01}^{(00)}-\varphi_{01}^{(01)}\varphi_{10}^{(00)}\right)+p_{01}^*\left(\varphi_{10}^{(11)}\varphi_{00}^{(00)}-\varphi_{00}^{(11)}\varphi_{10}^{(00)}\right)-\overline{p}_{00}^*\left(\varphi_{10}^{(11)}\varphi_{01}^{(00)}-\varphi_{01}^{(11)}\varphi_{10}^{(00)}\right)}{\sum_{r,s=0}^{1} w_{11}^{(rs)} p_{rs}^*}$$

$$+\frac{\left(m_{00}+n_{00}^*\right)\Big[p_{11}^*\left(\varphi_{01}^{(11)}\varphi_{01}^{(00)}-\varphi_{00}^{(11)}\varphi_{00}^{(01)}\right)-p_{01}^*\left(\varphi_{10}^{(11)}\varphi_{01}^{(00)}-\varphi_{01}^{(11)}\varphi_{10}^{(00)}\right)-\overline{p}_{00}^*\left(\varphi_{10}^{(11)}\varphi_{01}^{(01)}-\varphi_{01}^{(10)}\varphi_{10}^{(01)}\right)}{\sum_{r,s=0}^{1} w_{11}^{(rs)} p_{rs}^*}=0, \quad (9.75)$$

$$\frac{\partial \ln(\mathcal{L})}{\partial \varphi_{11}^{(01)}} = \frac{n_{11}^{(01)}}{\varphi_{11}^{(01)}} - \frac{n_{11}^{(00)}}{\overline{\varphi}_{01}^{(00)}}$$

$$+\frac{\left(m_{10}+n_{10}^*\right)\Big[p_{11}^*\left(\varphi_{01}^{(10)}\varphi_{00}^{(00)}-\varphi_{00}^{(10)}\varphi_{01}^{(00)}\right)-p_{10}^*\left(\varphi_{10}^{(10)}\varphi_{00}^{(00)}-\varphi_{00}^{(10)}\varphi_{10}^{(00)}\right)+\overline{p}_{00}^*\left(\varphi_{10}^{(10)}\varphi_{01}^{(00)}-\varphi_{10}^{(00)}\varphi_{01}^{(10)}\right)}{\sum_{r,s=0}^{1} w_{11}^{(rs)} p_{rs}^*}$$

$$+\frac{\left(m_{01}+n_{01}^*\right)\Big[-p_{11}^*\left(\varphi_{01}^{(11)}\varphi_{00}^{(00)}-\varphi_{01}^{(00)}\varphi_{00}^{(11)}\right)+p_{10}^*\left(\varphi_{10}^{(11)}\varphi_{00}^{(00)}-\varphi_{00}^{(11)}\varphi_{10}^{(00)}\right)-\overline{p}_{00}^*\left(\varphi_{10}^{(11)}\varphi_{01}^{(00)}-\varphi_{01}^{(11)}\varphi_{10}^{(00)}\right)}{\sum_{r,s=0}^{1} w_{11}^{(rs)} p_{rs}^*}$$

$$+\frac{\left(m_{00}+n_{00}^*\right)\Big[p_{11}^*\left(\varphi_{00}^{(10)}\varphi_{01}^{(11)}-\varphi_{01}^{(10)}\varphi_{10}^{(00)}\right)-p_{10}^*\left(\varphi_{10}^{(11)}\varphi_{00}^{(10)}-\varphi_{00}^{(11)}\varphi_{10}^{(10)}\right)+\overline{p}_{00}^*\left(\varphi_{10}^{(11)}\varphi_{01}^{(10)}-\varphi_{01}^{(11)}\varphi_{10}^{(10)}\right)}{\sum_{r,s=0}^{1} w_{11}^{(rs)} p_{rs}^*}=0, \quad (9.76)$$

$$\frac{\partial \ln(\mathcal{L})}{\partial \varphi_{10}^{(11)}} = \frac{n_{10}^{(11)}}{\varphi_{10}^{(11)}} - \frac{n_{10}^{(00)}}{\overline{\varphi}_{10}^{(00)}}$$

$$+\frac{\left(m_{11}+n_{11}^*\right)\Big[-p_{11}^*\left(\varphi_{01}^{(01)}\varphi_{00}^{(00)}-\varphi_{01}^{(00)}\varphi_{00}^{(01)}\right)-p_{01}^*\left(\varphi_{11}^{(01)}\varphi_{00}^{(00)}-\varphi_{00}^{(01)}\varphi_{11}^{(00)}\right)-\overline{p}_{00}^*\left(\varphi_{11}^{(01)}\varphi_{01}^{(00)}-\varphi_{11}^{(00)}\varphi_{01}^{(01)}\right)}{\sum_{r,s=0}^{1} w_{11}^{(rs)} p_{rs}^*}$$

$$+\frac{(m_{01}+n_{01}^{*})\left[p_{11}^{*}\left(\varphi_{11}^{(01)}\varphi_{00}^{(00)}-\varphi_{11}^{(00)}\varphi_{00}^{(10)}\right)-p_{01}^{*}\left(\varphi_{10}^{(11)}\varphi_{00}^{(00)}-\varphi_{11}^{(00)}\varphi_{00}^{(10)}\right)+\overline{p}_{00}^{*}\left(\varphi_{11}^{(10)}\varphi_{01}^{(00)}-\varphi_{11}^{(00)}\varphi_{01}^{(10)}\right)\right.}{\sum_{r,s=0}^{1}w_{11}^{(rs)}p_{rs}^{*}}$$

$$+\frac{(m_{00}+n_{00}^{*})\left[-p_{11}^{*}\left(\varphi_{01}^{(10)}\varphi_{00}^{(01)}-\varphi_{01}^{(01)}\varphi_{00}^{(10)}\right)+p_{01}^{*}\left(\varphi_{11}^{(10)}\varphi_{00}^{(01)}-\varphi_{11}^{(01)}\varphi_{00}^{(10)}\right)-\overline{p}_{00}^{*}\left(\varphi_{11}^{(10)}\varphi_{01}^{(01)}-\varphi_{11}^{(01)}\varphi_{01}^{(10)}\right)\right.}{\sum_{r,s=0}^{1}w_{11}^{(rs)}p_{rs}^{*}}=0, \quad (9.77)$$

$$\frac{\partial\ln(\mathcal{L})}{\partial\varphi_{01}^{(11)}}=\frac{n_{01}^{(11)}}{\varphi_{01}^{(11)}}-\frac{n_{01}^{(00)}}{\overline{\varphi}_{01}^{(00)}}$$

$$+\frac{(m_{10}+n_{10}^{*})\left[p_{11}^{*}\left(\varphi_{10}^{(01)}\varphi_{00}^{(00)}-\varphi_{00}^{(01)}\varphi_{10}^{(00)}\right)-p_{10}^{*}\left(\varphi_{11}^{(01)}\varphi_{00}^{(00)}-\varphi_{00}^{(01)}\varphi_{11}^{(00)}\right)+\overline{p}_{00}^{*}\left(\varphi_{11}^{(01)}\varphi_{10}^{(00)}-\varphi_{11}^{(00)}\varphi_{10}^{(01)}\right)\right.}{\sum_{r,s=0}^{1}w_{11}^{(rs)}p_{rs}^{*}}$$

$$+\frac{(m_{01}+n_{01}^{*})\left[-p_{11}^{*}\left(\varphi_{10}^{(10)}\varphi_{00}^{(00)}-\varphi_{10}^{(00)}\varphi_{00}^{(10)}\right)-p_{10}^{*}\left(\varphi_{11}^{(10)}\varphi_{00}^{(00)}-\varphi_{00}^{(10)}\varphi_{11}^{(00)}\right)-\overline{p}_{00}^{*}\left(\varphi_{11}^{(10)}\varphi_{10}^{(00)}-\varphi_{10}^{(10)}\varphi_{11}^{(00)}\right)\right.}{\sum_{r,s=0}^{1}w_{11}^{(rs)}p_{rs}^{*}}$$

$$+\frac{(m_{00}+n_{00}^{*})\left[p_{11}^{*}\left(\varphi_{10}^{(10)}\varphi_{00}^{(01)}-\varphi_{00}^{(10)}\varphi_{10}^{(01)}\right)-p_{10}^{*}\left(\varphi_{11}^{(10)}\varphi_{00}^{(01)}-\varphi_{11}^{(01)}\varphi_{00}^{(10)}\right)+\overline{p}_{00}^{*}\left(\varphi_{10}^{(01)}\varphi_{11}^{(10)}-\varphi_{11}^{(01)}\varphi_{10}^{(10)}\right)\right.}{\sum_{r,s=0}^{1}w_{11}^{(rs)}p_{rs}^{*}}=0, \quad (9.78)$$

$$\frac{\partial\ln(\mathcal{L})}{\partial\varphi_{00}^{(11)}}=\frac{n_{00}^{(11)}}{\varphi_{00}^{(11)}}-\frac{n_{00}^{(00)}}{\overline{\varphi}_{00}^{(00)}}$$

$$+\frac{(m_{10}+n_{10}^{*})\left[p_{11}^{*}\left(\varphi_{10}^{(01)}\varphi_{01}^{(00)}-\varphi_{01}^{(01)}\varphi_{10}^{(00)}\right)+p_{10}^{*}\left(\varphi_{11}^{(01)}\varphi_{01}^{(00)}-\varphi_{01}^{(01)}\varphi_{11}^{(00)}\right)-p_{01}^{*}\left(\varphi_{11}^{(01)}\varphi_{10}^{(00)}-\varphi_{11}^{(00)}\varphi_{10}^{(01)}\right)\right.}{\sum_{r,s=0}^{1}w_{11}^{(rs)}p_{rs}^{*}}$$

$$+\frac{(m_{01}+n_{01}^{*})\left[p_{11}^{*}\left(\varphi_{10}^{(10)}\varphi_{01}^{(00)}-\varphi_{10}^{(00)}\varphi_{01}^{(10)}\right)-p_{10}^{*}\left(\varphi_{11}^{(10)}\varphi_{01}^{(00)}-\varphi_{01}^{(10)}\varphi_{11}^{(00)}\right)+p_{01}^{*}\left(\varphi_{11}^{(10)}\varphi_{10}^{(00)}-\varphi_{10}^{(10)}\varphi_{11}^{(00)}\right)\right.}{\sum_{r,s=0}^{1}w_{11}^{(rs)}p_{rs}^{*}}$$

$$+\frac{(m_{00}+n_{00}^{*})\left[-p_{11}^{*}\left(\varphi_{10}^{(10)}\varphi_{01}^{(01)}-\varphi_{01}^{(10)}\varphi_{10}^{(01)}\right)+p_{10}^{*}\left(\varphi_{11}^{(00)}\varphi_{01}^{(01)}-\varphi_{11}^{(01)}\varphi_{01}^{(00)}\right)-p_{01}^{*}\left(\varphi_{10}^{(01)}\varphi_{11}^{(10)}-\varphi_{11}^{(01)}\varphi_{10}^{(10)}\right)\right.}{\sum_{r,s=0}^{1}w_{11}^{(rs)}p_{rs}^{*}}=0, \quad (9.79)$$

$$\frac{\partial\ln(\mathcal{L})}{\partial\varphi_{10}^{(10)}}=\frac{n_{10}^{(10)}}{\varphi_{10}^{(10)}}-\frac{n_{10}^{(00)}}{\overline{\varphi}_{10}^{(00)}}$$

$$+\frac{(m_{11}+n_{11}^{*})\left[p_{11}^{*}\left(\varphi_{01}^{(01)}\varphi_{00}^{(00)}-\varphi_{01}^{(00)}\varphi_{00}^{(01)}\right)-p_{01}^{*}\left(\varphi_{11}^{(01)}\varphi_{00}^{(00)}-\varphi_{00}^{(01)}\varphi_{11}^{(00)}\right)+\overline{p}_{00}^{*}\left(\varphi_{11}^{(01)}\varphi_{01}^{(00)}-\varphi_{01}^{(01)}\varphi_{11}^{(00)}\right)\right.}{\sum_{r,s=0}^{1}w_{11}^{(rs)}p_{rs}^{*}}$$

$$+\frac{(m_{01}+n_{01}^{*})\left[-p_{11}^{*}\left(\varphi_{01}^{(11)}\varphi_{00}^{(00)}-\varphi_{01}^{(00)}\varphi_{00}^{(11)}\right)+p_{01}^{*}\left(\varphi_{11}^{(11)}\varphi_{00}^{(00)}-\varphi_{00}^{(11)}\varphi_{11}^{(00)}\right)-\overline{p}_{00}^{*}\left(\varphi_{11}^{(11)}\varphi_{01}^{(00)}-\varphi_{01}^{(11)}\varphi_{11}^{(00)}\right)\right.}{\sum_{r,s=0}^{1}w_{11}^{(rs)}p_{rs}^{*}}$$

$$+\frac{(m_{00}+n_{00}^{*})\left[p_{11}^{*}\left(\varphi_{01}^{(11)}\varphi_{00}^{(01)}-\varphi_{01}^{(01)}\varphi_{00}^{(11)}\right)-p_{01}^{*}\left(\varphi_{10}^{(11)}\varphi_{00}^{(01)}-\varphi_{10}^{(01)}\varphi_{00}^{(11)}\right)+\overline{p}_{00}^{*}\left(\varphi_{11}^{(11)}\varphi_{01}^{(01)}-\varphi_{11}^{(01)}\varphi_{01}^{(11)}\right)\right.}{\sum_{r,s=0}^{1}w_{11}^{(rs)}p_{rs}^{*}}=0, \quad (9.80)$$

$$\frac{\partial\ln(\mathcal{L})}{\partial\varphi_{01}^{(10)}}=\frac{n_{01}^{(10)}}{\varphi_{01}^{(10)}}-\frac{n_{01}^{(00)}}{\overline{\varphi}_{01}^{(00)}}$$

$$
+\frac{(m_{11}+n_{11}^*)\left[-p_{11}^*\left(\varphi_{10}^{(01)}\varphi_{00}^{(00)}-\varphi_{10}^{(00)}\varphi_{00}^{(01)}\right)+p_{10}^*\left(\varphi_{11}^{(01)}\varphi_{00}^{(00)}-\varphi_{00}^{(01)}\varphi_{11}^{(00)}\right)-\overline{p}_{00}^*\left(\varphi_{11}^{(01)}\varphi_{10}^{(00)}-\varphi_{10}^{(01)}\varphi_{11}^{(00)}\right)\right.}{\sum_{r,s=0}^{1}w_{11}^{(rs)}p_{rs}^*}
$$

$$
+\frac{(m_{01}+n_{01}^*)\left[p_{11}^*\left(\varphi_{10}^{(11)}\varphi_{00}^{(00)}-\varphi_{10}^{(00)}\varphi_{00}^{(11)}\right)-p_{10}^*\left(\varphi_{11}^{(11)}\varphi_{00}^{(00)}-\varphi_{00}^{(11)}\varphi_{11}^{(00)}\right)+\overline{p}_{00}^*\left(\varphi_{11}^{(11)}\varphi_{10}^{(00)}-\varphi_{10}^{(11)}\varphi_{11}^{(00)}\right)\right.}{\sum_{r,s=0}^{1}w_{11}^{(rs)}p_{rs}^*}
$$

$$
+\frac{(m_{00}+n_{00}^*)\left[-p_{11}^*\left(\varphi_{10}^{(11)}\varphi_{00}^{(01)}-\varphi_{10}^{(01)}\varphi_{00}^{(11)}\right)+p_{10}^*\left(\varphi_{11}^{(11)}\varphi_{00}^{(01)}-\varphi_{11}^{(01)}\varphi_{00}^{(11)}\right)-p_{00}^*\left(\varphi_{11}^{(11)}\varphi_{01}^{(01)}-\varphi_{11}^{(01)}\varphi_{01}^{(11)}\right)\right.}{\sum_{r,s=0}^{1}w_{11}^{(rs)}p_{rs}^*}=0, \quad (9.81)
$$

$$
\frac{\partial\ln(\mathcal{L})}{\partial\varphi_{00}^{(10)}}=\frac{n_{00}^{(10)}}{\varphi_{00}^{(10)}}-\frac{n_{00}^{(00)}}{\overline{\varphi}_{00}^{(00)}}
$$

$$
+\frac{(m_{11}+n_{11}^*)\left[p_{11}^*\left(\varphi_{10}^{(01)}\varphi_{01}^{(00)}-\varphi_{01}^{(01)}\varphi_{10}^{(00)}\right)-p_{10}^*\left(\varphi_{11}^{(01)}\varphi_{01}^{(00)}-\varphi_{01}^{(01)}\varphi_{11}^{(00)}\right)+p_{01}^*\left(\varphi_{11}^{(01)}\varphi_{10}^{(00)}-\varphi_{11}^{(00)}\varphi_{10}^{(01)}\right)\right.}{\sum_{r,s=0}^{1}w_{11}^{(rs)}p_{rs}^*}
$$

$$
+\frac{(m_{01}+n_{01}^*)\left[-p_{11}^*\left(\varphi_{10}^{(11)}\varphi_{01}^{(00)}-\varphi_{10}^{(00)}\varphi_{01}^{(11)}\right)+p_{10}^*\left(\varphi_{11}^{(11)}\varphi_{01}^{(00)}-\varphi_{01}^{(11)}\varphi_{11}^{(00)}\right)-p_{01}^*\left(\varphi_{11}^{(11)}\varphi_{10}^{(00)}-\varphi_{10}^{(11)}\varphi_{11}^{(00)}\right)\right.}{\sum_{r,s=0}^{1}w_{11}^{(rs)}p_{rs}^*}
$$

$$
+\frac{(m_{00}+n_{00}^*)\left[p_{11}^*\left(\varphi_{10}^{(11)}\varphi_{01}^{(01)}-\varphi_{01}^{(11)}\varphi_{10}^{(01)}\right)-p_{10}^*\left(\varphi_{11}^{(11)}\varphi_{01}^{(01)}-\varphi_{11}^{(01)}\varphi_{01}^{(11)}\right)+p_{01}^*\left(\varphi_{10}^{(01)}\varphi_{11}^{(11)}-\varphi_{11}^{(01)}\varphi_{10}^{(11)}\right)\right.}{\sum_{r,s=0}^{1}w_{11}^{(rs)}p_{rs}^*}=0, \quad (9.82)
$$

$$
\frac{\partial\ln(\mathcal{L})}{\partial\varphi_{10}^{(01)}}=\frac{n_{10}^{(01)}}{\varphi_{10}^{(01)}}-\frac{n_{10}^{(00)}}{\overline{\varphi}_{10}^{(00)}}
$$

$$
+\frac{(m_{11}+n_{11}^*)\left[-p_{11}^*\left(\varphi_{01}^{(10)}\varphi_{00}^{(00)}-\varphi_{01}^{(00)}\varphi_{00}^{(10)}\right)-p_{01}^*\left(\varphi_{11}^{(10)}\varphi_{10}^{(00)}-\varphi_{01}^{(10)}\varphi_{11}^{(00)}\right)-\overline{p}_{00}^*\left(\varphi_{11}^{(10)}\varphi_{00}^{(00)}-\varphi_{01}^{(10)}\varphi_{11}^{(00)}\right)\right.}{\sum_{r,s=0}^{1}w_{11}^{(rs)}p_{rs}^*}
$$

$$
+\frac{(m_{10}+n_{10}^*)\left[p_{11}^*\left(\varphi_{01}^{(11)}\varphi_{00}^{(00)}-\varphi_{11}^{(00)}\varphi_{00}^{(11)}\right)-p_{01}^*\left(\varphi_{11}^{(11)}\varphi_{00}^{(00)}-\varphi_{00}^{(11)}\varphi_{11}^{(00)}\right)+\overline{p}_{00}^*\left(\varphi_{11}^{(11)}\varphi_{01}^{(00)}-\varphi_{01}^{(11)}\varphi_{11}^{(00)}\right)\right.}{\sum_{r,s=0}^{1}w_{11}^{(rs)}p_{rs}^*}
$$

$$
+\frac{(m_{00}+n_{00}^*)\left[-p_{11}^*\left(\varphi_{01}^{(11)}\varphi_{00}^{(10)}-\varphi_{01}^{(10)}\varphi_{00}^{(11)}\right)+p_{01}^*\left(\varphi_{11}^{(11)}\varphi_{00}^{(10)}-\varphi_{10}^{(10)}\varphi_{00}^{(11)}\right)-\overline{p}_{00}^*\left(\varphi_{11}^{(11)}\varphi_{01}^{(10)}-\varphi_{11}^{(10)}\varphi_{01}^{(11)}\right)\right.}{\sum_{r,s=0}^{1}w_{11}^{(rs)}p_{rs}^*}=0, \quad (9.83)
$$

$$
\frac{\partial\ln(\mathcal{L})}{\partial\varphi_{01}^{(01)}}=\frac{n_{01}^{(01)}}{\varphi_{01}^{(01)}}-\frac{n_{01}^{(00)}}{\overline{\varphi}_{01}^{(00)}}
$$

$$
+\frac{(m_{11}+n_{11}^*)\left[p_{11}^*\left(\varphi_{01}^{(10)}\varphi_{00}^{(00)}-\varphi_{10}^{(00)}\varphi_{00}^{(10)}\right)-p_{10}^*\left(\varphi_{11}^{(10)}\varphi_{00}^{(00)}-\varphi_{00}^{(10)}\varphi_{11}^{(00)}\right)-\overline{p}_{00}^*\left(\varphi_{11}^{(10)}\varphi_{10}^{(00)}-\varphi_{01}^{(10)}\varphi_{11}^{(00)}\right)\right.}{\sum_{r,s=0}^{1}w_{11}^{(rs)}p_{rs}^*}
$$

$$
+\frac{(m_{10}+n_{10}^*)\left[-p_{11}^*\left(\varphi_{10}^{(11)}\varphi_{00}^{(00)}-\varphi_{10}^{(00)}\varphi_{00}^{(11)}\right)+p_{10}^*\left(\varphi_{11}^{(11)}\varphi_{00}^{(00)}-\varphi_{00}^{(11)}\varphi_{11}^{(00)}\right)-\overline{p}_{00}^*\left(\varphi_{11}^{(11)}\varphi_{10}^{(00)}-\varphi_{10}^{(11)}\varphi_{11}^{(00)}\right)\right.}{\sum_{r,s=0}^{1}w_{11}^{(rs)}p_{rs}^*}
$$

$$
+\frac{(m_{00}+n_{00}^*)\left[p_{11}^*\left(\varphi_{10}^{(11)}\varphi_{00}^{(10)}-\varphi_{10}^{(10)}\varphi_{00}^{(11)}\right)-p_{10}^*\left(\varphi_{11}^{(11)}\varphi_{00}^{(10)}-\varphi_{11}^{(10)}\varphi_{00}^{(11)}\right)+\overline{p}_{00}^*\left(\varphi_{11}^{(11)}\varphi_{10}^{(10)}-\varphi_{10}^{(11)}\varphi_{11}^{(10)}\right)\right.}{\sum_{r,s=0}^{1}w_{11}^{(rs)}p_{rs}^*}=0, \quad (9.84)
$$

$$\frac{\partial \ln(\mathcal{L})}{\partial \varphi_{00}^{(01)}} = \frac{\mathrm{n}_{00}^{(01)}}{\varphi_{00}^{(01)}} - \frac{n_{00}^{(00)}}{\overline{\varphi}_{00}^{(00)}}$$

$$+\frac{\left(m_{11}+n_{11}^{*}\right)\left[-p_{11}^{*}\left(\varphi_{10}^{(10)}\varphi_{01}^{(00)}-\varphi_{01}^{(10)}\varphi_{10}^{(00)}\right)+p_{10}^{*}\left(\varphi_{11}^{(10)}\varphi_{00}^{(01)}-\varphi_{00}^{(10)}\varphi_{11}^{(01)}\right)-p_{01}^{*}\left(\varphi_{11}^{(10)}\varphi_{10}^{(00)}-\varphi_{11}^{(00)}\varphi_{10}^{(10)}\right)\right.}{\sum_{r,s=0}^{1} w_{11}^{(rs)} p_{rs}^{*}}$$

$$+\frac{\left(m_{10}+n_{10}^{*}\right)\left[p_{11}^{*}\left(\varphi_{10}^{(11)}\varphi_{01}^{(00)}-\varphi_{10}^{(00)}\varphi_{01}^{(11)}\right)-p_{10}^{*}\left(\varphi_{11}^{(11)}\varphi_{01}^{(00)}-\varphi_{01}^{(11)}\varphi_{11}^{(00)}\right)+p_{01}^{*}\left(\varphi_{11}^{(11)}\varphi_{10}^{(00)}-\varphi_{10}^{(11)}\varphi_{11}^{(00)}\right)\right.}{\sum_{r,s=0}^{1} w_{11}^{(rs)} p_{rs}^{*}}$$

$$+\frac{\left(m_{00}+n_{00}^{*}\right)\left[-p_{11}^{*}\left(\varphi_{10}^{(11)}\varphi_{01}^{(10)}-\varphi_{01}^{(11)}\varphi_{10}^{(10)}\right)+p_{10}^{*}\left(\varphi_{11}^{(11)}\varphi_{01}^{(10)}-\varphi_{11}^{(10)}\varphi_{01}^{(11)}\right)-p_{01}^{*}\left(\varphi_{10}^{(10)}\varphi_{11}^{(11)}-\varphi_{11}^{(10)}\varphi_{10}^{(11)}\right)\right.}{\sum_{r,s=0}^{1} w_{11}^{(rs)} p_{rs}^{*}} = 0, \quad (9.85)$$

By applying the Newton-Raphson method to solve the system of nonlinear equations of (9.67) and from (9.70) to (9.84), the maximum likelihood estimators $\left\{\tilde{p}_{ij}^{*}\right\}_{i,j=0}^{1}$ and $\left\{\tilde{\varphi}_{ij}^{(k\ell)}\right\}_{i,j,k,\ell=0}^{1}$ are obtained accordingly.

The likelihood ratio statistic for testing H_0 versus H_1 is given by

$$\lambda = \frac{\prod_{i,j=0}^{1}\sum_{r,s=0}^{1}\left(\det\left(\tilde{\mathcal{W}}\right)\right)^{-1}\tilde{w}_{ij}^{rs}\prod_{k,\ell=0}^{1}\tilde{\varphi}_{ij}^{(k\ell)}}{\prod_{i,j=0}^{1}\sum_{r,s=0}^{1}\left(\det\left(\widehat{\mathcal{W}}\right)\right)^{-1}\widehat{w}_{ij}^{rs}\prod_{k,\ell=0}^{1}\widehat{\varphi}_{ij}^{(k\ell)}}, \tag{9.86}$$

where $\widehat{()}$ and $\tilde{()}$ denote estimates under no restriction and under H_0, respectively.

Theorem 9.1
The statistic defined by

$$C^2 = -2\ln(\lambda), \tag{9.87}$$

where λ is given by Eq. (9.85) is asymptotically distributed as a chi-square random variable with one degree of freedom when $0 < \varphi_{ij}^{(k\ell)}, p_{ij}^{*}, p_{k\ell} < 1$, and N, n → + ∞, but n/N $\rightarrow \gamma > 0$.

Proof: The proof is rather straightforward and given in Chiacchierini-Arnold [1].

9.3 Log-Linear Models

In this section, we are going to build the log-linear model as a misclassification model for the adjustment of misclassification in the data. Let X be a categorical variable with t possible categories. Assume that using a fallible and inexpensive device, we observe a different variable X^* with same t categories. A two-dimensional t × t contingency table is used to represent the situation: The first dimension is the fallible classification, while the second dimension is the true classification. Let the probability of the (i, j)[th] observation be p_{ij}, where $\sum_{i,j=1}^{t} p_{ij} = 1,\ 0 < p_{ij} < 0$. The elements $\{\varphi_{ij}\}$ of a misclassification matrix W are defined as

$$\varphi_{ij} = \frac{p_{ij}}{p_{+j}}, \tag{9.88}$$

which is the conditional probability of any observation having i as the fallible classification given that it has j as the true classification. If the φ_{ij}'s do not depend on j, then we have a random misclassification and $p_{ij} = p_{i+}p_{+j}$. This random misclassification model can be represented by a log-linear model [2]: for all i, j,

$$\ln\left(p_{ij}\right) = u + u_{1(i)} + u_{2(j)} \tag{9.89}$$

where $\sum_{i=1}^{t} u_{1(i)} = 0$, and $\sum_{j=1}^{t} u_{2(j)} = 0$. We will use the notation $H_{[1,2]}$ to denote this model because the highest u terms in the model are $\{u_{1(i)}\}$ and $\{u_{2(j)}\}$. If we wish to analyze a categorical variable with misclassification and double sampling, our approach is to analyze a three-dimensional contingency table with the first dimension being the observed counts, the second dimension representing the fallible and the true X, and the third dimension representing the true Y variable. Let t and s be the numbers of categories for X and Y. Suppose that n subjects are observed on all three dimensions and N—n subjects on the first and the third denote dimensions. Let n_{ijk}denote the observed counts in the full table and v_{ik} denote the supplemental observed counts in the 13 marginal. We assume that all n_{ijk} are positive.

The first unrestricted (saturated) model ($H_{[1,2,3]}$) is expressed as for all i, j, k

$$\ln\left(p_{ijk}\right) = u + u_{1(i)} + u_{2(j)} + u_{3(k)} + u_{12(ij)} + u_{13(ik)} + u_{23(jk)} + u_{123(ijk)}, \tag{9.90}$$

where $\sum_i\sum_j\sum_k p_{ijk} = 1$, with each set of subscripted u terms adding to zero when summed over its subscript. Under the unrestricted model $H_{[123]}$, the iterative proportional fitting of the maximum likelihood (ML) estimators are given by for all i, j, k

$$\widehat{p}_{ijk}^{(\ell+1)} = \frac{1}{N}\left(n_{ijk} + \frac{v_{ik}\widehat{p}_{ijk}^{(\ell)}}{\widehat{p}_{i+k}^{(\ell)}}\right). \tag{9.91}$$

The second model is a model of no second-order interaction with $u_{123(ijk)} = 0$ in Eq. (9.89). The third and fourth models are models of conditional independence in Eq. (9.89). If $\varphi_{i,\,jk}$'s do not depend on k, then the misclassification is the same for any Y value, and we have for all i, j, k

$$p_{ijk} = \frac{n_{ij+}n_{+jk}}{n_{+j+}}. \tag{9.92}$$

Equation (9.89) is to be expressed as for all i, j, k

$$\ln(p_{ijk}) = u + u_{1(i)} + u_{2(j)} + u_{3(k)} + u_{12(ij)} + +u_{23(jk)}. \qquad (9.93)$$

Here each set of subscripted u terms adds to zero when summed over its subscript. We will denote this model by $H_{[12,23]}$.

Because we have double sampling data, the expected counts for n_{ijk} and v_{ik} are nn_{ijk} and $(N - n)n_{i+k}$, respectively. Under the unrestricted model $H_{[123]}$ and independent multinomial distributions for $\{n_{ijk}\}$ and $\{v_{ik}\}$, we have the following ML equation for all i, j, k

$$N\widehat{p}_{ijk} = n_{ijk} + \frac{v_{ik}\widehat{p}_{ijk}}{\widehat{p}_{i+k}}. \qquad (9.94)$$

For the no second-order interaction model, $H_{[12,13,23]}$, the ML equations are given by.

$$N\widehat{p}_{ij+} = n_{ij+} + \sum\nolimits_k \frac{v_{ik}\widehat{p}_{ijk}}{\widehat{p}_{i+k}}, \text{ for all i, j} \qquad (9.95)$$

$$N\widehat{p}_{i+k} = n_{i+k} + v_{ik}, \text{ for all i, k} \qquad (9.96)$$

and

$$N\widehat{p}_{+jk} = n_{+jk} + \sum\nolimits_i \frac{v_{ik}\widehat{p}_{ijk}}{\widehat{p}_{i+k}}, \text{ for all j, k} \qquad (9.97)$$

We can use the procedure of the iterative proportional fitting method to calculate the ML estimation of the cell proportions [4]. For all models, the initial value is taken the same as $n_{ijk}^{(0)} = \frac{1}{st^2}$ for all i, j, k. For a given log-linear model, each cycle consists of a set of pairs of steps, each pair corresponding to one of the sets of ML equations for the model. For $H_{[12,13.23]}$, each cycle of the iterative procedure consists of the following six steps:

$$p_{ij+}^{(m+1)} = \frac{1}{N}\left(n_{ij+} + \sum\nolimits_k \frac{v_{ik}p_{ijk}^{(m)}}{p_{i+k}^{(m)}}\right), \text{ for all i, j,} \qquad (9.98)$$

$$p_{ijk}^{(m+1)} = \frac{p_{ijk}^{(m)}p_{ij+}^{(m+1)}}{p_{ij+}^{(m)}}, \text{ for all i, j, k,} \qquad (9.99)$$

$$p_{i+k}^{(m+2)} = \frac{n_{i+k} + v_{ik}}{N}, \text{ for all i, k,} \qquad (9.100)$$

$$p_{ijk}^{(m+2)} = \frac{p_{ijk}^{(m+1)} p_{i+k}^{(m+2)}}{p_{i+k}^{(m+1)}}, \text{ for all i, j, k,} \tag{9.101}$$

$$p_{+jk}^{(m+3)} = \frac{1}{N}\left(n_{+jk} + \sum\nolimits_i \frac{v_{ik} p_{ijk}^{(m+2)}}{p_{i+k}^{(m+2)}}, \text{ for all j, k,} \right. \tag{9.102}$$

and

$$p_{ijk}^{(m+3)} = \frac{p_{ijk}^{(m+2)} p_{+jk}^{(m+2)}}{p_{+jk}^{(m+2)}}, \text{ for all i, j, k.} \tag{9.103}$$

For $H_{[12, 23]}$, each cycle of the iterative procedure consists of the four steps given by Eqs. (9.97), (9.98), (9.101), and (9.102) with $p_{ijk}^{(m+2)} = p_{ijk}^{(m+1)}$ for all i, j, k.

Once we have the MLE's $\widehat{p}_{ijk}$ for the cell probabilities, we can test the goodness of fit of the misclassification model $H_{[123]}$ ($H_{[12, 23, 13]}$ or $H_{[12, 23]}$) by applying the Pearson chi-square statistics

$$x^2 = \sum\nolimits_{i,j,k} \frac{\left(n_{ijk} - n \cdot \widehat{p}_{ijk}\right)^2}{n \cdot \widehat{p}_{ijk}} + \sum\nolimits_{i,k} \frac{\left[v_{ik} - (N-n) \cdot \widehat{p}_{i+k}\right]^2}{(N-n) \cdot \widehat{p}_{i+k}} \tag{9.104}$$

with the one (four or five) degrees of freedom.

Example 9.2

The data given in Table 9.4 is the same study as in Example 9.1 except with the addition of the gender data.

The supplemental data of a second sample for the interview results with the variable of gender:

Table 9.4 The number of persons having joint pain by physician's examination versus by nonmedical interviews

		Physician's examination		
		Yes	No	Gender
Interview result	Yes	124	23	Males
	No	37	53	
	Yes	123	12	Females
	No	40	66	

		Gender	
Interview result (a second supplement sample)		Males	Females
	Yes	139	133
	No	103	103

Find the appropriate log-linear model as a misclassification model that fits the double sampling data given by Table 9.4.

Solution

The physician examinations data are error-free, but the interview data are error-prone. From Table 9.4, the cell observations are $n_{111} = 124$, $n_{121} = 23$, $n_{211} = 37$, $n_{221} = 53$, $n_{112} = 123$, $n_{122} = 12$, $n_{212} = 40$, and $n_{222} = 66$, while the second doble sampling data are $v_{11} = 139$, $v_{12} = 133$, $v_{21} = 103$, and $v_{22} = 103$.

By choosing the saturated model $H_{[123]}$, we use Eq. (9.90) to calculate the iterative maximum likelihood estimators of the cell proportions given in Table 9.5.

Table 9.5 Iterations of the MLEs of the cell proportions for the log-linear misclassification model $H_{[123]}$

ℓ	$\left(\widehat{p}_{111}^{(\ell)}, \widehat{p}_{121}^{(\ell)}, \widehat{p}_{211}^{(\ell)}, \widehat{p}_{221}^{(\ell)}, \widehat{p}_{112}^{(\ell)}, \widehat{p}_{122}^{(\ell)}, \widehat{p}_{212}^{(\ell)}, \widehat{p}_{222}^{(\ell)}\right)$
1	(0.202, 0.097, 0.093, 0.109, 0.198, 0.082, 0.096, 0.123)
2	(0.228, 0.071, 0.088, 0.109, 0.227, 0.053, 0.089, 0.130)
3	(0.241, 0.059, 0.087, 0.115, 0.241, 0.026, 0.086, 0.133)
4	(0.247, 0.053, 0.085, 0.117, 0.254, 0.026, 0.084, 0.135)
5	(0.250, 0.050, 0.084, 0.118, 0.255, 0.026, 0.083, 0.135)
6	(0.251, 0.048, 0.084, 0.118, 0.255, 0.025, 0.083, 0.136)

The iteration stops at $\ell = 6$ because the MLEs of p_{ijk} are almost the same. The Pearson's chi-square statistics for $H_{[123]}$ calculated by Eq. (9.103) is $X^2 = 1.19$ which is insignificant at the 0.05 level

Table 9.6 Iterations of the MLEs of the cell proportions for the log-linear misclassification model $H_{[12,23,13]}$

m	$\left(\widehat{p}_{111}^{(m)}, \widehat{p}_{121}^{(m)}, \widehat{p}_{211}^{(m)}, \widehat{p}_{221}^{(m)}, \widehat{p}_{112}^{(m)}, \widehat{p}_{122}^{(m)}, \widehat{p}_{212}^{(m)}, \widehat{p}_{222}^{(m)}\right)$
3	(0.201, 0.054, 0.117, 0.109, 0.192, 0.066, 0.123, 0.118)
6	(0.229, 0.029, 0.111, 0.090, 0.210, 0.067, 0.116, 0.186)
9	(0.233, 0.024, 0.119, 0.081, 0.217, 0.044, 0.107, 0.131)
12	(0.205, 0.009, 0.107, 0.039, 0.203, 0.035, 0.096, 0.126)
15	(0.230, 0.050, 0.153, 0.062, 0.224, 0.036, 0.106, 0.132)
18	(0.210, 0.032, 0.143, 0.066, 0.235, 0.027, 0.097, 0.140)
21	(0.175, 0.053, 0.137, 0.068, 0.219, 0.049, 0.096, 0.135)
24	(0.204, 0.043, 0.143, 0.068, 0.227, 0.037, 0.096, 0.138)
27	(0.217, 0.030, 0.141, 0.070, 0.237, 0.026, 0.093, 0.142)
30	(0.229, 0.027, 0.145, 0.073, 0.241, 0.024, 0.091, 0.144)

The iteration stops at m = 30. The Pearson's chi-square statistics for $H_{[123]}$ calculated by Eq. (9.103) is $X^2 = 36.6$ which is significant at the 0.05 level

To consider the no second-order interaction model $H_{[12,23,13]}$, we apply Eqs. (9.97) to (9.102) to calculate the maximum likelihood estimators of the cell proportions given in Table 9.6.

As a conclusion, the saturated model $H_{[123]}$ is the appropriate misclassification model for the data of Table 9.4. The estimated MLE of the cell proportions are

$$\begin{aligned}&\widehat{p}_{111} = 0.251, \widehat{p}_{121} = 0.048, \widehat{p}_{211} = 0.084, \widehat{p}_{221} = 0.118, \widehat{p}_{112}\\ &\quad = 0.255, \widehat{p}_{122} = 0.025, \widehat{p}_{212} = 0.083, \text{and } \widehat{p}_{222} = 0.136.\end{aligned} \tag{9.105}$$

The misclassification probabilities are given by a modification of Eq. (9.87):

$$\widehat{\varphi}_{i,jk} = \frac{\widehat{\mathrm{p}}_{ijk}}{\widehat{p}_{+jk}}. \tag{9.106}$$

By substituting the above MLE estimators $\widehat{p}_{ijk}$ of Eq. (9.104) into Eq, (9.105), the misclassification probabilities are given by Eq. (9.106):

$$\begin{aligned}
\widehat{\varphi}_{1,11} &= \frac{0.251}{0.251 + 0.084} = 0.749 \approx 0.75,\\
\widehat{\varphi}_{1,12} &= \frac{0.255}{0.255 + 0.083} = 0.754 \approx 0.75,\\
\widehat{\varphi}_{1,21} &= \frac{0.048}{0.048 + 0.118} = 0.289 \approx 0.29,\\
\widehat{\varphi}_{1,22} &= \frac{0.025}{0.025 + 0.136} = 0.155 \approx 0.16,\\
\widehat{\varphi}_{2,11} &= \frac{0.084}{0.251 + 0.084} = 0.251 \approx 0.25,\\
\widehat{\varphi}_{2,12} &= \frac{0.083}{0.255 + 0.083} = 0.245 \approx 0.25,\\
\widehat{\varphi}_{2,21} &= \frac{0.118}{0.118 + 0.048} = 0.711 \approx 0.71, \text{and}\\
\widehat{\varphi}_{2,22} &= \frac{0.136}{0.025 + 0.136} = 0.844 \approx 0.84.
\end{aligned} \tag{9.107}$$

References

1. Chiacchierini, R. P., & Arnold, J. C. (1977). A two sample test for independence in 2 × 2 contingency tables with both margins subject to misclassification. *Journal of the American Statistical Association, 72*, 170–174.
2. Chen, T. T. (1979). Log-linear models for categorical data with misclassification and double sampling. *Journal of the American Statistical Association, 74*, 481–488.
3. Cobb, S., & Rosenbaum, J. (1956). A comparison of specific symptom data obtained by nonmedical interviews and by physicians. *Journal of Chronic Diseases, 4*, 245–252.

4. Haberman, S. J. (1974). *The analysis of frequency data*. University of Chicago Press.
5. Strang, G. (1976). *Linear algebra and its applications*. Academic Press, Inc.
6. Tenenbein, A. (1970). A double sampling scheme for estimating from binomial data with misclassification. *Journal of the American Statistical Association, 65*, 1350–1361.
7. Tenenbein, A. (1972). A double sampling scheme for estimating from misclassified multinomial data with application to sampling inspection. *Technometrics, 14*, 187–202.

Part VI
Other Studies

Chapter 10
Misclassification in Two Cohort Groups

10.1 Estimating the Risk Ratio

Assume that we have data from two independent binomial populations given in Table 10.1.

Let p_1 and p_2 be the respective failure probabilities and the risk ratio be $\pi = \frac{p_1}{p_2}$. If the observed data in Table 10.1 are not misclassified, the classical estimate of π is given by

$$\widehat{\pi} = \frac{\widehat{p}_1}{\widehat{p}_2} = \frac{xN_2}{yN_1}. \tag{10.1}$$

If Table 10.1 was misclassified, the misclassification error probability for group i is defined by

$$\varphi_i = \Pr(\text{he is classified as unexposed} | \text{a subject is truly exposed}) \tag{10.2}$$

and

$$\psi_i = \Pr(\text{he is classified as exposed} | \text{a subject is truly unexposed}) \tag{10.3}$$

Since it is a cohort study, it is reasonable to assume that an assumption of nondifferential misclassification holds, that is, $\varphi_1 = \varphi_2 \equiv \varphi$ and $\psi_1 = \psi_2 \equiv \psi$. Thus, the expected probability of failure for cohort group i is given by

$$E(\widehat{p}_i) = (1 - \varphi)p_i + \psi q_i, \tag{10.4}$$

where $q_i = 1 - p_i$, $i = 1, 2$.

Evidently, $\widehat{p}_i$ is not an unbiased estimator of p_i, if $\varphi \neq 0$ or $\psi \neq 0$. A bias-adjusted estimate of p_i s given by

T.-S. Lee, *Misclassification in Epidemiology*, Emerging Topics in Statistics and Biostatistics, https://doi.org/10.1007/978-3-032-12563-7_10

Table 10.1 Observed data from two binomial distributions

	Cohort Group 1	Cohort Group 2
Exposed	x	y
Unexposed	$N_1 - x$	$N_2 - y$
Total	N_1	N_2

Where N_1 or N_2 are assumed to be fixed

$$\tilde{p}_i = \frac{\widehat{p}_i - \psi}{\Delta}, \tag{10.5}$$

where Δ and ψ satisfy

$$\Delta \equiv 1 - \varphi - \psi > 0, \tag{10.6}$$

and

$$\psi < \widehat{p}_i. \tag{10.7}$$

As a result, a bias-adjusted risk ratio is given by

$$\tilde{\pi} = \frac{\tilde{p}_1}{\tilde{p}_2} = \frac{\widehat{p}_1 - \psi}{\widehat{p}_2 - \psi}. \tag{10.8}$$

It can be shown that the large-sample asymptotic variance of the logarithm of $\tilde{\pi}$ is given by (Exercise 10.1)

$$\sigma^2(\ln(\tilde{\pi})) = \sigma^2(\ln(\tilde{p}_1)) + \sigma^2(\ln(\tilde{p}_2)) = \frac{x(N_1 - x)}{\Delta^2 p_1^2 N_1^3} + \frac{y(N_2 - y)}{\Delta^2 p_2^2 N_2^3}, \tag{10.9}$$

where Δ is given by Eq. (10.6).

A 100% confidence interval for the risk ratio π is given by

$$\exp\left[\ln(\tilde{\pi}) - z_{1-\frac{\alpha}{2}} \cdot \widehat{\sigma}(\ln(\tilde{\pi}))\right] \le \pi \le \exp\left[\ln(\tilde{\pi}) + z_{1-\frac{\alpha}{2}} \cdot \widehat{\sigma}(\ln(\tilde{\pi}))\right], \tag{10.10}$$

where $z_{1-\frac{\alpha}{2}}$ is the $100\left(1-\frac{\alpha}{2}\right)$th percentile of a standard normal distribution, and $\widehat{\sigma}(\ln(\tilde{\pi}))$ is the square root of Eq. (10.9) with the true unknown p_i being replaced by the bias-adjusted estimator $\widehat{p}_i$, i = 1, 2.

Remark

The unknown misclassification error probabilities φ or ψ are estimated by using the validation sample data or the data from counterfactual true tables.

Table 10.2 Selected medical histories in DES-exposed (G_1) and DES-unexposed (G_2) males

Medical history	G_1 (n = 225)	G_2 (n = 111)	Risk ratio ($\widehat{\pi}$)
D_1:Urogenital tract symptoms or abnormalities	55	17	1.60
D_2:infections	14	3	2.30
D_3:Problems passing urine	29	2	7.15
D_4:Abnormality of penile urethra	10	0	–
D_5:Other physical abnormality	8	3	1.32
D_6:Kidney or bladder pain	16	5	1.58
D_7:Penile bleeding or discharge	11	2	2.71

This table is adapted from Table 1 in Henderson et al.

Example 10.1

After 1971 linking diethystilbestrol (DES) therapy in mothers with vaginal adenocarcinoma in their daughter was noticed. A registry of DES-exposed male and female offspring was established. It appears that male urogenital tract abnormalities are also associated with DES therapy.

In November 1971, a mail inquiry regarding the past and current use of DES was made of the members of the Los Angeles County Obstetrical and Gynecological Society. From the replies, 30 physicians were identified who had used DES in the past. From this group, we were able to identify 18 physicians who still had record of office visits back to 1945, and who agreed to participate in this study. A cohort study was performed. Of the 500 DES-exposed and 389 unexposed males identified in office records, it was able to locate mothers of 306 (61%) and 231 (60%) and obtained complete questionnaires from 225 (45%) and 111 (29%). Information pertaining to the siblings of exposed offspring on the urogenital tract symptoms or abnormalities are given Table 10.2.

The values of risk ratio in Table 10.2 were computed by using Eq. (10.1). Since there is no validation sample data, we are going to obtain the counterfactual (CF) true table to calculate the misclassification error probabilities. For the six immune disorders in Table 10.2, only the first disorder D_1 has nine feasible CF true tables so that misclassification error probabilities are able to be computed as given in Table 10.3. Note that the fifth over-reporting CF true table for D_1 is not feasible because the value of $\tilde{p}_2$ is negative as shown with boldface. The way to calculate misclassification error probabilities from the observed and CF true frequency tables is described in Sect. 10.3 (Table 10.4).

The values of $\tilde{\pi}$, $\widehat{\sigma}(\ln(\tilde{\pi}))$ and its 95% confidence interval for π were computed by using Eqs. (10.8) to (10.10). Note that all bias-adjusted risk ratios for both over- and under-reporting CF true tables for urogenital tract symptoms are significant and greater than the classical odds ratio.

Remarks

1. Although the classical risk ratio for urogenital is not significant (Exercise 10.2), all bias-adjusted risk ratios for all counterfactual true models are significant.
2. Not all observed immune disorder in DES-exposed subjects have feasible counterfactual true frequency tables as shown in this example (Exercise 10.3).

Table 10.3 Feasible CF true tables for D_1 CF true tables and bias-adjusted failure probabilities

Immune disorder	G_1	G_2	φ	ψ	$\tilde{p}_1$	$\tilde{p}_2$
D_1: Observed	55	17	–	–	0.244	0.153
D_1: CF true tables (over-reporting)	54	16	0.009	0.03	0.223	0.128
	53	15	0.019	0.063	0.198	0.099
	52	14	0.028	0.097	0.169	0.064
	51	13	0.038	0.133	0.134	0.024
	50	12	0.048	0.172	0.092	**−0.025**
D_1: CF true tables (under-reporting)	56	18	0.009	0.029	0.224	0.129
	57	19	0.018	0.056	0.204	0.105
	58	20	0.027	0.081	0.183	0.081
	59	21	0.035	0.105	0.162	0.056
	60	22	0.043	0.128	0.140	0.030

Table 10.4 Bias-adjusted risk ratio $\tilde{\pi}$ for D_1 CF true tables and its 95% confidence interval for π

Immune disorder	G_1	G_2	$\tilde{\pi}$	$\hat{\sigma}(\ln(\tilde{\pi}))$	95% CI for π
D_1: CF true tables (over-reporting)	54	16	1.74	0.257	1.05–2.88
	53	15	2.01	0.263	1.20–3.36
	52	14	2.62	0.269	1.54–4.44
	51	13	5.61	0.277	3.26–9.65
D_1: CF true tables (under-reporting)	56	18	1.73	0.267	1.03–2.92
	57	19	1.94	0.283	1.11–3.37
	58	20	2.27	0.296	1.26–4.07
	59	21	2.91	0.315	1.57–5.39
	60	22	4.66	0.332	2.43–8.93

10.2 Correlated Misclassifications in Cross-Sectional Studies

Given a cross-sectional study, let D and E denote the disease and the exposure variables of a subject, in which D = 1 if a subject is diseased, = 0 otherwise and E = 1 if a subject is exposed, = 0 otherwise. Let p_{ij} be the proportions of D = i and E = j of a subject in a population. Then the true odds ratio is $R = \frac{p_{11}p_{00}}{p_{01}p_{10}}$. But the observed odds ratio in the population given by $R^* = \frac{p^*_{11}p^*_{00}}{p^*_{01}p^*_{10}}$, where $p^*_{ij} = \Pr(D^* = i, E^* = j)$, D^* and E^*, surrogate variables of D and E, which depend on the answers, accurate or wrong, given by the subjects. Let the sensitivity and specificity be defined, respectively, by

Table 10.5 Probability of answers for the four categories of subjects assuming nondifferential correlated misclassifications by over-reporting

	$E^* = 0$	$E^* = 1$		$E^* = 0$	$E^* = 1$	
$D^* = 0$	q	$Sp_D - q$	Sp_D	0	Sp_D	Sp_D
$D^* = 1$	$Sp_E - q$	$Sp_D - Sp_E + q$	Sp_D	0	Sp_D	Sp_D
	Sp_E	Sp_E		0	1	
	p_{00}			p_{01}		
	$E^* = 0$	$E^* = 1$		$E^* = 0$	$E^* = 1$	
$D^* = 0$	0	0	0	0	0	0
$D^* = 1$	Sp_E	Sp_E	1	0	1	1
	Sp_E	Sp_E		0	1	
	p_{10}			p_{11}		

Where $\overline{X} = 1 - X, X = Sp_D \text{ or } Sp_E$. This table is adapted from adapted from Table 1 in Chavance et al. [1]

$$Se_D = \Pr(D^* = 1|D = 1), \tag{10.11}$$

$$Sp_D = \Pr(D^* = 0|D = 0), \tag{10.12}$$

$$Se_E = \Pr(E^* = 1|E = 1), \tag{10.13}$$

and

$$Sp_E = \Pr(E^* = 0|E = 0). \tag{10.14}$$

Assume that the data are collected by a self-administered survey. Furthermore, assume that there are over-reporting and under-reporting errors are allowed in a single direction in the data, that is, assume that all exposed (respectively diseased) subjects are correctly classified for exposure (respectively diseased), or $Se_D = Se_E = 1$. If misclassification is assumed to be nondifferential, $Sp_D = Sp_E$. In the absence of any relation between exposure and disease and if over-reporting of exposure and over-reporting of disease are independent among healthy nonexposed subjects, the misclassification errors will not bias the measure of odds ratio, $R^* = R = 1$. However, if among healthy nonexposed subjects the measure of odds ratio will be biased if these events are related.

Under the assumption of nondifferential over-reporting, Table 10.5 provides the probabilities of answers for the four categories of subjects, according to the specificities Sp_D and Sp_E and of the probability q that healthy nonexposed subjects answer correctly the two questions D and E.

Table 10.5 provides that healthy nonexposed subjects will be classified as diseased and exposed with a probability $1 - Sp_D - Sp_E + q$, while healthy exposed subjects will be classified as diseased and exposed with a probability $1 - Sp_D$. The total proportion of subjects who will be classified as diseased and exposed is $p_{00}(1 - Sp_D - Sp_E + q) + p_{01}(1 - Sp_D) + p_{10}(1 - Sp_E) + p_{11}$. Finally, the odds ratio is adjusted by over-reporting as

Table 10.6 Odds ratio adjusted by nondifferential correlated misclassifications assuming that its true value is unity and that only over-reporting, only under-reporting, or both occur some values of disease prevalence (p_D), prevalence of exposure (p_E), marginal probability of giving correct answers (π), probability of correct classification for subjects at risk of correlated misclassifications (q)

p_D	p_E	π	q	R_O^* [a]	R_U^* [b]	R^* [c]
0.1	0.2	0.9	0.82	1.25	1.02	1.29
0.1	0.2	0.9	0.83	1.55	1.03	1.63
0.1	0.1	0.8	0.65	1.22	1.02	1.24
0.1	0.1	0.8	0.67	1.77	1.06	1.87
0.1	0.1	0.8	0.69	2.56	1.09	2.79
0.05	0.2	0.9	0.82	1.34	1.02	1.37
0.05	0.2	0.9	0.83	1.76	1.03	1.84
0.05	0.1	0.8	0.65	1.25	1.02	1.28
0.05	0.1	0.8	0.67	1.93	1.05	2.02
0.05	0.1	0.8	0.69	2.93	1.09	3.15
0.01	0.2	0.9	0.82	1.46	1.02	1.49
1.49	0.2	0.9	0.83	2.08	1.03	2.15
0.01	0.1	0.8	0.65	1.30	1.02	1.31
0.01	0.1	0.8	0.67	2.11	1.05	2.19
0.01	0.1	0.8	0.69	3.39	1.09	3.56

[a]Over-reporting with $Sp_D = Sp_E = \pi$
[b]Under-reporting with $Se_D = Se_E = \pi$
[c]Over- and under- reporting with $Se_D = Sp_D = Se_E = Sp_E = \pi$
This table is adapted from Table 2 in Chavance et al. [1]

$$R_O^* = \frac{p_{00} q [p_{00}(1 - Sp_D - Sp_E + q) + p_{01}(1 - Sp_D) + p_{10}(1 - Sp_E) + p_{11}]}{[p_{00}(Sp_D - q) + p_{01} Sp_D][p_{00}(Sp_E - q) + p_{10} Sp_E]}. \tag{10.15}$$

Under the hypothesis that D and E are unrelated (R = 1), we have that $p_{00} = (1 - p_D)(1 - p_E)$, $p_{01} = (1 - p_D)p_E$, $p_{10} = p_D(1 - p_E)$, and $p_{11} = p_D p_E$, where p_D and p_E represent, respectively, the prevalence of disease and exposure. As a result, Eq. (10.15) may be written as

$$R_O^* = 1 + \frac{q - Sp_D Sp_E}{[Sp_D - (1 - p_E)q][Sp_E - (1 - p_D)q]}. \tag{10.16}$$

Similarly, under the assumption that misclassification arise only from under-reporting, the adjusted odds ratio is given by

$$R_U^* = 1 + \frac{q^* - Se_D Se_E}{(Se_D - p_E q^*)(Se_E - p_D q^*)}, \tag{10.17}$$

where q^* is the probability of being correctly classified for diseased, exposed subjects (Table 10.6).

Table 10.7 Probability of answers for the four categories of subjects assuming nondifferential correlated misclassifications by over- and under-reporting

	$E^* = 0$	$E^* = 1$		$E^* = 0$	$E^* = 1$	
$D^* = 0$	q	$Sp_D - q$	Sp_D	$Sp_D\overline{Sp_E}$	Sp_DSp_E	Sp_D
$D^* = 1$	$Sp_E - q$	$\overline{Sp_D} - Sp_E + q$	$\overline{Sp_D}$	$\overline{Sp_D}\,\overline{Sp_E}$	$Sp_E\overline{Sp_D}$	$\overline{Sp_D}$
	Sp_E	$\overline{Sp_E}$		$\overline{Sp_E}$	Sp_E	
	p_{00}			p_{01}		
	$E^* = 0$	$E^* = 1$		$E^* = 0$	$E^* = 1$	
$D^* = 0$	$\overline{Sp_D}Sp_E$	$\overline{Sp_D}\,\overline{Sp_E}$	$\overline{Sp_D}$	$\overline{Sp_D} - Sp_E + q$	$Sp_E - q$	$\overline{Sp_D}$
$D^* = 1$	Sp_DSp_E	$Sp_D\overline{Sp_E}$	Sp_D	$Sp_D - q$	q	Sp_D
	Sp_E	$\overline{Sp_E}$		$\overline{Sp_E}$	Sp_E	
	p_{10}			p_{11}		

where $\overline{X} = 1 - X, X = Sp_D$ *or* Sp_E. This table is adapted from Table 3 in Chavance et al. [1]

Table 10.7 gives the probabilities of the different possible answers according to the true status of the subjects under the following assumptions: (1) misclassifications according to the subjects' answers are nondifferential; (2) for each criterium, the sensitivity of the classification is equal to its specificity, that is, $Se_D = Sp_D$, $Se_E = Sp_E$; (3) for healthy exposed and diseased nonexposed subjects, misclassifications according to the two questions are independent events; (4) for healthy nonexposed and diseased exposed subjects, misclassifications according to the two questions may be related, and the probability of being correctly classified is the same for these two categories, $q = q^*$. If exposure and disease are independent, the adjusted odds ratio for both over- and under-reporting is given by

$$R^* = 1 + \frac{2p_Dp_E(q - Sp_DSp_E) + (p_D + p_E)(Sp_DSp_E - q) + q - Sp_DSp_E}{BC}, \quad (10.18)$$

where B and C are given, respectively, by

$$\begin{aligned} B = {} & p_Dp_E(2Sp_D + 2Sp_E - 2Sp_DSp_E - 2q - 1) + p_D \\ & \cdot (1 - 2Sp_D - Sp_E + Sp_DSp_E + q) + p_E(-Sp_D + Sp_DSp_E + q) \\ & + Sp_D - q, \end{aligned} \quad (10.19)$$

and

$$\begin{aligned} C = {} & p_Dp_E[2(Sp_D + Sp_E - Sp_DSp_E - q) - 1] + p_D(-Sp_E + Sp_DSp_E + q) \\ & + p_E(1 - Sp_D - 2Sp_E + Sp_DSp_E + q) + Sp_E - q. \end{aligned} \quad (10.20)$$

Example 10.2
The associations between nonright-handedness (E) and several aspects of health status (D) were observed in a sample of objects from a general population. All

subjects were inhabitants of Savignyle-Temple, a small town located 35 km from Paris. One adult (18 years and over) was randomly selected from each household. From the 2817 households contacted, 979 refused to participate and 168 subjects failed to send back or to correctly complete the self-administered questionnaire. An analysis of the answers from the first 744 respondents has already presented.

For assessment of handedness, a ten-item self-administered questionnaire was completed by subjects. The ten questions pertained to hand preference (right, left, or either) for throwing, using a tennis racket, shaving or making up, combing one's hair, tooth brushing, cutting bread with a knife, using a hammer, using a screwdriver, striking a match, and using a spoon. These ten activities were shown, in a previous study performed on a sample of 882 French subjects, to be the ones with the highest loadings on the first factor (identified as the handedness factor) of a principal component analysis. A score of one was given for each "right" answer, two for each "either," and three for each "left" answer. The subjects who did not answer four questions or more were excluded. The handedness index was computed as HI = 10·(sum of scores)/(number of answers). The higher the handedness index, the more left-handed (or the least right-handed) the subject. Left-hand shift was defined as HI > 10.

The handedness index was available for 1674 subjects, 645 men and 1029 women. Most of them (1615, 89.4%) answered all questions about handedness. There were 1174 (70%) pure right-handers (HI = 10), 347 (20.8%) other right-handers ($11 \leq HI \leq 19$) and 155 (9.2%) left-handers ($HI \geq 20$). Left-hand shift ($HI \geq 11$) was less frequent among subjects born up to 1946 (23.1%) than among subjects born later (32.8%, $\chi_1^2 = 15.4, p < 0.001$). It was significantly related to education ($p < 0.05$), with a frequency of 26.8% for university level, 27.6% for high-school level, 29.6% for primary level, and 41.9% for technical studies. Left-hand shift was slightly less frequent among women (28.5%) than among men (32.4%, $\chi_1^2 = 2.87, p < 0.1$). The answers to questions about health were strongly related to gender. Women were more likely than men to answer positively to at least one of the questions about diseases (78.8% versus 71.3%, $p < 0.001$), to at least one question about use of drugs (80.7% versus 68.7%, $p < 0.001$) or to at least one question about the use of health services (69.3% versus 56.3%, $p < 0.001$).

Table 10.8 gives the odds ratio measuring the association between left-hand shift and the answers to the various questions about health, after adjustment for sex, education, and age. It was significantly greater than one for 4 out of 12 questions. The odds ratio was also significantly greater than 1 when considering the experience of any of the health problems encompassed in the questionnaire, odds ratio = 1.36, 95% CI: 1.02–1.79.

When over-reporting of exposure and of disease are correlated events among sick nonexposed subjects, the measurement of the odds ratio is biased. For a real odds ratio equal to 1, the modeling showed that the increase in the odds ratio may be modest, it is easy to find a spurious but significant relation. The partial derivatives show that the bias induced for an odds ratio equal to unity by over-reporting increases with the proportion of subjects for which over-reporting may occur with

Table 10.8 Odds ratio adjusted for sex, education, and years of birth (≤1946 versus >1946) between left-hand shift ($HI \geq 10$ versus HI = 10) and health disorders

Type of disorder	Answer	No.	Odds ratio	95% CI
Migraine headache	No	750	1.15	0.91–1.44
	Yes	790		
Migraine headache in the family	No	809	1.08	0.85–1.38
	Yes	541		
Allergy to drugs	No	1200	1.21	0.91–1.61
	Yes	287		
Asthma	No	1420	1.14	0.86–1.70
	Yes	122		
Eczema during childhood	No	1339	1.45*	1.03–2.04
	Yes	169		
Urticaria	No	1168	1.33*	1.03–1.74
	Yes	341		
Hay fever	No	1130	1.02	0.79–1.32
	Yes	395		
Diabetes	No	1411	1.69	0.65–4.45
	Yes	18		
Epilepsy	No	1514	0.71	0.19–2.63
	Yes	13		
Hypertension	No	1297	1.07	0.78–1.48
	Yes	224		
Serious health problem (present)	No	1371	1.66**	1.14–2.44
	Yes	131		
Serious health problem (in the past)	No	1120	1.21*	1.07–1.81
	Yes	358		

This table is adapted from Table 4 in Chavance et al. [1]

the misclassification error probability, and with the strength of the association between the two types of misclassifications [1].

When under-reporting of disease is correlated with under-reporting of exposure among sick exposed subjects, the odds ratio is also biased, but in most cross-sectional studies healthy nonexposed subjects are dozens of hundreds of times more numerous than diseased exposed subjects, and the influence of under-reporting is negligible as compared to that of over-reporting. The model that encompasses both under- and over-reporting shows that, for reasonable values of the parameters, bias induced by bidirectional errors is not very different from that induced by over-reporting only.

Remarks

1. The bidirectional model presented here is not totally realistic: a) assuming the equality of the sensitivities and of the specificities is a very strong hypothesis; b) the strength of the association between misclassifications is assumed to be the

same for over- and under-reporting. But a model with two or three more parameters would be awkward to handle.

2. Several significant relations were found between left hand shift and the answers about experience of common diseases, use of drugs or consultation of medical services.
3. Tables that give the odds ratio measuring the associations between left-hand shift and the answers about the use of drugs or of health services are omitted here but can be found in Chavance et al. [1].

10.3 Joint Misclassification of Exposure and Disease

Let D and E be the dichotomous disease and exposure variable in a cohort study, in which D = 1 if a subject is diseased; otherwise, = 0; E = 1 if a subject is exposed; otherwise, = 0. We are going to study the problem of joint misclassification of exposure and disease that allows for correlation of classification errors of exposure and disease. We consider the situation in which overall misclassification of the disease is independent of true exposure status (nondifferential). However, we allow for variation in accuracy of disease classification among strata defined by accuracy of the exposure measurement within the true exposure categories to reflect misclassification dependencies.

The total number of study participants in a cohort is N and p is the prevalence of exposure in the cohort. The cumulative incidence of disease in the unexposed is CI_0 and CIR is the cumulative incidence ratio. Subgroup of the truly exposed individuals of size $N \cdot p \cdot CIR \cdot CI_0$ with the disease are given in Table 10.10, where p is the exposure prevalence and the incidence ratio at the base-line. The sensitivity and specificity of disease and exposure are defined by

$$Se_D = \Pr(D^* = 1 | D = 1), \tag{10.21}$$

$$Sp_D = \Pr(D^* = 0 | D = 0), \tag{10.22}$$

$$Se_E = \Pr(E^* = 1 | E = 1), \tag{10.23}$$

and

$$Sp_E = \Pr(E^* = 0 | E = 0), \tag{10.24}$$

where D^* and E^* are classified surrogate variables of D and E. Assume that (Se_D, Sp_D) and (Se_E, Sp_E) are independent of true exposure and disease status respectively. The relation between Se_D, Sp_D, Se_E, Sp_E, Se_{dik}, and Sp_{dik} is given in Table 10.9.

In Table 10.9, all correct classification probabilities are computed as follows.

Table 10.9 Correct classification probabilities within the observed sample data

	Exposure classification		
Disease classification	E^*: Correct	$\overline{E}^*$: Incorrect	Total
D^*: Correct	$s_{11}=Se_{d11}Se_E$	$s_{12}=Se_{d10}(1-Se_E)$	Se_D
$\overline{D}^*$incorrect	$s_{21}=\overline{Se}_{d11}Se_E$	$s_{22}=\overline{Se}_{d10}\overline{Se}_E$	$\overline{Se}_D$
Total	Se_E	$\overline{Se}_E$	

Where $\overline{X}=1-X, X=Se_D, Se_E, Se_{dik}$, Se_{dik}, and Sp_{dik} are sensitivity and specificity of disease classification in the subgroup with true exposure level i and observed exposure level k

$$s_{11}=\Pr(D^*E^*|DE)=\Pr(D^*|DEE^*)\Pr(E^*|DE)=Se_{D|EE^*}Se_{E|D}=Se_{d11}Se_E;$$

$$s_{12}=\Pr\left(D^*\overline{E}^*|D\overline{E}\right)=\Pr\left(D^*|D\overline{E}\overline{E}^*\right)\Pr\left(\overline{E}^*|D\overline{E}\right)=Se_{D|\overline{E}\overline{E}^*}Se_{\overline{E}|D}=Se_{d10}(1-Se_E);$$

$$s_{21}=\Pr\left(\overline{D}^*E^*|\overline{D}E\right)=\Pr\left(\overline{D}^*|\overline{D}EE^*\right)\Pr\left(E^*|\overline{D}E\right)=Se_{\overline{D}|EE^*}Se_{E|\overline{D}}=(1-Se_{d11})Se_E;$$

$$s_{22}=\Pr\left(\overline{D}^*\overline{E}^*|\overline{D}\overline{E}\right)=\Pr\left(\overline{D}^*|\overline{D}\overline{E}\overline{E}^*\right)\Pr\left(\overline{E}^*|\overline{D}\overline{E}\right)=Se_{\overline{D}|\overline{E}\overline{E}^*}Se_{\overline{E}|\overline{D}}=(1-Se_{d10})\times(1-Se_E).$$

Let a and b denote the true (unobservable) numbers of exposed and unexposed persons with the disease, and c and d denote the true numbers of exposed and unexposed persons without the disease. Then the observed data $\vec{y}^T=\left(\hat{a},\hat{b},\hat{c},\hat{d}\right)$ are related to the true person counts $\vec{x}^T=$(a, b, c, d) by

$$E(\vec{y})=\mathcal{W}\vec{x}, \tag{10.25}$$

where $\mathcal{W}$ is given by

$$\mathcal{W}=\begin{bmatrix} w_{11} & w_{12} & w_{13} & w_{14} \\ w_{21} & w_{22} & w_{23} & w_{24} \\ w_{31} & w_{32} & w_{33} & w_{34} \\ w_{41} & w_{42} & w_{43} & w_{44} \end{bmatrix},$$

$w_{11}=s_{11}, w_{12}=Se_{d01}\overline{Sp}_E, w_{13}=\overline{Sp}_{d11}Se_E, w_{14}=\overline{Sp}_{d01}\overline{Sp}_E;$
$w_{21}=s_{12}, w_{22}=Se_{d00}Sp_E, w_{23}=s_{22}, w_{24}=\overline{Sp}_{d00}Sp_E;$
$w_{31}=s_{21}, w_{32}=\overline{Se}_{d01}\overline{Sp}_E, w_{33}=Sp_{d11}Se_E, w_{34}=Sp_{d01}\overline{Sp}_E;$
$w_{41}=s_{22}, w_{42}=\overline{Se}_{d00}Sp_E, w_{43}=Sp_{d10}\overline{Se}_E, w_{44}=Sp_{d00}Sp_E.$

By using the approximate relation $\vec{y}\approx E(\vec{y})$, the bias-adjusted true person counts are solved from Eq. (10.25)

Table 10.10 Follow-up study sample data

	$E^* = 1$	$E^* = 0$	Total
$D^* = 1$	38	24	62
$D^* = 0$	62	76	138
Total	100	100	200

Where D^* and E^* are the observed surrogate variables of D and E

$$\tilde{\vec{x}} = \mathcal{W}^{-1}\vec{y} = \mathcal{V}\vec{y}, \tag{10.26}$$

where $\widetilde{\vec{x}} = \left(\tilde{a}, \tilde{b}, \tilde{c}, \tilde{d}\right)^T$, provided that $\mathcal{W}$ is invertible, and $\mathcal{V} = \mathcal{W}^{-1}$.

Incidentally, the bias-adjusted cumulative confidence ratio is given by [5]

$$\widetilde{CIR} = \frac{\tilde{a}\left(\tilde{b} + \tilde{d}\right)}{\tilde{b}(\tilde{a} + \tilde{c})}, \tag{10.27}$$

where $\tilde{a}, \tilde{b}, \tilde{c}, \tilde{d}$ are given by Eq. (10.26).

Example 10.3

Consider a cohort study with the disease and exposure variable D and E, where D = 1 if a subject is diseased, = 0 otherwise and E = 1 if exposed, = 0 otherwise. The following hypothetical data (Table 10.10) are taken from Table 12.12 in Kleinbaum et al. [5].

Find the bias-adjusted cumulative incidence ratio from Table 10.10.

Solution

Assume that the misclassification in Table 10.10 is nondifferential with $Se_D = 0.8$, $Sp_D = 0.9$, $Se_E = 0.9$, and $Sp_E = 0.7$. Furthermore, assume that $Se_{d11} = 0.75$, $Se_{d10} = 0.85$, $Se_{d00} = 0.8$, $Sp_{d11} = 0.65$, $Sp_{d10} = 0.7$, $Se_{p01} = 0.8$, and $Se_{d00} = 0.9$. By substituting the above assumed sensitivities and specificities with $\widehat{a} = 38, \widehat{b} = 24, \widehat{c} = 62, \widehat{d} = 76$ into Eq. (10.26), we have

$$\widetilde{\vec{x}} = \begin{bmatrix} 25.65 & 6.48 & 19.53 & 0.06 \\ 3.23 & 13.44 & 1.86 & 5.32 \\ 8.55 & 0.72 & 36.27 & 18.24 \\ 0.57 & 3.36 & 13.02 & 47.88 \end{bmatrix}^{-1} \begin{bmatrix} 38 \\ 24 \\ 62 \\ 76 \end{bmatrix} = \begin{bmatrix} 0.50 \\ 1.04 \\ 0.94 \\ 1.25 \end{bmatrix}. \tag{10.28}$$

By substituting Eq. (10.28) into Eq. (10.27),

$$\widetilde{CIR} = \frac{0.5(1.04 + 1.25)}{1.04(0.5 + 0.94)} = 0.764557 \approx 0.76. \tag{10.29}$$

By comparing Eq. (10.29) with the classical cumulative incidence ratio that is 1.58 (= 38(24 + 76)/(24(38 + 62)), the bias-adjusted cumulative incidence ratio is biased toward the value of the null hypothesis.

10.4 Misclassification in Evaluating the Subgroup Means

Assume that a large population are distributed over m classes. The classes are disjoint and each element belongs to one and only one class. The probability that a certain element belongs to the ith class is assumed constant and equal to z_i ($z_i \geq 0, \sum_{i=1}^{m} z_i = 1$). We are interested in estimating the class means μ_i of a response random variable Y. At our disposal are $N^* = N + n$ elements obtained through simple random sampling. Through an imperfect classification device, these elements have been assigned to different classes. By the way, we also know the true classes for a random subsample of n elements. The probability that an element belonging to the ith class is classified to the jth class is thus $\psi_{ji} = z_i \varphi_{ji}$. The distribution of the N^* elements over the m^2 cells, defined by the different alternatives of true and recorded class, is a multinomial random variable with N^* and the $\psi_{ji}^{'}s$ as parameters. We assume that the probability of misclassification is independent of the random variable of analysis Y.

For the sample, n_{ji} denotes that the number of i elements are recorded as j elements, and $\overline{y}_{ji}$ the arithmetic average of these elements. The marginal distribution of the elements over the true classes is denoted by the column vector $\vec{n}_t = (n_1^t, n_2^t, \ldots, n_m^t)$, where $n_i^t = \sum_{j=1}^{m} n_{ji}$; the corresponding distribution over the recorded classes is denoted by $\vec{n}_r = (n_1^r, n_2^r, \ldots, n_m^r)$, where $n_j^r = \sum_{i=1}^{m} n_{ji}$ (Table 10.11).

To demonstrate that misclassification results in biased subgroup means, we consider the elements classified to the jth class. The average $\overline{y}_j$ of those n_j^r elements is written as a weighted average of the cell average $\overline{y}_{ji}$ given as

$$\overline{y}_j = \sum_{i=1}^{m} \frac{n_{ji}\overline{y}_{ji}}{n_j^r} = \sum_{i=1}^{m} \frac{n_{ji}\left(\overline{y}_{ji} - \overline{y}_{jj} + \overline{y}_{jj}\right)}{n_j^r} = \sum_{i=1}^{m} \frac{n_{ji}\overline{y}_{jj}}{n_j^r}$$
$$+ \sum_{i=1, i \neq j}^{m} \frac{n_{ji}\left(\overline{y}_{ji} - \overline{y}_{jj}\right)}{n_j^r} = \overline{y}_{jj} + \sum_{i=1, i \neq j}^{m} \frac{n_{ji}\left(\overline{y}_{ji} - \overline{y}_{jj}\right)}{n_j^r}, \tag{10.30}$$

where $\sum_{i=1}^{m} n_{ji} = n_j^r$.

Table 10.11 The marginal distribution of the jth classified assignment

		ith class				Marginal total
		1	2	…	m	
	1	n_{11}	n_{12}	…	n_{1m}	n_1^r
jth class	2	n_{21}	n_{22}	…	n_{2m}	n_2^r
	…	…	…		…	
	m	n_{m1}	n_{m2}	…	n_{mm}	n_m^r
Marginal total		n_1^t	n_2^t		n_m^t	$N^* = n + N$

The expectation of Eq. (10.30) with respect to the response random variable Y is given by

$$E_Y(\overline{y}_j) = \mu_j + \sum_{i=1, i \neq j}^{m} \frac{n_{ji}(\mu_i - \mu_j)}{n_j^r}, \tag{10.31}$$

where $E(\overline{y}_{ji}) = \mu_i$, which means that misclassification from i to j is independent of the y value. Eq. (10.31) implies that $\overline{y}_j$ is a biased estimator of μ_j. In the formula, the distribution of the elements over the m^2 cells is regarded as fixed. For large samples, the bias is

$$E(\overline{y}_j) = E_N(E_Y(\overline{y}_j)) \approx \mu_j + \frac{\sum_{i=1, i \neq j}^{m} \Psi_{ji}(\mu_i - \mu_j)}{\sum_{i=1}^{m} \Psi_{ji}}, \tag{10.32}$$

where E_N denotes the expectation with respect to the marginal distribution of the elements over the cells.

The variance of $\overline{y}_j$ can be derived with the help of the identity $\sigma^2(\overline{y}_j) = \sigma_N^2(E_Y(\overline{y}_j)) + E_N(\sigma_Y^2(\overline{y}_j))$, where σ_N^2 denotes the variance with respect to the marginal distribution of the elements over the cells and σ_Y^2 denotes the variance with respect to the response variable Y when the $n_{ji}'s$ are regarded as fixed. We get

$$\sigma^2(\overline{y}_j) = \sigma_N^2\left(\sum_{i=1}^{m} \frac{n_{ji}\mu_i}{n_j^r}\right) + E_N\left(\frac{\sum_{i=1}^{m} n_{ji}\sigma_i^2}{\left(n_j^r\right)^2}\right)$$

$$\approx \left[\sum_{i=1}^{m} \frac{\psi_{ji}}{\psi_{j+}}\left(\mu_i^2 - \sum_{k=1}^{m} \frac{\psi_{jk}\mu_i\mu_k}{\psi_{j+}}\right) + \sum_{i=1}^{m} \frac{\psi_{ji}\sigma_i^2}{N^*\psi_{j+}}, \tag{10.33}$$

where $\psi_{j+} = \sum_{i=1}^{m} \psi_{ji}$, $\sigma_N^2\left(\sum_{i=1}^{m} \frac{n_{ji}\mu_i}{n_j^r}\right)$ is approximated through a linear expansion [4]. The expansion for E_N here and in Eq. (10.32) also relies on this expansion, and σ_i^2 denotes the variance of Y in the ith class.

Remarks

1. From Eqs. (10.31) to (10.33), it implies that both the expectation and the variance are affected by the possibility of misclassification.
2. The effects depend on the probability of misclassification, the proportions of elements belonging to the different classes, and the differences between the true means.
3. For the variance, the true class variances are also of importance. From standard sampling theory results it follows that $\frac{s_j^2}{n_j^r}$ is an unbiased estimator of the variance

$\sigma^2(\overline{y}_j)$, where $\left(n_j^r - 1\right)s_j^2 = \sum_{i,k=1}^{m}\left(y_{jik} - \overline{y}_j\right)^2$, y_{jik} denotes the kth observation in cell ji.

To adjust for misclassification when the probabilities of classification by the imperfect device from a random subsample, we form the linear combination of the $\overline{y}_j$'s, the averages of the recorded classes. Thus, we obtain the expectation of the column vector $\overrightarrow{\overline{y}} = (\overline{y}_1, \overline{y}_2, \ldots, \overline{y}_m)^T$

$$E\left(\overrightarrow{\overline{y}}\right) = \left[diag\left(\Phi\vec{z}\right)\right]^{-1} \cdot \Phi \cdot diag(\mathcal{Z}) \cdot \vec{\mu}, \tag{10.34}$$

where $\vec{\mu} = (\mu_1, \mu_2, \ldots, \mu_m)^T$ is the column vector of true means, $\vec{z} = (z_1, z_2, \ldots, z_m)^T$ denotes the column vector of class proportions in the population, $\Phi = \left[\varphi_{ji}\right]_{i,j=1}^{m}$ is the matrix of classification probabilities, "diag" is the diagonalization operator, and diag($\mathcal{Z}$) is the m × m matrix with z_i as the ith diagonal entry.

From Eq. (10.34), it is easily shown that the unbiased estimator of $\vec{\mu}$ is given by

$$\widehat{\vec{\mu}} = \mathcal{W}^{-1}\overrightarrow{\overline{y}}, \tag{10.35}$$

where $\mathcal{W} = \left[diag\left(\Phi\vec{z}\right)\right]^{-1}\Phi diag(\mathcal{Z})$ is assumed to be nonsingular. The variance of $\widehat{\vec{\mu}}$ is given by

$$\sigma^2\left(\widehat{\vec{\mu}}\right) = \mathcal{W}^{-1}\sigma^2\left(\overrightarrow{\overline{y}}\right)\left(\mathcal{W}^{-1}\right)^T. \tag{10.36}$$

In fact, neither $\vec{z}$ nor Φ are known, what is always known, is the number of elements classified to different classes that can be used to estimate $\vec{z}$. These numbers are assembled in $\vec{n}^r$. The expected value of $\vec{n}^r$, given the number of elements $\vec{n}^t$ and the misclassification matrix Φ is

$$E\left(\vec{n}^r \mid \vec{n}^t, \Phi\right) = \Phi\vec{n}^t. \tag{10.37}$$

The expected value of $N^{-1}\vec{n}^t$ is $\vec{z}$, and $N^{-1}\vec{n}^r$ can be viewed as a biased estimator of both $N^{-1}\vec{n}^t$ and $\vec{z}$.

The estimator $\widehat{\vec{n}^t} = \Phi^{-1}\vec{n}^r$ then is an unbiased estimator of $\vec{n}^t$, and $N^{-1}\widehat{\vec{n}^t}$ is an unbiased estimator of $\vec{z}$. With $\vec{z}$ replaced by this estimator, $\mathcal{W}$ in Eq. (10.35) is written as

$$\tilde{\mathcal{W}} = \left[diag\left(\vec{n}^{r}\right)\right]^{-1} \Phi \left[diag\left(\Phi^{-1}\vec{n}^{r}\right)\right]. \tag{10.38}$$

$\tilde{W}^{-1}\vec{\overline{y}}$ is an adjusted estimator of $\vec{\mu}$, where $\tilde{W}^{-1}$ is a corrected matrix for $\vec{\overline{y}}$.

To estimate Φ we assume that an independent double sampling subsample is available, where the elements are classified both by the unexpensive device of and by an expansive device that gives the true class. For such a sample it is known that the maximum likelihood estimator of φ_{ij} is given by $\widehat{\varphi}_{ij} = n_{ij}/n_{i\cdot}^{t}$. The final corrected matrix is

$$\tilde{\mathcal{W}}^{-1} = \left[diag\left(\widehat{\mathcal{W}}^{-1}\vec{n}^{r}\right)\right]^{-1} \widehat{\mathcal{W}}^{-1} diag\left(\vec{n}^{r}\right), \tag{10.39}$$

and $\tilde{\mathcal{W}}^{-1}\vec{\overline{y}}$ is the final estimator of the unknown true means $\vec{\mu}$, where $\tilde{\mathcal{W}}^{-1}$ is given by Eq. (10.39).

When we take account of the fact that we know the true classes for the double-sampled n elements, an estimator of the true numbers $\vec{n}^{t}$ is $\widehat{\vec{n}}^{t}_{d} = \widehat{\Phi}^{-1}\vec{n}^{r}_{s} + \vec{n}^{t}_{d}$, where $\vec{n}^{t}_{d}$ denotes the true number of doubled-sampled elements, $\vec{n}^{r}_{s}$ denotes the recorded numbers for the non-double-sampled elements. A modified final estimator is

$$\vec{\tilde{\mu}} = \frac{N}{N^{*}} \widehat{\mathcal{W}}_{d}^{-1} \vec{\overline{y}}_{s} + \frac{n}{N^{*}} \vec{\overline{y}}_{d}, \tag{10.40}$$

where $\vec{\overline{y}}_{d}$ contains the means for the double-sampled elements, $\vec{\overline{y}}_{s}$ the means for the other elements, and the correction matrix $\widehat{\mathcal{W}}_{d}^{-1}$ is obtained as the inverse of $\mathcal{W}$ in Eq. (10.35) with $\vec{z}$ replaced by $(N^{*})^{-1}\widehat{\vec{n}}^{t}_{d}$ and Φ by $\widehat{\Phi}$.

Remarks

1. The corrected matrix $\widehat{\mathcal{W}}$ is random and maybe singular, in which case the inverse and the correction do not exist. To make life easier, we assume that the classification procedure and the sample for estimation of Φ are such that the probability that $\widehat{\mathcal{W}}$ is singular is negligible.
2. We further assume that $\widehat{\mathcal{W}}^{-1}\vec{\overline{y}}$ as a vector function of the estimated φ_{ij} probabilities obeying regularity conditions required for linear expansion. Then $\widehat{\mathcal{W}}^{-1}\vec{\overline{y}}$ is an unbiased estimator of $\vec{\mu}$ to the first order and the variance is to the first order [6]

$$\sigma^2\left(\widehat{\mathcal{W}}^{-1}\overrightarrow{\mathrm{y}}\right)=\sigma_N^2\left[E_Y\left(\widehat{\mathcal{W}}^{-1}\overrightarrow{\mathrm{y}}\right)\right]+E_N\left[\sigma_Y^2\left(\widehat{\mathcal{W}}^{-1}\overrightarrow{\mathrm{y}}\right)\right]$$
$$\approx\sigma_N^2\left[\widehat{\mathcal{W}}^{-1}E_Y\left(\overrightarrow{\mathrm{y}}\right)\right]+\mathcal{W}^{-1}\sigma_N^2\left(\overrightarrow{\mathrm{y}}\right)\left(\mathcal{W}^{-1}\right)^T. \tag{10.41}$$

Since the y values and the classification are independent, the variance of Eq. (10.40) is obtained through obvious modifications of Eq. (10.41).

Assume that Y is a dichotomous response variable having an error. Also, we assume that the assignment of class is independent of the true response. Let the true proportions of responses belonging to the first and second categories of the 1–0 Y for the ith class be denoted by p_i^Y and $1-p_i^Y$ $(0\leq p_i^Y\leq 1)$. The probabilities of correct assignment for the response variable are denoted by $p_{ji}^{Y1\,|\,1}$ $\left(0\leq p_{ji}^{Y1\,|\,1}\leq 1\right)$ and $p_{ji}^{Y0\,|\,0}$ $\left(0\leq p_{ji}^{Y0\,|\,0}\leq 1\right)$ for the jith cell of elements. The probabilities of incorrect classification are $p_{ji}^{Y1\,|\,0}=1-p_{ji}^{Y1\,|\,1}$ and $p_{ji}^{Y0\,|\,1}=1-p_{ji}^{Y0\,|\,0}$. The probability of a specific response that is assigned to a specific category is easily derived. For example, the probability of obtaining and correctly classifying the response 1 is equal to $p_i^Y p_{ji}^{Y1\,|\,1}$.

The expectation of the cell average is accordingly given by normal

$$E_Y\left(\overline{y}_{ji}\right)=p_{ji}^{Y1\,|\,1}p_i^Y+\left(1-p_{ji}^{Y0\,|\,0}\right)\left(1-p_i^Y\right). \tag{10.42}$$

Remark

Equation (10.42) holds provided that misclassification is independent of the response.

By using Eq. (10.42) for Eq. (10.32) we obtain large-sample expression for $E\left(\overrightarrow{\mathrm{y}}\right)$ which is given by

$$E\left(\overrightarrow{\mathrm{y}}\right)\approx\mathbb{Q}\vec{\mu}+\mathbb{R}, \tag{10.43}$$

where $\mathbb{Q}=\mathbb{S}\odot\left(\mathbb{P}^{Y1\,|\,1}-\mathbb{P}^{Y1\,|\,0}\right)$ and $\mathbb{R}=\mathbb{S}\odot\mathbb{P}^{Y1\,|\,0}\overrightarrow{\mathrm{e}}$, $\overrightarrow{\mathrm{e}}$ denoting the unit vector, and $\mathbb{S}=\left[diag\left(\mathbb{P}\vec{p}\right)\right]^{-1}\mathbb{P}diag\left(\vec{p}\right)$, $\mathbb{P}^{Y1\,|\,1}$ is the matrix of the $p_{ji}^{Y1\,|\,1}$ elements, $\mathbb{P}^{Y1\,|\,0}$ is the matrix of the $p_{ji}^{Y1\,|\,0}$ elements, and "$\odot$" denotes the elementwise or Hadamard matrix product.

A correction of the biased $\vec{\mu}$ estimator is $\overrightarrow{\mathrm{y}}=\mathbb{Q}^{-1}\left(\overrightarrow{\mathrm{y}}-\mathcal{R}\right)$. When the misclassification error probabilities and the population proportions are unknown, the final estimator of $\vec{y}$ is given by

Table 10.12 The number (percentage) of the heart-diseased variable in the 1968 Swedish Level of Living Survey

		H		
		1	0	Total
H^*	1	173 (0.03)	47 (0.008)	220 (0.038)
	0	13 (0.002)?	5627 (0.9603)?	5640 (0.9625)
Total		186 (0.0322)?	5674 (0.9683)?	5860 (1.0)

$$\overrightarrow{\overline{y}} = \widehat{\mathbb{Q}}^{-1}\left(\overrightarrow{\overline{y}} - \widehat{\mathbb{R}}\right), \tag{10.44}$$

where $\widehat{\mathbb{Q}} = \widehat{\mathbb{S}} \odot \left(\widehat{\mathbb{P}}^{Y1|1} - \widehat{\mathbb{P}}^{Y1|0}\right)$ and $\widehat{\mathbb{R}} = \widehat{\mathbb{S}} \odot \widehat{\mathbb{P}}^{Y1|0}\overrightarrow{e}$ with $\widehat{\mathbb{P}}^{Y1|1}$ and $\widehat{\mathbb{P}}^{Y1|0}$ denotes estimates of the corresponding matrices of the misclassification error probabilities.

Remarks

1. It can be proved that Eq. (10.44) is an unbiased estimator of $\overrightarrow{\overline{y}}$.
2. The variance can be obtained according to three-stage sampling as follows:

$$\sigma^2_{\overrightarrow{\overline{y}}} = E_1E_2\sigma_3^2\left(\overrightarrow{\overline{y}}\right) + E_1\sigma_2^2E_3\left(\overrightarrow{\overline{y}}\right) + \sigma_1^2E_2E_3\left(\overrightarrow{\overline{y}}\right), \tag{10.45}$$

where E_3 denotes the expectation with respect to the errors in Y given the true Y values and the distribution of the elements over the m^2 cells, E_2 denotes the expectation of the marginal distribution of the elements, and E_1 denotes the expectation with respect to the marginal distribution of the elements. σ_3^2, σ_2^2, and σ_1^2 denote the corresponding variances. From Eq. (10.45) we may obtain the approximations [6].

The empirical illustration that followed are based on data from the 1968 Swedish level of Living Survey and its replication in 1974 [2].

Example 10.4

A number of 220 out of the 5860 individuals in the 1968 survey were originally classified as heart disease. This classification was based on the answers to questions concerning symptoms thought relevant [6]. After expert evaluation of the complete evidence for these 220 individuals, their number was reduced to 173 which are regarded as truly heart disease. Let H be a dichotomous truly heart disease variable defined by H = 1, if a subject is truly heart disease; otherwise, = 0. Similarly, H^* is denoted by the classified heart-diseased variable defined accordingly. The data are summarized in Table 10.12.

We thus have

$$p_1^{H^*} = \Pr(H^* = 1) = \frac{220}{5860} \approx 0.038, \tag{10.46}$$

whereas

$$p_0^{H^*} = \Pr(H^* = 0) = 1 - p_1^{H^*} = 0.962. \tag{10.47}$$

Also,

$$p_{11}^{H^*1|1} = \Pr[(H^* = 1) \cap (H = 1)] = \frac{173}{5860} \approx 0.03. \tag{10.48}$$

and

$$p_{10}^{H^*1|1} = \Pr[(H^* = 1) \cap (H = 0)] = \frac{47}{5860} \approx 0.008. \tag{10.49}$$

Unfortunately, there was no quality control for those classified as $\{H^* = 0\}$ (Table 10.12). The additional specifications are arbitrarily chosen as

$$n_{01} = 13 \text{ and } n_{00} = 5627 \tag{10.50}$$

After substituting Eq. (10.50) for the "?" mark in the 01th and the 00th cell in Table 10.12, we have Table 10.12 as shown in the current form.

By taking the values of $\widehat{\mathbb{P}}$ and $\widehat{p}$ from Table 10.12, we have

$$\widehat{\mathbb{P}} = \begin{bmatrix} 0.03 & 0.008 \\ 0.002 & 0.9603 \end{bmatrix} \text{ and } \widehat{p} = \begin{bmatrix} 0.0322 \\ 0.9683 \end{bmatrix}. \tag{10.51}$$

By substituting Eq. (10.51) into Eq. (10.43),

$$\mathbb{S} = \begin{bmatrix} 0.129 & 0.871 \\ 8.2 \cdot 10^{-5} & 1.0 \end{bmatrix}. \tag{10.52}$$

Furthermore, the matrices $\widehat{\mathbb{P}}^{H^*1|1}$ and $\widehat{\mathbb{P}}^{H^*1|0}$ are obtained as follows:

$$\widehat{\mathbb{P}}^{H^*1|1} = \begin{bmatrix} 0.03 & 0.04 \\ 0.97 & 0.96 \end{bmatrix}, \text{ and}$$
$$\widehat{\mathbb{P}}^{H^*1|0} = \begin{bmatrix} 0.998 & 0.008 \\ 0.002 & 0.96 \end{bmatrix}. \tag{10.53}$$

By substituting Eqs. (10.52) and (10.53) into Eq. (10.43),

$$\widehat{\mathbb{Q}} = \begin{bmatrix} -0.125 & 0.028 \\ 8.0 \cdot 10^{-5} & 0 \end{bmatrix}, \tag{10.54}$$

and

$$\widehat{\mathbb{R}} = \begin{bmatrix} 0.14 \\ 0.96 \end{bmatrix}. \tag{10.55}$$

Since $\det\left(\widehat{\mathbb{Q}}\right) = -2.2 \cdot 10^{-6}$ is not zero, the inverse of $\widehat{\mathbb{Q}}$ is given by

$$\widehat{\mathbb{Q}}^{-1} = \begin{bmatrix} 0 & 12573.9 \\ 36.2 & 56804.8 \end{bmatrix}. \tag{10.56}$$

From Table 10.12,

$$\overrightarrow{y} = \begin{bmatrix} 0.032 \\ 0.968 \end{bmatrix}. \tag{10.57}$$

By substituting Eqs. (10.55) to (10.57) into Eq. (10.44), the final corrected estimator of the mean of the subcategories is given by

$$\overrightarrow{\hat{y}} = \begin{bmatrix} 100 \\ 442.6 \end{bmatrix}.$$

10.5 Exercise

1. Show that Eq. (10.9) holds.
2. Show that the classical risk ratio estimator $\hat{\pi}$ in Table 10.2 for D_1 is not statistically significant.
3. Show that all counterfactual true frequency tables for the immune disorder diseases D_2 to D_7 in Table 10.2 are not feasible.

References

1. Chavance, M., Dellatolas, G., & Lellouch, J. (1992). Correlated nondifferential misclassifications of disease and exposure: Application to a cross-sectional study of the relation between handedness and immune disorders. *International Journal of Epidemiology, 21*, 537–546.
2. Johansson, S. (1973). The level of living survey. *Acta Sociologica, 3*, 211–219.
3. Katz, D., Baptista, J., Azen, S. P., & Pike, M. C. (1978). Obtaining confidence intervals for the risk ratio in cohort studies. *Biometrics, 34*, 469–474.
4. Kendall, M. G., & Stuart, A. (1961). *The Advaced theory of statistics* (Vol. 2). Hafner Publishing Company.

5. Kleinbaum, D. G., Kupper, L. L., & Morgenstern, H. (1982). *Epidemiologic research: Principles and quantitative methods*. Wiley.
6. Selen, J. (1986). Adjusting for errors in classification and measurement in the analysis of partly and purely categorical data. *Journal of the American Statistical Association, 81*, 75–81.
7. Henderson, B. E., Benton, B., Cosgrov, M., et al. (1976.): Urogenital tract abnormalities in sons of women treated with diethylstilbestrol). *Pediatrics, 58*, 505–507.

Chapter 11
Latent Class Models for Misclassified Data

11.1 Latent Class Models

Consider four observed dichotomous variables (A, B, C, D) and one unobserved (or latent) dichotomous variable X. We say that variable X explains the relationship among A, B, C, and D if these relationships disappear when the level of variable X is held constant, that is, the four variables (A, B, C, D) becomes mutually independent when we examine the conditional relationship among the four variables in the four-way cross-classification table {ABCD} at each level of X. If these apparent relationships disappear, we say they are "spurious." In this situation, the four variables (A, B, C, D) are not directly related to each other, but each of the four variables may be affected by variable X; and when the level of X is not held constant, then these effects may produce the apparent relationships among the four variables.

Let variables A, B, C, and D consist of I, J, K, L classes, where I = J = K = L = 2. Let $\pi^{ijk\ell}$denote the probability that an individual will be at level (i, j, k, ℓ) with respect to the joint variables (A, B, C, D). Suppose the hypothesis H_1 is that a latent variable X can explain the relationship among the manifest variables (A, B, C, D). For the tth laten class, let π_{X_t} denote the probability that an individual is in class t, and let $\pi_{ABCDX_{ijk\ell t}}$ denote the probability that an individual is at level (i, j, k, ℓ, t) with respect to the joint variable (A, B, C, D, X). Let $\pi_{\overline{A}X_{it}}$ denote the conditional probability that an individual is at level i with respect to variable A, given that he is at latent level t on variable X; and let the conditional probability $\pi_{\overline{A}X_{it}}, \pi_{\overline{A}X_{it}}, \pi_{\overline{A}X_{it}}$ be similarly defined. The hypothesis H_1 states that

$$\pi_{ABCDX_{ijk\ell t}} = \pi_{X_t} \cdot \pi_{\overline{A}X_{it}} \cdot \pi_{\overline{B}X_{jt}} \cdot \pi_{\overline{C}X_{kt}} \cdot \pi_{\overline{D}X_{\ell t}} \tag{11.1}$$

and

T.-S. Lee, *Misclassification in Epidemiology*, Emerging Topics in Statistics and Biostatistics, https://doi.org/10.1007/978-3-032-12563-7_11

$$\pi^{ijk\ell} = \sum\nolimits_{t=1}^{2} \pi_{ABCDX_{ijk\ell t}}. \tag{11.2}$$

Remarks

1. Equation (11.1) states that, given an individual is at a latent class t with respect to variable X, his responses on the manifest variable (A, B, C, D) will be mutually independent.
2. Equation (11.2) describes the fact that each individual in the population under consideration is in one and only one of the two latent classes.

The conditional probability $\pi_{ABCD\overline{X}_{ijk\ell t}}$ can be expressed as

$$\pi_{ABCD\overline{X}_{ijk\ell t}} = \left(\pi^{ijk\ell}\right)^{-1} \pi_{ABCDX_{ijk\ell t}}. \tag{11.3}$$

From the definition of the probability π_{X_t} and $\pi_{ABCDX_{ijk\ell t}}$, we have

$$\pi_{X_t} = \sum\nolimits_{i,j,k,\ell=1}^{2} \pi_{ABCDX_{ijk\ell t}}, \tag{11.4}$$

and from the definition of the conditional probability $\pi_{\overline{A}X_{it}}$, we have

$$\pi_{X_t} \cdot \pi_{\overline{A}X_{it}} = \sum\nolimits_{j,k,\ell=1}^{2} \pi_{ABCDX_{ijk\ell t}}. \tag{11.5}$$

Formulas similar in form to Eq. (11.5) can be obtained for π_{X_t} multiplied by $\pi_{\overline{B}X_{jt}}$, $\pi_{\overline{C}X_{kt}}$, and $\pi_{\overline{D}X_{\ell t}}$. From Eqs. (11.3) and (11.4) can be written as

$$\pi_{X_t} = \sum\nolimits_{i,j,k,\ell=1}^{2} \pi^{ijk\ell} \pi_{ABCD\overline{X}_{ijk\ell t}}. \tag{11.6}$$

Similarly, Eq. (11.5) can be written as

$$\pi_{\overline{A}X_{it}} = \sum\nolimits_{j,k,\ell=1}^{2} \pi_{X_t}^{-1} \cdot \pi^{ijk\ell} \cdot \pi_{ABCD\overline{X}_{ijk\ell t}}, \tag{11.7}$$

and we can also obtain the following formulas:

$$\pi_{\overline{B}X_{jt}} = \sum\nolimits_{i,k,\ell=1}^{2} \pi_{X_t}^{-1} \cdot \pi^{ijk\ell} \cdot \pi_{ABCD\overline{X}_{ijk\ell t}}, \tag{11.8}$$

$$\pi_{\overline{C}X_{kt}} = \sum\nolimits_{i,j,\ell=1}^{2} \pi_{X_t}^{-1} \cdot \pi^{ijk\ell} \cdot \pi_{ABCD\overline{X}_{ijk\ell t}}, \tag{11.9}$$

$$\pi_{\overline{D}X_{\ell t}} = \sum\nolimits_{i,j,k=1}^{2} \pi_{X_t}^{-1} \cdot \pi^{ijk\ell} \cdot \pi_{ABCD\overline{X}_{ijk\ell t}}. \tag{11.10}$$

Suppose for a moment that the numerical values of the conditional probabilities $\pi_{ABCD\overline{X}_{ijk\ell t}}$ were available. In this case, we could estimate the parameters in the model, namely, π_{X_t}, $\pi_{\overline{A}X_{it}}$, $\pi_{\overline{B}X_{it}}$, $\pi_{\overline{C}X_{it}}$, $\pi_{\overline{D}X_{it}}$, in the following way, using the observed proportion $p^{ijk\ell}$ ($=f^{ijk\ell}/n$) of individuals at level (i, j, k, ℓ) with respect to the manifest variables (A, B, C, D). We would replace Eqs. (11.6) to (11.10) by

$$\widehat{\pi}_{X_t} = \sum\nolimits_{i,j,k,\ell=1}^{2} p^{ijk\ell} \pi_{ABCD\overline{X}_{ijk\ell t}}, \tag{11.11}$$

$$\widehat{\pi}_{\overline{A}X_{it}} = \sum\nolimits_{j,k,\ell=1}^{2} \widehat{\pi}_{X_t}^{-1} \cdot p^{ijk\ell} \cdot \pi_{ABCD\overline{X}_{ijk\ell t}}, \tag{11.12}$$

$$\widehat{\pi}_{\overline{B}X_{Jt}} = \sum\nolimits_{i,k,\ell=1}^{2} \widehat{\pi}_{X_t}^{-1} \cdot p^{ijk\ell} \cdot \pi_{ABCD\overline{X}_{ijk\ell t}}, \tag{11.13}$$

$$\widehat{\pi}_{\overline{C}X_{kt}} = \sum\nolimits_{i,j,\ell=1}^{2} \widehat{\pi}_{X_t}^{-1} \cdot p^{ijk\ell} \cdot \pi_{ABCD\overline{X}_{ijk\ell t}}, \tag{11.14}$$

$$\widehat{\pi}_{\overline{D}X_{\ell t}} = \sum\nolimits_{i,j,k=1}^{2} \widehat{\pi}_{X_t}^{-1} \cdot p^{ijk\ell} \cdot \pi_{ABCD\overline{X}_{ijk\ell t}}, \tag{11.15}$$

For a given set of numerical values for the $\pi_{ABCD\overline{X}_{ijk\ell t}}$, we can use Eqs. (11.11) to (11.15) to obtain tentative estimates of the parameters, and these tentative estimates can be inserted in Eqs. (11.1) to (11.3); and the new estimate of $\pi_{ABCD\overline{X}_{ijkt}}$ thus obtained can be again inserted in Eqs. (11.11) to (11.15) to obtain new estimates of the parameters in the model. This procedure is iterated until the estimates of the parameters in the model remain unchanged. If the parameters in this latent structure model have maximum likelihood estimates, it is possible to prove that the maximum likelihood estimates will satisfy this same system of equations. In this case, the iterative procedure described above can be used to obtain the maximum likelihood estimates.

To test whether hypothesis H_1 is congruent with the data, we compare the observed $f^{ijk\ell}$ with the corresponding estimated $\widehat{f}^{ijk\ell}$ under H_1 using the usual goodness-of-fit χ^2 statistic,

$$\mathfrak{X}^2 = \sum\nolimits_{i,j,k,\ell=1}^{2} \left(f^{ijk\ell} - \widehat{f}^{ijk\ell}\right)^2 / \widehat{f}^{ijk\ell}, \tag{11.16}$$

or the corresponding χ^2 based upon the likelihood -ratio statistic:

$$\mathfrak{L}^2 = 2 \cdot \sum\nolimits_{i,j,k,\ell=1}^{2} f^{ijk\ell} \cdot \ln\left(\frac{f^{ijk\ell}}{\widehat{f}^{ijk\ell}}\right), \tag{11.17}$$

where $f^{ijk\ell} = n \cdot p^{ijkl}$, $\widehat{f}^{ijk\ell} = n \cdot \sum_{t=1}^{2} \left(\widehat{\pi}_{X_t} \cdot \widehat{\pi}_{\overline{A}X_{1t}} \cdot \widehat{\pi}_{\overline{B}X_{1t}} \cdot \widehat{\pi}_{\overline{C}X_{1t}} \cdot \widehat{\pi}_{\overline{D}X_{1t}}\right)$, $\widehat{\pi}_{X_t}, \widehat{\pi}_{\overline{A}X_{1t}}, \widehat{\pi}_{\overline{B}X_{1t}}, \widehat{\pi}_{\overline{C}X_{1t}}$ and $\widehat{\pi}_{\overline{D}X_{1t}}$ are the maximum likelihood estimates of the parameters of $\pi_{X_t}, \pi_{\overline{A}X_{1t}}, \pi_{\overline{B}X_{1t}}, \pi_{\overline{C}X_{1t}}$ and $\pi_{\overline{D}X_{1t}}$. The χ^2 value obtained from $\mathfrak{X}^2$ of

Eqs. (11.16) or $\mathfrak{L}^2$ of (11.17) can be assessed by comparing its numerical value with the percentiles of the tabulated χ^2 distribution. The degrees of freedom for testing hypothesis H_1 are $16 - 1 - 9 = 6$.

Remarks

1. The entire theory considered in this section can be easily extended the polytomous variables [2].
2. For the polytomous variables the issue of the identifiability has to be carefully addressed [3].

Example 11.1

Let A, B, C, and D denote the four variables in Table 11.1 (membership at the first interview, attitudes at the first interview, membership at the second interview, attitudes at the second interview, respectively). A positive (+) response on a given variable is denoted by the number 1, and a negative (−) response by the number 2. Let (i, j, k, ℓ) denote the cell in the four-way table corresponding to the case where the respondent is classified as i on variable A (i = 1 or 2), j on variable B (j = 1 or 2), k on variable C (k = 1 or 2), and ℓ on variable D (ℓ = 1 or 2). Let $f^{ijk\ell}$ denote the observed frequency in cell (i, j, k, ℓ).

Solution

(a) Since the initial value of $\pi_{ABCD\overline{X}_{ijk\ell t}}$ is not available and

$$\sum\nolimits_{i=1}^{2} \pi_{\overline{A}X_{it}} = 1 = \sum\nolimits_{j=1}^{2} \pi_{\overline{B}X_{jt}} = \sum\nolimits_{k=1}^{2} \pi_{\overline{C}X_{kt}} = \sum\nolimits_{\ell=1}^{2} \pi_{\overline{D}X_{\ell t}} \tag{11.18}$$

we merely need to set up the trial values for nine independent variables π_{X_1}, $\pi_{\overline{A}X_{1t}}$, $\pi_{\overline{B}X_{1t}}$, $\pi_{\overline{C}X_{1t}}$, and $\pi_{\overline{D}X_{1t}}$ (t = 1 or 2) to be substituted in Eq. (11.1). After that, using Eqs. (11.2) to (11.3) and (11.11) to (11.15) to calculate $\pi_{ABCDX_{ijk\ell t}}$, $\pi^{ijk\ell}$, $\pi_{ABCD\overline{X}_{ijk\ell t}}$ and $\widehat{\pi}_{X_t}$, $\widehat{\pi}_{\overline{A}X_{1t}}$, $\widehat{\pi}_{\overline{B}X_{1t}}$, $\widehat{\pi}_{\overline{C}X_{1t}}$, $\widehat{\pi}_{\overline{D}X_{1t}}$. Then reiterate the entire procedure

Table 11.1 Observed cross-classification frequency ($f^{ijk\ell}$) of 3398 schoolboys, in interview at two successive points in time, with respect to dichotomous variables

		Second interview			
	Membership	+	+	−	−
	Attitude	+	−	+	−
First interview					
Membership	Attitude				
+	+	458	140	110	49
+	−	171	182	56	87
−	+	184	75	531	281
−	−	85	97	338	554

This table is taken from Coleman [1]

(a) Find the maximum likelihood estimators of the nine parameters of π_{X_1}, $\pi_{\overline{A}X_{1t}}$, $\pi_{\overline{B}X_{1t}}$, $\pi_{\overline{C}X_{1t}}$, and $\pi_{\overline{D}X_{1t}}$ (t = 1 or 2)

(b) Testing if hypothesis H_1 is congruent to the observed data in Table 11.1

Table 11.2 The iteration step (n) of the calculation

n	t	$\widehat{\pi}_{X_t}$	$\widehat{\pi}_{\overline{A}X_{1t}}$	$\widehat{\pi}_{\overline{B}X_{1t}}$	$\widehat{\pi}_{\overline{C}X_{1t}}$	$\widehat{\pi}_{\overline{D}X_{1t}}$
0	1	0.3	0.4	0.5	0.2	0.3
	2	0.2	0.2	0.3	0.3	0.4
1	1	0.002840	0.488924	0.644946	0.410027	0.538606
	2	0.001853	0.511076	0.355054	0.589973	0.461394
2	1	0.605183	0.368746	0.537964	0.409653	0.568864
	2	0.394817	0.631254	0.462036	0.590347	0.431136
3	1	0.605183	0.368746	0.537964	0.409653	0.568864
	2	0.394817	0.631254	0.462036	0.590347	0.431136

until the values of $\widehat{\pi}_{X_t}$, $\widehat{\pi}_{\overline{A}X_{it}}$, $\widehat{\pi}_{\overline{A}X_{it}}$, $\widehat{\pi}_{\overline{A}X_{it}}$, $\widehat{\pi}_{\overline{A}X_{it}}$ remain unchanged as shown in Table 11.2.

From the fourth iteration of Table 11.2, we have

$$\begin{aligned} \widehat{\pi}_{X_1} &= 0.605183 \approx 0.61, \\ \widehat{\pi}_{X_2} &= 0.394817 \approx 0.39. \end{aligned} \tag{11.19}$$

From both the fourth iteration of Table 11.2 and Eq. (11.18), we have

$$\begin{aligned} \widehat{\pi}_{\overline{A}X_{11}} &= 0.368746 \approx 0.37, \\ \widehat{\pi}_{\overline{A}X_{21}} &= 0.631254 \approx 0.63, \\ \widehat{\pi}_{\overline{B}X_{11}} &= 0.537964 \approx 0.54, \\ \widehat{\pi}_{\overline{B}X_{21}} &= 0.462036 \approx 0.46, \\ \widehat{\pi}_{\overline{C}X_{11}} &= 0.590347 \approx 0.59, \\ \widehat{\pi}_{\overline{C}X_{21}} &= 0.409653 \approx 0.41, \\ \widehat{\pi}_{\overline{D}X_{11}} &= 0.568864 \approx 0.57 \text{ and} \\ \widehat{\pi}_{\overline{D}X_{21}} &= 0.431136 \approx 0.43. \end{aligned} \tag{11.20}$$

From Eqs. (11.19) and (11.20), the maximum likelihood estimators for Table 11.1 are given by

$$\begin{aligned} &(\widehat{\pi}_{X_1}, \widehat{\pi}_{X_2}) = (0.61, 0.39), \\ &\left(\widehat{\pi}_{\overline{A}X_{11}}, \widehat{\pi}_{\overline{A}X_{21}}\right) = (0.37, 0.63), \\ &\left(\widehat{\pi}_{\overline{B}X_{11}}, \widehat{\pi}_{\overline{B}X_{21}}\right) = (0.54, 0.46), \\ &\left(\widehat{\pi}_{\overline{C}X_{11}}, \widehat{\pi}_{\overline{C}X_{21}}\right) = (0.59, 0.41) \text{ and} \\ &\left(\widehat{\pi}_{\overline{D}X_{11}}, \widehat{\pi}_{\overline{D}X_{21}}\right) = (0.57, 0.43). \end{aligned} \tag{11.21}$$

Table 11.3 The observed and expected frequency of 3398 schoolboys at the first and second interviews

$ijk\ell$	$f^{ijk\ell}$	$\widehat{f}^{ijk\ell}$	$\mathfrak{X}^2$ (Eq. (11.16))	$\mathfrak{L}^2$ (Eq. (11.17))
1111	458	164.5	523.4	468.9
1112	140	124.1	2.0	16.8
1121	110	236.8	67.9	−84.3
1122	49	178.6	94.1	−63.4
1211	171	129.3	13.5	47.8
1212	182	97.5	73.2	113.5
1221	56	186.0	90.9	−67.2
1222	87	140.3	20.3	−41.6
2111	184	280.2	33.0	−77.7
2112	75	211.4	88.0	−77.7
2121	531	403.2	40.5	146.3
2122	281	304.1	1.8	−22.2
2211	85	220.1	82.9	−80.9
2212	97	166.1	28.7	−52.2
2221	338	316.8	1.4	21.9
2222	554	239.0	415.3	465.8
Total	3398	3398	1576.8	1428.4

(b) From Eq. (11.21) obtained in part (a), we calculate the expected observed frequency $\widehat{f}^{ijk\ell}$ as follows:

$$\widehat{f}^{ijk\ell} = n \cdot \widehat{\pi}_{\overline{A}X_{i1}} \cdot \widehat{\pi}_{\overline{B}X_{j1}} \cdot \widehat{\pi}_{\overline{C}X_{k1}} \cdot \widehat{\pi}_{\overline{D}X_{\ell 1}}, \tag{11.22}$$

and their values are given in the third column of Table 11.3.

From the fourth and fifth columns of Table 11.3, both the values of the chi-square statistic ($\mathfrak{X}^2 = 1576.8$) and the log likelihood ratio statistic ($\mathfrak{L}^2 = 1428.4$) are greater than critical value of $\chi^2_{6;0.95} = 14.45$. Therefore, hypothesis H_1 is not congruent to the observed data.

Remark

Goodman [2] considered other models of two latent variables that are congruent for the interview data of schoolboys.

11.2 Latent Class Model in Medical Diagnosis [5]

In this section, we are going to learn how to apply the latent class analysis in determining the sensitivity (the probability that an indicator is positive when a particular disease is present), specificity (the probability that an indicator is negative when a particular disease is absent), efficiency (the total probability of making a correct statement about the presence or absence of a particular disease) and predictive positive (or negative) value (the probability that an person is positive (or negative) for an indicator actually has (or does not have) a particular disease). Calculation of these statistics depends on knowledge of whether each patient in a study actually does or does not have the disease. Error in this determination leads to inaccuracies in the above quantities. In those cases where one cannot determine the correct diagnosis, we must use methods such as latent class analysis. Latent class analysis will even test the validity of the diagnosis even when the diagnosis is presumed correct. We will use the data from Galen and Gambino on myocardial infarction (MI) to demonstrate the method involved in the following example.

Example 11.2
The data used are taken from Table 5 in chapter 13 of Galen-Gambino [4]. It pertains to a study of patients in the Coronary Care Unit of the Presbyterian Hospital in New York City. The patients were admitted for the purpose of ruling out myocardial infarction. Each of 94 patients had the following information available on five diagnostic indicators, we only use the first four of them: (i) A: presence or absence of a positive Q-wave in the ECG, (ii) B: presence or absence of a classical clinical history, (iii) C: presence or absence of high CPK-MB, and (iv) D: whether or not the patient had flipped LDH (Table 11.4).

The latent variable X is defined as whether the patient has MI. The variables here are similar to that of Example 11.1. As a result, we apply the technique in Example 11.1 to Table 11.4. The results of iteration obtained from Table 11.4 are given in Table 11.5.

Table 11.4 Frequencies of observed data, probabilities of correct classification

Indicator				Frequencies		
A	B	C	D	Observed	Class	Prob of correct classification
1	1	1	1	24	2	1.000
2	1	1	1	5	2	0.992
1	2	1	1	4	2	1.000
2	2	1	1	3	2	0.889
1	1	2	1	3	2	1.000
2	1	2	1	5	1	0.580
1	2	2	1	2	2	1.000
2	2	2	1	7	1	0.956
1	1	1	2	0	–	–
2	1	1	2	0	1	1.000
1	2	1	2	0	–	–
2	2	1	2	1	1	1.000
1	1	2	2	0	–	–
2	1	2	2	7	1	1.000
1	2	2	2	0	–	–
2	2	2	2	33	1	1.000

Where yes: = "1," no: = "2"

Table 11.5 The iteration step (n) of the calculation

n	t	$\hat{\pi}_{X_t}$	$\hat{\pi}_{\bar{A}X_{1t}}$	$\hat{\pi}_{\bar{B}X_{1t}}$	$\hat{\pi}_{\bar{C}X_{1t}}$	$\hat{\pi}_{\bar{D}X_{1t}}$
0	1	0.2	0.4	0.5	0.7	0.3
	2	0.8	0.6	0.5	0.3	0.7
1	1	0.01013	0.265911	0.410208	0.282294	0.439824
	2	0.04052	0.734089	0.589792	0.616257	0.560176
2	1	0.2	0.351064	0.468085	0.393617	0.56383
	2	0.8	0.648936	0.531915	0.606383	0.43617
3	1	0.2	0.351064	0.468085	0.393617	0.56383
	2	0.8	0.648936	0.531915	0.606383	0.43617

Table 11.6 The observed and expected frequency of 94 patients in a study of ruling out MI

$ijk\ell$	$f^{ijk\ell}$	$\hat{f}^{ijk\ell}$	$\mathfrak{X}^2$ (Eq. (10.16))	$\mathfrak{L}^2$ (Eq. (10.17))
1111	24	3.43	123.45	−39.31
2111	5	6.34	0.28	14.38
1211	4	3.90	0.003	29.06
2211	3	7.20	2.45	0.61
1121	3	5.28	0.99	3.34
2121	5	9.76	2.32	3.83
1221	2	6.00	2.67	−0.58
2221	7	11.01	1.51	10.73
1112	0	2.65	2.65	–
2112	0	4.90	4.90	–
1212	0	3.01	3.01	–
2212	1	5.57	3.75	−1.32
1122	0	4.09	4.08	–
2122	7	7.55	0.04	36.09
1222	0	4.64	4.64	–
2222	33	8.58	69.48	−24.57
Total	94	93.91	226.22	32.26

The compute value of Eq. (11.16) (or (11.17)) is $\mathfrak{X}^2 = 226.22$ (or $\mathfrak{L}^2 = 32.26$) that is greater than the critical value of $\chi^2_{6;0.95} = 14.45$ (or $\chi^2_{1;0.95} = 5.024$). Consequently, the hypothesis that four indicators A, B, C, and D are independent is rejected, that is, there are relationships among these four indicators (Table 11.6).

References

1. Coleman, J. S. (1964). *Introduction to mathematical sociology*. Free Press.
2. Goodman, L. A. (1974a). The analysis of systems of qualitative variables when some of the variables are unobservable. Part I- A modified latent structure approach. *American Journal of Sociology, 79*, 1179–1259.

3. Goodman, L. A. (1974b). Exploratory latent structure analysis using both identifiable and unidentifiable models. *Biometrika, 61*, 215–231.
4. Galen, R. S., & Gambino, S. R. (1975). *Beyond normality: The predictive value and efficiency of medical diagnosis*. Wiley.
5. Rindskopf, D., & Rindskopf, W. (1986). The value of latent class analysis in medical diagnosis. *Statistics in Medicine, 5*, 21–27.

Appendix

Table A1 Standard Normal Distribution (Z) $\Pr(Z \le z) = \Phi(z) = \int_{-\infty}^{z} \frac{1}{\sqrt{2\pi}} e^{-x^2/2} dx$ $[\Phi(-z) = 1 - \Phi(z)]$

z	0.00 0.05	0.01 0.06	0.02 0.07	0.03 0.08	0.04 0.09
0.0	0.5000 0.5199	0.5040 0.5239	0.5080 0.5279	0.5120 0.5319	0.5160 0.5359
0.1	0.5398 0.5596	0.5438 0.5636	0.5478 0.5675	0.5517 0.5714	0.5557 0.5753
0.2	0.5793 0.5987	0.5832 0.6026	0.5871 0.6064	0.5910 0.6103	0.5948 0.6141
0.3	0.6179 0.6368	0.6217 0.6406	0.6255 0.6443	0.6293 0.6480	0.6331 0.6517
0.4	0.6554 0.6736	0.6591 0.6772	0.6628 0.6808	0.6664 0.6844	0.6700 0.6879
0.5	0.6915 0.7088	0.6950 0.7123	0.6985 0.7157	0.7019 0.7190	0.7054 0.7224
0.6	0.7257 0.7422	0.7291 0.7454	0.7324 0.7486	0.7357 0.7517	0.7389 0.7549
0.7	0.7580 0.7734	0.7611 0.7764	0.7642 0.7794	0.7673 0.7823	0.7703 0.7852
0.8	0.7881 0.8023	0.7910 0.8051	0.7939 0.8078	0.7967 0.8106	0.7995 0.8133
0.9	0.8159 0.8289	0.8186 0.8315	0.8212 0.8340	0.8238 0.8365	0.8264 0.8389
1.0	0.8413 0.8531	0.8438 0.8554	0.8461 0.8577	0.8485 0.8599	0.8508 0.8621
1.1	0.8643 0.8749	0.8665 0.8770	0.8686 0.8790	0.8708 0.8810	0.8729 0.8830
1.2	0.8849 0.8944	0.8869 0.8962	0.8888 0.8980	0.8907 0.8997	0.8925 0.9015
1.3	0.9032 0.9115	0.9049 0.9131	0.9066 0.9147	0.9082 0.9162	0.9099 0.9177
1.4	0.9192 0.9265	0.9207 0.9279	0.9222 0.9292	0.9236 0.9306	0.9251 0.9319
1.5	0.9332 0.9394	0.9345 0.9406	0.9357 0.9418	0.9370 0.9429	0.9382 0.9441
1.6	0.9452 0.9505	0.9463 0.9515	0.9474 0.9525	0.9484 0.9535	0.9495 0.9545

(continued)

T.-S. Lee, *Misclassification in Epidemiology*, Emerging Topics in Statistics and Biostatistics, https://doi.org/10.1007/978-3-032-12563-7

Table A1 (continued)

z	0.00 0.05	0.01 0.06	0.02 0.07	0.03 0.08	0.04 0.09
1.7	0.9554 0.9599	0.9564 0.9608	0.9573 0.9616	0.9582 0.9625	0.9591 0.9633
1.8	0.9641 0.9678	0.9649 0.9686	0.9656 0.9693	0.9664 0.9699	0.9671 0.9706
1.9	0.9713 0.9744	0.9719 0.9750	0.9726 0.9756	0.9732 0.9761	0.9738 0.9767
2.0	0.9772 0.9798	0.9778 0.9803	0.9783 0.9808	0.9788 0.9812	0.9793 0.9817
2.1	0.9821 0.9842	0.9826 0.9846	0.9830 0.9850	0.9834 0.9854	0.9838 0.9857
2.2	0.9861 0.9878	0.9864 0.9881	0.9868 0.9884	0.9871 0.9887	0.9875 0.9890
2.3	0.9893 0.9906	0.9896 0.9909	0.9898 0.9911	0.9901 0.9913	0.9904 0.9916
2.4	0.9918 0.9929	0.9920 0.9931	0.9922 0.9932	0.9925 0.9934	0.9927 0.9936
2.5	0.9938 0.9946	0.9940 0.9948	0.9941 0.9949	0.9943 0.9951	0.9945 0.9952
2.6	0.9953 0.9960	0.9955 0.9961	0.9956 0.9962	0.9957 0.9963	0.9959 0.9964
2.7	0.9965 0.9970	0.9966 0.9971	0.9967 0.9972	0.9968 0.9973	0.9969 0.9974
2.8	0.9974 0.9978	0.9975 0.9979	0.9976 0.9979	0.9977 0.9980	0.9977 0.9981
2.9	0.9981 0.9984	0.9982 0.9985	0.9982 0.9985	0.9983 0.9986	0.9984 0.9986
3.0	0.9987 0.9989	0.9987 0.9989	0.9987 0.9989	0.9988 0.9990	0.9988 0.9990
α	0.001 0.100	0.005 0.200	0.010 0.300	0.025 0.400	0.050
$z_{1-\frac{\alpha}{2}}$	3.291 1.645	2.807 1.282	2.576 1.036	2.240 0.842	1.960
$z_{1-\alpha}$	3.090 1.282	2.576 0.842	2.326 0.524	1.960 0.253	1.645

Table A2 Percentiles in Kolmogorov-Smirnov Statistics $Pr(\sup_x|S_n(x) - F_0(x)| \leq d_{n;\,1-\alpha}) = 1 - \alpha$

		α			
	0.20	0.10	0.05	0.02	0.01
n		$d_{n;1-\alpha}$			
1	0.9000	0.9500	0.9750	0.9900	0.9950
2	0.6838	0.7764	0.8419	0.9000	0.9293
3	0.5648	0.6360	0.7076	0.7846	0.8290
4	0.4927	0.5652	0.6239	0.6889	0.7342
5	0.4470	0.5095	0.5633	0.6272	0.6685
6	0.4104	0.4680	0.5193	0.5774	0.6166
7	0.3815	0.4361	0.4834	0.5384	0.5758
8	0.3583	0.4096	0.4543	0.5065	0.5418
9	0.3391	0.3875	0.4300	0.4796	0.5133
10	0.3226	0.3687	0.4093	0.4566	0.4889
11	0.3083	0.3524	0.3912	0.4367	0.4677
12	0.2958	0.3382	0.3754	0.4192	0.4491
13	0.2847	0.3255	0.3614	0.4036	0.4325
14	0.2748	0.3142	0.3489	0.3897	0.4176
15	0.2659	0.3040	0.3376	0.3771	0.4042
16	0.2578	0.2947	0.3273	0.3657	0.3920
17	0.2504	0.2863	0.3180	0.3553	0.3809
18	0.2446	0.2785	0.3094	0.3457	0.3706
19	0.2374	0.2714	0.3014	0.3369	0.3612
20	0.2316	0.2647	0.2941	0.3287	0.3524
21	0.2262	0.2586	0.2872	0.3210	0.3443
22	0.2212	0.2528	0.2809	0.3139	0.3367
23	0.2165	0.2475	0.2749	0.3073	0.3295
24	0.2121	0.2424	0.2693	0.3010	0.3229
25	0.2079	0.2377	0.2640	0.2952	0.3166
26	0.2040	0.2332	0.2591	0.2896	0.3106
27	0.2003	0.2290	0.2544	0.2844	0.3050
28	0.1968	0.2250	0.2500	0.2794	0.2997
29	0.1935	0.2212	0.2457	0.2747	0.2947
30	0.1903	0.2176	0.2417	0.2702	0.2899
31	0.1873	0.2141	0.2379	0.2660	0.2853
32	0.1845	0.2109	0.2342	0.2619	0.2809
33	0.1817	0.2077	0.2308	0.2580	0.2768
34	0.1791	0.2047	0.2274	0.2543	0.2728
35	0.1766	0.2019	0.2243	0.2507	0.2690
36	0.1742	0.1991	0.2212	0.2473	0.2653
37	0.1719	0.1965	0.2183	0.2440	0.2618
38	0.1697	0.1939	0.2154	0.2409	0.2584
39	0.1675	0.1915	0.2127	0.2379	0.2552
40	0.1655	0.1891	0.2101	0.2349	0.2521

(continued)

Table A2 (continued)

		α			
41	0.1635	0.1869	0.2076	0.2321	0.2490
42	0.1616	0.1847	0.2052	0.2294	0.2461
43	0.1597	0.1826	0.2028	0.2268	0.2433
44	0.1580	0.1805	0.2006	0.2243	0.2406
45	0.1562	0.1786	0.1984	0.2218	0.2380
46	0.1546	0.1767	0.1963	0.2194	0.2354
47	0.1530	0.1748	0.1942	0.2172	0.2330
48	0.1514	0.1730	0.1922	0.2149	0.2306
49	0.1499	0.1713	0.1903	0.2128	0.2283
50	0.1484	0.1696	0.1884	0.2107	0.2260
51	0.1470	0.1680	0.1866	0.2086	0.2239
52	0.1456	0.1664	0.1848	0.2067	0.2217
53	0.1442	0.1648	0.1831	0.2048	0.2197
54	0.1429	0.1633	0.1814	0.2029	0.2177
55	0.1416	0.1619	0.1798	0.2011	0.2157
56	0.1404	0.1604	0.1782	0.1993	0.2138
57	0.1392	0.1591	0.1767	0.1976	0.2120
58	0.1380	0.1577	0.1752	0.1959	0.2102
59	0.1369	0.1564	0.1737	0.1943	0.2084
60	0.1357	0.1551	0.1723	0.1927	0.2067
61	0.1346	0.1539	0.1709	0.1911	0.2051
62	0.1336	0.1526	0.1696	0.1896	0.2034
63	0.1325	0.1514	0.1682	0.1881	0.2018
64	0.1315	0.1503	0.1669	0.1867	0.2003
65	0.1305	0.1491	0.1657	0.1853	0.1988
66	0.1295	0.1480	0.1644	0.1839	0.1973
67	0.1286	0.1469	0.1632	0.1825	0.1958
68	0.1277	0.1459	0.1620	0.1812	0.1944
69	0.1268	0.1448	0.1609	0.1799	0.1930
70	0.1259	0.1438	0.1598	0.1786	0.1917
71	0.1250	0.1428	0.1586	0.1774	0.1903
72	0.1241	0.1418	0.1576	0.1762	0.1890
73	0.1233	0.1409	0.1565	0.1750	0.1878
74	0.1225	0.1399	0.1554	0.1738	0.1865
75	0.1217	0.1390	0.1544	0.1727	0.1853
76	0.1209	0.1381	0.1534	0.1716	0.1841
77	0.1201	0.1372	0.1524	0.1705	0.1829
78	0.1194	0.1364	0.1515	0.1694	0.1817
79	0.1186	0.1355	0.1505	0.1683	0.1806
80	0.1179	0.1347	0.1496	0.1673	0.1795
81	0.1172	0.1339	0.1487	0.1663	0.1784
82	0.1165	0.1331	0.1478	0.1653	0.1773

(continued)

Table A2 (continued)

		α			
83	0.1158	0.1323	0.1469	0.1643	0.1763
84	0.1151	0.1315	0.1461	0.1633	0.1752
85	0.1144	0.1307	0.1452	0.1624	0.1742
86	0.1138	0.1300	0.1444	0.1614	0.1732
87	0.1131	0.1292	0.1436	0.1605	0.1722
88	0.1125	0.1285	0.1427	0.1596	0.1713
89	0.1119	0.1278	0.1420	0.1587	0.1703
90	0.1113	0.1271	0.1412	0.1579	0.1694
91	0.1106	0.1264	0.1404	0.1570	0.1685
92	0.1101	0.1257	0.1397	0.1562	0.1676
93	0.1095	01251	0.1389	0.1553	0.1667
94	0.1089	0.1244	0.1382	0.1545	0.1658
95	0.1083	0.1238	0.1375	0.1537	0.1649
96	0.1078	0.1231	0.1368	0.1529	0.1641
97	0.1072	0.1225	0.1361	0.1521	0.1632
98	0.1067	0.1219	0.1354	0.1514	0.1624
99	0.1062	0.1213	0.1347	0.1506	0.1616
100	0.1056	0.1207	0.1340	0.1499	0.1608

This table is taken with the copyright clearance permission from the JASA Journal in Miller L.H.: Table of percentage points of Kolmogorov statistics, J Am Statist Assoc 51: 111–121, 1956. https://doi.org/10.1080/01621459.1956.10501314

Index

T.-S. Lee, *Misclassification in Epidemiology*, Emerging Topics in Statistics and Biostatistics, https://doi.org/10.1007/978-3-032-12563-7

MIX
Papier aus verantwortungsvollen Quellen
Paper from responsible sources
FSC® C105338

If you have any concerns about our products,
you can contact us on
ProductSafety@springernature.com

In case Publisher is established outside the EU,
the EU authorized representative is:
Springer Nature Customer Service Center GmbH
Europaplatz 3, 69115 Heidelberg, Germany

Printed by Libri Plureos GmbH
in Hamburg, Germany